INTRINSIC and SKULL BASE TUMORS

NEUROSURGERY: CASE MANAGEMENT COMPARISON SERIES

INTRINSIC and SKULL BASE TUMORS

NEUROSURGERY: CASE MANAGEMENT COMPARISON SERIES

Kaisorn L. Chaichana, MD, FAANS, FACS

Professor of Neurosurgery
Vice Chair of Education
Director of Brain Tumor Surgery
Director of Skull Base and Minimally Invasive Cranial Surgery
Neurosurgery Residency Program Director
Mayo Clinic
Jacksonville, Florida, USA

Alfredo Quiñones-Hinojosa, MD, FAANS, FACS

William J. and Charles H. Mayo Professor
Chair, Neurologic Surgery
Mayo Clinic
Jacksonville, Florida, USA

ELSEVIER

Elsevier
1600 John F. Kennedy Blvd.
Ste. 1800
Philadelphia, PA 19103-2899

INTRINSIC AND SKULL BASE TUMORS:
NEUROSURGERY: CASE MANAGEMENT COMPARISON SERIES ISBN: 978-0-323-69642-5

Library of Congress Control Number: 2020938474

Director, Content Development: Ellen Wurm-Cutter
Content Strategist: Humayra Khan
Content Development Specialist: Dominque McPherson
Publishing Services Manager: Shereen Jameel
Senior Project Manager: Karthikeyan Murthy
Design: Patrick Ferguson

Working together
to grow libraries in
developing countries

www.elsevier.com • www.bookaid.org

Printed in China
Last digit is the print number: 9 8 7 6 5 4 3 2 1

Expert Case Reviewers

Isaac J. Abecassis, MD
Resident Physician
Neurological Surgery
University of Washington
Seattle, WA, USA

Lucas Alverne Freitas de Albuquerque, MD
Medical Doctor
Department of Neurosurgery
Hospital Geral de Fortaleza
Fortaleza/Ceará, Brazil

Joao Paulo Almeida, MD
Advanced Endoscopic and Open Skull Base
    Clinical Fellow
Department of Neurosurgery
Cleveland Clinic
Cleveland, OH, USA

Román Pablo Arévalo, MD
Neurological Surgeon
Department of Neurosurgery
Hospital Alta Complejidad En Red El Cruce
Buenos Aires, Argentina

Omar Arnaout, MD
Assistant Professor
Neurological Surgery
Brigham and Women's Hospital
Harvard School of Medicine
Boston, MA, USA

Miguel A. Arraez, MD, PhD
Professor and Chairman
Carlos Haya University Hospital
Malaga, Spain

Arturo Ayala-Arcipreste, MD
Head of Skull Base Clinic
Neurosurgery Department
Hospital Juárez de México
Universidad Nacional Autónoma de México (UNAM)
México City, México

Juan A. Barcia, MD, PhD
Professor and Head
Department of Neurosurgery
Hospital Clínico San Carlos
Chair of Neurosurgery
Universidad Complutense de Madrid
Madrid, Spain

Bernard R. Bendok, MD, MSCI, FAANS, FACS, FAHA
Consultant and Chair, Neurological Surgery in
    Arizona, Professor of Neurosurgery, William J.
    and Charles H. Mayo Professor
Department of Neurological Surgery
Department of Radiology
Department of Otolaryngology
Mayo Clinic
Phoenix, AZ, USA

Massimiliano Del Bene, MD
Resident in Neurosurgery
Department of Neurosurgery, Fondazione
    IRCCS Istituto Neurologico Carlo Besta
Department of Experimental Oncology, IEO,
    European Institute of Oncology IRCCS
Milan, Italy

Mitchel S. Berger, MD, FACS, FAANS
Berthold and Belle N. Guggenhime Professor
Chairman, Department of Neurological Surgery
Director, Brain Tumor Center
University of California, San Francisco
San Francisco, CA, USA
Adjunct Consultant
Philippine General Hospital
University of Philippines
Department of Neurosciences
Manila, Republic of the Philippines

Mark Bernstein, BSc, MD, FRCSC, MHSc (Bioethics)
Professor
Department of Surgery, Division of
    Neurosurgery
Greg-Wilkins Barrick Chair in Global Surgery
University of Toronto
Toronto, Ontario, Canada

Chetan Bettegowda, MD, PhD
Jennison and Nowak Families Professor of
    Neurosurgery and Oncology
Neurosurgery
Johns Hopkins University School of Medicine
Baltimore, MD, USA

Orin Bloch, MD, FAANS
Associate Professor and Director of
    Neurosurgical Oncology
Department of Neurological Surgery
University of California–Davis
Sacramento, CA, USA

Henry Brem, MD
Harvey Cushing Professor
Director Department of Neurosurgery
Director, Hunterian Neurosurgery Laboratory
Professor of Neurosurgery, Oncology
    Ophthalmology and Biomedical Engineering
Neurosurgeon in Chief
Johns Hopkins University School of Medicine
Baltimore, Maryland

Steven Brem, MD
Professor and Chief, Neurosurgical Oncology
Department of Neurosurgery, Hospital of the
    University of Pennsylvania
Co-Director, Penn Brain Tumor Center,
    Abramson Cancer Center
Perelman, School of Medicine, University of
    Pennsylvania
Philadelphia, PA, USA

Carlos E. Briceno, MD
Neurosurgeon
Neurosurgery
Centro Medico Paitilla
Panama, Republic of Panama

Jeffrey N. Bruce, MD
Edgar M. Housepian Professor of
    Neurological Surgery
Neurological Surgery
Columbia University Vagelos College of
    Physicians and Surgeons
New York, NY, USA

Peter Bullock, MB, ChB, FRCS, MRCP
Consultant Neurosurgeon
The London Clinic
London, UK

Bob S. Carter, MD, PhD, FAANS
Professor and Chief of Neurosurgery
Department of Neurosurgery
Massachusetts General Hospital and Harvard
    Medical School
Boston, MA, USA

Luigi Maria Cavallo, MD, PhD
Associate Professor
Division of Neurosurgery
University of Naples Federico II
Naples, Italy

Fernando Hakim, MD
Chairman Neurosurgery, Associate Professor of
    Neurosurgery, Director of Normal Pressure
    Hydrocephalus Program
Neurosurgical Service, Department of Surgery
Hospital Universitario Fundación Santafe de
    Bogota
Universidad de Los Andes, Universidad del
    Bosque
Bogota DC, Colombia, South America

Tony Van Havenbergh, MD, PhD
Neurosurgeon, Chairman
Department of Neurosurgery
GZA Hospitals Antwerp
Antwerp, Belgium

Shawn L. Hervey-Jumper, MD
Associate Professor
Neurological Surgery
UCSF Weill Institute for Neurosciences
San Francisco, CA, USA

**Eslam Mohsen Mahmoud Hussein, MBBS,
    MSc, MRCS**
Assistant Lecturer of Neurological and Spine
    surgery
Neurosurgery Department, Ain Shams
    University
Cairo, Egypt
Neurosurgery Senior Clinical Fellow
King's College Hospital
London, United Kingdom

George I. Jallo, MD
Director, Institute for Brain Protection Sciences;
    Professor, Neurosurgery, Oncology and
    Pediatrics
Division of Pediatric Neurosurgery
Johns Hopkins All Children's Hospital, Johns
    Hopkins University
St. Petersburg, FL, USA

Randy L. Jensen, MD, PhD
Professor of Neurosurgery, Radiation Oncology,
    and Oncological Sciences
Department of Neurosurgery
University of Utah
Salt Lake City, UT, USA

Chae-Yong Kim, MD, PhD
Professor
Neurosurgery
Seoul National University Bundang Hospital,
    Seoul National University College of Medicine
Seoul, South Korea

Matthew A. Kirkman, MEd, FRCS
Specialty Registrar
Victor Horsley Department of Neurosurgery
The National Hospital for Neurology and
    Neurosurgery, Queen Square
London, UK

Ricardo J. Komotar, MD, FAANS, FACS
Professor & Program Director
Director of UM Brain Tumor Initiative
Director of Surgical Neurooncology
University of Miami School of Medicine
Miami, FL, USA

Danil A. Kozyrev, MD
Pediatric Neurosurgical Fellow
Department of Pediatric Neurosurgery
Tel Aviv Sourasky Medical Center
Tel Aviv, Israel

John S. Kuo, MD, PhD, FAANS, FACS
Inaugural Chair and Professor of Neurosurgery
    and Oncology
Department of Neurosurgery
Dell Medical School, Surgical Director, Mulva
    Neurosciences
The University of Texas at Austin
Austin, TX, USA

**Frederick F. Lang, MD, FACS, FAANS,
    FAAAS**
Professor & Chairman, Department of
    Neurosurgery
Beau Biden Endowed Chair for Brain Cancer
    Research
Director, Brain Tumor Center
The Univeristy of Texas MD Anderson Cancer
    Center
Houston, TX, USA

Edward R. Laws, Jr., MD, FACS
Professor, Director
Neurosurgery, Pituitary/Neuroendocrine Center
Harvard Medical School, Brigham and
    Women's Hospital
Boston, MA, USA

Michael T. Lawton, MD
Professor & Chairman, Department of
    Neurological Surgery President & CEO,
    Barrow Neurological Institute
Chief of Vascular & Skull Base Neurosurgery,
    The Robert F. Spetzler Endowed Chair in
    Neurosciences
Phoenix, AZ, USA

Gerardo D. Legaspi, MD
Director and Chief of Neurosurgery
University of the Philippines – Philippine
    General Hospital
Manila, Philippines

Maciej S. Lesniak, MD, MHCM
Professor and Chair
Neurological Surgery
Northwestern University
Chicago, IL, USA

Gordon Li, MD
Professor
Department of Neurosurgery
Stanford University School of Medicine
Stanford, CA, USA

Linda M. Liau, MD, PhD, MBA, FAANS
Professor and Chair
Department of Neurosurgery
David Geffen School of Medicine at UCLA
Los Angeles, CA, USA

Michael Lim, MD
Professor and Chair
Department of Neurosurgery
Stanford University School of Medicine
Stanford, CA, USA

Harry Van Loveren, MD
Associate Dean, College of Medicine
    Neurosurgery
Vice-Chairman, Executive Management
    Committee
David W. Cahill Professor and Chair,
    Department of Neurosurgery and
    Brain Repair
Professor, Chair & Assoc. Dean, College of
    Medicine Neurosurgery
University of South Florida, Tampa, FL, USA

Larry B. Lundy, MD
Associate Professor
Otolaryngology Head and Neck Surgery
Mayo Clinic Florida
Jacksonville, FL, USA

Michael W. McDermott, MD
Chief Physician Executive, Miami Neuroscience
    Institute
Professor of Neurosurgery
Chair, Division of Neuroscience
Herbert Wertheim College of Medicine
Florida International University
Miami, FL, USA

José Hinojosa Mena-Bernal, MD, PhD
Chairman, Department of Neurosurgery
Hospital Sant Joan de Dèu
Barcelona, Spain

Javier Avendano Mendez-Padilla, MD
Vice-chair of education, Professor of
    Neurosurgery, Director of Neuro-Oncology
    program
Professor of spine surgery
National Institute of Neurology and
    Neurosurgery
Medica Sur Hospital
Tlalpan, Mexico

**Fredric B. Meyer, MD, FAANS, ABNS
    certified, licensed in Minnesota, Florida,
    and Arizona**
Uihlein Family Professor of Neurological
    Surgery
Mayo Clinic Enterprise Chair of Neurological
    Surgery
Executive Dean, Mayo Clinic College of
    Medicine and Science
Dean, Mayo Clinic Alix School of Medicine
Executive Director, American Board of
    Neurological Surgery
Department of Neurological Surgery
Mayo Clinic
Rochester, MN, USA

Basant K. Misra, MBBS, MS, MCh
Diplomate National Board Head, Department
    of Surgery
Head, Department of Neurosurgery & Gamma
    Knife Radiosurgery
PD Hinduja National Hospital and MRC
Mumbai, Maharashtra, India

**Jacques J. Morcos, MD, FRCS(Eng),
    FRCS(Ed), FAANS**
Professor and Co-Chairman
Department of Neurosurgery
University of Miami
Miami, FL, USA

Peter Nakaji, MD, FAANS, FACS
Professor and Chair
Department of Neurosurgery
University of Arizona College of Medicine–
    Phoenix
Banner University Medical Center–Phoenix
Phoenix, AZ, USA

Hirofumi Nakatomi, MD, PhD
University of Tokyo
Tokyo, Japan

Farshad Nassiri, MD
Resident Physician, Division of Neurosurgery,
    University of Toronto
Toronto, Ontario, Canada

Manabu Natsumeda, MD, PhD
Assistant Professor
Department of Neurosurgery
Brain Research Institute, Niigata University
Niigata, Japan

Jorge Navarro-Bonnet, MD
Oncology Neurosurgeon, Neurosurgery
    Department, Medica Sur Clinical Foundation
Director of Neurosurgery, Sedna Hospital
Associate Professor, La Salle University
Investigator, Anahuac University
Mexico City, Mexico

Kenji Ohata, MD, PhD
Specially Appointed Professor
Department of Minimally Invasive Neurosurgery
Osaka City University Graduate School of
    Medicine
Osaka, Japan

Evandro de Oliveira, MD, PhD
Adjunct Professor of Neurological Surgery
Department of Neurosurgery
Mayo Clinic, Jacksonville, FL, USA
Neurosurgeon
Institute of Neurological Sciences
Hospital BP – Beneficencia Portuguesa de
    São Paulo, São Paulo, SP. Brazil

Alessandro Olivi, MD
Professor and Chair
Institute of Neurosurgery
Fondazione Universitaria "Agostino Gemelli"
Università Cattolica del Sacro Cuore, Rome, Italy
Professor Emeritus of Neurosurgery
The Johns Hopkins University
Baltimore, Maryland, USA

**Nelson M. Oyesiku, MD, MSc (Lond),
    PhD, FACS**
Al Lerner Chair and Vice-Chairman
Professor, Neurosurgery and Medicine
    (Endocrinology)
Co-Director, Emory Pituitary Center
Residency Program Director, Department of
    Neurosurgery, Emory University School of
    Medicine
Editor-in-Chief, NEUROSURGERY
Department of Neurosurgery
Emory University School of Medicine
Atlanta, GA, USA

Ian F. Parney, MD, PhD, FRCS(C), FAANS
Professor and Vice-Chair
Neurological Surgery
Mayo Clinic
Rochester, MN, USA

Devi Prasad Patra, MD, MCh, MRCSEd
Clinical Fellow, Neurovascular, Cranial Base and
    Endovascular
Department of Neurological Surgery
Mayo Clinic
Phoenix, AZ, USA

Gustavo Pradilla, MD, FAANS
Associate Professor, Department of
    Neurological Surgery, Emory University
    School of Medicine
Chief of Neurosurgery, Grady Memorial Hospital
Director Cerebrovascular Research Laboratory
Atlanta, GA, USA

Daniel M. Prevedello, MD, FACS
Professor
Department of Neurological Surgery
The Ohio State University, Wexner Medical
    Center, School of Medicine
Columbus, OH, USA

Stephen J. Price, BSc, MBBS, PhD, FRCS
Honorary Consultant Neurosurgeon and
    Principal Research Associate (NIHR Career
    Development Fellow)
Neurosurgery Division, Department of Clinical
    Neurosciences
University of Cambridge and Addenbrooke's
    Hospital
Cambridge, UK

Vicent Quilis-Quesada, MD, PhD
Neurosurgeon, Department of Neurosurgery,
    University Hospital Clinic of València, Spain
Adjunct Assistant Professor of Neurosurgery,
    College of Medicine and Science,
    Mayo Clinic, Jacksonville, USA
Associate Professor of Neuroanatomy,
    Department of Human Anatomy and
    Embryology, Faculty of Medicine, University
    of Valencia, Spain

Joseph Quillin, MD
Neurosurgery Resident, Department of
    Neurosurgery, Emory University School of
    Medicine
Atlanta, GA, USA

Andreas Raabe, MD
Director and Chairman
Department of Neurosurgery
Inselspital, University of Bern
Bern, Switzerland

Maryam Rahman, MD, MS, FAANS
Assistant Professor
Lillian S. Wells Department of Neurosurgery
University of Florida
Gainesville, FL, USA

Zvi Ram, MD
Neurosurgeon, Chairman
Department of Neurosurgery
Tel Aviv University Sackler School of Medicine
Tel Aviv Medical Center
Tel Aviv, Israel

**Rodrigo Ramos-Zúñiga, MD, PhD, AANS,
    EANS**
Professor, Head Doctor
Institute of Translational Neurosciences
Universidad de Guadalajara
Guadalajara, México

Ganesh Rao, MD
Marc J. Shapiro Professor and Chairman
Department of Neurosurgery
Baylor College of Medicine
Houston, TX, USA

Shaan M. Raza, MD, FAANS
Associate Professor of Neurosurgery and Head
    and Neck Surgery
Skull Base Tumor Program, Department of
    Neurosurgery
The University of Texas MD Anderson Cancer
    Center
Houston, TX, USA

Mateus Reghin Neto, MD
Institute of Neurological Sciences
Hospital Beneficencia Portuguesa Sao Paulo
São Paulo, Brazil

Preface

Neurosurgical expertise, technology, resources, and access to information continue to evolve around the globe, but there is no concise body of literature that shows how experts throughout the world would manage a similar disease, patient, or case. To our knowledge, this book is the first attempt to look at this very important question to bring diversity of experts, ideas, and management of similar conditions and to explore how different experts around the world with different resources, technology, and cultural backgrounds would approach a similar patient. This book is part of a neurosurgical series that focuses on the most common intrinsic and skull base tumors cases. Each case is a chapter, in which the patient's chief complaint, history of presenting illness, past medical and surgical history, medications and allergies, social and family history, physical examination findings, and neuroimaging are presented. Four international experts are presented with a case and each expert provides information on how they would handle that particular case. This will be a reference to any health care provider, trainee, and surgeon treating brain tumors by being able to delve into the minds of experts from around the world on how they manage their patients despite geographic differences, as well as differences sometimes in access to resources/technology and at times cultures that can potentially influence management. This book is the first of its kind to show the similarities and differences in the management of neurosurgical cases among international experts from preoperative workup to operative approaches to postoperative care. We hope you enjoy it and we hope to bring you more of these types of series in the years to come.

Kaisorn Chaichana and Alfredo Quiñones-Hinojosa

Acknowledgments

We would like to acknowledge our families, patients, and colleagues. Our families have been patient with us as we take away time from them to continue to push ways to advance neurosurgical education and research. Without them, nothing is possible. We would also like to acknowledge our patients. All the cases presented in this book are our patients and they have trusted us to care for them. Although many physicians would handle the cases differently, every case was treated with the utmost concern for their well-being. Finally, we would like to acknowledge our colleagues at the Mayo Clinic; not just our colleagues in Jacksonville, Florida, but also Rochester, Minnesota, and Phoenix, Arizona. This includes consultants, trainees, and nurses. These works, and others, would not have been possible without their support, collegiality, guidance, and friendship.

Contents

1

Right frontal low-grade glioma

Case reviewed by Sunit Das, Hugues Duffau, John S. Kuo, Nader Sanai

Introduction

Low-grade gliomas (LGGs) represent a heterogenous group of intrinsic brain neoplasms that typically occur in younger, healthier individuals.[1] In 2012, there were approximately 66,000 new primary central nervous system tumors that were diagnosed, in which 20,000 of these cases were gliomas.[1] LGGs are typically diagnosed between the second and fourth decade of life, and seizures are seen in 80% of patients.[1] Magnetic resonance imaging (MRI) scans typically reveal a nonenhancing lesion that is hyperintense on T2-weighted imaging, but approximately 33% have some enhancement.[2] The majority of these lesions have frontal lobe involvement that ranges from 40% to 70% in several series.[3–8] In recent years, it has been shown that aggressive surgical resection with avoidance of neurologic deficits is far superior to observation, biopsies, or lesser resections in prolonging survival, delaying recurrence, and delaying malignant degeneration.[3–8] A common location for these lesions is the frontal lobe, in which presenting symptoms can include seizures, headaches, cognitive disabilities, incoordination, and personality changes, among others.[3–8] Tumors located in the right frontal lobe are often erroneously considered as minimal risk surgeries because this region is devoid of language and motor function.[9–11] However, with improvement in brain mapping, functional MRI, and tractography, surgery for lesions in this region can be as dangerous as lesions in the dominant hemisphere.[9–11] In this chapter, we present a right frontal likely LGG.

Example case

Chief complaint: syncopal event
History of present illness
A 51-year-old, right-handed woman with a history of anemia who presented after a syncopal event. She was working when she had a sudden loss of consciousness for an unspecified amount of time. She was started on levetiracetam, and imaging revealed a brain tumor (Fig. 1.1).

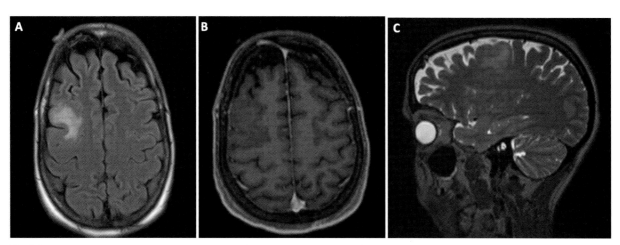

Fig. 1.1 **Preoperative magnetic resonance imaging. (A)** T2 axial fluid attenuation inversion recovery image; **(B)** T1 axial image with gadolinium contrast; **(C)** T2 sagittal magnetic resonance imaging scan demonstrating a right posterior middle frontal gyrus nonenhancing lesion that primarily involves the subcortical white matter and follows the subcortical U-fibers of the premotor region.

1

Medications: Levetiracetam.
Allergies: No known drug allergies.
Past medical and surgical history: Anemia.
Family history: No history of intracranial malignancies.

Social history: Cashier, no smoking history, occasional alcohol.
Physical examination: Awake, alert, oriented to person, place, and time; cranial nerves II-XII intact; no drift, moves all extremities with full strength.

	Sunit Das, MD, PhD, St. Michael's Hospital, University of Toronto, Toronto, Canada	Hugues Duffau, MD, PhD, University Hospital of Montpellier, Montpellier, France	John S. Kuo, MD, PhD, University of Texas at Austin, Austin, TX, United States	Nader Sanai, MD, Barrow Neurological Institute, Phoenix, AZ, United States
Preoperative				
Additional tests requested	Functional MRI (motor, speech laterality) DTI MRI perfusion Neuropsychological assessment (research)	Neuropsychological assessment Repeat MRI for growth rate Functional MRI (research) DTI (research)	Functional MRI	DTI	DTI
Surgical approach selected	Right frontal craniotomy with awake cortical/ subcortical mapping	Right frontal and central craniotomy with awake cortical/subcortical mapping	Right frontal craniotomy	Right frontal craniotomy with asleep cortical/ subcortical motor mapping
Anatomic corridor	Right frontal	Dorsolateral prefrontal cortex	Right frontal	Right frontal
Goal of surgery	Gross total resection of FLAIR	Extensive resection (GTR or NTR) with preservation of neurologic and cognitive functions	Diagnosis, maximal resection of FLAIR abnormality and adjacent gyrus	Gross total resection of FLAIR
Perioperative				
Positioning	Right supine with slight rotation	Lateral	Right supine with left rotation	Right supine
Surgical equipment	Surgical navigation Brain stimulator Surgical microscope Ultrasonic aspirator Ultrasound EEG	Brain stimulator Dedicated team (anesthesia, neuropsychological, speech pathology) No neuronavigation, intraoperative MRI, microscope, or functional neuroimaging	Surgical navigation IOM (EEG, phase reversal) Surgical microscope	Surgical navigation Brain stimulator Surgical microscope
Medications	Steroids	Steroids Antiepileptic drugs	Steroids Mannitol, furosemide Antiepileptic drugs	Steroids Mannitol
Anatomic considerations	Motor cortex CST	SFS medially, PCS posteriorly, FST, SLF, IFOF, oculomotor tract, CST	Central sulcus, white matter tracts deep to tumor	CST
Complications feared with approach chosen	Motor deficit	Motor deficit, executive function, semantic process, theory of mind	Motor deficit, residual/ resectable tumor	Motor deficit
Intraoperative				
Anesthesia	Asleep-awake	Asleep-awake-asleep	General	General
Skin incision	Reverse question mark	Reverse question mark	Horseshoe or curvilinear	Linear
Bone opening	Right frontal and parietal	Right frontal and central	Right frontal	Right frontal
Brain exposure	Right frontal and precentral	Right frontal and central area	Right frontal	Right frontal

	Sunit Das, MD, PhD, St. Michael's Hospital, University of Toronto, Toronto, Canada	Hugues Duffau, MD, PhD, University Hospital of Montpellier, Montpellier, France	John S. Kuo, MD, PhD, University of Texas at Austin, Austin, TX, United States	Nader Sanai, MD, Barrow Neurological Institute, Phoenix, AZ, United States
Method of resection	Craniotomy to encompass lesion, ultrasound to visualize lesion, dura opened, patient awakened for testing, motor cortex identified and used as posterior extent of resection, subpial dissection to mobilize tumor from adjacent structures, at depth use ultrasound and biopsy to determine if beyond area of tumor involvement, inspect cavity with microscope and ultrasound	Bone flap to include IFG and perirolandic area for positive mapping, patient awoken prior to dural opening, cortical mapping at low intensity (1.5–3 mA) with counting/left upper extremity movement/naming/semantic association/mentalizing tasks, subpial dissection concurrent with mapping and functional testing, resection up to functional boundaries of FST/SLF/IFOF/oculomotor tract/CST, avoidance of coagulation, general anesthesia for closure	Craniotomy based on surgical navigation, center dural opening over lesion, antibiotic-impregnated irrigation during dural opening, place EEG strip electrode to identify central sulcus based on phase reversal, removal of lesion en bloc based on navigation and location of central sulcus, watertight dural closure	Craniotomy to include lesion, stimulation of cortical and subcortical pathways monitoring for EMG firing in face and arm, resection of negatively mapped areas
Complication avoidance	Cortical and subcortical mapping with motor movement, subpial dissection, ultrasound, biopsies to determine if beyond tumor	Cortical and subcortical mapping with counting, left upper extremity movement, naming, semantic association task, and mentalizing	Identification of central sulcus, en bloc resection	Asleep cortical and subcortical mapping
Postoperative				
Admission	Step-down unit	ICU	ICU	ICU
Postoperative complications feared	Motor deficit	Movement execution and control, executive function, semantic processing, theory of mind	Seizure, motor deficit	Motor deficit
Follow-up testing	MRI within 48 hours after surgery	MRI within 24 hours after surgery Neuropsychological testing 2 days after surgery	MRI within 24 hours after surgery	MRI within 24 hours after surgery
Follow-up visits	1 month after surgery	Cognitive rehabilitation, MRI 3 months and then every 3–6 months throughout lifetime	2 weeks after surgery	7–10 days after surgery
Adjuvant therapies recommended				
Diffuse astrocytoma (IDH mutant, retain 1p19q)	STR–radiation/temozolomide GTR–radiation/temozolomide	STR–growth rate observation GTR–growth rate observation	STR–second look surgery if resectable, neuro and radiation oncology evaluation if not resectable GTR–observation	STR–radiation/temozolomide GTR–radiation/temozolomide

(continued on next page)

	Sunit Das, MD, PhD, St. Michael's Hospital, University of Toronto, Toronto, Canada	Hugues Duffau, MD, PhD, University Hospital of Montpellier, Montpellier, France	John S. Kuo, MD, PhD, University of Texas at Austin, Austin, TX, United States	Nader Sanai, MD, Barrow Neurological Institute, Phoenix, AZ, United States
Oligodendroglioma (IDH mutant, 1p19q LOH)	STR–radiation/PCV GTR–observation	STR–growth rate observation GTR–growth rate observation	STR–second look surgery if resectable, neuro and radiation oncology evaluation if not resectable GTR–observation	STR–radiation/ temozolomide GTR–observation
Anaplastic astrocytoma (IDH-wild type)	STR–radiation/ temozolomide GTR–radiation/ temozolomide	Homogenous AA–temozolomide AA foci removal and GTR of FLAIR abnormality–treatment as for diffuse astrocytoma	STR–second look surgery if resectable, radiation/ chemotherapy GTR–radiation/ chemotherapy	STR–radiation/ temozolomide GTR–radiation/ temozolomide

AA, anaplastic astrocytoma; *CST*, corticospinal tracts; *DTI*, diffusion tensor imaging; *EEG*, electroencephalogram; *EMG*, electromyogram; *FLAIR*, fluid attenuation inversion recovery; *FST*, frontostriatal tract; *GTR*, gross total resection; *ICU*, intensive care unit; *IFG*, inferior frontal gyrus; *IFOF*, inferior fronto-occipital fasciculus; *IOM*, intraoperative monitoring; *LOH*, loss of heterozygosity; *MRI*, magnetic resonance imaging; *NTR*, near total resection; *PCS*, precentral sulcus; *PCV*, procarbazine, lomustine, and vincristine; *SFS*, superior frontal sulcus; *SLF*, superior longitudinal fasciculus; *STR*, subtotal resection.

Differential diagnosis

- LGG (astrocytoma, oligodendroglioma)
- High-grade glioma
- Demyelinating disease (i.e., multiple sclerosis)

Important anatomic considerations

The right frontal lobe has typically been considered a safe surgical zone for extensive resection.[10,11] However, regardless of patient handedness, it houses critical cortical and subcortical structures.[10,11] The posterior boundary of the frontal lobe is the precentral sulcus, and its inferior boundary is the Sylvian fissure.[10,11] It is divided into superior, middle, and inferior frontal gyri by the superior and inferior frontal sulcus.[10,11] This lesion is located in the middle frontal gyrus below the banks of the superior frontal sulcus. It is bounded posteriorly by the precentral gyrus, which can be identified by the omega sign of the precentral gyrus hand-region, the gyrus posterior to the superior frontal sulcus, and identification of the pars marginalis.[10,11] The lesion is bounded medially by the supplementary motor area (SMA) and inferiorly by the inferior frontal gyrus in close juxtaposition to the ventral premotor cortex and dorsolateral prefrontal cortex.[10,11] Although the lesion is located in the right frontal lobe, there are several adjacent structures that can cause significant morbidity if injured.[10,11] Damage to the precentral gyrus and corticospinal tracts can result in contralateral weakness; the supplementary motor cortex can lead to contralateral weakness, akinesia, and motor incoordination; ventral premotor cortex can result in difficulty with speech initiation; and dorsolateral prefrontal cortex can lead to emotional lability, disorders in executive function, and problems with working memory.[10,11] Besides the corticospinal tract, injury to the superior longitudinal fasciculus, which is deep and medial to this lesion, can lead to phonetic paraphasias and difficulties with spatial orientation.[10,11] This lesion most likely involves the pre-SMA, SMA, and dorsolateral prefrontal cortex.

Approaches to this lesion

The primary surgical approaches for right frontal LGGs can be divided into either asleep or awake surgery (Fig. 1.2).[6,12–16] Asleep surgery involves general anesthesia in which the patient does not actively participate in intraoperative examinations, and can be done with or without monitoring.[15,16] This monitoring involves some combination of somatosensory evoked potentials (SSEPs), motor evoked potentials (MEPs), and/or electroencephalogram that passively monitor specific neurologic pathways.[15,16] SSEPs monitor the sensory pathway, MEPs monitor the motor pathway, and electroencephalograms monitor the general electrical activity of the brain.[15,16] The advantage of these asleep intraoperative monitoring modalities is that they provide feedback about the motor and somatosensory pathways without the need for patient cooperation.[6,12,14,15] However, the primary disadvantages are that they only identify changes after deficits occur, sensitivities are affected by anesthetic regimens, only assess motor and sensory pathways, and lack sensitivity and specificity.[6,12,14,15] Motor and sensory mapping, however, can be done while asleep, in which the cortex or subcortical regions can be stimulated, and electrical activity is monitored in distal muscles groups.[16] This provides more real-time information than SSEPs and MEPs, but is prone to false positives because of cortical and subcortical spread.[16] Awake surgery with brain mapping, unlike asleep surgery, can be used to provide real-time information of the motor and somatosensory pathways, as well as other functions including language, executive function, and proprioception, among others.[6,12,14] However, it requires patient cooperation and can be prone to intraoperative seizures.[13] In addition, there are several surgical adjuncts that can facilitate more extensive resection. These includes ultrasound, surgical navigation, and intraoperative MRI, among others.[17]

In terms of directionality of approach, this lesion primarily involves the pre-SMA and extends along the subcortical U-fiber posteriorly to likely the SMA. Based on identification of eloquence, the craniotomy and cortisectomy should be centered over this lesion.

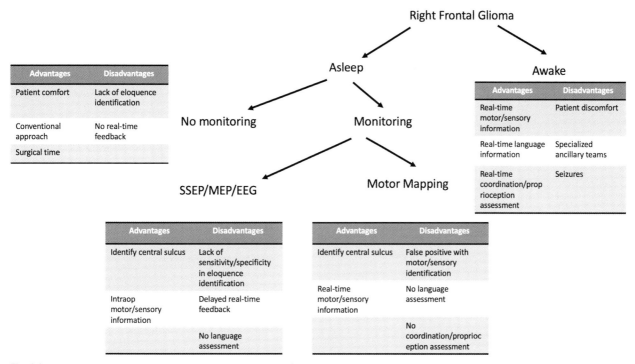

Fig. 1.2 **Diagram of typical approaches for right frontal gliomas.** *EEG,* Electroencephalogram; *MEP,* motor evoked potential; *SSEP,* somatosensory evoked potential.

What was actually done

The patient underwent a neuropsychological evaluation that showed no deficits. The patient was taken to surgery for a right frontal craniotomy with awake language and motor mapping for resection of the lesion. The patient was intubated with a laryngeal mask airway. The scalp was blocked bilaterally with local anesthetic, and the head was fixed in pins, with two pins straddling the inion and one pin on the left forehead in the midpupillary line. The head was turned 30 degrees to the left. A curved incision posterior to the lesion that extended from the superior temporal line to the vertex was planned with the aid of preoperative MRI navigation. The patient was draped in the usual standard fashion and given dexamethasone, levetiracetam, and cefazolin. A myocutaneous flap was made, and the flap was held in place with fishhooks attached to the drapes. A standard craniotomy was done to encompass the lesion plus one gyrus in each dimension. Ultrasound and surgical navigation were used to confirm lesion boundaries, and the boundaries were designated with letter tags once the dura was opened. The dura was anesthetized with local anesthetics between the leaflets adjacent to the middle meningeal vessels. The patient was awakened, and the dura was opened once the patient followed commands consistently. Strip electrodes were placed in the subdural space for after discharge monitoring. The cortex was stimulated with an Ojemann stimulator (Integra, Princeton, NJ) starting at 2 mA while the patient underwent a battery of motor tests involving the left face, arm, and leg concurrently with picture naming. The patient had speech motor arrest at 4 mA near the ventral premotor area, and the rest of the cortical and subcortical mapping took place at 4 mA. Positive mapping sites were designated with number tags.

Negative mapping occurred over the tumor, and the cortical boundaries that were identified with cortical mapping were the motor cortex posteriorly (decreased strength), supplementary motor cortex medially (decreased dexterity), and ventral premotor cortex laterally (speech arrest). The subcortical boundaries that were identified were the corticospinal tract (decreased strength) posteriorly and superior longitudinal fasciculus (phonetic paraphasias) deep and medial to the lesion. Preliminary diagnosis was infiltrating glioma. Once the resection was complete, the patient was put back to sleep with deep sedation without a laryngeal mask airway. The dura, bone, and skin were closed in standard fashion.

The patient awoke at their neurologic baseline with intact speech and full strength bilaterally and taken to the intensive care unit for recovery. An MRI scan was done within 48 hours that showed gross total resection of the lesion (Fig. 1.3). The patient participated with physical and occupational therapy and was discharged to home on postoperative day 2. The patient was discharged on 3 months of levetiracetam, and the dexamethasone was tapered to off over 5 days. The patient was seen at 2 weeks postoperatively for staple removal. Pathology was a World Health Organization grade II astrocytoma (IDH-wild type, 1p/19q wild type). After a discussion with neurooncology and radiation oncology, the patient underwent concurrent temozolomide and radiation therapy for 6 weeks followed by six adjuvant cycles. The lesion was observed with serial MRI examinations at 3 months, followed by 6-month intervals, and has been without recurrence for 18 months. The patient had a repeat neuropsychological evaluation at 3 months postoperatively that showed no change from preoperative evaluation. The patient returned to work 4 weeks postoperatively and remains without neurologic deficits.

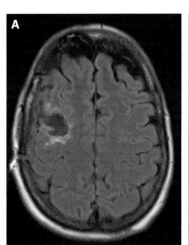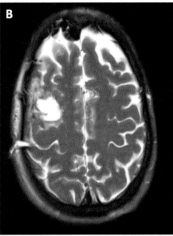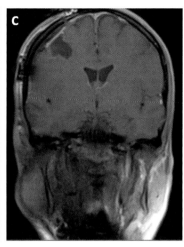

Fig. 1.3 Postoperative magnetic resonance imaging. (A) T2 axial fluid attenuation inversion recovery image; **(B)** T2 axial image; **(C)** T1 coronal magnetic resonance imaging scan with gadolinium contrast demonstrating gross total resection of the lesion.

Commonalities among the experts

The majority of the surgeons preferred to obtain functional MRI and diffusion tensor imaging for eloquent localization and white matter tract anatomy prior to surgery. Despite the tumor being in the nondominant hemisphere, the majority of the surgeons elected to perform the surgery with cortical and subcortical mapping, in which two physicians chose awake and one physician chose asleep mapping. The goal was typically to achieve gross total, if not more extensive, resection of this likely LGG. Most were cognizant of the corticospinal tract, and the approach was through the superficial aspect of the lesion. The most feared complication was motor deficit with injury to the corticospinal tract. Surgery was pursued with surgical navigation, brain stimulation, and surgical microscope, with perioperative steroids and antiepileptics. The majority favored cortical and subcortical mapping with subpial resection to avoid iatrogenic injuries. Following surgery, patients were admitted to the intensive care unit and MRI scans were obtained within 48 hours after surgery. If the diagnosis was a diffuse astrocytoma, radiation and temozolomide for both subtotal and gross total resection were preferred by most. If the diagnosis was an oligodendroglioma, observation was typically preferred for gross total resection, and radiation and chemotherapy for subtotal resections. If the diagnosis was an anaplastic astrocytoma, radiation and chemotherapy were preferred.

SUMMARY OF QUALITY OF EVIDENCE TO GUIDE SPECIFIC INTERVENTIONS FOR THIS CASE

- Surgery as opposed to biopsy or observation for LGGs— Class II-1.
- Increasing extent of resection associated with improved outcomes for LGGs—Class II-2.
- Awake mapping versus asleep surgery for noneloquent LGGs—Class II-3.
- Neuropsychological testing for LGGs—Class III.
- Supratotal resection for noneloquent lesions—Class III.

REFERENCES

1. Forst DA, Nahed BV, Loeffler JS, Batchelor TT. Low-grade gliomas. *Oncologist*. 2014;19:403–413.
2. Chaichana KL, McGirt MJ, Niranjan A, Olivi A, Burger PC, Quinones-Hinojosa A. Prognostic significance of contrast-enhancing low-grade gliomas in adults and a review of the literature. *Neurol Res*. 2009;31:931–939.
3. Chaichana KL, McGirt MJ, Laterra J, Olivi A, Quinones-Hinojosa A. Recurrence and malignant degeneration after resection of adult hemispheric low-grade gliomas. *J Neurosurg*. 2010;112:10–17.
4. Chaichana KL, McGirt MJ, Woodworth GF, et al. Persistent outpatient hyperglycemia is independently associated with survival, recurrence and malignant degeneration following surgery for hemispheric low grade gliomas. *Neurol Res*. 2010;32:442–448.
5. Duffau H. Long-term outcomes after supratotal resection of diffuse low-grade gliomas: a consecutive series with 11-year follow-up. *Acta Neurochir (Wien)*. 2016;158:51–58.
6. Eseonu CI, Eguia F, ReFaey K, et al. Comparative volumetric analysis of the extent of resection of molecularly and histologically distinct low grade gliomas and its role on survival. *J Neurooncol*. 2017;134:65–74.
7. Jakola AS, Myrmel KS, Kloster R, et al. Comparison of a strategy favoring early surgical resection vs a strategy favoring watchful waiting in low-grade gliomas. *JAMA*. 2010;308:1881–1888.
8. McGirt MJ, Chaichana KL, Attenello FJ, et al. Extent of surgical resection is independently associated with survival in patients with hemispheric infiltrating low-grade gliomas. *Neurosurgery*. 2008;63:700–707; author reply 707–708.
9. Duffau H, Mandonnet E. The "onco-functional balance" in surgery for diffuse low-grade glioma: integrating the extent of resection with quality of life. *Acta Neurochir (Wien)*. 2013;155:951–957.
10. Fernandez-Miranda JC, Rhoton AL, Jr., Alvarez-Linera J, Kakizawa Y, Choi C, de Oliveira EP. Three-dimensional microsurgical and tractographic anatomy of the white matter of the human brain. *Neurosurgery*. 2008;62:989–1026; discussion 1026–1028.
11. Rhoton AL, Jr. The cerebrum. Anatomy. *Neurosurgery*. 2007; 61:37–118; discussion 118–119.
12. Duffau H. The reliability of asleep-awake-asleep protocol for intraoperative functional mapping and cognitive monitoring in glioma surgery. *Acta Neurochir (Wien)*. 2013;155:1803–1804.
13. Eseonu CI, Eguia F, Garcia O, Kaplan PW, Quinones-Hinojosa A. Comparative analysis of monotherapy versus duotherapy antiseizure drug management for postoperative seizure control in patients undergoing an awake craniotomy. *J Neurosurg*. 2018;128:1661–1667.

14. Eseonu CI, Rincon-Torroella J, ReFaey K, et al. Awake craniotomy vs craniotomy under general anesthesia for perirolandic gliomas: evaluating perioperative complications and extent of resection. *Neurosurgery.* 2017;81:481–489.
15. Bertani G, Fava E, Casaceli G, et al. Intraoperative mapping and monitoring of brain functions for the resection of low-grade gliomas: technical considerations. *Neurosurg Focus.* 2009;27:E4.
16. Nossek E, Korn A, Shahar T, et al. Intraoperative mapping and monitoring of the corticospinal tracts with neurophysiological assessment and 3-dimensional ultrasonography-based navigation. Clinical article. *J Neurosurg.* 2011;114:738–746.
17. Garzon-Muvdi T, Kut C, Li X, Chaichana KL. Intraoperative imaging techniques for glioma surgery. *Future Oncol.* 2017;13:1731–1745.

2

Left frontal low-grade glioma

Case reviewed by Randy L. Jensen, Andreas Raabe, George Samandouras, Matthew A. Kirkman, Andrew E. Sloan

Introduction

Gliomas account for 27% of all brain tumors, and the overwhelming majority of gliomas are malignant.[1] Low-grade gliomas (LGGs) represent approximately 30% of glioma cases and include World Health Organization grade I and II tumors.[1] The most common location for these gliomas to occur is in the frontal lobe, which many have speculated is because of the increased size of the frontal lobe as compared with other lobes and/or close proximity to neurogenic niches, such as the subventricular zone.[2,3] The incidence of frontal lobe involvement for LGGs ranges from 40% to 70% in several series, and at least one-half occur in the dominant hemisphere.[4–9] Left-sided or dominant-hemisphere lesions are considered to carry more surgical risk as a result of close proximity to language functions and control of dominant hand functions. In this chapter, we present a left frontal LGG not adjacent to cortical language regions.

Example case

Chief complaint: seizure
History of present illness
A 40-year-old, right-handed woman with no significant past medical history who presented after a seizure event. While driving, she developed uncontrolled right arm shaking with loss of consciousness. She was seen at a local emergency room where imaging revealed a brain tumor (Fig. 2.1).
Medications: Levetiracetam.
Allergies: No known drug allergies.
Past medical and surgical history: None.
Family history: No history of intracranial malignancies.
Social history: Teacher. No smoking or alcohol history.
Physical examination: Awake, alert, oriented to person, place, and time; Cranial nerves II to XII intact; No drift, moves all extremities with full strength.

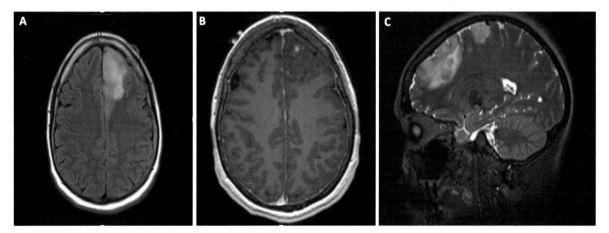

Fig. 2.1 Preoperative magnetic resonance imaging. (A) T2 axial fluid attenuation inversion recovery image; **(B)** T1 axial image with gadolinium contrast; **(C)** T2 sagittal magnetic resonance imaging scan demonstrating left anterior superior and partial middle frontal gyrus minimally enhancing lesion and left supplementary motor nonenhancing lesion that appear noncontiguous.

	Randy L. Jensen, MD, PhD, University of Utah, Salt Lake City, UT, United States	Andreas Raabe, MD, University Hospital at Inselspital, Bern, Switzerland	George Samandouras, MD, Matthew A. Kirkman, MEd, National Hospital for Neurology and Neurosurgery, Queen Square, London, United Kingdom	Andrew E. Sloan, MD, University Hospital, Case Western Reserve, Cleveland, OH, United States
Preoperative				
Additional tests requested	None	DTI Functional MRI Neuropsychological assessment	DTI Functional MRI MRS and perfusion MRI	CT chest, abdomen, pelvis Functional MRI
Surgical approach selected	Left frontal craniotomy with asleep motor mapping and intraoperative MRI confirmation	Left frontal craniotomy with asleep motor mapping	Left frontal craniotomy with awake motor and language mapping	Left fronto-parietal craniotomy with asleep motor mapping
Anatomic corridor	Left frontal	Left SFG, MFG	Left SFG, MFG	Left frontal
Goal of surgery	Diagnosis	99% resection with possible residual in left subcallosal	Maximal safe resection of both lesions	Diagnosis and maximal resection
Perioperative				
Positioning	Left supine 10-degree rotation	Left supine	Supine neutral	Supine neutral
Surgical equipment	Surgical navigation IOM (MEPs) Brain stimulator Surgical microscope Ultrasonic aspirator Intraoeprative MRI	Surgical navigation IOM (MEPs) Brain stimulator Surgical microscope with 5-ALA Intraoperative MRI	Surgical navigation IOM (ECoG) Brain stimulator Surgical microscope Ultrasonic aspirator	Surgical navigation IOM Brain stimulator Surgical microscope Ultrasonic aspirator
Medications	Steroids	Antiepileptics	Steroids	Mannitol Steroids Antiepileptics
Anatomic considerations	SMA posteriorly, Broca laterally	M1, ACA, hypothalamus	Pre-SMA, SMA, motor cingulate, corpus callosum, primary motor cortex, AF	Lateral ventricle, primary motor cortex, ACA branches (pericallosal, callosomarginal)
Complications feared with approach chosen	Speech difficulty, injury to ACA vessels, SMA syndrome	Moor deficit, SMA syndrome, vascular injury	Motor deficit, language deficit, SMA syndrome	Motor deficit, ACA injury, ventricular penetration
Intraoperative				
Anesthesia	General	General	Awake-awake-awake	General
Skin incision	Linear, bifrontal	Curvilinear, modified bicoronal	Semibicoronal	Modified bicoronal
Bone opening	Left anterior frontal	Left frontal encompassing both lesions	Left frontal encompassing both lesions and MFG	Left frontal encompassing both lesions
Brain exposure	Left anterior frontal	Left frontal encompassing both lesions	Left frontal encompassing both lesions and MFG	Left frontal encompassing both lesions

(continued on next page)

	Randy L. Jensen, MD, PhD, University of Utah, Salt Lake City, UT, United States	Andreas Raabe, MD, University Hospital at Inselspital, Bern, Switzerland	George Samandouras, MD, Matthew A. Kirkman, MEd, National Hospital for Neurology and Neurosurgery, Queen Square, London, United Kingdom	Andrew E. Sloan, MD, University Hospital, Case Western Reserve, Cleveland, OH, United States
Method of resection	Left frontal craniotomy to encompass lesion, navigation to identify lesion, cortical motor mapping, cortisectomy over negative mapping site with tumor biopsy, microscopic dissection and tumor resection, continuous MEP, intraoperative MRI to confirm resection and supplement, update neuronavigation if further resection is needed	Craniotomy extending at least over posterior aspect of tumor and allowing anterior access, placement of grids over motor leg and arm, perform mapping, subpial resection of dorsal tumor, resect anterior tumor up to frontal superior sulcus, follow tumor to resect part of cingulate gyrus, perform subcortical mapping to identify CST, intraoperative MRI to evaluate need for further resection	Scalp block, patient remains awake, left frontal craniotomy to encompass both lesions and MFG, open dura, map primary motor cortex adjacent to posterior lesion, test language in SFG and MFG with likely negative language mapping, target anterior lesion first identifying distal ACA/genu of corpus callosum/frontal horn of lateral ventricle, subpial resection leaving pia covering falx and protecting pericallosal and callosomarginal arteries, deroof the ventricle if ependyma involved and leave EVD for 24 hours, target posterior lesion that abuts primary motor cortex, cortical motor mapping, resect lesion based on functional boundaries, debulk tumor with ultrasonic aspirator (tissue select medium and amplitude 40%), preserve all vessels including small caliber arteries and veins	Craniotomy to encompass lesion, biopsy enhancing portion of anterior lesion, place grid and map posterior lesion for primary motor cortex, resect anterior component of lesion and identify and preserve ACA branches, resect posterior lesion if anterior to primary motor cortex with continuous monopolar stimulation looking for CST, biopsy lesion if in primary motor cortex, ultrasound to help assess resection cavity
Complication avoidance	Cortical mapping, continuous MEP, focus on anterior portion of tumor, intraoperative MRI	Cortical and subcortical mapping, subpial resection, intraoperative MRI	Cortical and subcortical motor and language mapping, subpial resection, preserve all arteries and veins	Grid placement to identify functional areas, focus on anterior portion of tumor, identify and preserve ACA branches, ultrasound to assess resection cavity
Postoperative				
Admission	ICU	ICU	Floor	Intermediate care
Postoperative complications feared	Speech difficulty, SMA syndrome	Motor or language deficit, SMA syndrome	Motor deficit, SMA syndrome, language deficit	Motor deficit, ventriculitis
Follow-up testing	None	MRI within 48 hours after surgery Neuropsychological assessment 2 months after surgery	MRI within 24 hours after surgery Speech and language assessment within 48 hours after surgery	CT immediately after surgery MRI within 72 hours after surgery

	Randy L. Jensen, MD, PhD, University of Utah, Salt Lake City, UT, United States	Andreas Raabe, MD, University Hospital at Inselspital, Bern, Switzerland	George Samandouras, MD, Matthew A. Kirkman, MEd, National Hospital for Neurology and Neurosurgery, Queen Square, London, United Kingdom	Andrew E. Sloan, MD, University Hospital, Case Western Reserve, Cleveland, OH, United States
Follow-up visits	2–4 weeks with neurooncology 4–6 weeks postoperative	4 weeks after surgery	1 week after surgery with neurooncology multidisciplinary clinic	10–14 days after surgery
Adjuvant therapies recommended				
Diffuse astrocytoma (IDH mutant, retain 1p19q)	STR–radiation/ temozolomide GTR–radiation/ temozolomide	STR–radiation/ temozolomide GTR–radiation/ temozolomide	STR–radiation/temozolomide GTR–observation	STR–radiation/ temozolomide or PCV GTR–radiation/ temozolomide or PCV
Oligodendroglioma (IDH mutant, 1p19q LOH)	STR–radiation/ temozolomide GTR–observation	STR–radiation/PCV GTR–observation	STR–temozolomide +/− radiation GTR–observation	STR–radiation/ temozolomide GTR–observation
Anaplastic astrocytoma (IDH wildtype)	STR–radiation/ temozolomide GTR–radiation/ temozolomide	STR–radiation/ temozolomide GTR–radiation	STR–radiation GTR–radiation	STR–radiation/ temozolomide GTR–radiation/ temozolomide

5-ALA, 5-aminolevulinic acid; *ACA*, anterior cerebral artery; *AF*, arcuate fasciculus; *CST*, corticospinal tract; *CT*, computed tomography; *DTI*, diffusion tensor imaging; *ECoG*, electrocorticography; *EVD*, external ventricular drain; *GTR*, gross total resection; *ICU*, intensive care unit; *IOM*, intraoperative monitoring; *LOH*, loss of heterozygosity; *MEP*, motor evoked potential; *MFG*, middle frontal gyrus; *MRI*, magnetic resonance imaging; *MRS*, magnetic resonance spectroscopy; *PCV*, procarbazine, lomustine, vincristine; *SFG*, superior frontal gyrus; *SMA*, supplementary motor area; *STR*, subtotal resection.

Differential diagnosis and actual diagnosis

- LGG (astrocytoma, oligodendroglioma)
- Gliomatosis cerebri
- High-grade glioma
- Demyelinating disease (i.e., multiple sclerosis)

Important anatomic and preoperative considerations

The frontal lobe consists of superior, middle, and inferior frontal gyri on the lateral surface, the orbital and rectus gyri on the inferior surface, and the superior frontal gyrus on the medial surface.[10,11] On the lateral surface, the frontal lobe is bounded posteriorly by the precentral sulcus and inferiorly by the Sylvian fissure.[10,11] The frontal lobe itself is divided by two longitudinal sulci (superior and inferior frontal sulci) that divides it into three gyri (superior, middle, and inferior frontal gyri).[10,11] The superior frontal sulcus has its posterior portion near the omega of the precentral gyrus, and the superior frontal gyrus runs parallel to the midline between the interhemispheric fissure and the superior frontal sulcus.[10,11] The middle frontal gyrus is located between the superior frontal sulcus and the inferior frontal sulcus, is the most prominent of the frontal gyri, and is typically continuous with the precentral gyrus and can be used as a landmark for identifying the precentral gyrus.[10,11] On the medial aspect, the frontal lobe is continuous with the superior frontal gyrus and is limited by the paracentral sulcus posteriorly and the

cingulate sulcus inferiorly.[10,11] The region anterior to the precentral gyrus at the posterior aspect of the superior frontal gyrus is the supplementary motor area (SMA), whereas at the posterior aspect of the middle frontal gyrus is the premotor cortex.[10,11] Anterior to the SMA is the pre-SMA that plays a role in conflict decision-making, and the ventral part of the premotor cortex is involved with speech initiation.[10,11] Injury to precentral gyrus and corticospinal tracts can result in contralateral weakness; the supplementary motor cortex can lead to contralateral weakness, akinesia, and motor incoordination; and ventral premotor cortex can result in difficulty with speech initiation.[10,11] Besides the corticospinal tract, injury to the superior longitudinal fasciculus (SLF), which is deep and medial lateral to this lesion, can lead to phonetic paraphasias and difficulties with spatial orientation, and to the frontal aslant tract, which is medial to the SLF, which can result in speech hesitancy and stuttering.[10,11] This lesion likely involves the pre-SMA, SMA, and frontal aslant tract.

Approaches to this lesion

As discussed in Chapter 1, the approaches to this lesion can be divided into asleep and awake procedures (Fig. 1.2). The asleep procedure is done under general anesthesia, and monitoring of the motor tracts can be done passively with motor evoked potentials or actively with motor cortex stimulation.[12,13] The advantages of the asleep approach is that is the conventional approach, does not require patient cooperation, and decreases surgery time, whereas the disadvantages include lack of real-time feedback about the neurologic status, unable to assess nonmotor functions (i.e., language), and is associated with potentially increased risk of neurologic injury.[12,13] The alternative is an awake approach, whereby multiple neurologic functions can be assessed simultaneously, including phonetics, semantics, motor strength, and motor coordination, among others.[7,12,14,15] The advantages of the awake approach is real-time neurologic feedback, ability to assess several different neurologic functions, and it is associated with improved resections and less morbidity; however, it requires surgeon experience, patient participation, and can potentially be associated with an increased risk of seizures.[7,12,14,15] In addition, the use of intraoperative magnetic resonance imaging (MRI) can be associated with improved resection.[16] If residual lesion is seen with intraoperative MRI, the additional lesion can be resected.[16] However, without real-time feedback, this may be associated with increased neurologic risk.

Given that this lesion is multifocal, possible approaches include biopsy versus extensive resection of one or both lesions. The goal of a biopsy is to obtain tissue for diagnosis to guide possible adjuvant therapy, but this would be associated with potential sampling error, poorer prognosis, and inability to improve symptoms directly. Resection can focus on one or both lesions. If one lesion is targeted, the anterior lesion is larger with more mass effect, likely less eloquent as the posterior lesion, and likely involves the SMA. The advantage of targeting both lesions is that it may potentially improve prognosis by reducing tumor burden, improving mass effect, and increasing susceptibility to adjuvant therapies. The best trajectory into this lesion would likely be an anterior frontal approach over the superior frontal gyrus, thus avoiding the laterally positioned Broca area, as well as the SLF and arcuate fasciculus (AF). An alternative approach is laterally, but this could potentially endanger Broca area, SLF, and AF by traversing through uninvolved cortical and subcortical tissue.

What was actually done

The patient underwent a neuropsychological evaluation that showed no deficits. The patient was taken to surgery for a left frontal craniotomy with awake language and motor mapping for resection of the lesion with intraoperative MRI. The patient was intubated with a laryngeal mask airway. The scalp was blocked bilaterally with local anesthetic, and the head was fixed in pins, with two pins straddling the inion and one pin on the right forehead in the midpupillary line. The head was positioned with a 30-degree turn to the right. A curved incision posterior to the lesion that extended from the ipsilateral superior temporal line to the anterior hair line of the contralateral pupil was planned with the aid of preoperative MRI navigation. The patient was draped in the usual standard fashion and given dexamethasone, levetiracetam, and cefazolin. A myocutaneous flap was made and was held in place with fishhooks attached to the drapes. A standard craniotomy was done to encompass both lesions and remained ipsilateral to the sagittal sinus and extended anterior, posterior, and lateral to both lesions. Ultrasound and surgical navigation were used to confirm lesion boundaries, and the boundaries were designated with letter tags once the dura was opened. The dura was anesthetized with local anesthetics between the leaflets adjacent to the middle meningeal vessels. The patient was awakened, and the dura was opened once the patient followed commands consistently. Strip electrodes were placed in the subdural space for after-discharge monitoring. The cortex was initially stimulated at 2 mA, and the ventral premotor cortex was identified and resulted in speech arrest with counting at 3 mA with an Ojemann stimulator (Integra, Princeton, NJ). The rest of the cortical and subcortical mapping took place at 3 mA and involved continuous contralateral face, arm, and leg examinations with picture naming. Positive mapping sites were designated with number tags. Negative mapping occurred over the tumor. The positive cortical sites that were obtained were the motor cortex posteriorly to the posterior lesion (decreased strength), supplementary motor cortex in between both lesions (decreased dexterity), and ventral premotor cortex laterally (speech arrest). The subcortical boundaries that were identified were the corticospinal tract (decreased strength) posteriorly to the posterior lesion and the frontal aslant tract (speech hesitancy) deep and lateral to the lesion. Preliminary diagnosis was infiltrating glioma. Once the resection was complete, the patient was put back to sleep with a laryngeal mask airway, and an intraoperative MRI scan confirmed gross total resection and no more tissue was resected (Fig. 2.2). The dura, bone, and skin were closed in standard fashion.

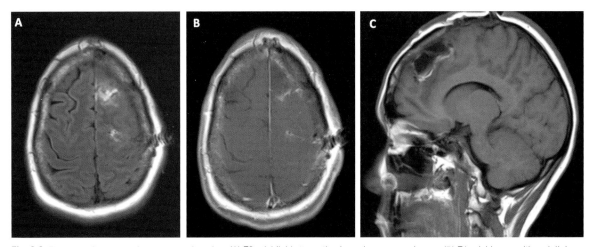

Fig. 2.2 Postoperative magnetic resonance imaging. (A) T2 axial fluid attenuation inversion recovery image; **(B)** T1 axial image with gadolinium contrast; **(C)** T1 sagittal magnetic resonance imaging scan with gadolinium contrast demonstrating gross total resection of both lesions.

The patient awoke at their neurologic baseline with intact speech and full strength bilaterally, and was taken to the intensive care unit for recovery. The patient participated with physical, occupational, and speech therapy and was discharged to home on postoperative day 2. The patient was discharged on 3 months of levetiracetam, and the dexamethasone was tapered to off over 5 days. The patient was seen at 2 weeks postoperatively for staple removal. Pathology was a World Health Organization grade II oligodendroglioma (IDH mutant, 1p/19q codeletion). After a discussion with neurooncology and radiation oncology, the patient was observed with serial imaging. The lesion was observed with serial MRI examinations at 3 months, followed by 6-month intervals, and has been without recurrence for 24 months. The patient had a repeat neuropsychological evaluation at 3 months postoperatively that showed no change from preoperative evaluation. The patient returned to work at 3 weeks postoperatively and remains without neurologic deficits.

Commonalities among the experts

The majority of the surgeons preferred to obtain functional MRI and diffusion tensor imaging for eloquent localization and white matter tract anatomy prior to surgery. All surgeons elected to perform the surgery with cortical and subcortical mapping, of which three chose asleep and one chose awake mapping. The general goal was typically to achieve maximal safe resection of this likely multifocal LGG by working through the left superior and middle frontal gyri. Most were cognizant of the pre-SMA, SMA, motor cortex, and anterior cerebral artery and its branches, and the most feared complication was language and motor deficit, as well as SMA syndrome with injury to Broca area laterally, motor cortex and corticospinal tracts posteriorly, and SMA. Surgery was generally pursued with surgical navigation, brain stimulation, and surgical microscope, with perioperative steroids and/or antiepileptics. Most surgeons performed cortical and subcortical mapping, subpial resection, and avoidance of arterial injury to avoid iatrogenic injury. Following surgery, patients were admitted to the intensive care unit, and MRIs were obtained within 72 hours after surgery. If the diagnosis was a diffuse astrocytoma, radiation and temozolomide for both subtotal and gross total resection were chosen. If the diagnosis was an oligodendroglioma, observation was typically preferred for gross total resection, and radiation and chemotherapy for subtotal resections. If the diagnosis was an anaplastic astrocytoma, radiation and chemotherapy were chosen.

SUMMARY OF QUALITY OF EVIDENCE TO GUIDE SPECIFIC INTERVENTIONS FOR THIS CASE

- Surgery as opposed to biopsy or observation for LGGs—Class II-1.
- Increasing extent of resection associated with improved outcomes—Class II-2.
- Awake mapping versus asleep surgery for LGGs—Class II-2.
- Use of intraoperative MRI to facilitate extent of resection—Class I.

REFERENCES

1. Forst DA, Nahed BV, Loeffler JS, Batchelor TT. Low-grade gliomas. *Oncologist.* 2014;19:403–413.
2. Chaichana KL, McGirt MJ, Frazier J, Attenello F, Guerrero-Cazares H, Quinones-Hinojosa A. Relationship of glioblastoma multiforme to the lateral ventricles predicts survival following tumor resection. *J neurooncol.* 2008;89:219–224.
3. Keles GE, Lamborn KR, Berger MS. Low-grade hemispheric gliomas in adults: a critical review of extent of resection as a factor influencing outcome. *J Neurosurg.* 2001;95:735–745.
4. Chaichana KL, McGirt MJ, Laterra J, Olivi A, Quinones-Hinojosa A. Recurrence and malignant degeneration after resection of adult hemispheric low-grade gliomas. *J Neurosurg.* 2010;112:10–17.
5. Chaichana KL, McGirt MJ, Woodworth GF, et al. Persistent outpatient hyperglycemia is independently associated with survival, recurrence and malignant degeneration following surgery for hemispheric low grade gliomas. *Neurol Res.* 2010;32:442–448.
6. Duffau H. Long-term outcomes after supratotal resection of diffuse low-grade gliomas: a consecutive series with 11-year follow-up. *Acta Neurochir (Wien).* 2016;158:51–58.
7. Eseonu CI, Eguia F, ReFaey K, et al. Comparative volumetric analysis of the extent of resection of molecularly and histologically distinct low grade gliomas and its role on survival. *J Neurooncol.* 2017;134:65–74.
8. Jakola AS, Myrmel KS, Kloster R, et al. Comparison of a strategy favoring early surgical resection vs a strategy favoring watchful waiting in low-grade gliomas. *JAMA.* 2012;308:1881–1888.
9. McGirt MJ, Chaichana KL, Attenello FJ, et al. Extent of surgical resection is independently associated with survival in patients with hemispheric infiltrating low-grade gliomas. *Neurosurgery.* 2008;63:700–707; author reply 707–708.
10. Fernandez-Miranda JC, Rhoton Jr AL. Alvarez-Linera J, Kakizawa Y, Choi C, de Oliveira EP. Three-dimensional microsurgical and tractographic anatomy of the white matter of the human brain. *Neurosurgery.* 2008;62:989–1026; discussion 1026–1028.
11. Rhoton AL Jr. The cerebrum. Anatomy. *Neurosurgery.* 2007;61:37–118; discussion 118–119.
12. Bertani G, Fava E, Casaceli G, et al. Intraoperative mapping and monitoring of brain functions for the resection of low-grade gliomas: technical considerations. *Neurosurg Focus.* 2009;27:E4.
13. Nossek E, Korn A, Shahar T, et al. Intraoperative mapping and monitoring of the corticospinal tracts with neurophysiological assessment and 3-dimensional ultrasonography-based navigation. Clinical article. *J Neurosurg.* 2011;114:738–746.
14. Duffau H. The reliability of asleep-awake-asleep protocol for intraoperative functional mapping and cognitive monitoring in glioma surgery. *Acta Neurochir (Wien).* 2013;155:1803–1804.
15. Eseonu CI, Rincon-Torroella J, ReFaey K, et al. Awake craniotomy vs craniotomy under general anesthesia for perirolandic gliomas: evaluating perioperative complications and extent of resection. *Neurosurgery.* 2017;81:481–489.
16. Senft C, Bink A, Franz K, Vatter H, Gasser T, Seifert V. Intraoperative MRI guidance and extent of resection in glioma surgery: a randomised, controlled trial. *Lancet Oncol.* 2011;12:997–1003.

3

Right perirolandic low-grade glioma

Case reviewed by Miguel A. Arraez, Juan A. Barcia, Mitchel S. Berger, Shawn L. Hervey-Jumper

Introduction

Low-grade gliomas (LGGs) are characterized by the presence of mutations in the isocitrate dehydrogenase (IDH) gene, in which low-grade oligodendrogliomas also possess codeletion of chromosomes 1p and 19q, whereas astrocytomas lack this codeletion.[1,2] In addition to genetic makeup, the prognosis for these lesions is dependent on patient age, neurologic status, and extent of resection.[3–6] Among these factors, the only modifiable risk factor is the extent of resection.[3–6] The challenge is that these lesions infiltrate along white matter tracts and involve eloquent cortical and subcortical structures that can preclude extensive resection.[3–6] In this chapter, we present an LGG that is in close proximity and possibly involves the precentral gyrus in the nondominant hemisphere.

Example case

Chief complaint: seizure
History of present illness
A 44-year-old, right-handed male with no significant past medical history who presented after a seizure event. He was at work and was standing, when he had an acute loss of consciousness accompanied by diffuse body shaking, and a fall in which he struck his head. He underwent imaging that revealed a brain lesion (Fig. 3.1).
Medications: Levetiracetam.
Allergies: No known drug allergies.
Past medical and surgical history: None.
Family history: No history of intracranial malignancies.
Social history: Works as an accountant. No smoking history or alcohol.
Physical examination: Awake, alert, oriented to person, place, and time; Cranial nerves II to XII intact; No drift, moves all extremities with full strength.

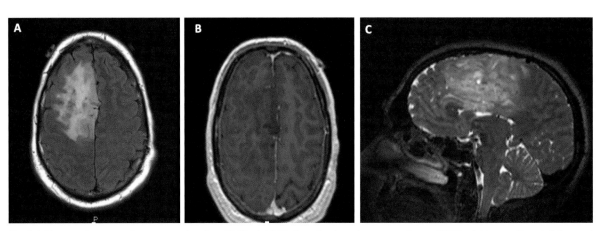

Fig. 3.1 Preoperative magnetic resonance imaging. (A) T2 axial fluid attenuation inversion recovery image; **(B)** T1 axial image with gadolinium contrast; **(C)** T2 sagittal magnetic resonance imaging scan demonstrating a right frontal and perirolandic, nonenhancing lesion involving the presupplementary motor, supplementary motor, and perirolandic areas.

	Miguel A. Arraez, MD, PhD, Carlos Haya University Hospital, Malaga, Spain	Juan A. Barcia, MD, PhD, Hospital Clínico San Carlos, Complutense University, Madrid, Spain	Mitchel S. Berger, MD, University of California at San Francisco, San Francisco, CA	Shawn L. Hervey-Jumper, MD, University of California at San Francisco, San Francisco, CA
Preoperative				
Additional tests requested	MRS DTI fMRI	DTI fMRI Neuropsychological assessment	MEG DTI	MEG DTI Neuropsychological assessment
Surgical approach selected	Right fronto-temporal craniotomy with asleep motor mapping and intraoperative MRI	Right frontal craniotomy with cortical and subcortical mapping	Right frontal craniotomy with asleep motor mapping	Right frontal craniotomy with asleep motor mapping
Anatomic corridor	Right frontal	Right frontal	Right frontal	Right frontal
Goal of surgery	Maximal resection	Cytoreduction with functional preservation, diagnosis	Maximal resection with preservation of motor function	Maximal resection with preservation of motor function
Perioperative				
Positioning	Right supine with left rotation	Right supine neutral	Right supine	Right supine
Surgical equipment	IOM Brain stimulator Surgical navigation Surgical microscope with 5-ALA Ultrasonic aspirator Intraoperative MRI	IOM Surgical navigation Brain stimulator Ultrasonic aspirator	IOM Transcranial motor stimulation Bipolar and monopolar brain stimulators Surgical microscope	IOM (EMG) Surgical navigation Brain stimulation Surgical microscope Ultrasonic aspirator
Medications	Steroids Antiepileptics	Steroids Antiepileptics	Mannitol Steroids Antiepileptics	Mannitol Steroids Antiepileptics
Anatomic considerations	Frontal and parietal sulci, primary motor cortex, CST, interhemispheric region, bridging veins	Sagittal suture, sagittal sinus and veins, central sulcus, precentral gyrus, SMA, MFG, IFG, cingulate gyrus, corpus callosum, pericallosal arteries	Sagittal sinus and draining veins, primary motor cortex, CST	SMA, premotor cortex, primary motor cortex, primary sensory cortex, callosomarginal and pericallosal arteries
Complications feared with approach chosen	Injury to superior sagittal sinus and bridging veins, motor deficit	Motor deficit, venous injury	Motor deficit, expect SMA syndrome	Motor deficit, expect SMA syndrome
Intraoperative				
Anesthesia	General	Asleep-awake-asleep	General	General
Skin incision	Fronto-parieto-temporal	Pterional	Pterional	L-shaped
Bone opening	Bifrontal craniotomy eccentric to the right	Right frontal craniotomy up to sagittal sinus	Right frontal ipsilateral to sagittal sinus	Right frontal
Brain exposure	Right frontal	Right frontal (SFG, MFG), and central sulcus	Right frontal	Right frontal

(continued on next page)

	Miguel A. Arraez, MD, PhD, Carlos Haya University Hospital, Malaga, Spain	Juan A. Barcia, MD, PhD, Hospital Clínico San Carlos, Complutense University, Madrid, Spain	Mitchel S. Berger, MD, University of California at San Francisco, San Francisco, CA	Shawn L. Hervey-Jumper, MD, University of California at San Francisco, San Francisco, CA
Method of resection	Right frontal dural opening up to midline with preservation of bridging veins, cortical mapping to identify motor area, identify boundaries of lesion, removal of tumor along safe regions, subcortical stimulation in vicinity of CST, intraoperative MRI to guide further resection, insertion of subgaleal drain with low pressure	Right frontal craniotomy up to sagittal sinus with wide enough exposure of SFG/MFG/ interhemispheric/central sulcus, awake patient, SMA and motor cortex mapping, subpial tumor resection within SFG/ MFG/cingulate gyrus/ corpus callosum with preservation of the motor cortex/CST by subcortical stimulation/ventricular ependymal lining	Exposure up to sagittal sinus, cortical and subcortical brain mapping with intermittent TMS, continue resection until motor cortex encountered, dural tack up suture, insertion of subgaleal drain	Cortical brain stimulation up to 16 mA to identify primary motor cortex, resect just anterior to primary motor cortex, resect along anterior and medial margins via subpial resections up to lateral margin, expose falx/cingulate sulcus/ callosomarginal arteries and anterior margin of primary motor cortex, subcortical stimulation to 5 mm from CST
Complication avoidance	Large bony opening, cortical and subcortical mapping	Large bony opening, cortical and subcortical motor mapping, subpial dissection	Large bony opening, cortical and subcortical brain mapping with intermittent TMS	Cortical and subcortical stimulation, leaving posterior margin for last
Postoperative				
Admission	ICU	ICU	ICU	ICU
Postoperative complications feared	Motor deficit, cognitive dysfunction	CSF leak, expected SMA syndrome	Transient SMA, motor deficit	SMA syndrome
Follow-up testing	MRI within 72 hours after surgery	CT immediately after surgery MRI within 1 month after surgery Rehabilitation if SMA syndrome	MRI with DWI and DTI within 48 hours after surgery	MRI within 48 hours after surgery
Follow-up visits	7 days after surgery	7 days after surgery 1 month after surgery	Dependent on lesion type	14 days after surgery
Adjuvant therapies recommended				
Diffuse astrocytoma (IDH mutant, retain 1p19q)	STR–radiation/ temozolomide GTR–radiation/ temozolomide	STR–radiation/temozolomide GTR–radiation (unmethylated), radiation/temozolomide (methylated)	STR–radiation/ temozolomide GTR–observation	STR–radiation/ temozolomide GTR–observation
Oligodendroglioma (IDH mutant, 1p19q LOH)	STR–radiation/PCV GTR–radiation/PCV	STR–radiation/PCV GTR–radiation/PCV	STR–chemotherapy GTR–observation	STR–tumor board discussion but likely chemoradiation GTR–observation
Anaplastic astrocytoma (IDH wildtype)	STR–radiation/ temozolomide GTR–radiation/ temozolomide	STR–radiation/temozolomide GTR–radiation/ temozolomide	STR–radiation/ temozolomide GTR–radiation/ temozolomide	STR–radiation/ temozolomide GTR–radiation/ temozolomide

5-ALA, 5-aminolevulinic acid; CSF, cerebrospinal fluid; CST, corticospinal tracts; CT, computed tomography; DTI, diffusion tensor imaging; DWI, diffusion-weighted imaging; EMG, electromyography; fMRI, functional magnetic resonance imaging; GTR, gross total resection; ICU, intensive care unit; IFG, interior frontal gyrus; IOM, intraoperative monitoring; LOH, loss of heterozygosity; MEG, magnetoencephalogram; MFG, middle frontal gyrus; MRI, magnetic resonance imaging; MRS, magnetic resonance spectroscopy; PCV, procarbazine, lomustine, vincristine; SFG, superior frontal gyrus; SMA, supplementary motor area; STR, subtotal resection; TMS, transcranial magnetic stimulation.

Differential diagnosis and actual diagnosis

- LGG (astrocytoma, oligodendroglioma)
- High-grade glioma
- Demyelinating disease (i.e., multiple sclerosis)

Important anatomic and preoperative considerations

The central lobe has a lateral and a medial surface.[7,8] The precentral and postcentral gyri that are divided by the central sulcus lie on the lateral surface, and the paracentral lobule lies on the medial surface.[7,8] The precentral gyrus corresponds to the primary motor cortex, and the postcentral gyrus corresponds to the primary sensory area.[7,8] This area is bounded anteriorly and posteriorly by the precentral and postcentral sulci, respectively.[7,8] The central sulcus extends from the medial aspect of the hemisphere and runs on the lateral surface from a posterior to anterior direction toward the Sylvian fissure, where it makes contact via the subcentral gyrus that connects the pre- and postcentral gyri.[7,8] Anterior to the central lobe above the Sylvian fissure is the frontal lobe.[7,8] At the level of the middle frontal gyrus is the premotor cortex, and at the level of the superior frontal gyrus is the supplementary motor area (SMA).[7,8] The central sulcus as three curves, in which the superior curve is near the midline and its convexity faces anteriorly, the middle curve has its convexity facing posteriorly, and the inferior curve has its convexity facing anteriorly.[7,8] These curves make the precentral gyrus appear as an omega shape centered on the second curve, and is the motor representation of the hand.[7,8] Additionally, the superior frontal sulcus ends at the level of the omega. Finally, the postcentral sulcus has a bifurcation at its superior end that caps the marginal ramus of the cingulate gyrus.[7,8] On the medial surface of the central lobe is the quadrangular-shaped paracentral lobule, which is limited by the paracentral sulcus anteriorly, the marginal ramus posteriorly, and the cingulate sulcus inferiorly.[7,8] The marginal ramus can be identified as lying within the middle of the bifurcation of the postcentral sulcus. Stimulation of the motor cortex can inhibit motor movement, whereas stimulation of the SMA can cause complex postural movement, incoordination, and motor or speech arrest.[7,8] The lesion spans the pre-SMA, SMA, premotor, and motor cortex, as well as the corticospinal tract based on preoperative magnetic resonance imaging (MRI).

Approaches to this lesion

As discussed in Chapter 1, the approaches to this lesion can be divided into asleep and awake procedures (Fig. 1.2). The general approaches to this lesion are biopsy versus extensive surgical resection. When extensive resection is pursued, the goal is maximal percent resection and minimal residual volume, while avoiding neurologic deficits.[9–11] One way of minimizing neurologic deficits is by identifying and minimizing damage to eloquent cortical and subcortical areas. This can be done through indirect and direct cortical and subcortical identification, which can be done outside and within the operating room (Fig. 3.2). Passive means of identifying eloquent cortex extraoperatively (outside of the operating room) includes functional MRI, which relies on changes in blood flow with specific neuronal activity, and diffusion tensor imaging (DTI), which relies on the anisotropic diffusion of water molecules along white matter facts.[12] The problem with these extraoperative modalities is that they are associated with false-positive and false-negative identification that can lead to reduced resections and/or iatrogenic neurologic deficits, and intraoperatively because of brain shifts that can lose accurate localization

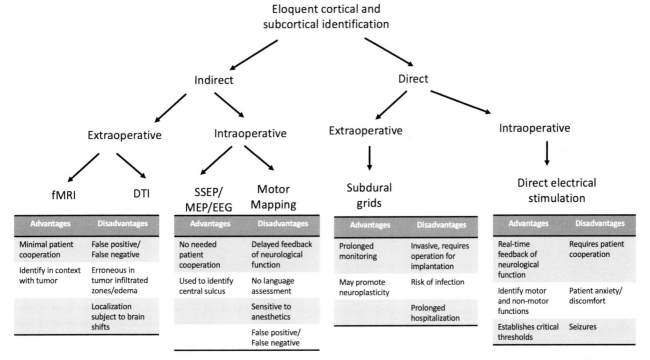

Fig. 3.2 Diagram of different direct and indirect methods of identifying eloquent cortical and subcortical structures. DTI, Diffusion tensor imaging; EEG, electroencephalogram; fMRI, functional magnetic resonance imaging; MEP, motor evoked potential; SSEP, somatosensory evoked potential.

intraoperatively. Direct methods of identifying cortical and subcortical areas involves awake brain mapping, in which cortical and subcortical structures are stimulated to guide resection based on avoiding eloquently identified regions.

In terms of directionality of approach, this lesion involves the superficial cortex of the superior frontal gyrus and precentral gyrus along the interhemispheric fissure, and therefore the most practical approach would be to center the approach over this area. Approaching from a more lateral trajectory would require traversing uninvolved cortex and subcortical tissue and, more specifically, white matter tracts, such as the superior longitudinal fasciculus.

What was actually done

The patient underwent a neuropsychological evaluation that showed mild deficits in attention and working memory. The patient was taken to surgery for a right frontal craniotomy with awake language and motor mapping for resection of the lesion. The patient was intubated with a laryngeal mask airway. The scalp was blocked bilaterally with local anesthetic, and the head was fixed in pins, with two pins oriented coronally on the left with the inferior pin near the mastoid process and the contralateral pin posterior to the external auditory meatus on the right side. The head was positioned neutral and slightly flexed to minimize patient discomfort. A bicoronal incision at the midpoint of the lesion was planned based on preoperative MRI navigation, and spanned from the superior temporal line on the left to below this point on the right. The patient was draped in the usual standard fashion and given dexamethasone, levetiracetam, and cefazolin. The flap was made and held in place with self-retaining cerebellar retractors. A right frontal-parietal craniotomy was done to encompass the lesion, as well as extend at least one gyrus anterior, posterior, and lateral to the lesion, and remained just ipsilateral to the sagittal sinus. Ultrasound and surgical navigation were used to confirm lesion boundaries, and the boundaries were designated with letter tags once the dura was opened. The dura was anesthetized with local anesthetics between the leaflets adjacent to the middle meningeal vessels. The patient was awakened, and the dura was opened once the patient followed commands consistently. Strip electrodes were placed in the subdural space for after

discharge monitoring. The cortex was initially stimulated at 2 mA, and speech motor arrest was achieved with counting at 3 mA with an Ojemann stimulator (Integra, Princeton, NJ) over the precentral gyrus. The rest of the cortical and subcortical mapping took place at 3 mA. The patient participated in continuous motor movement of the left face, arm, and leg, as well as participated in picture naming. Positive mapping sites were designated with number tags. Negative mapping occurred over the anterior portion of the tumor. The positive cortical sites that were obtained were the motor cortex posteriorly within the lesion (decreased strength), whereas the positive subcortical boundary was the corticospinal tract (decreased strength) along the posterior and deep portion of the lesion. Preliminary diagnosis was infiltrating glioma. Once the lesion was disconnected from the positive motor cortical and subcortical sites, the patient was put back to sleep with a laryngeal mask airway, and the remaining tumor tissue was resected. The dura, bone, and skin were closed in standard fashion.

The patient awoke at their neurologic baseline with full strength bilaterally and taken to the intensive care unit for recovery. On postoperative day 1, the patient developed some apraxia in their left lower extremity. Postoperative MRI done 48 hours after surgery showed near total resection with expected residual in the precentral gyrus and corticospinal tract (Fig. 3.3). The patient participated with physical and occupational therapy and was discharged to home on postoperative day 3 with left lower extremity apraxia. The patient was prescribed 3 months of levetiracetam, and dexamethasone was tapered to off over 5 days after surgery. The patient was seen at 2 weeks postoperatively for staple removal and was full strength without apraxia with continued physical therapy. Pathology was a World Health Organization grade II oligodendroglioma (IDH mutant, 1p/19q codeletion). The patient underwent procarbazine, lomustine, and vincristine chemotherapy with radiation therapy. The lesion was observed with serial MRI examinations at 3 months, followed by 6-month intervals, and has been without recurrence for 36 months. The patient had a repeat neuropsychological evaluation at 3 months postoperatively that showed no change from preoperative evaluation. The patient returned to work at 4 weeks postoperatively and remains without neurologic deficits.

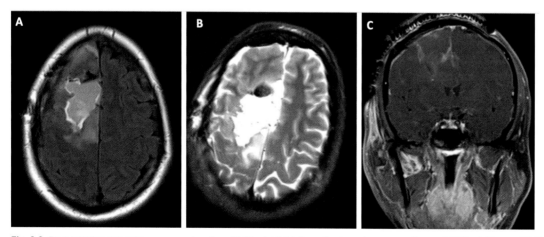

Fig. 3.3 Postoperative magnetic resonance imaging. (A) T2 axial fluid attenuation inversion recovery image; **(B)** T2 axial image; **(C)** T1 coronal magnetic resonance imaging scan with gadolinium contrast demonstrating near total resection of the tumor with residual tumor within the precentral gyrus.

Commonalities among the experts

For this diffuse lesion, the majority of the surgeons preferred to obtain fMRI and DTI for eloquent localization and white matter tract anatomy prior to surgery, and even magnetoencephalogram in two surgeons. All of the surgeons elected to perform asleep surgery with cortical and subcortical mapping. The general goal was typically to achieve maximal safe resection. Most surgeons were cognizant of the perirolandic area (precentral, central, and postcentral sulci), sagittal sinus and draining veins, and pericallosal and callosomarginal arteries, and the most feared complication was a motor deficit and/or SMA syndrome with injury to motor cortex and corticospinal tracts posteriorly, as well as the SMA. Surgery was generally pursued with surgical navigation, brain stimulation, and surgical microscope, with perioperative steroids and/or antiepileptics. Most surgeons favored the use of large bony openings, cortical and subcortical mapping, and subpial dissection to avoid iatrogenic injury. Following surgery, patients were admitted to the intensive care unit, and MRIs were obtained within 72 hours after surgery. If the diagnosis was a diffuse astrocytoma, radiation and temozolomide for both subtotal and gross total resection were chosen. If the diagnosis was an oligodendroglioma, observation versus radiation and chemotherapy were both chosen for gross total resection, whereas radiation and chemotherapy was chosen for subtotal resections. If the diagnosis was an anaplastic astrocytoma, radiation and chemotherapy were chosen.

SUMMARY OF QUALITY OF EVIDENCE TO GUIDE SPECIFIC INTERVENTIONS FOR THIS CASE

- Surgery as opposed to biopsy or observation for LGGs—Class II-1.
- Surgery for LGGs in perirolandic regions—Class II-2.
- Increasing extent of resection associated with improved outcomes—Class II-2.
- Awake mapping versus asleep surgery for LGGs—Class II-2.
- Procarbazine, lomustine, and vincristine chemotherapy and radiation therapy for oligodendrogliomas—Class I.

REFERENCES

1. Parsons DW, Jones S, Zhang X, et al. An integrated genomic analysis of human glioblastoma multiforme. *Science.* 2008;321:1807–1812.
2. Leeper HE, Caron AA, Decker PA, Jenkins RB, Lachance DH, Giannini C. IDH mutation, 1p19q codeletion and ATRX loss in WHO grade II gliomas. *Oncotarget.* 2015;6:30295–30305.
3. Chaichana KL, McGirt MJ, Laterra J, Olivi A, Quinones-Hinojosa A. Recurrence and malignant degeneration after resection of adult hemispheric low-grade gliomas. *J Neurosurg.* 2010;112:10–17.
4. Chaichana KL, McGirt MJ, Niranjan A, Olivi A, Burger PC, Quinones-Hinojosa A. Prognostic significance of contrast-enhancing low-grade gliomas in adults and a review of the literature. *Neurol Res.* 2009;31:931–939.
5. Eseonu CI, Eguia F, ReFaey K. et al: Comparative volumetric analysis of the extent of resection of molecularly and histologically distinct low grade gliomas and its role on survival. *J Neurooncol.* 2017;134:65–74.
6. Jakola AS, Myrmel KS, Kloster R, et al. Comparison of a strategy favoring early surgical resection vs a strategy favoring watchful waiting in low-grade gliomas. *JAMA.* 2012;308:1881–1888.
7. Fernandez-Miranda JC, Rhoton AL Jr., Alvarez-Linera J, Kakizawa Y, Choi C, de Oliveira EP. Three-dimensional microsurgical and tractographic anatomy of the white matter of the human brain. *Neurosurgery.* 2008;62:989–1026; discussion 1026–1028.
8. Rhoton AL Jr. The cerebrum. Anatomy. *Neurosurgery.* 2007;61:37–118; discussion 118–119.
9. Duffau H, Mandonnet E. The "onco-functional balance" in surgery for diffuse low-grade glioma: integrating the extent of resection with quality of life. *Acta Neurochir (Wien).* 2013;155:951–957.
10. Keles GE, Lamborn KR, Berger MS. Low-grade hemispheric gliomas in adults: a critical review of extent of resection as a factor influencing outcome. *J Neurosurg.* 2011;95:736–745.
11. McGirt MJ, Chaichana KL, Attenello FJ, et al. Extent of surgical resection is independently associated with survival in patients with hemispheric infiltrating low-grade gliomas. *Neurosurgery.* 2008;63:700–707.
12. Duffau H. The dangers of magnetic resonance imaging diffusion tensor tractography in brain surgery. *World Neurosurg.* 2014;81:56–58.

4

Left perirolandic low-grade glioma

Case reviewed by Steven Brem, Jeffrey N. Bruce, Ricardo Díez Valle, Santiago Gil-Robles

Introduction

Gliomas are known to infiltrate cortical areas and white matter tracts.[1,2] In low-grade gliomas (LGGs), there can be interspersing tumor with nontumor tissue.[3] Therefore when LGGs involve eloquent regions, surgical resection can result in significant neurologic morbidity.[4–6] A common location for LGGs is the perirolandic region, where surgery is associated with risk of motor weakness and sensory loss that can be debilitating and significantly affect quality of life.[6] Dominant versus nondominant perirolandic involvement can alter management. In this chapter, we present an LGG that is in close proximity and possibly involves the precentral gyrus in the dominant hemisphere.

Example case

Chief complaint: headaches

History of present illness

A 46-year-old, right-handed woman with a history of anxiety and depression with a known lesion is being followed with serial imaging. Her history dates back to 5 years prior when she complained of headaches and underwent imaging that revealed the left-sided brain tumor. It was followed with serial imaging, and the lesion had increased in size (Fig. 4.1). She remains with headaches that are responsive to acetaminophen, and was referred for further evaluation and management.

Medications: Alprazolam, clonazepam.

Allergies: No known drug allergies.

Past medical and surgical history: Anxiety and depression.

Family history: No history of intracranial malignancies.

Social history: Homemaker. No smoking history or alcohol.

Physical examination: Awake, alert, oriented to person, place, and time; Cranial nerves II to XII intact; No drift, moves all extremities with full strength.

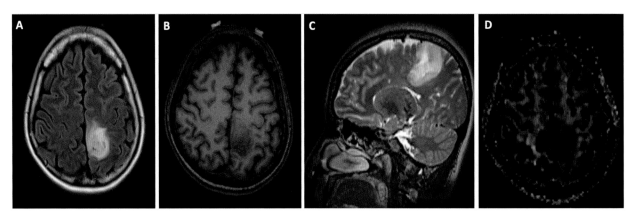

Fig. 4.1 Preoperative magnetic resonance imaging. (A) T2 axial fluid attenuation inversion recovery image; **(B)** T1 axial image with gadolinium contrast; **(C)** T2 sagittal image; **(D)** diffusion tractography magnetic resonance imaging scan demonstrating a left perirolandic, nonenhancing lesion involving the pre- and postcentral gyri.

	Steven Brem, MD, University of Pennsylvania, Philadelphia, PA, United States	Jeffrey N. Bruce, MD, Columbia University, New York City, NY, United States	Ricardo Díez Valle, MD, PhD, Fundación Jimenez Díaz University Clinic, Madrid, Spain	Santiago Gil-Robles, MD, PhD, Universidad Europea de Madrid, Madrid, Spain
Preoperative				
Additional tests requested	DTI fMRI Perfusion MRI MRS Neuropsychological assessment		DTI	DTI fMRI or MEG Neuropsychological assessment
Surgical approach selected	Left fronto-parietal craniotomy	Left fronto-parietal craniotomy with awake motor mapping	Left fronto-parietal craniotomy with IOM and iMRI with asleep mapping	Left paracentral craniotomy with awake mapping
Anatomic corridor	Fronto-parietal lobe over tumor surface	Fronto-parietal lobe over tumor surface	Fronto-parietal lobe over tumor surface	Left paracentral/ precuneus
Goal of surgery	Maximal safe resection (80%–95%)	Extensive resection with functional preservation	Diagnosis, reduction of tumor mass	Extensive resection with functional preservation
Perioperative				
Positioning	Supine neutral	Left supine with slight rotation	Prone vs. left lateral	Left supine 45-degree rotation
Surgical equipment	Surgical navigation IOM (SSEP) Brain stimulator Surgical microscope Ultrasonic aspirator	Surgical navigation IOM (ECoG) Brain stimulator Ultrasound Ultrasonic aspirator Surgical microscope	Surgical navigation IOM Brain stimulator Surgical microscope with 5-ALA iMRI	Brain stimulator Surgical navigation Ultrasonic aspirator Speech therapist
Medications	Steroids Antiepileptics	Steroids Antiepileptics	Steroids	Steroids Antiepileptics
Anatomic considerations	Motor cortex, CST	Motor cortex	Motor and sensory cortex, terminal branches of ACA, sagittal sinus	Primary motor cortex (especially lower limb), IPL (language, reading, calculation), sensory cortex, thalamocortical pathway, CST, SLF I and II
Complications feared with approach chosen	Motor deficit	Motor deficit	Sagittal sinus and/or ACA injury, motor or somatosensory deficits	Motor, language, reading, calculation, and sensory deficits
Intraoperative				
Anesthesia	General	Asleep-awake-asleep	General	Asleep-awake-asleep
Skin incision	Linear parasagittal	Linear coronal	Linear	Horseshoe
Bone opening	Left fronto-parietal	Left fronto-parietal	Left fronto-parietal	Left frontal-parietal
Brain exposure	Left fronto-parietal	Left fronto-parietal	Left fronto-parietal	Paracentral and SPL/IPL

(continued on next page)

	Steven Brem, MD, University of Pennsylvania, Philadelphia, PA, United States	Jeffrey N. Bruce, MD, Columbia University, New York City, NY, United States	Ricardo Díez Valle, MD, PhD, Fundación Jimenez Díaz University Clinic, Madrid, Spain	Santiago Gil-Robles, MD, PhD, Universidad Europea de Madrid, Madrid, Spain
Method of resection	Keyhole craniotomy (~3 cm) ipsilateral to sagittal sinus, curvilinear dural opening, phase reversal to identify rolandic fissure, stimulate cortex with brain stimulator from 3–20 mA or higher to identify and avoid motor cortex, cortical entry where negative stimulation sites, transsulcal if eloquent, maximal safe resection with goal 80%–95%	Monitored anesthesia care, craniotomy ipsilateral to sagittal sinus, U-shaped dural opening based on sagittal sinus, grid placed for cortical mapping, awaken patient to map for motor cortex, resection based on motor mapping, internal debulking, ultrasound to determine if residual present	Craniotomy centered over lesion ipsilateral to sagittal sinus, dura opened to midline, mapping with monopolar and strip electrode to monitor MEP, dissection of tumor border and internal debulking with bipolar and forceps, iMRI to assess completeness of resection and need for further resection	Left parietal craniotomy, dural anesthesia, patient awoken, detection of boundaries based on navigation, identify motor cortex with low threshold stimulation (1.5–3 mA) with limb contraction, cortical mapping for motor/ somatosensory/ cognitive and language function, subpial resection of the postcentral sulcus and interparietal sulcus, alternate resection and stimulation until functional boundaries reached (medial primary motor of lower limb/ thalamocortical pathway/SLF laterally
Complication avoidance	Phase reversal, cortical stimulation, transsulcal entry if eloquent, goal resection 80%–95%	ECoG and cortical and subcortical brain mapping, ultrasound	Cortical and subcortical mapping, MEP, iMRI	Cortical and subcortical mapping of motor/ somatosensory cortex, IPL, thalamocortical/CST/ SLF I and II
Postoperative				
Admission	ICU	ICU	ICU	ICU
Postoperative complications feared	Motor deficit, aphasia, seizures	Motor deficit, seizures	Right lower extremity motor or sensory deficit	Transient ataxia, lower limb palsy, aphasia
Follow-up testing	MRI within 24 hours after surgery Next generation sequencing	MRI within 48 hours after surgery	MRI within 72 hours after surgery	MRI within 24 hours after surgery Neuropsychological assessment Physical/cognitive therapy
Follow-up visits	1 month after surgery	7 days after surgery	7 days after surgery	7–10 days after surgery
Adjuvant therapies recommended				
Diffuse astrocytoma (IDH mutant, retain 1p19q)	GTR–radiation +/– temozolomide STR–radiation +/– temozolomide	GTR–radiation/ temozolomide STR–radiation/ temozolomide	GTR–radiation/ temozolomide STR–radiation/ temozolomide	<4 mm/year growth rate–observation >4 mm/year growth rate–radiation/ temozolomide

	Steven Brem, MD, University of Pennsylvania, Philadelphia, PA, United States	Jeffrey N. Bruce, MD, Columbia University, New York City, NY, United States	Ricardo Díez Valle, MD, PhD, Fundación Jimenez Díaz University Clinic, Madrid, Spain	Santiago Gil-Robles, MD, PhD, Universidad Europea de Madrid, Madrid, Spain
Oligodendroglioma (IDH mutant, 1p19q LOH)	Pending positive TERT status, GTR–PCV or temozolomide STR–PCV or temozolomide	GTR–observation STR–radiation/ temozolomide because of preop growth	GTR–radiation/PCV STR–radiation/PCV	GTR–observation STR–<4 mm/year growth rate– observation; >4 mm/ year growth rate–PCV
Anaplastic astrocytoma (IDH wildtype)	GTR–radiation/ temozolomide STR–radiation/ temozolomide	GTR–radiation/ temozolomide STR–radiation/ temozolomide	GTR–radiation/ temozolomide STR–radiation/ temozolomide	Homogenous AA–radiation/ temozolomide AA foci removal– treatment as for diffuse astrocytoma

5-ALA, 5-aminolevulinic acid; *AA*, anaplastic astrocytoma; *ACA*, anterior cerebral artery; *CST*, corticospinal tract; *DTI*, diffusion tensor imaging; *ECoG*, electrocorticography; *fMRI*, functional magnetic resonance imaging; *ICU*, intensive care unit; *iMRI*, intraoperative magnetic resonance imaging; *IPL*, inferior parietal lobule; *IOM*, intraoperative monitoring; *LOH*, loss of heterozygosity; *MEG*, magnetoencephalogram; *MEP*, motor evoked potential; *MRI*, magnetic resonance imaging; *MRS*, magnetic resonance spectroscopy; *PCV*, procarbazine, lomustine, vincristine; *SEEP*, somatosensory evoked potential; *SLF*, superior longitudinal fasciculus; *SPL*, superior parietal lobule; *TERT*, telomerase reverse transcriptase.

Differential diagnosis and actual diagnosis

- LGG (astrocytoma, oligodendroglioma)
- High-grade glioma
- Demyelinating disease (i.e., multiple sclerosis)

Important anatomic and preoperative considerations

See Chapter 3 for a full detailed description of the central lobe with pre- and postcentral gyri. There are several different ways to identify the pre- and postcentral gyri based on preoperative imaging.[7,8] A common method is to identify the superior frontal sulcus, which is located immediately paramedian to the anterior interhemispheric fissure, and tracing it posteriorly on axial images to where it joins the precentral sulcus that runs immediately anterior and parallel to the central sulcus.[7,8] The central sulcus can then be confirmed by its anterior to posterior trajectory from inferior to superior as it courses toward the interhemispheric fissure, and typically ends by pointing at the horizontal bracket formed by pars marginalis.[7,8] In addition, the central sulcus can be identified by the omega shape of the precentral gyrus, in which the knob portion at the axial level of the superior frontal sulcus corresponds to the hand motor region.[7,8] Furthermore, the anteroposterior thickness of the precentral gyrus is always greater than that of the postcentral gyrus.[7,8] The lesion in this case spans the dominant hemisphere primary motor and somatosensory cortices, with involvement of the corticospinal tract based on preoperative magnetic resonance imaging (MRI) and diffusion tractography imaging (DTI).

Approaches to this lesion

The approaches to this lesion can be divided into asleep and awake procedures (see Chapter 1, Fig. 1.2), and the identification of eloquent cortical and subcortical structures by direct and indirect methods (see Chapter 3, Fig. 3.2). As this lesion primarily involves the pre- and postcentral gyri, it is important to be able to monitor the motor and sensory cortices and corticospinal tracts. Asleep surgery with motor evoked potentials and somatosensory evoked potentials record these areas passively.[9,10] This passive monitoring only records changes after potentially irreversible damage occurs, is not sensitive or specific, and is sensitive to anesthetics.[9,10] It can be supplemented with brain mapping to identify potential eloquent areas, but does not provide feedback on neurologic function.[9,10] As opposed to asleep surgery, awake mapping allows active evaluation of motor and sensory pathways with real-time feedback, but requires patient cooperation, surgeon experience, increased surgical time, and potentially increased risk of seizures.[9,11–13]

In terms of the directionality of approach, this lesion involves the primary motor and somatosensory cortices adjacent to the interhemispheric fissure. The craniotomy and corticectomy should be centered over this area, as the lesion itself abuts the cortical surface. A more laterally positioned approach could potential endanger uninvolved cortical and subcortical areas of the motor and sensory cortices and corticospinal tract.

What was actually done

The patient underwent a neuropsychological evaluation that showed no significant deficits. The patient was taken to surgery for a left frontal-parietal craniotomy with awake motor mapping for resection of the lesion. The patient was intubated with a laryngeal mask airway. The scalp was blocked bilaterally with local anesthetic, and the head was fixed in pins, with two pins centered on the right external auditory meatus at the level of the superior temporal line and one pin over the left external auditory meatus just below superior temporal line. The head was positioned neutral and slightly flexed to minimize patient discomfort. A bicoronal incision at the midpoint of the lesion was planned based on preoperative MRI navigation. The patient was draped in the usual standard fashion and given dexamethasone, levetiracetam, and cefazolin. The flap was made and held in place with self-retaining cerebellar retractors. A left frontal-parietal craniotomy was done to encompass the lesion, as well as extend at least one gyrus anterior, posterior, and lateral to the lesion, and remained just ipsilateral to the sagittal sinus. Ultrasound and surgical navigation were used to confirm lesion boundaries, and the boundaries were designated with letter tags once the dura was opened. The dura was anesthetized with local anesthetics between the leaflets adjacent to the middle meningeal vessels. The patient was awakened, and the dura was opened once the patient followed commands consistently. Strip electrodes were placed in the subdural space for after discharge monitoring. The cortex was initially stimulated at 2 mA, and hand dysfunction was achieved at 3 mA with an Ojemann stimulator (Integra, Princeton, NJ) over the precentral gyrus. The rest of the cortical and subcortical mapping took place at 3 mA. The patient participated in continuous motor movement of the right face, arm, and leg. Positive mapping sites were designated with number tags. Negative mapping occurred over the tumor, but positive cortical sites were obtained laterally with decreased hand strength (hand motor cortex), anteriorly with decreased coordination (supplementary motor area), and paresthesias posteriorly over the leg (sensory cortex). Positive subcortical sites were obtained laterally and deep with hand dysfunction and spasticity (corticospinal tract). Preliminary diagnosis was infiltrating glioma. The dura, bone, and skin were closed in standard fashion.

The patient awoke at their neurologic baseline with full strength bilaterally and was taken to the intensive care unit for recovery. Postoperative MRI done within 48 hours after surgery showed gross total resection (Fig. 4.2). The patient participated with physical and occupational therapy and was discharged to home on postoperative day 2 with an intact neurologic examination. The patient was prescribed 3 months of levetiracetam, and dexamethasone was tapered to off over 5 days after surgery. The patient was seen at 2 weeks postoperatively for staple removal and was at full strength. Pathology was a World Health Organization grade II oligodendroglioma (IDH mutant, 1p/19q codeletion). The lesion was observed with serial MRI examinations at 3 months, followed by 6-month intervals, and has been without recurrence for 24 months. The patient had a repeat neuropsychological evaluation at 3 months postoperatively that showed no change from preoperative evaluation. The patient returned to work at 3 weeks postoperatively and remains without neurologic deficits.

Commonalities among the experts

For this lesion, the majority of the surgeons preferred to obtain functional MRI and DTI for eloquent localization and white matter tract anatomy prior to surgery. Neuropsychiatry evaluation was also chosen by two surgeons. The majority of surgeons elected to perform surgery with cortical and subcortical motor mapping (two awake, one asleep). The general goal was typically to achieve extensive resection with functional preservation. Most surgeons were cognizant of the motor and sensory cortices, as well as the corticospinal tract, and the most feared complication was a motor deficit with injury to motor cortex and corticospinal tracts. Surgery was generally pursued with surgical navigation, brain stimulation, surgical microscope, and ultrasonic aspirator, with perioperative steroids and/or antiepileptics. Most surgeons favored the use of cortical and subcortical mapping to avoid iatrogenic injury. Following surgery, patients were admitted to the intensive care unit, and MRIs were obtained within 72 hours after surgery. If the diagnosis was a diffuse astrocytoma, radiation and temozolomide for both subtotal and gross total resection were chosen. If the diagnosis was an oligodendroglioma, observation versus radiation and chemotherapy were both chosen for gross total resection, whereas radiation and chemotherapy were chosen for subtotal resections. If the diagnosis was an anaplastic astrocytoma, radiation and chemotherapy were chosen.

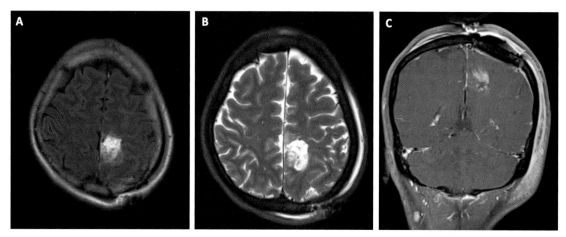

Fig. 4.2 Postoperative magnetic resonance imaging. (A) T2 axial fluid attenuation inversion recovery image; **(B)** T2 axial image; **(C)** T1 coronal magnetic resonance imaging scan with gadolinium contrast demonstrating gross total resection of the tumor involving the perirolandic regions.

SUMMARY OF QUALITY OF EVIDENCE TO GUIDE SPECIFIC INTERVENTIONS FOR THIS CASE

- Surgery as opposed to biopsy or observation for LGGs—Class II-1.
- Surgery for LGGs in eloquent perirolandic regions—Class II-2.
- Increasing extent of resection associated with improved outcomes—Class II-2.
- Awake mapping versus asleep surgery for LGGs—Class II-2.
- DTI to avoid deficits from white matter tract injury—Class III.

REFERENCES

1. Chaichana KL, Guerrero-Cazares H, Capilla-Gonzalez V, et al. Intra-operatively obtained human tissue: protocols and techniques for the study of neural stem cells. *J Neurosci Methods.* 2009;180:116–125.
2. Li Q, Wijeseekera O, Salas SJ, et al. Mesenchymal stem cells from human fat engineered to secrete BMP4 are nononcogenic, suppress brain cancer, and prolong survival. *Clin Cancer Res.* 2014;20:2375–2387.
3. Kut C, Chaichana KL, Xi J, et al. Detection of human brain cancer infiltration ex vivo and in vivo using quantitative optical coherence tomography. *Sci Transl Med.* 2015;7:292ra100.
4. Chaichana KL, McGirt MJ, Laterra J, Olivi A, Quinones-Hinojosa A. Recurrence and malignant degeneration after resection of adult hemispheric low-grade gliomas. *J Neurosurg.* 2010;112:10–17.
5. Chaichana KL, McGirt MJ, Niranjan A, Olivi A, Burger PC, Quinones-Hinojosa A. Prognostic significance of contrast-enhancing low-grade gliomas in adults and a review of the literature. *Neurol Res.* 2009;31:931–939.
6. McGirt MJ, Mukherjee D, Chaichana KL, Than KD, Weingart JD, Quinones-Hinojosa A. Association of surgically acquired motor and language deficits on overall survival after resection of glioblastoma multiforme. *Neurosurgery.* 2009;65:463–469; discussion 469–470.
7. Fernandez-Miranda JC, Rhoton AL Jr. Alvarez-Linera J, Kakizawa Y, Choi C, de Oliveira EP. Three-dimensional microsurgical and tractographic anatomy of the white matter of the human brain. *Neurosurgery.* 2008;62:989–1026; discussion 1026–1028.
8. Rhoton AL Jr. The cerebrum. Anatomy. *Neurosurgery.* 2007;61:37–118; discussion 118–119.
9. Bertani G, Fava E, Casaceli G, et al. Intraoperative mapping and monitoring of brain functions for the resection of low-grade gliomas: technical considerations. *Neurosurg Focus.* 2009;27:E4.
10. Nossek E, Korn A, Shahar T, et al. Intraoperative mapping and monitoring of the corticospinal tracts with neurophysiological assessment and 3-dimensional ultrasonography-based navigation. Clinical article. *J Neurosurg.* 2011;114:738–746.
11. Duffau H. The reliability of asleep-awake-asleep protocol for intraoperative functional mapping and cognitive monitoring in glioma surgery. *Acta Neurochir (Wien).* 2013;155:1803–1804.
12. Eseonu CI, Eguia F, ReFaey K, et al. Comparative volumetric analysis of the extent of resection of molecularly and histologically distinct low grade gliomas and its role on survival. *J Neurooncol.* 2017;134:65–74.
13. Eseonu CI, Rincon-Torroella J, ReFaey K. et al: Awake craniotomy vs craniotomy under general anesthesia for perirolandic gliomas: evaluating perioperative complications and extent of resection. *Neurosurgery.* 2017;81:481–489.

5

Broca area low-grade glioma

Case reviewed by Bob S. Carter, Clark C. Chen, Jorge Navarro-Bonnet, George Samandouras, Matthew A. Kirkman

Introduction

The goal of achieving extensive resection for low-grade gliomas (LGGs) in eloquent regions is a relatively new paradigm, as many recent studies are now showing that observation and lesser resections are associated with poorer outcomes.[1–7] Jakola et al.[7] evaluated outcomes from a Norwegian population-based parallel cohort study where one hospital performed diagnostic biopsies followed by observation and another hospital advocated early resection. They found that estimated 5-year overall survival was 74% in the surgery cohort as compared with 60% in the biopsy and observation cohort.[7] However, although surgery in the Broca region can be associated with significant risk of neurologic deficits, namely speech function, it can be done.[1] In this chapter, we present a case of an LGG involving the Broca area.

Example case

Chief complaint: right-hand paresthesias and speech disturbances
History of present illness
A 47-year-old, right-handed man with no significant past medical history who presented with right-hand numbness and paresthesias and speech disturbances. He was running when he developed intermittent right-hand numbness, and shortly thereafter developed difficulties with getting his words out. His symptoms resolved shortly thereafter, but he was concerned because of his family history of strokes. He was evaluated in the emergency room, where a magnetic resonance imaging (MRI) scan showed a brain lesion (Fig. 5.1).
Medications: Levetiracetam.
Allergies: No known drug allergies.
Past medical and surgical history: None.
Family history: No history of intracranial malignancies.
Social history: Business executive. No smoking history or alcohol.
Physical examination: Awake, alert, oriented to person, place, and time; Language: intact naming and repetition; Cranial nerves II to XII intact; No drift, moves all extremities with full strength.

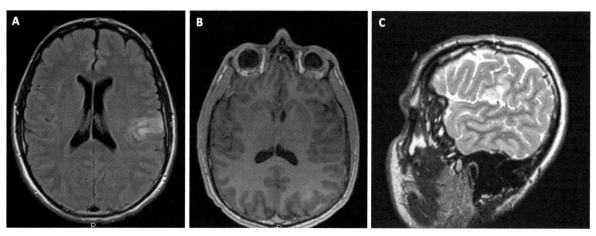

Fig. 5.1 Preoperative magnetic resonance imaging. (A) T2 axial fluid attenuation inversion recovery image; **(B)** T1 axial image with gadolinium contrast; **(C)** T2 sagittal magnetic resonance imaging scan demonstrating a nonenhancing lesion involving the left inferior frontal gyrus or Broca region.

	Bob S. Carter, MD, PhD, Massachusetts General Hospital, Boston, MA, United States	Clark C. Chen, MD, PhD, University of Minnesota, Minneapolis, MN, United States	Jorge Navarro-Bonnet, MD, Oncologic Neurosurgery, Medica Sur, Tlalpan, Mexico	George Samandouras, MD, Matthew A. Kirkman, MEd, National Hospital for Neurology and Neurosurgery, Queen Square, London, United Kingdom
Preoperative				
Additional tests requested	fMRI DTI Neuropsychological assessment	fMRI DTI Medical evaluation	Neuropsychological assessment fMRI DTI EEG	fMRI DTI Perfusion MRI, MRS Dopamine PET Speech and language therapist evaluation Neurooncology multidisciplinary meeting
Surgical approach selected	Left frontal stereotactic biopsy, possible awake craniotomy with speech mapping pending pathological diagnosis	Left awake craniotomy with cortical and subcortical mapping and intraoperative MRI	Left frontal awake craniotomy with cortical and subcortical mapping and 5-ALA	Left fronto-temporo-parietal awake craniotomy with cortical and subcortical mapping
Anatomic corridor	Left frontal	Left frontal through negative mapping sites	Left frontal through negative mapping sites	Left fronto-parietal through negative mapping site
Goal of surgery	Diagnosis	Safe maximal tumor resection	Safe maximal tumor resection	Safe maximal tumor resection
Perioperative				
Positioning	Left supine	Left supine with right rotation	Left lateral decubitus	Left supine with right rotation
Surgical equipment	Surgical navigation Biopsy kit	Surgical navigation IOM Brain stimulator Surgical microscope with 5-ALA Intraoperative MRI	Surgical navigation Ultrasound Brain stimulator Surgical microscope with 5-ALA	Surgical navigation Brain stimulator IOM (ECoG) Surgical microscope Ultrasonic aspirator
Medications	Antiepileptics	Steroids Antiepileptics Mannitol	Steroids Antiepileptics	Steroids
Anatomic considerations	Sylvian fissure vessels, Broca area	Sylvian fissure and veins, central sulcus, pre- and postcentral gyri, AF	Broca, Wernicke, AF, face and hand motor	Distal MCA, AF, SLF III
Complications feared with approach chosen	Hemorrhage, speech deficit	Motor and speech deficit	Motor and speech deficit	MCA stroke, AF injury (phonological paraphasias and repetition disorders), SLF III injury (articulatory disorder)
Intraoperative				
Anesthesia	General	Asleep-awake-asleep	Awake	Awake-awake-awake
Skin incision	Linear	Pterional	C-shaped	Inverted U
Bone opening	Left frontal	Left frontal-temporal-parietal	Left frontal	Left frontal-parietal
Brain exposure	Left frontal	Left frontal-temporal-parietal	Left frontal	Left frontal-parietal

(continued on next page)

	Bob S. Carter, MD, PhD, Massachusetts General Hospital, Boston, MA, United States	Clark C. Chen, MD, PhD, University of Minnesota, Minneapolis, MN, United States	Jorge Navarro-Bonnet, MD, Oncologic Neurosurgery, Medica Sur, Tlalpan, Mexico	George Samandouras, MD, Matthew A. Kirkman, MEd, National Hospital for Neurology and Neurosurgery, Queen Square, London, United Kingdom
Method of resection	Left frontal linear incision, burr hole, dural opening, pass needle biopsy under navigation guidance into center of lesion, 2–3 core biopsies, confirm lesional by pathology	Preoperatively identify tumor and motor strip based on navigation, myocutaneous flap, C-shaped dural opening based on sphenoid wing and exposing Sylvian fissure, awake patient, ECoG to identify areas of eloquence, biopsy of negative mapping sites, maximal safe resection guided by 5-ALA and eloquence, intraoperative MRI to assess for further resection, watertight dural closure	Larger craniotomy for potential recurrence, local anesthetics including dura, cortical stimulation to find positive sites, enter cortex through negative mapping sites, extensive resection guided by cortical and subcortical mapping, avoid coagulation if necessary, resection also guided by ultrasound and 5-ALA	Scalp block, smaller craniotomy based on navigation with exposure of inferior parietal lobule and distal Sylvian fissure, map face sensory area knowing that little measurable disturbances will be elicited, small corticectomy at inferior part of primary sensory cortex, regulate suction to remove parts of tumor, switch to ultrasonic aspirator using low settings (tissue select medium or high and amplitude 40%), subcortical mapping with phonology/articulation/repetition (error acceptance rate of 40%), avoid distal MCA injury with subpial resection, skeletonize vessels if pia breached
Complication avoidance	Needle biopsy	5-ALA, cortical and subcortical mapping, intraoperative MRI	Cortical and subcortical mapping, minimize bipolar cautery	Cortical and subcortical mapping, small corticectomy in sensory region, minimize bipolar cautery
Postoperative				
Admission	ICU	ICU	Floor, possible discharge	Floor
Postoperative complications feared	Speech deficit	Speech and motor deficit	Cerebral edema, neurologic deficit	MCA injury, phonological paraphasias, articulatory and repetition disorders
Follow-up testing	MRI within 4 weeks after surgery	MRI within 48 hours after surgery Physical and occupational therapy	CT immediately after surgery MRI within 48 hours after surgery	MRI within 24 hours after surgery Neuropsychological assessment within 48 hours after surgery

	Bob S. Carter, MD, PhD, Massachusetts General Hospital, Boston, MA, United States	Clark C. Chen, MD, PhD, University of Minnesota, Minneapolis, MN, United States	Jorge Navarro-Bonnet, MD, Oncologic Neurosurgery, Medica Sur, Tlalpan, Mexico	George Samandouras, MD, Matthew A. Kirkman, MEd, National Hospital for Neurology and Neurosurgery, Queen Square, London, United Kingdom
Follow-up visits	7–10 days after surgery	2 weeks after surgery along with radiation oncology and neurooncology Radiation and chemotherapy 4–6 weeks after surgery	10 days after surgery	7 days after surgery with neurooncology multidisciplinary clinic
Adjuvant therapies recommended				
Diffuse astrocytoma (IDH mutant, retain 1p19q)	Radiation/temozolomide	GTR–observation STR–temozolomide/ radiation	GTR–radiation/ temozolomide STR–radiation/ temozolomide	GTR–observation STR–radiation/ temozolomide
Oligodendroglioma (IDH mutant, 1p19q LOH)	Radiation/PCV	GTR–observation STR–radiation/PCV	GTR–radiation, radiation/ PCV, or radiation/ temozolomide STR–radiation, radiation/ PCV, or radiation/ temozolomide	GTR–observation STR–temozolomide +/− radiation
Anaplastic astrocytoma (IDH wildtype)	GTR–radiation/ temozolomide STR–radiation/ temozolomide	GTR–radiation/ temozolomide STR–radiation/ temozolomide	GTR–radiation/ temozolomide STR–radiation/ temozolomide	GTR–radiation/ temozolomide STR–radiation/ temozolomide

5-ALA, 5-aminolevulinic acid; *AF*, arcuate fasciculus; *CT*, computed tomography; *DTI*, diffusion tensor imaging; *ECoG*, electrocorticography; *EEG*, electroencephalogram; *fMRI*, functional magnetic resonance imaging; *GTR*, gross total resection; *ICU*, intensive care unit; *IOM*, intraoperative monitoring; *LOH*, loss of heterozygosity; *MCA*, middle cerebral artery; *MRI*, magnetic resonance imaging; *MRS*, magnetic resonance spectroscopy; *PCV*, procarbazine, lomustine, vincristine; *PET*, positron emission tomography; *SLF*, superior longitudinal fasciculus, *STR*, subtotal resection.

Differential diagnosis and actual diagnosis

- LGG (astrocytoma, oligodendroglioma)
- High-grade glioma
- Demyelinating disease (i.e., multiple sclerosis)

Important anatomic and preoperative considerations

As stated in Chapters 1 and 2, the frontal lobe on the lateral surface is limited posteriorly by the precentral sulcus and inferiorly by the Sylvian fissure.[8,9] The lateral surface of the frontal lobe is divided by two longitudinal sulci (superior and inferior frontal sulci) into three gyri (superior, middle, and inferior frontal gyri).[8,9] These two sulci end near the precentral sulci.[8,9] The superior frontal gyrus runs parallel to the midline between the interhemispheric fissure and the superior frontal sulcus, the middle frontal gyrus is between the superior and inferior frontal sulcus, and the inferior frontal gyrus is between the inferior frontal sulcus and the Sylvian fissure.[8,9]

The inferior frontal gyrus is divided by the horizonal and ascending rami of the Sylvian fissure into the pars orbitalis, pars triangularis, and pars opercularis, in which the latter is frequently divided by the diagonal sulcus.[8,9] The Broca area, by convention, typically consists of the pars triangularis and pars opercularis on the dominant hemisphere.[8,9] Superior to the Broca area is the ventral premotor cortex that plays a role in speech initiation and functions in both hemispheres.[4,5] Posterior to the Broca is the precentral gyrus that controls contralateral motor movement primarily of the face.[8,9] There are several white matter tracts that terminate in the vicinity of the Broca area, and include the superior longitudinal fasciculus (phonetics), arcuate fasciculus (phonetics and repetition), frontal aslant tract (speech initiation), and inferior frontal occipital fasciculus (semantics).[8,9]

Approaches to this lesion

The general approaches to this lesion are observation versus biopsy versus extensive surgical resection. Because of the high risk of neurologic morbidity, some may opt for observation, even though recent studies show that surgery for LGGs is associated with prolonged survival, delayed recurrence, and delayed malignant degeneration.[2–4,7,10] An alternative to observation is a needle biopsy for diagnosis to guide possible adjuvant therapy.[7] However, increasing extent of resection is associated with improved outcomes.[2–4,7,10] For surgery, this can be done asleep or awake with mapping as discussed in Chapter 1 (Fig. 1.2), and eloquent structure identification can be done with direct and indirect methods as discussed in

Chapter 3 (Fig. 3.2).[6,11–13] The risk of asleep surgery in this region is high because monitoring will not be useful, as it is designed to monitor motor and somatosensory tracts and not language functions or white matter tracts associated with nonmotor functions, such as language.[6,11–13] For surgical resection, the most commonly employed method is awake brain mapping with an attempt to identify all adjacent eloquent cortical (Broca, ventral premotor, and motor) and subcortical (superior longitudinal fasciculus, arcuate fasciculus, frontal aslant tract, and inferior frontal occipital fasciculus) regions to guide resection.[6,11–13]

In terms of directionality of approach, the conventional surgical approach is lateral to the lesion as the lesion approaches the cortical surface and is the shortest working distance. A more anterior or posterior approach may compromise normal brain parenchyma but can be done if eloquence of the tissue within and around the lesion is established.

What was actually done

The patient underwent a neuropsychological evaluation that showed no significant deficits. The patient was taken to surgery for a left pterional craniotomy with awake motor and language mapping for resection of the lesion. The patient was intubated with a laryngeal mask airway. The scalp was blocked bilaterally with local anesthetic, and the head was fixed in pins, with two pins centered on the inion, and one on the right forehead in the midpupillary line. The head was turned 45 degrees to the right, and a bump was placed under the left shoulder and hip to facilitate turning. A pterional incision was then planned that spanned from the root of the zygoma to the vertex, and incorporated the lesion based on preoperative MRI navigation. The patient was draped in the usual standard fashion and given dexamethasone, levetiracetam, and cefazolin. A myocutaneous flap was formed and held in place with fishhooks attached to a retracting arm. A left pterional craniotomy was done to encompass the lesion. Ultrasound and surgical navigation were used to confirm lesion boundaries, and the boundaries were designated with letter tags once the dura was opened. The dura was anesthetized with local anesthetics between the leaflets adjacent

to the middle meningeal vessels. The patient was awakened, and the dura was opened once the patient followed commands consistently. Strip electrodes were placed in the subdural space for after-discharge monitoring. The cortex was initially stimulated at 2 mA, and speech arrest occurred with stimulating the ventral premotor cortex superior to the lesion at 4 mA with an Ojemann stimulator (Integra, Princeton, NJ). The rest of the cortical and subcortical mapping took place at 4 mA. The patient participated in continuous language testing with picture naming, phonetic tests, and repetition, with concurrent motor movement of the right face and arm. Positive mapping sites were designated with number tags. Negative mapping occurred over the anterior but not the posterior aspect of the tumor. Positive cortical mapping sites were obtained anteriorly and superiorly to the lesion with speech arrest (ventral premotor cortex), posteriorly and superiorly with mouth and hand weakness (motor cortex), medial and superior with phonetic paraphasias and repetition errors (superior longitudinal and arcuate fasciculus), and medial and inferior with semantic paraphasias (inferior frontal occipital fasciculus). In addition, the posterior aspect of the lesion resulted in inconsistent naming errors and was not resected. Preliminary diagnosis was infiltrating glioma. The dura, bone, and skin were closed in standard fashion.

The patient awoke at their neurologic baseline with intact speech and full strength bilaterally and was taken to the intensive care unit for recovery. On postoperative day 1, they developed some mild dysarthria. Postoperative MRI done within 48 hours after surgery showed near total resection with expected residual posteriorly (Fig. 5.2). The patient participated with physical, occupational, and speech therapy and was discharged to home on postoperative day 2 with an intact neurologic examination, except for some dysarthria. The patient was prescribed 3 months of levetiracetam, and dexamethasone was tapered to off over 5 days after surgery. The patient was seen at 2 weeks postoperatively for staple removal and was full strength with intact speech. Pathology was a World Health Organization grade II astrocytoma (IDH mutant, 1p/19q wildtype). The patient underwent radiation and temozolomide chemotherapy. The lesion was observed with serial MRI examinations at 3 months, followed by 6-month

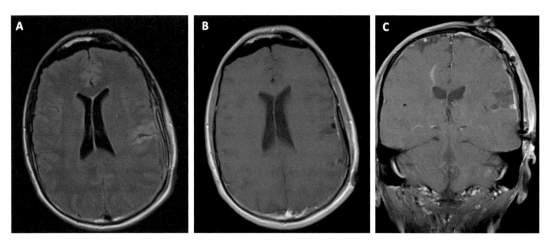

Fig. 5.2 Postoperative magnetic resonance imaging. (A) T2 axial fluid attenuation inversion recovery image; **(B)** T1 axial image with gadolinium contrast; **(C)** T1 coronal with gadolinium contrast magnetic resonance imaging scan demonstrating near total resection of the tumor involving the Broca region with residual posteriorly along the resection cavity.

intervals, and has been without recurrence for 18 months. The patient had a repeat neuropsychological evaluation at 3 months postoperatively that showed no change from pre-operative evaluation. The patient returned to work at 3 weeks postoperatively and remains without neurologic deficits.

Commonalities among the experts

For this lesion, all the surgeons preferred to obtain function-al MRI and DTI for eloquent localization and white matter tract anatomy prior to surgery. All the surgeons elected to perform awake surgery with cortical and subcortical lan-guage and motor mapping. The general goal was typically to achieve extensive resection with functional preservation. Most surgeons were cognizant of the Broca and Wernicke areas, as well as the Sylvian fissure and its vessels, in which the most feared complication was a motor deficit with injury to motor cortex, and language deficits to language cortical areas and white matter tracts. Surgery was gener-ally pursued with surgical navigation, brain stimulation, surgical microscope, and ultrasonic aspirator, with periop-erative steroids and/or antiepileptics. Two surgeons opted for 5-aminolevulinic acid (5-ALA) to help guide resection. To avoid iatrogenic injuries, most surgeons used cortical and subcortical mapping, and most stressed the need to avoid bipolar cauterization as much as possible. Following surgery, patients were admitted to the intensive care unit or floor, and MRIs were obtained within 48 hours after sur-gery. If the diagnosis was a diffuse astrocytoma, radiation and temozolomide for both subtotal and gross total resec-tion were chosen by most surgeon. If the diagnosis was an oligodendroglioma, most opted for radiation and chemo-therapy. If the diagnosis was an anaplastic astrocytoma, radiation and temozolomide were chosen.

SUMMARY OF QUALITY OF EVIDENCE TO GUIDE SPECIFIC INTERVENTIONS FOR THIS CASE

- Surgery as opposed to biopsy or observation for LGGs—Class II-1.
- Surgery for LGGs in eloquent language regions—Class II-2.
- Increasing extent of resection associated with improved outcomes—Class II-2.
- Awake mapping versus asleep surgery for LGGs—Class II-2.
- Functional MRI to avoid deficits from eloquent cortical injury—Class III.

REFERENCES

1. Benzagmout M, Gatignol P, Duffau H. Resection of World Health Organization Grade II gliomas involving Broca's area: methodological and functional considerations. *Neurosurgery*. 2007;61:741–752; discussion 752–743.
2. Chaichana KL, McGirt MJ, Laterra J, Olivi A, Quinones-Hinojosa A. Recurrence and malignant degeneration after resection of adult hemispheric low-grade gliomas. *J Neurosurg*. 2010;112:10–17.
3. Chaichana KL, McGirt MJ, Niranjan A, Olivi A, Burger PC, Quinones-Hinojosa A. Prognostic significance of contrast-enhancing low-grade gliomas in adults and a review of the literature. *Neurol Res*. 2009;31:931–939.
4. Duffau H. Long-term outcomes after supratotal resection of diffuse low-grade gliomas: a consecutive series with 11-year follow-up. *Acta Neurochir (Wien)*. 2016;158:51–58.
5. Duffau H, Mandonnet E. The "onco-functional balance" in surgery for diffuse low-grade glioma: integrating the extent of resection with quality of life. *Acta Neurochir (Wien)*. 2013;155:951–957.
6. Eseonu CI, Eguia F, ReFaey K, et al. Comparative volumetric analysis of the extent of resection of molecularly and histologically distinct low grade gliomas and its role on survival. *J Neurooncol*. 2017;134:65–74.
7. Jakola AS, Myrmel KS, Kloster R, et al. Comparison of a strategy favoring early surgical resection vs a strategy favoring watchful waiting in low-grade gliomas. *JAMA*. 2012;308:1881–1888.
8. Rhoton AL Jr. The cerebrum. Anatomy. *Neurosurgery*. 2007;61:37–118; discussion 118–119.
9. Fernandez-Miranda JC, Rhoton AL Jr. Alvarez-Linera J, Kakizawa Y, Choi C, de Oliveira EP. Three-dimensional microsurgical and tractographic anatomy of the white matter of the human brain. *Neurosurgery*. 2008;62:989–1026; discussion 1026–1028.
10. McGirt MJ, Chaichana KL, Attenello FJ, et al. Extent of surgical resection is independently associated with survival in patients with hemispheric infiltrating low-grade gliomas. *Neurosurgery*. 2008;63:700–707; author reply 707–708.
11. Bertani G, Fava E, Casaceli G, et al. Intraoperative mapping and monitoring of brain functions for the resection of low-grade gliomas: technical considerations. *Neurosurg Focus*. 2009;27:E4.
12. Duffau H. The reliability of asleep-awake-asleep protocol for intraoperative functional mapping and cognitive monitoring in glioma surgery. *Acta Neurochir (Wien)*. 2013;155:1803–1804.
13. Eseonu CI, Rincon-Torroella J, ReFaey K, et al. Awake craniotomy vs craniotomy under general anesthesia for perirolandic gliomas: evaluating perioperative complications and extent of resection. *Neurosurgery*. 2017;81:481–489.

6

Wernicke area low-grade glioma

Case reviewed by Mark Bernstein, Henry Brem, Guilherme C. Ribas, Michael E. Sughrue

Introduction

Lesions in close proximity to essential cortical language functions, namely the Broca and Wernicke areas, have long been considered to not be amenable to surgical resection.[1] Unlike in strokes, the brain can undergo reshaping of the language networks and allow for resection to occur, especially in chronic conditions, such as low-grade gliomas (LGGs).[2,3] Moreover, surface anatomy is not always reliable in identifying these areas intraoperatively.[2,3] Surgical resection can occur in these regions with minimal morbidity, as long as the surrounding eloquent cortical and subcortical structures can readily be identified and avoided.[2–8] In this chapter, we present a case of an LGG in close proximity to the Wernicke area.

Example case

Chief complaint: seizures
History of present illness
A 47-year-old, right-handed man with hypertension and hyperlipidemia who presented with seizures. He was in his usual state of health until he developed intermittent episodes of right facial drooping and tingling, right-hand weakness, and inability to get any words out. These episodes have happened three to four times in the past month. He was evaluated in the emergency room where a magnetic resonance imaging (MRI) scan showed a brain lesion, and was referred for care (Fig. 6.1).
Medications: Levetiracetam.
Allergies: No known drug allergies.
Past medical and surgical history: Hypertension, hyperlipidemia.
Family history: No history of intracranial malignancies.

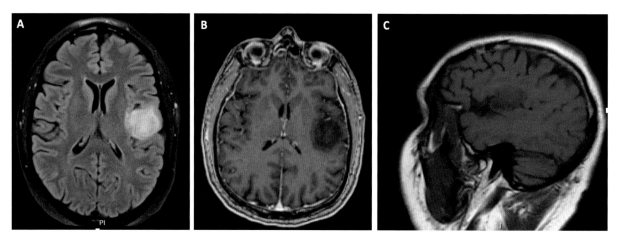

Fig. 6.1 Preoperative magnetic resonance imaging. (A) T2 axial fluid attenuation inversion recovery image; **(B)** T1 axial image with gadolinium contrast; **(C)** T2 sagittal magnetic resonance imaging scan demonstrating a nonenhancing lesion involving the Heschl gyrus and Wernicke area.

Social history: Accountant. Occasional smoking (smokes socially) and occasional alcohol.

Physical examination: Awake, alert, oriented to person, place, and time; Language: intact naming and repetition; Cranial nerves II to XII intact; No drift, moves all extremities with full strength.

	Mark Bernstein, MD, University of Toronto, Toronto, Canada	Henry Brem, MD, Johns Hopkins University, Baltimore, MD, United States	Guilherme C. Ribas, MD, PhD, Hospital Israelita Albert Einstein, São Paulo, Brazil	Michael E. Sughrue, MD, Prince of Wales Hospital, Sydney, Australia
Preoperative				
Additional tests requested	fMRI Neuropsychological assessment	fMRI MRA	fMRI DTI Language evaluation	fMRI with connectome analysis DTI
Surgical approach selected	Left fronto-temporal awake craniotomy (as opposed to wait-and-see approach based on the MEAN score)	Left fronto-temporal craniotomy with intraoperative MRI	Left awake craniotomy with cortical and subcortical mapping	Left keyhole temporo-parietal craniotomy with awake cortical and subcortical mapping
Anatomic corridor	Left frontal	Left fronto-temporal	Left subcentral gyrus	Left posterior temporal
Goal of surgery	Maximal safe resection	Maximal safe resection with preservation of neurologic function	Maximal safe resection without permanent deficit	Gross total resection
Perioperative				
Positioning	Left supine with right rotation	Left supine with 60-degree right rotation	Left lateral	Left lateral
Surgical equipment	Surgical navigation Brain mapping Surgical microscope Ultrasonic aspirator	Surgical navigation IOM (SSEP/MEP) Ultrasound Surgical microscope Ultrasonic aspirator Intraoperative MRI	Surgical navigation Ultrasound Brain stimulator Ultrasonic aspirator	Surgical navigation Brain stimulator Surgical microscope
Medications	Steroids Antiepileptics	Mannitol Steroids Antiepileptic	Antiepileptics	Mannitol Steroids Antiepileptic
Anatomic considerations	Speech cortex	Sylvian fissure, MCA, vein of Labbé, superior temporal gyrus	Sylvian fissure, fronto-opercular convolutions and sulci	Opercular MCA branches, CST AF/SLF
Complications feared with approach chosen	Speech dysfunction	Speech dysfunction, motor deficit, visual field deficit	Speech dysfunction	Speech dysfunction, motor deficit
Intraoperative				
Anesthesia	Awake	General	Asleep-awake-asleep	Asleep-awake-asleep
Skin incision	Linear	Linear	Question mark	Linear
Bone opening	Left frontal	Left fronto-temporal	Left fronto-temporal	Left keyhole temporo-parietal
Brain exposure	Left frontal	Left fronto-temporal	Left fronto-temporal	Left supramarginal gyrus

(continued on next page)

	Mark Bernstein, MD, University of Toronto, Toronto, Canada	Henry Brem, MD, Johns Hopkins University, Baltimore, MD, United States	Guilherme C. Ribas, MD, PhD, Hospital Israelita Albert Einstein, São Paulo, Brazil	Michael E. Sughrue, MD, Prince of Wales Hospital, Sydney, Australia
Method of resection	Regional field block with local anesthetic, bone flap to encompass lesion, cruciate dural opening, motor and speech mapping with brain stimulator, bring in operative microscope, find tumor pseudoplane, exploit pseudoplane as much as possible, keep resection 1 cm away from positive mapping sites, periodic confirmation with navigation	Left fronto-temporal craniotomy with bone soaked in betadine during operation, dural opening, surgical navigation to identify point where tumor comes closest to the surface, biopsy for frozen section (if high-grade glioma then carmustine wafers), internal debulking to normal white matter borders, watertight dural closure, reapproximate skull and scalp, intraoperative MRI for potential additional resection, watertight dural closure with fibrin glue, subgaleal drain	Wide left fronto-temporal craniotomy with drilling of sphenoid wing, large dural opening, expose frontal and temporal operculi, anatomic identification of exposed sulci and gyri with aid of surgical navigation and ultrasound, awaken patient, language mapping, open Sylvian fissure to expose basal aspect of tumor which projects toward subcentral gyrus, dissection anterior/superior/posterior margins while patient awake, remove with aid of ultrasonic aspirator from outer aspect toward center, resect based on anatomic boundaries	Craniotomy and dural opening adjacent to Sylvian fissure at inferior aspect, map cortex for motor/speech arrest/anomia, subpial dissection with microscope visualization inferiorly to locate fissure, identify insula based on periinsular sulci, superior cut of tumor in cortical and subcortical regions, subpial resection anterior and posterior sulcal boundaries, amputate tumor at its base based on continuous awake cortical and subcortical motor and language mapping
Complication avoidance	Awake cortical motor and speech mapping, staying away from positive sites	Closest point to cortical surface, intraoperative MRI	Wide bony opening, anatomic landmarks, awake language mapping, anatomic boundary-based resection	Awake cortical and subcortical mapping with motor and speech mapping, subpial dissection
Postoperative				
Admission	Outpatient	ICU	ICU	ICU
Postoperative complications feared	Language dysfunction	Language dysfunction, visual field deficit, headaches, lethargy	Language dysfunction	MCA artery injury or vasospasm Motor deficit Language deficit
Follow-up testing	CT or MRI same day of surgery prior to discharge	MRI within 24 hours after surgery	MRI within 48 hours after surgery Language evaluation after surgery	MRI within 24 hours after surgery
Follow-up visits	10–14 days after surgery	14 days after surgery 3 months and then every 6 months after surgery	2–3 months after surgery	14 days after surgery
Adjuvant therapies recommended				
Diffuse astrocytoma (IDH mutant, retain 1p19q)	STR–observation or radiation GTR–observation or radiation	STR–radiation/temozolomide GTR–observation	STR–radiation/temozolomide GTR–radiation/temozolomide	STR–observation GTR–observation
Oligodendroglioma (IDH mutant, 1p19q LOH)	STR–temozolomide +/– radiation GTR–observation	STR–temozolomide or PCV +/– radiation GTR–observation	STR–temozolomide GTR–observation	STR–patient selection GTR–patient selection
Anaplastic astrocytoma (IDH wildtype)	STR–radiation/temozolomide GTR–radiation/temozolomide	STR–radiation/temozolomide GTR–radiation/temozolomide	STR–radiation/temozolomide GTR–radiation/temozolomide	STR–radiation/temozolomide GTR–radiation/temozolomide

AF, arcuate fasciculus; *CST,* corticospinal tract; *CT,* computed tomography; *DTI,* diffusion tensor imaging; *fMRI,* functional magnetic resonance imaging; ***GTR***, gross total resection; *ICA,* internal carotid artery; *ICU,* intensive care unit; *IOM,* intraoperative monitoring; *LOH,* loss of heterozygosity; *MCA,* middle cerebral artery; *MEAN,* (M = mass effect, E = enhancement, A = age >40, N = neurologic deficits more than seizures); *MEP,* motor evoked potential; *MRA,* magnetic resonance angiogram; *MRI,* magnetic resonance imaging; *PCV,* procarbazine, lomustine, vincristine; *SEEP,* somatosensory evoked potential; *SLF,* superior longitudinal fasciculus; *STR,* subtotal resection.

Differential diagnosis and actual diagnosis

- LGG (astrocytoma, oligodendroglioma)
- High-grade glioma
- Demyelinating disease (i.e., multiple sclerosis)

Important anatomic and preoperative considerations

This lesion is in close proximity to the language networks and, more specifically, the Heschl gyrus and the Wernicke area.[9,10] The transverse temporal gyrus or the Heschl gyrus is the primary auditory cortex that extends anterolaterally from the posterior end of the insula, and can be identified on sagittal images as a protuberance between the posterior insula and superior temporal gyrus.[9,10] The planum temporale, which is involved in language processing, is the area in-between the posterior end of the Sylvian fissure and the Heschl gyrus.[9,10] The initial cortical processing of speech takes place along the Heschl gyrus, where it then projects to the posterior half of the superior temporal sulcus for phonological processing or the Wernicke area. From here, language processing is distributed along the dorsal-phonetic (superior longitudinal fasciculus [SLF] and arcuate fasciculus [AF]) and the ventral-semantic stream (inferior frontal occipital fasciculus [IFOF]).[11] For this lesion, it is located in close proximity to the Heschl gyrus, where superiorly is the precentral gyrus, anteriorly and superiorly are the Broca area and the ventral premotor cortex, and posteriorly and inferiorly are the Wernicke area and the superior temporal sulcus.[9,10] The SLF and AF reside on the deep, medial surface of the lesion.[9,10]

Approaches to this lesion

As stated in Chapter 5, the general approaches to this lesion are observation, biopsy, or extensive surgical resection. Because of the high risk of neurologic morbidity, some may opt for observation, even though recent studies show that surgery for LGGs is associated with prolonged survival, delayed recurrence, and delayed malignant degeneration as compared with observation and/or biopsy followed by observation.[2,5,6,8,12] For surgery, this can be done asleep or awake with mapping as discussed in Chapter 1 (Fig. 1.2), whereas the direct and indirect methods of identifying eloquent cortical and subcortical structures are discussed in Chapter 3 (Fig. 3.2).[7,13–15] The risk of asleep surgery in this region is high because monitoring will not be useful, as it is designed to monitor motor and somatosensory tracts and not language functions or white matter tracts associated with nonmotor functions.[7,13–15] For surgical resection, the most commonly employed method is awake brain mapping, with an attempt to identify all adjacent eloquent cortical (Broca, ventral premotor, and motor) and subcortical (SLF, AF, frontal aslant tract, IFOF) regions to guide resection.[7,13–15] Although awake brain mapping is the most commonly used direct method of identifying eloquent cortical and subcortical structures, there are also other direct (including subdural grids) and indirect methods (functional MRI, diffusion tensor imaging, and intraoperative monitoring) (see Chapter 3, Fig. 3.2).

In terms of directionality of approach, the conventional surgical approach is lateral to the lesion, as the lesion approaches the cortical surface and is the shortest working distance. A more anterior or posterior approach may compromise normal brain parenchyma but can be done if eloquence of the tissue within and around the lesion is established.

What was actually done

The patient underwent a neuropsychological evaluation that showed mild disorders in attention and working memory. The patient was taken to surgery for a left pterional craniotomy with awake motor and language mapping for resection of the lesion. The patient was intubated with a laryngeal mask airway. The scalp was blocked bilaterally with local anesthetic, and the head was fixed in pins, with two pins centered on the inion and one on the right forehead in the midpupillary line. The head was turned 45 degrees to the right, and a bump was placed under the left shoulder and hip to facilitate turning. A pterional incision was then planned that spanned from the root of the zygoma to the vertex and incorporated the lesion based on preoperative MRI navigation. The patient was draped in the usual standard fashion and given dexamethasone, levetiracetam, and cefazolin. A myocutaneous flap was formed and held in place with fishhooks attached to a retracting arm. A left pterional craniotomy was done to encompass the lesion. Ultrasound and surgical navigation were used to confirm lesion boundaries, and the boundaries were designated with letter tags once the dura was opened. The dura was anesthetized with local anesthetics between the leaflets adjacent to the middle meningeal vessels. The patient was awakened, and the dura was opened once the patient followed commands consistently. Strip electrodes were placed in the subdural space for after-discharge monitoring. The cortex was initially stimulated at 2 mA, and speech arrest occurred with stimulating the ventral premotor cortex superior and anterior to the lesion at this setting with an Ojemann stimulator (Integra, Princeton, NJ). The rest of the cortical and subcortical mapping took place at 2 mA. The patient participated in continuous language testing with picture naming, phonetic tests, and repetition, with concurrent motor movement of the right face and arm. Positive mapping sites were designated with number tags. Negative mapping occurred over cortical surface of the tumor. Positive cortical mapping sites were obtained anteriorly and superiorly to the lesion with speech arrest (ventral premotor cortex), posteriorly and superiorly with mouth and hand weakness (motor cortex), medial and superior with phonetic paraphasias and repetition errors (SLF and AF), and medial and inferior with semantic paraphasias (IFOF). At the tumor depth, positive subcortical mapping occurred with stimulation of the SLF and AF that resulted in phonetic paraphasias precluding gross total resection. Preliminary diagnosis was infiltrating glioma. The dura, bone, and skin were closed in standard fashion.

The patient awoke at their neurologic baseline with intact speech and full strength bilaterally and was taken to the intensive care unit for recovery. On postoperative day 2, he developed dysarthria but with intact naming and repetition. Postoperative MRI done within 48 hours after surgery showed near total resection with expected residual anteromedially (Fig. 6.2). The patient participated with physical,

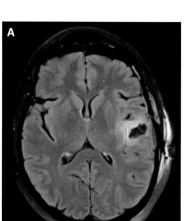 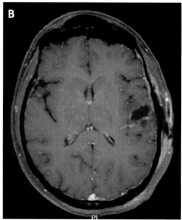 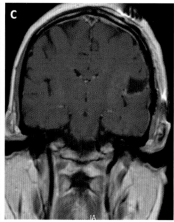

Fig. 6.2 Postoperative magnetic resonance imaging. (A) T2 axial fluid attenuation inversion recovery image; **(B)** T1 axial image with gadolinium contrast; **(C)** T1 coronal with gadolinium contrast magnetic resonance imaging scan demonstrating near total resection of the tumor involving the Heschl gyrus and Wernicke area, with residual anteromedially along the resection cavity.

occupational, and speech therapy and was discharged to home on postoperative day 3 with an intact neurologic examination, except for some dysarthria. The patient was prescribed 3 months of levetiracetam, and dexamethasone was tapered to off over 5 days after surgery. The patient was seen at 2 weeks postoperatively for staple removal and was full strength with improved dysarthria that resolved with speech therapy at 3 months postoperatively. Pathology was a World Health Organization grade II astrocytoma (IDH mutant, 1p/19q wildtype). The patient underwent 6 weeks of concurrent temozolomide and radiation therapy, followed by 6 adjuvant temozolomide cycles. The lesion was observed with serial MRI examinations at 3 months, followed by 6-month intervals, and has been without recurrence for 18 months. The patient had a repeat neuropsychological evaluation at 3 months postoperatively that showed no change from preoperative evaluation. The patient returned to work at 3 weeks postoperatively and remains without neurologic deficits.

Commonalities among the experts

For this lesion in close juxtaposition to language cortical and subcortical areas, all surgeons preferred to obtain functional MRI for eloquent localization, and half requested diffusion tensor imaging for white matter tract anatomy prior to surgery. The majority of surgeons elected to perform the surgery with awake cortical and subcortical mapping, in which the goal was maximal safe resection. Most surgeons were cognizant of the speech cortices involving the frontal and temporal opercula, as well as the Sylvian fissure and its vessels. The most feared complication was speech dysfunction shared by all surgeons, and half were concerned about a motor deficit. Surgery was generally pursued with surgical navigation, brain stimulation, and surgical microscope, with perioperative steroids and antiepileptics. Most surgeons favored the use of cortical and subcortical mapping to avoid iatrogenic injury. Following surgery, most patients were admitted to the intensive care unit, and MRIs were obtained within 48 hours after surgery. If the diagnosis was a diffuse astrocytoma, radiation and temozolomide were chosen by

half of the surgeons for subtotal resection, and most preferred observation for gross total resection. If the diagnosis was an oligodendroglioma, chemotherapy (temozolomide or procarbazine, lomustine, vincristine) was typically chosen for subtotal resection and observation for gross total resection. If the diagnosis was an anaplastic astrocytoma, radiation and/or temozolomide was chosen by all.

SUMMARY OF QUALITY OF EVIDENCE TO GUIDE SPECIFIC INTERVENTIONS FOR THIS CASE

- Surgery as opposed to biopsy or observation for LGGs—Class II-1.
- Surgery for LGGs in eloquent language regions—Class II-2.
- Increasing extent of resection associated with improved outcomes—Class II-2.
- Awake mapping versus asleep surgery for LGGs—Class II-2.
- Functional MRI to avoid deficits from eloquent cortical injury—Class III.

REFERENCES

1. Sarubbo S, Latini F, Sette E, et al. Is the resection of gliomas in Wernicke's area reliable?: Wernicke's area resection. *Acta Neurochir (Wien)*. 2012;154:1653–1662.
2. Duffau H. Long-term outcomes after supratotal resection of diffuse low-grade gliomas: a consecutive series with 11-year follow-up. *Acta Neurochir (Wien)*. 2016;158:51–58.
3. Duffau H, Mandonnet E. The "onco-functional balance" in surgery for diffuse low-grade glioma: integrating the extent of resection with quality of life. *Acta Neurochir (Wien)*. 2013;155:951–957.
4. Benzagmout M, Gatignol P, Duffau H. Resection of World Health Organization Grade II gliomas involving Broca's area: methodological and functional considerations. *Neurosurgery*. 2007;61:741–752; discussion 752–753.
5. Chaichana KL, McGirt MJ, Laterra J, Olivi A, Quinones-Hinojosa A. Recurrence and malignant degeneration after resection of adult hemispheric low-grade gliomas. *J Neurosurg*. 2010;112:10–17.
6. Chaichana KL, McGirt MJ, Niranjan A, Olivi A, Burger PC, Quinones-Hinojosa A. Prognostic significance of contrast-enhancing low-grade gliomas in adults and a review of the literature. *Neurol Res*. 2009;31:931–939.

7. Eseonu CI, Eguia F, ReFaey K, et al. Comparative volumetric analysis of the extent of resection of molecularly and histologically distinct low grade gliomas and its role on survival. *J Neurooncol.* 2017;134:65–74.

8. Jakola AS, Myrmel KS, Kloster R, et al. Comparison of a strategy favoring early surgical resection vs a strategy favoring watchful waiting in low-grade gliomas. *JAMA.* 2012;308:1881–1888.

9. Fernandez-Miranda JC, Rhoton AL Jr., Alvarez-Linera J, Kakizawa Y, Choi C, de Oliveira EP. Three-dimensional microsurgical and tractographic anatomy of the white matter of the human brain. *Neurosurgery.* 2008;62:989–1026; discussion 1026–1028.

10. Rhoton AL Jr. The cerebrum. Anatomy. *Neurosurgery.* 2007;61:37–118; discussion 118–119.

11. Hickok G, Poeppel D. Dorsal and ventral streams: a framework for understanding aspects of the functional anatomy of language. *Cognition.* 2004;92:67–99.

12. McGirt MJ, Chaichana KL, Attenello FJ, et al. Extent of surgical resection is independently associated with survival in patients with hemispheric infiltrating low-grade gliomas. *Neurosurgery.* 2008;63:700–707; author reply 707–708.

13. Bertani G, Fava E, Casaceli G, et al. Intraoperative mapping and monitoring of brain functions for the resection of low-grade gliomas: technical considerations. *Neurosurg Focus.* 2009;27:E4.

14. Duffau H. The reliability of asleep-awake-asleep protocol for intraoperative functional mapping and cognitive monitoring in glioma surgery. *Acta Neurochir (Wien).* 2013;155:1803–1804.

15. Eseonu CI, Rincon-Torroella J, ReFaey K, et al. Awake craniotomy vs craniotomy under general anesthesia for perirolandic gliomas: evaluating perioperative complications and extent of resection. *Neurosurgery.* 2017;81:481–489.

7

Right insular low-grade glioma

Case reviewed by Steven Brem, Hugues Duffau, Frederick F. Lang, Manabu Natsumeda

Introduction

The insula is considered the fifth lobe and is a complex structure both anatomically and functionally.[1–3] Functionally, the insula is thought to play critical roles in memory, executive function, taste, olfaction, memory, motor integration, and motor planning, among others.[1–3] Gliomas, namely low-grade gliomas (LGGs), are the most common lesions within this region, in which they account for almost 30% of the lesions that involve the insula.[4–6] Surgery in this region is challenging because of its complex anatomic location, in which morbidity rates are as high as 60%, and subtotal resection rates range from 62% to 100% in several series.[4–7] Therefore surgery in this region can be associated with significant morbidity with little efficacy.[4–6] The case in this chapter is a nondominant insular LGG.

Example case

Chief complaint: headaches

History of present illness

A 19-year-old, right-handed man with rheumatoid arthritis who presented with worsening headaches. He was in his usual state of health until he had an acute exacerbation of joint pain from his rheumatoid arthritis and concomitant headaches. These headaches were more severe and prolonged than usual, but not associated with vision changes, nausea, and/or vomiting. Imaging was done that showed a brain lesion, and he was referred for evaluation and management (Fig. 7.1).

Medications: Prednisone, methotrexate.

Allergies: No known drug allergies.

Past medical and surgical history: Rheumatoid arthritis.

Family history: No history of intracranial malignancies.

Social history: Engineering student and avid hunter. No smoking or alcohol.

Physical examination: Awake, alert, oriented to person, place, and time; Language: intact naming and repetition; Cranial nerves II to XII intact; No drift, moves all extremities with full strength.

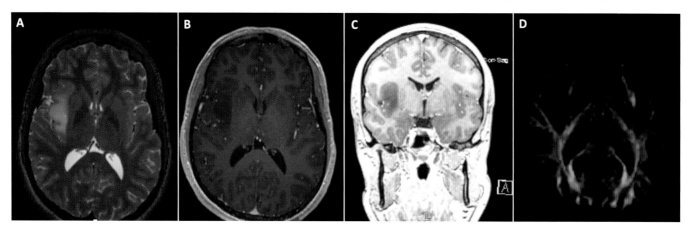

Fig. 7.1 Preoperative magnetic resonance imaging. (A) T2 axial fluid attenuation inversion recovery image; **(B)** T1 axial image with gadolinium contrast; **(C)** T1 coronal image with gadolinium contrast; **(D)** diffusion tensor magnetic resonance imaging scan demonstrating a nonenhancing lesion involving the right insular region.

	Steven Brem, MD, University of Pennsylvania, Philadelphia, PA, United States	Hugues Duffau, MD, PhD, University Hospital of Montpellier, Montpellier, France	Frederick F. Lang, MD, MD Anderson Cancer Center, Houston, TX, United States	Manabu Natsumeda, MD, PhD, Niigata University, Niigata, Japan
Preoperative				
Additional tests requested	DTI fMRI MRS Perfusion MRI Neuropsychological assessment	Repeat MRI for growth rate DTI (research) fMRI (research) Neuropsychological assessment	MRA/MRV fMRI DTI Neuropsychological assessment	Angiography MRA DTI MRS Neuropsychological assessment
Surgical approach selected	Right awake fronto-temporal craniotomy	Right fronto-temporal-parietal craniotomy with awake cortical/subcortical mapping	Right fronto-temporal craniotomy with awake cortical/subcortical mapping	Right frontal-temporal-parietal craniotomy with trans-Sylvian approach
Anatomic corridor	Right trans-Sylvian	Right frontal operculum	Right trans-Sylvian	Right trans-Sylvian
Goal of surgery	Maximal safe resection (>80%)	Extensive resection (GTR or NTR) with preservation of neurologic and cognitive functions	Complete removal of FLAIR abnormality	Complete removal of FLAIR abnormality
Perioperative				
Positioning	Right supine with 45-degree left rotation	Lateral	Right supine 45-degree rotation	Right supine 45-degree rotation
Surgical equipment	Surgical navigation Surgical microscope Ultrasonic aspirator	Brain stimulator Dedicated team (anesthesia, neuropsychological, speech pathology) No neuronavigation, intraoperative MRI, microscope, or functional neuroimaging	Surgical navigation Brain stimulator Ultrasonic aspirator	Surgical navigation Intraoperative monitoring (MEP/SSEP) Intraoperative CT/MRI Ultrasonic aspirator
Medications	Steroids Antiepileptics	Steroids Antiepileptics	Steroids Antiepileptics Milrinone for vasospasm	Mannitol Steroids Antiepileptics
Anatomic considerations	MCA branches laterally, CST medially	IFOF (temporal stem), negative motor network, CST, sensory thalamocortical tract	Sylvian fissure veins, M1 and M2 branches, lenticulostriates, IFOF, UF, AF	Insular cortex, long insular artery, MCA M1–3, LSA, insular sulci
Complications feared with approach chosen	Motor deficit	Motor deficit, movement control, executive function, semantic processing, and mentalizing	Injury to lenticulostriate and M2 branches	Motor deficit, cognitive dysfunction
Intraoperative				
Anesthesia	Asleep-awake-asleep	Asleep-awake-asleep	Asleep-awake-asleep	General
Skin incision	Pterional	Question mark	Question mark	Question mark
Bone opening	Right fronto-temporal	Right frontal-temporal	Right frontal-temporal-parietal	Right frontal-temporal-parietal-temporal
Brain exposure	Right fronto-temporal	Right frontal-temporal	Right frontal-temporal-parietal	Right frontal-temporal-parietal-temporal

(continued on next page)

	Steven Brem, MD, University of Pennsylvania, Philadelphia, PA, United States	Hugues Duffau, MD, PhD, University Hospital of Montpellier, Montpellier, France	Frederick F. Lang, MD, MD Anderson Cancer Center, Houston, TX, United States	Manabu Natsumeda, MD, PhD, Niigata University, Niigata, Japan
Method of resection	Keyhole (~3 cm) craniotomy centered over Sylvian fissure, curvilinear dural opening. Sylvian fissure opening under microscopic visualization, awaken patient, cortical stimulation, cortical entry on negative mapping sites with preference to anterior entry sites (pars orbitalis as opposed to pars opercularis), subpial dissection, maximal safe resection (80%–95%), avoid lateral lenticulostriate arteries, functional observation, map posterior aspect for CST, put patient asleep for closure	Bone flap to include IFG and perirolandic area for positive mapping, patient awoken prior to dural opening, cortical mapping at low intensity (1.5–3 mA) with counting/left upper extremity movement/ naming /semantic association tasks/ mentalizing tasks, cortical resection in right frontal operculum to access insula, subpial dissection concurrent with mapping and functional testing, resection up to functional boundaries of IFOF for semantics/mentalizing/ negative motor network/ sensorimotor pathways, avoidance of coagulation, general anesthesia for closure	Location of tumor identified, Sylvian fissure opened, inferior followed by superior and anterior insular sulcus dissected, MCA vessels dissected from tumor and small perforators to the tumor are cut, tumor internally debulked, dissection continues until medial edge of circular sulci reached, follow M2 perforators branches to define deep part of the tumor, tumor removed from front to back, patient awakened at most posterior part of tumor to stimulate for motor areas and IFOF/AF, ultrasound and navigation used to dictate location	Two layered skin flap, right craniotomy, SSEP/MEP analysis, Sylvian fissure opening from distal to carotid cistern, identify M1/M2 junction with M2 branches and insular cortex, dissection of superior periinsular sulcus, dissection along M1 to most lateral LSA, corticectomy in insular cortex, subpial removal of tumor, most lateral LSA defines medial boundary, insertion subgaleal drain, intraoperative CT, additional removal if necessary
Complication avoidance	Awake mapping, trans-Sylvian opening, subpial dissection, lateral lenticulostriate arteries as medial boundary, 80%–95% goal resection	Cortical and subcortical mapping with counting, left upper extremity movement, naming, semantic association task, and mentalizing, avoidance of coagulation, subpial dissection, resection up to functional boundaries	Trans-Sylvian opening, identify insular sulci to guide deep part of resection, awake subcortical mapping at posterior aspect of tumor in close proximity to CST	Trans-Sylvian opening, identification of M1/M2, insular cortex, dissection of periinsular sulci, resection to lateral most LSA, intraoperative CT
Postoperative				
Admission	ICU	ICU	ICU	ICU
Postoperative complications feared	Motor deficit, seizures	Motor deficit, executive function, semantic processing, theory of mind	Stroke, weakness, seizures	Motor deficit, cognitive dysfunction
Follow-up testing	MRI within 24 hours after surgery Next-generation sequencing	MRI within 24 hours after surgery Neuropsychological assessment 48 hours after surgery	MRI within 24 hours after surgery	CT immediately after surgery MRI within 24 hours after surgery Neuropsychological assessment 1 week postoperative
Follow-up visits	1 month after surgery	Cognitive rehabilitation, MRI 3 months and then every 3–6 months throughout lifetime	10 days after surgery	2 weeks after surgery
Adjuvant therapies recommended				
Diffuse astrocytoma (IDH mutant, retain 1p19q)	GTR–radiation +/– temozolomide STR–radiation +/– temozolomide	STR–observation for growth rate GTR–observation for growth rate	STR–radiation followed by temozolomide GTR–observation	STR–radiation/ temozolomide GTR–observation

	Steven Brem, MD, University of Pennsylvania, Philadelphia, PA, United States	Hugues Duffau, MD, PhD, University Hospital of Montpellier, Montpellier, France	Frederick F. Lang, MD, MD Anderson Cancer Center, Houston, TX, United States	Manabu Natsumeda, MD, PhD, Niigata University, Niigata, Japan
Oligodendroglioma (IDH mutant, 1p19q LOH)	Pending positive TERT status, GTR–PCV or temozolomide STR–PCV or temozolomide	STR–observation for growth rate GTR–observation for growth rate	STR–radiation followed by PCV GTR–observation	STR–radiation/PAV or temozolomide GTR–observation
Anaplastic astrocytoma (IDH wildtype)	GTR–radiation/ temozolomide STR–radiation/ temozolomide	Homogenous AA– temozolomide AA foci removal and GTR of FLAIR abnormality– treatment as for diffuse astrocytoma	STR–radiation/ temozolomide GTR–radiation/ temozolomide	STR–radiation/ temozolomide GTR–radiation/ temozolomide

AA, anaplastic astrocytoma; *AF*, arcuate fasciculus; *CST*, corticospinal tract; *CT*, computed tomography; *DTI*, diffusion tensor imaging; *FLAIR*, fluid attenuation inversion recovery; *fMRI*, functional magnetic resonance imaging; *GTR*, gross total resection; *ICU*, intensive care unit; *IFG*, inferior frontal gyrus; *IFOF*, inferior frontal-occipital fasciculus; *LOH*, loss of heterozygosity; *LSA*, lenticulostriate artery; *MCA*, middle cerebral artery; *MEP*, motor evoked potential; *MRA*, magnetic resonance angiography; *MRI*, magnetic resonance imaging; *MRS*, magnetic resonance spectroscopy; *MRV*, magnetic resonance venography; *PAV*, procarbazine, *ACNU*, vincristine; *PCV*, procarbazine, lomustine, vincristine; *NTR*, near total resection; *SSEP*, somatosensory evoked potential; *STR*, subtotal resection; *TERT*, telomerase reverse transcriptase; *UF*, uncinate fasciculus.

Differential diagnosis and actual diagnosis

- LGG (astrocytoma, oligodendroglioma)
- High-grade glioma
- Demyelinating disease (i.e., multiple sclerosis)

Important anatomic and preoperative considerations

The insula is a pyramidal-shaped structure that lies deep to the Sylvian fissure with its apex being located under the Sylvian point.[1] On its lateral surface lies the frontal, parietal, and temporal opercula, and is typically 9 to 16 mm below the cortical surface, and extends from the anterior perforated substance to the supramarginal gyrus in the anterior-posterior dimension.[1–3] The insula is separated from the adjoining cortical structures by the anterior, superior, and inferior sulci, also known as the circular sulcus of Reil.[1–3] The insular cortex can be divided into the larger anterior insula and smaller posterior insula by the central insular sulcus that mirrors the rolandic fissure, in which the anterior part can be subdivided into three to four short (anterior, middle, and posterior short) gyri, and the posterior part consists of two (anterior and posterior) long gyri.[1–3] The anterior insula is covered by the orbito-fontal operculum and receives direct projections from the ventral medial nucleus of the thalamus and connects reciprocally with the amygdala.[1–3] The posterior insula is covered superiorly by the fronto-parietal operculum and inferiorly by the temporal opercula and receives direct input from the ventral posterior inferior thalamus and connects reciprocally with the secondary somatosensory cortex.[1–3] The base of the insular

pyramid and central portion of the insula lies lateral to the extreme capsule, claustrum, external capsule, putamen, globus pallidus, internal capsule, and thalamus in that order from lateral to medial.[1–3]

In regard to its orientation with the vasculature, the middle cerebral artery (MCA) lies directly lateral on the insular cortex, and short M2 perforators supply the insula and long M2 perforators course through the insula to supply the corona radiata.[1–3] The lenticulostriate arteries from the M1 segment of the MCA represent the anterior and mesial limits of the insula.[1–3] The insular veins drain superficially into the Sylvian fissure veins.[1–3] Critical white matter tracts lie deep to the insula.[1–3] The arcuate fasciculus (AF) and superior longitudinal fasciculus (SLF) of the dorsal language stream lie deep, anterior and superior to the insula, where these pathways are involved in articulation, phonetics, and repetition.[1–3] The inferior frontal occipital fasciculus (IFOF) and uncinate fasciculus of the ventral language stream lie deep, inferior, and anterior to the insula and are involved with semantics and executive processing, respectively.[1–3] Medial and posterior to the insula is the posterior limb of the internal capsule, and medial and superior to the insula is the corticospinal tract within the centrum semiovale.[1–3]

There are several classification schemes for tumors involving the insula.[8–10] For the full description scheme, see Chapter 8.

Approaches to this lesion

The approaches for this lesion can be divided into observation, biopsy, or surgical resection. If surgery is pursued, the options include awake versus asleep surgery (Chapter 1, Fig. 1.2). In terms of surgical approach, this lesion can be accessed either anteriorly from a Kocher point or laterally through the Sylvian fissure or frontal/temporal opercula. The anterior approach is typically reserved for needle biopsies because of the long working corridor but avoids the MCAs within the Sylvian fissure, as well as the MCA perforators. Surgical resection or excisional biopsy can also be done from a lateral approach. The case presented in this chapter is a Yasargil type 3A, Berger zone 1 and 2, Duffau AF and IFOF insular glioma. This lesion is different than other insular lesions because it does not extend to the opercula surface. This lack of extension makes the approach to this lesion somewhat controversial. A lateral surgical approach can be either through a trans-Sylvian or transopercular route. The traditional surgical approach, originally advocated by Yasargil, was a trans-Sylvian approach. In this approach, the Sylvian fissure is split widely, and resection proceeds between the perforating vessels from M2 of the MCA.[10] The advantages of the trans-Sylvian approach are direct access to the insula without having to directly compromise the overlying frontal, parietal, and/or temporal opercula, as well as direct identification of these perforating vessels.[10] The disadvantages of the trans-Sylvian approach are risk of vascular damage to these perforating vessels either from direct injury or vasospasm, and small working corridors between each of these vessels.[10] An alternative to the trans-Sylvian approach for nonbiopsy surgery is a transcortical or transopercular approach.[4] This approach involves accessing the insula through the overlying opercula by a subpial dissection, which involves transgressing the cortex of the overlying opercula followed by entering the cortex of the insula.[4] The specific opercula used depends on the lesion location and on eloquence.[4] The advantages of this approach is that it minimizes injury to and potential vasospasm of the MCA and its branches by preserving the pia around these vessels, avoids the use of retractors to hold the Sylvian fissure open, and allows easier access to lesions below the parietal operculum.[4] The disadvantage is that it involves transgressing the overlying opercula, which can have functional consequences.[4]

What was actually done

The patient underwent a neuropsychological evaluation that showed mild disorders in attention. The patient was taken to surgery for a right pterional craniotomy with awake motor and language mapping for resection of the lesion. The patient was intubated with a laryngeal mask airway. The scalp was blocked bilaterally with local anesthetic, and the head was fixed in pins, with two pins centered on the inion and one on the left forehead in the midpupillary line. The head was turned 45 degrees to the left, and a bump was placed under the right shoulder and hip to facilitate turning. A pterional incision was then planned that spanned from the root of the zygoma to the vertex and incorporated the lesion based on preoperative magnetic resonance imaging (MRI) navigation. The patient was draped in the usual standard fashion and given dexamethasone, levetiracetam, and cefazolin. A myocutaneous flap was formed and held in place with fishhooks attached to a retracting arm. A right pterional craniotomy was done to encompass the lesion. Ultrasound and surgical navigation were used to confirm lesion boundaries, and the boundaries were designated with letter tags once

the dura was opened. The dura was anesthetized with local anesthetics between the leaflets adjacent to the middle meningeal vessels. The patient was awakened, and the dura was opened once the patient followed commands consistently. Strip electrodes were placed in the subdural space for after discharge monitoring. The cortex was initially stimulated at 2 mA, and speech arrest occurred with stimulating the ventral premotor cortex at 3 mA with an Ojemann stimulator (Integra, Princeton, NJ). The rest of the cortical and subcortical mapping took place at 3 mA. The patient participated in continuous language testing with picture naming with concurrent motor movement of the left face, arm, and leg. Positive mapping sites were designated with number tags. Negative mapping occurred over the frontal operculum in the region of the pars opercularis and pars triangularis, and a corticectomy was done over this area to access the insula. Resection took place in the insula with continuous mapping until the lateral lenticulostriates were obtained anteromedially and numbness and tingling in the leg with stimulation designating the posterior limb of the internal capsule posteromedially. At the tumor depth, positive subcortical mapping occurred with stimulation of the SLF and AF that resulted in phonetic paraphasias anteromedial and superior to the tumor, and IFOF anteromedial and inferior to the tumor. Preliminary diagnosis was infiltrating glioma. The dura, bone, and skin were closed in standard fashion.

The patient awoke at their neurologic baseline with intact speech and full strength bilaterally and was taken to the intensive care unit for recovery. Postoperative MRI done within 48 hours after surgery showed gross total resection of the lesion (Fig. 7.2). The patient participated with physical and occupational therapy and was discharged to home on postoperative day 2 with an intact neurologic examination. The patient was prescribed 3 months of levetiracetam, and dexamethasone was tapered to off over 5 days after surgery. The patient was seen at 2 weeks postoperatively for staple removal and was at full strength. Pathology was a World Health Organization grade II oligodendroglioma (IDH mutant, 1p/19q loss of heterozygosity). The lesion was observed with serial MRI examinations at 3 months, followed by 6-month intervals, and has been without recurrence for 18 months. The patient had a repeat neuropsychological evaluation at 3 months postoperatively that showed no change from preoperative evaluation. The patient returned to school at 4 weeks postoperatively and remains without neurologic deficits.

Commonalities among the experts

For this lesion, the surgeons preferred to obtain functional MRI and diffusion tensor imaging for eloquent localization and white matter tract anatomy prior to surgery, as well as neuropsychiatry evaluation for assessing baseline neurocognitive function. Two surgeons also preferred to obtain magnetic resonance spectroscopy for lesion characterization. The majority of surgeons elected to perform awake surgery with cortical and subcortical language and motor mapping through an asleep-awake-asleep anesthetic approach. The transcortical approach selected was trans-Sylvian in three of the surgeons and transopercular in one surgeon. The general goal was typically to achieve maximal safe resection. Most surgeons were cognizant of the Sylvian fissure and its vessels, the corticospinal tract within the internal capsule,

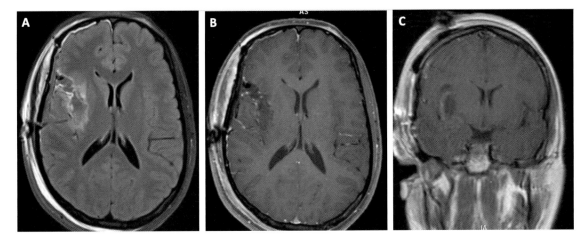

Fig. 7.2 Postoperative magnetic resonance imaging. (A) T2 axial fluid attenuation inversion recovery image; **(B)** T1 axial image with gadolinium contrast; **(C)** T1 coronal with gadolinium contrast magnetic resonance imaging scans demonstrating gross total resection of the insular tumor.

and the SLF and IFOF white matter tracts, and the most feared complication was motor deficit from injury to the internal capsule, as well as cognitive deficits. Surgery was generally pursued with surgical navigation, brain stimulation, surgical microscope, and ultrasonic aspirator, with perioperative steroids and/or antiepileptics. The main surgical techniques that were employed to avoid neurologic injury was to open the Sylvian fissure widely to identify lenticulostriate vessels, subpial dissection, subcortical mapping at the depths of the lesion, and use the lenticulostriate vessels as the medial boundary of the resection. Following surgery, the majority of patients were admitted to the intensive care unit, and MRIs were obtained within 24 hours after surgery. If the diagnosis was a diffuse astrocytoma, observation was chosen after gross total resection, and radiation and chemotherapy for subtotal resection. If the diagnosis was an oligodendroglioma, most surgeons opted for observation if gross total resection was achieved, and chemotherapy with or without radiation for subtotal resection. If the diagnosis was an anaplastic astrocytoma, radiation and temozolomide were chosen.

SUMMARY OF QUALITY OF EVIDENCE TO GUIDE SPECIFIC INTERVENTIONS FOR THIS CASE

- Surgery as opposed to biopsy or observation for LGGs—Class II-1.
- Surgery as opposed for biopsy for insular LGGs—Class II-3.
- Increasing extent of resection associated with improved outcomes—Class II-2.

- Awake mapping versus asleep surgery for LGGs—Class II-2.
- Transopercular versus trans-Sylvian access for insular gliomas—Class III.

REFERENCES

1. Ribas EC. Yagmurlu K, de Oliveira E, Ribas GC, Rhoton A Jr. Microsurgical anatomy of the central core of the brain. *J Neurosurg.* 2017:1–18.
2. Ture U, Yasargil DC, Al-Mefty O, Yasargil MG. Topographic anatomy of the insular region. *J Neurosurg.* 1999;90:720–733.
3. Ture U, Yasargil MG, Al-Mefty O, Yasargil DC. Arteries of the insula. *J Neurosurg.* 2000;92:676–687.
4. Duffau H. Surgery of insular gliomas. *Prog Neurol Surg.* 2018;30:173–185.
5. Eseonu CI, ReFaey K, Garcia O, Raghuraman G, Quinones-Hinojosa A. Volumetric analysis of extent of resection, survival, and surgical outcomes for insular gliomas. *World Neurosurg.* 2017;103:265–274.
6. Kim YH, Kim CY. Current surgical management of insular gliomas. *Neurosurg Clin N Am.* 2012;23:199–206, vii.
7. Lu VM, Goyal A, Quinones-Hinojosa A, Chaichana KL. Updated incidence of neurological deficits following insular glioma resection: a systematic review and meta-analysis. *Clin Neurol Neurosurg.* 2018;177:20–26.
8. Mandonnet E, Capelle L, Duffau H. Extension of paralimbic low grade gliomas: toward an anatomical classification based on white matter invasion patterns. *J Neurooncol.* 2006;78:179–185.
9. Sanai N, Polley MY, Berger MS. Insular glioma resection: assessment of patient morbidity, survival, and tumor progression. *J Neurosurg.* 2010;112:1–9.
10. Yasargil MG, von Ammon K, Cavazos E, Doczi T, Reeves JD, Roth P. Tumours of the limbic and paralimbic systems. *Acta Neurochir (Wien).* 1992;118:40–52.

8

Left insular low-grade glioma

Case reviewed by Santiago Gil-Robles, Zvi Ram, Nader Sanai, Andrew E. Sloan

Introduction

As with other low-grade gliomas (LGGs), the ideal management of these lesions involves extensive resection while avoiding iatrogenic deficits.[1–7] More extensive resection is associated with longer overall survival, delayed progression-free survival, and delayed malignant transformation.[1–7] This association for only insular gliomas, however, is limited.[6,7] In previous series, extensive resection (>90%) is only achieved 16% to 87% of the time, in which subtotal resection rates range from 62% to 100%.[1–7] Although the goal is extensive resection, there is a tremendous concern of iatrogenic deficits.[1–7] Immediate and permanent neurologic deficits (not taking into account neuropsychological evaluations) range from 14% to 59% and 0% to 20%, respectively.[6,7] The permanent deficits included hemiparesis, facial palsy, dysphasia, and dysarthria, and were a result of direct injury to the eloquent tissue and vascular compromise of the middle cerebral artery and its branches.[6,7] Because of concern of iatrogenic injury in this location, others have pursued use of less invasive treatment options, including needle biopsy followed by various forms of radiotherapy and chemotherapy.[8,9] Despite the low postoperative neurologic morbidity in these cases, 26% of patients experienced radiotherapy-related complications, which were more prevalent in larger tumors.[8,9] The case in this chapter is a dominant-hemisphere, left-sided insular LGG.

Example case

Chief complaint: seizures
History of present illness
A 36-year-old, right-handed man with no significant past medical history who presented with new-onset seizures. He was involved in an altercation in which he was struck on the head and had an acute onset of loss of consciousness with diffuse body shaking and bowel and bladder incontinence. He was taken to the emergency room where imaging revealed a brain lesion (Fig. 8.1).

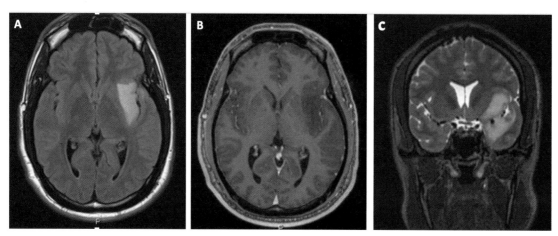

Fig. 8.1 Preoperative magnetic resonance imaging. (A) T2 axial fluid attenuation inversion recovery image; **(B)** T1 axial image with gadolinium contrast; **(C)** T2 coronal magnetic resonance imaging scan demonstrating a nonenhancing lesion involving the left insular region.

44

Medications: None.
Allergies: No known drug allergies.
Past medical and surgical history: None.
Family history: No history of intracranial malignancies.
Social history: Self-employed. No smoking and occasional alcohol.

Physical examination: Awake, alert, oriented to person, place, and time; Language: intact naming and repetition; Cranial nerves II to XII intact; No drift, moves all extremities with full strength.

	Santiago Gil-Robles, MD, PhD, Universidad Europea de Madrid, Madrid, Spain	Zvi Ram, MD, Tel Aviv Medical Center, Tel Aviv, Israel	Nader Sanai, MD, Barrow Neurological Institute, Phoenix, AZ, United States	Andrew E. Sloan, MD, University Hospital, Case Western Reserve, Cleveland, OH, United States
Preoperative				
Additional tests requested	DTI fMRI Neuropsychological assessment	DTI fMRI (research purposes) Neuropsychological assessment	DTI fMRI	DTI fMRI MR angiography Neuropsychological assessment
Surgical approach selected	Left pterional craniotomy with awake language and motor mapping	Left frontal-temporal craniotomy with awake motor mapping	Left frontal craniotomy with awake language and motor mapping	Left frontal-temporal craniotomy with awake language mapping
Anatomic corridor	Left frontal/temporal transopercular	Left frontal/temporal transopercular	Left frontal/temporal transopercular	Left frontal/temporal transopercular
Goal of surgery	Extensive resection with functional preservation	GTR	GTR	Maximal safe resection
Perioperative				
Positioning	Left lateral	Left lateral	Left supine	Left supine
Surgical equipment	Brain stimulator Ultrasonic aspirator Surgical navigation Speech therapist	5-ALA IOM (MEP) Brain stimulator Ultrasonic aspirator Surgical microscope Neuropsychologist	Brain stimulator Surgical navigation Surgical microscope	Stereotactic navigation Surgical microscope IOM (after-discharge) Brain stimulator
Medications	Steroids Antiepileptics	Steroids	Steroids Mannitol	Antiepileptics
Anatomic considerations	M1-M2, ventral premotor, primary motor, IFOF, SLF III, CST	Sylvian vessels CST and SLF	Frontal and temporal opercula Sylvian fissure Internal capsule	M2 vessels, lateral lenticulostriates, internal capsule
Complications feared with approach chosen	Stroke, aphasia, dysarthria, motor deficit, phonological disorders	Language deficit, motor deficit, vascular injury	Language deficit, motor deficit	M2/lateral lenticulostriate injury, retraction injury, venous obstruction
Intraoperative				
Anesthesia	Asleep-awake-asleep	Awake	Asleep-awake-asleep	Asleep-awake-asleep
Skin incision	Pterional	Pterional	Pterional	Pterional
Bone opening	Frontal-temporal-parietal craniotomy	Frontal-temporal craniotomy	Frontal-temporal craniotomy	Frontal-temporal craniotomy
Brain exposure	Frontal-temporal-parietal	Frontal-temporal	Frontal-temporal	Frontal-temporal

(continued on next page)

	Santiago Gil-Robles, MD, PhD, Universidad Europea de Madrid, Madrid, Spain	Zvi Ram, MD, Tel Aviv Medical Center, Tel Aviv, Israel	Nader Sanai, MD, Barrow Neurological Institute, Phoenix, AZ, United States	Andrew E. Sloan, MD, University Hospital, Case Western Reserve, Cleveland, OH, United States
Method of resection	Subfascial temporal muscle dissection, fronto-temporal craniotomy with posterior extension, intradural and muscle local anesthesia, dural opening, awaken patient, speech therapist for examinations, detection of anatomic tumor limits based on navigation, calibration of stimulation parameters (1.5–3 mA) based on anarthria over ventral premotor cortex, cortical mapping with naming and verb generation task, subpial dissection of both frontal and temporal operculi according to negative mapping until superior insular sulci, subcortical stimulation over SLF III anteriorly and CST posteriorly and IFOF with semantic paraphasias caudal to inferior insular sulcus, patient put back asleep once boundaries reached, debulking of tumor with ultrasonic aspirator keeping vessels over insular surface, intraoperative scan to determine if additional nonfunctional tissue can be resected	Standard craniotomy, dural opening, cortical mapping, insertion of strip electrode for MEP and after discharge, temporal opercular corticectomy, removal of temporal portion up to Sylvian fissure, followed by frontal opercular corticectomy, removal of insular portion with continuous motor monitoring, irrigate vessels with papaverine if exposed, sedation without LMA once language and cognitive monitoring is not needed	Craniotomy to encompass lesion, awaken patient prior to dural opening, language cortical mapping to identify frontal and/or temporal opercular corridors based on negative mapping, subpial dissection, motor mapping at posterior aspect of lesion	Sedate heavily, craniotomy to include 10-mm margin, open dura, confirm location of tumor based on navigation, indicate margin of tumor using suture, awaken patient, language mapping (2–10 mA) in cortical and subcortical regions, mark areas with speech arrest/dysarthria/word finding errors with tags, bring in surgical microscope to create cortical windows over negative mapping sites sparing sulcal vessels, debulk tumor with continuous language mapping and until internal capsule identified, biopsy if eloquence makes resection unsafe
Complication avoidance	Cortical and subcortical mapping of ventral premotor, SLF III anteriorly, CST posteriorly, IFOF inferiorly	Continuous motor monitoring with MEP; papaverine of Sylvian vessels	Cortical and subcortical language and motor mapping	Cortical and subcortical language and motor mapping, spare sulcal vessels
Postoperative				
Admission	ICU	ICU	ICU	ICU
Postoperative complications feared	Language deficit, motor deficit	Stroke, motor deficit, aphasia	Ischemic deficit	Seizures, stroke, aphasia
Follow-up testing	MRI within 24 hours after surgery Neuropsychological assessment Physical/cognitive therapy	CTA if deficits MRI within 48 hours after surgery	MRI within 24 hours after surgery	MRI within 48 hours after surgery
Follow-up visits	7–10 days after surgery	14 days after surgery	7–10 days after surgery	10–14 days after surgery
Adjuvant therapies recommended				
Diffuse astrocytoma (IDH mutant, retain 1p19q)	>10 cc – reresection + temozolomide, or radiation/temozolomide if cannot be resected GTR–observation	STR–radiation/temozolomide GTR–observation	STR–possible reresection GTR–observation	STR–radiation/temozolomide or PCV GTR–radiation/temozolomide or PCV

	Santiago Gil-Robles, MD, PhD, Universidad Europea de Madrid, Madrid, Spain	Zvi Ram, MD, Tel Aviv Medical Center, Tel Aviv, Israel	Nader Sanai, MD, Barrow Neurological Institute, Phoenix, AZ, United States	Andrew E. Sloan, MD, University Hospital, Case Western Reserve, Cleveland, OH, United States
Oligodendroglioma (IDH mutant, 1p19q LOH)	STR–PCV vs. reresection GTR–observation	STR–observation GTR–observation	STR–possible reresection GTR–observation	STR–radiation/ temozolomide GTR–observation vs. radiation/ temozolomide
Anaplastic astrocytoma (IDH wild type)	STR–radiation/temozolomide GTR–radiation/temozolomide	STR–radiation/ temozolomide GTR–radiation/ temozolomide	STR–radiation/ temozolomide GTR–radiation/ temozolomide	STR–radiation/ temozolomide GTR–radiation/ temozolomide

5-ALA, 5-aminolevulinic acid; *CST*, corticospinal tract; *CTA*, computed tomography angiography; *DTI*, diffusion tensor imaging; *fMRI*, functional magnetic resonance imaging; *GTR*, gross total resection; *ICU*, intensive care unit; *IFOF*, inferior frontal-occipital fasciculus; *IOM*, intraoperative monitoring; *MEP*, motor evoked potential; *MR*, magnetic resonance; *MRI*, magnetic resonance imaging; *PCV*, procarbazine, lomustine, vincristine; *SLF*, superior longitudinal fasciculus; *STR*, subtotal resection.

Differential diagnosis and actual diagnosis

- LGG (astrocytoma, oligodendroglioma)
- High-grade glioma
- Demyelinating disease (i.e., multiple sclerosis)

Important anatomic and preoperative considerations

For a full-detailed description of the insula, see Chapter 7. The insula is a pyramidal-shaped structure that lies deep to the Sylvian fissure with its apex being located under the Sylvian point, and is covered by the frontal, parietal, and temporal opercula.[10] There are several classification schemes for tumors involving the insula.[6,11,12] Yasargil et al.[12] classified gliomas limited to the insula as type 3A, gliomas that extend to the adjacent opercula as type 3B, gliomas that extend to the orbito-frontal and temporal-polar structures as type 5A, and gliomas that extend to the mesial temporal structures as type 5B. Sanai et al. classified insular tumors into four zones by the bisection in superior-inferior plane through the foramen of Monro, and the anterior-posterior plane along the Sylvian fissure.[6] Zone 1 represents the anterior-superior quadrant, zone 2 the posterior-superior quadrant, zone 3 the inferior-posterior quadrant, and zone 4 the anterior-inferior quadrant.[6] Duffau and colleagues described a classification system of insular gliomas based on white matter tract involvement (arcuate fasciculus, inferior frontal-occipital fasciculus, and/or UF).[11]

Approaches to this lesion

The case presented in this chapter is a Yasargil type 3B, Berger zone 1–4, Duffau superior longitudinal fasciculus, arcuate fasciculus, and inferior frontal-occipital fasciculus insular glioma. This lesion extends to the temporal operculum. As stated in Chapter 7, a nonbiopsy surgical approach can be either through a trans-Sylvian or transopercular route. The advantages of the trans-Sylvian approach are direct access to the insula without having to directly compromise the overlying opercula, and direct identification of perforating vessels.[12] The disadvantage of the trans-Sylvian approach is the risk of vascular damage to these perforating vessels and the small working corridors between these vessels.[12] An alternative to the trans-Sylvian approach is the transcortical or transopercular approach.[13] The advantage of this approach is that it minimizes injury to and potential vasospasm of the middle cerebral artery and its branches by preserving the pia around these vessels, avoids the use of retractors, and allows easier access to lesions below the parietal operculum.[13] The disadvantage is that it involves transgressing the overlying opercula, which can have functional consequences.[13]

In addition to the surgical approach through a trans-Sylvian or a transopercular route, the surgery can be done asleep under general anesthesia or awake with cortical and subcortical mapping (see Chapter 1, Fig. 1.2).[6,12–17] The advantages of an asleep craniotomy under general anesthesia is lack of need for patient cooperation and patient comfort.[12,17,18] The disadvantages are difficulty in identifying eloquent cortical and subcortical white matter tracts intraoperatively.[16,18]

What was actually done

The patient underwent a neuropsychological evaluation that showed mild deficits in attention, working memory, and phonetic paraphasias. The patient was offered an awake surgery with brain mapping, but after a lengthy discussion with the patient, the patient opted to not pursue an awake surgery because of anxiety. The patient was taken to surgery for a left temporal craniotomy for excisional biopsy of just the temporal component of the lesion. The patient was induced and intubated per routine, and no intraoperative monitoring was done. The head was fixed in pins, with two pins centered on the inion and one on the right forehead in the midpupillary line. The head was turned 90 degrees to the right, and a bump was placed under the left shoulder and hip to facilitate turning. A linear incision was then planned that spanned from the root of the zygoma to just below the superior temporal line based on preoperative magnetic resonance imaging (MRI) navigation. The patient was draped in the usual standard fashion and given

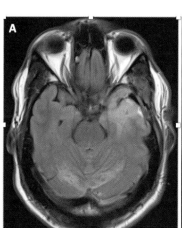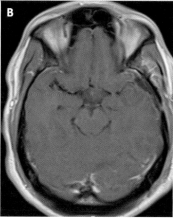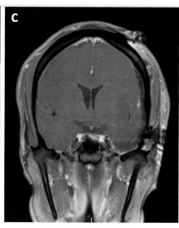

Fig. 8.2 Postoperative magnetic resonance imaging. (A) T2 axial fluid attenuation inversion recovery image; **(B)** T1 axial image with gadolinium contrast; **(C)** T1 coronal with gadolinium contrast magnetic resonance imaging scan demonstrating expected postoperative changes following excisional biopsy of the temporal component of the left insular tumor.

dexamethasone, levetiracetam, and cefazolin. A myocutaneous flap was formed, and the skin and temporalis muscles were retracted with a self-retaining retractor. A left temporal craniotomy was done to encompass the temporal component of the lesion. The dura was opened in a cruciate fashion, and several specimens were taken from the temporal component of the lesion. Preliminary pathology was consistent with an infiltrating glioma. The dura, bone, and skin were closed in standard fashion.

The patient awoke at their neurologic baseline with intact speech and full strength bilaterally and was taken to the intensive care unit for recovery. The patient participated with physical and occupational therapy and was discharged to home on postoperative day 1 with an intact neurologic examination. The patient continued on levetiracetam for his seizures, and dexamethasone was given for 24 hours. The patient was seen at 2 weeks postoperatively for staple removal and was full strength. Pathology was a World Health Organization grade II astrocytoma (IDH mutant, 1p/19q wild type), and underwent adjuvant radiation and temozolomide chemotherapy for 6 weeks followed by six adjuvant temozolomide cycles. A postoperative MRI was done prior to starting adjuvant therapy, which showed expected postoperative changes following excisional biopsy of the left temporal lesion (Fig. 8.2). The lesion was observed with serial MRI examinations at 3 months, followed by 6-month intervals, and has been without recurrence for 9 months and remains at neurologic baseline. The patient had a repeat neuropsychological evaluation at 3 months postoperatively that showed no change from preoperative evaluation.

Commonalities among the experts

For this lesion, the surgeons preferred to obtain functional MRI and diffusion tensor imaging for eloquent localization and white matter tract anatomy prior to surgery, as well as neuropsychiatry evaluation for assessing baseline neurocognitive function. All surgeons elected to perform surgery with cortical and subcortical mapping, in which all surgeons preferred to pursue surgery using an awake approach with motor mapping. The transcortical approach selected was transopercular in all. The general goal was typically to achieve maximal and gross total resection. Most surgeons were cognizant of the Sylvian fissure and its vessels, internal capsule, and superior longitudinal fasciculus, in which the most feared complications were language and motor deficits from injury to language cortical and subcortical areas, as well as the internal capsule. Surgery was generally pursued with surgical navigation, brain stimulation, surgical microscope, and ultrasonic aspirator, with perioperative steroids and/or antiepileptics. The main surgical technique that was employed to avoid complications was to perform subcortical mapping to identify deep-seated white matter tracts. Following surgery, all patients were admitted to the intensive care unit, and MRIs were obtained within 48 hours after surgery. If the diagnosis was a diffuse astrocytoma, observation was typically chosen after gross total resection, and radiation and chemotherapy for subtotal resection. If the diagnosis was an oligodendroglioma, most surgeons opted for observation if gross total resection was achieved, and potential reoperation for subtotal resection. If the diagnosis was an anaplastic astrocytoma, radiation and temozolomide were chosen.

SUMMARY OF QUALITY OF EVIDENCE TO GUIDE SPECIFIC INTERVENTIONS FOR THIS CASE

- Surgery as opposed to biopsy or observation for LGGs—Class II-1.
- Surgery as opposed to biopsy for insular LGGs—Class II-3.
- Increasing extent of resection associated with improved outcomes—Class II-2.
- Awake mapping versus asleep surgery for LGGs—Class II-2.
- Transopercular versus trans-Sylvian access for insular gliomas—Class III.

REFERENCES

1. Chaichana KL, McGirt MJ, Laterra J, Olivi A, Quinones-Hinojosa A. Recurrence and malignant degeneration after resection of adult hemispheric low-grade gliomas. *J Neurosurg.* 2010;112:10–17.
2. Chaichana KL, McGirt MJ, Niranjan A, Olivi A, Burger PC, Quinones-Hinojosa A. Prognostic significance of contrast-enhancing low-grade gliomas in adults and a review of the literature. *Neurol Res.* 2009;31:931–939.
3. Chaichana KL, McGirt MJ, Woodworth GF, et al. Persistent outpatient hyperglycemia is independently associated with survival, recurrence and malignant degeneration following surgery for hemispheric low grade gliomas. *Neurol Res.* 2010;32:442–448.
4. Jakola AS, Myrmel KS, Kloster R, et al. Comparison of a strategy favoring early surgical resection vs a strategy favoring watchful waiting in low-grade gliomas. *JAMA.* 2012;308:1881–1888.
5. Smith JS, Chang EF, Lamborn KR, et al. Role of extent of resection in the long-term outcome of low-grade hemispheric gliomas. *J Clin Oncol.* 2008;26:1338–1345.
6. Sanai N, Polley MY, Berger MS. Insular glioma resection: assessment of patient morbidity, survival, and tumor progression. *J Neurosurg.* 2010;112:1–9.
7. Simon M, Neuloh G, von Lehe M, Meyer B, Schramm J. Insular gliomas: the case for surgical management. *J Neurosurg.* 2009;110:685–695.
8. Shankar A, Rajshekhar V. Radiological and clinical outcome following stereotactic biopsy and radiotherapy for low-grade insular astrocytomas. *Neurol India.* 2003;51:503–506.
9. Mehrkens JH, Kreth FW, Muacevic A, Ostertag CB. Long term course of WHO grade II astrocytomas of the Insula of Reil after I-125 interstitial irradiation. *J Neurol.* 2004;251:1455–1464.
10. Ribas EC, Yagmurlu K, de Oliveira E, Ribas GC, Rhoton A Jr. Microsurgical anatomy of the central core of the brain. *J Neurosurg.* 2018;129:752–769.
11. Mandonnet E, Capelle L, Duffau H. Extension of paralimbic low grade gliomas: toward an anatomical classification based on white matter invasion patterns. *J Neurooncol.* 2006;78:179–185.
12. Yasargil MG, von Ammon K, Cavazos E, Doczi T, Reeves JD, Roth P. Tumours of the limbic and paralimbic systems. *Acta Neurochir (Wien).* 1992;118:40–52.
13. Duffau H. Surgery of insular gliomas. *Prog Neurol Surg.* 2018;30:173–185.
14. Eseonu CI, ReFaey K, Garcia O, Raghuraman G, Quinones-Hinojosa A. Volumetric analysis of extent of resection, survival, and surgical outcomes for insular gliomas. *World Neurosurg.* 2017;103:265–274.
15. Kim YH, Kim CY. Current surgical management of insular gliomas. *Neurosurg Clin N Am.* 2012;23:199–206, vii.
16. Duffau H. Long-term outcomes after supratotal resection of diffuse low-grade gliomas: a consecutive series with 11-year follow-up. *Acta Neurochir (Wien).* 2016;158:51–58.
17. Wu AS, Witgert ME, Lang FF, et al. Neurocognitive function before and after surgery for insular gliomas. *J Neurosurg.* 2011;115:1115–1125.
18. Eseonu CI, Eguia F, ReFaey K, et al. Comparative volumetric analysis of the extent of resection of molecularly and histologically distinct low grade gliomas and its role on survival. *J Neurooncol.* 2017;134:65–74.

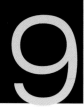

9

Parietal low-grade glioma

Case reviewed by Hugues Duffau, Shawn L. Hervey-Jumper, Randy L. Jensen, Stephen J. Price

Introduction

The parietal lobe is often considered a safe entry point for cortical and subcortical tumors because it avoids the somatosensory cortex anteriorly and the visual cortex posteriorly.[1] However, there are a variety of parietal lobe symptoms that can develop from accessing lesions in this region, which include Gerstmann syndrome (right-left confusion, agraphia, and acalculia), aphasia, and agnosia in the dominant hemisphere, as well as constructional apraxia, dressing apraxia, and anosognosia in the nondominant hemisphere.[1] In a study on parietal lobe gliomas, 34 of 119 (29%) parietal gliomas were low-grade gliomas (LGGs).[1] The most common deficits following parietal glioma surgery were dysphagia, sensory deficits, vision changes, and parietal lobe syndromes that occurred in 26% of patients.[1] In this chapter, we present a case of a nondominant-hemisphere, parieto-occipital, LGG.

Example case

Chief complaint: headaches
History of present illness
A 46-year-old, right-handed woman with hypertension presented with headaches. She has had intermittent episodes of excruciating headaches without nausea or vomiting that were different from her typical headaches. She was seen by her primary care physician who ordered imaging, which revealed a brain lesion (Fig. 9.1). She was referred for evaluation and management.
Medications: Lisinopril.
Allergies: No known drug allergies.
Past medical and surgical history: Hypertension.
Family history: No history of intracranial malignancies.
Social history: Cashier. No smoking, occasional alcohol.
Physical examination: Awake, alert, oriented to person, place, and time; Language: intact naming and repetition; Cranial nerves II to XII intact; No drift, moves all extremities with full strength.

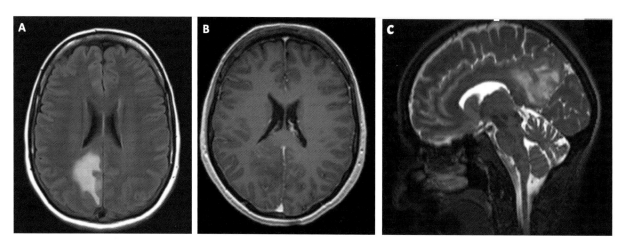

Fig. 9.1 Preoperative magnetic resonance imaging. (A) T2 axial fluid attenuation inversion recovery image; **(B)** T1 axial image with gadolinium contrast; **(C)** T2 sagittal (diffusion tensor imaging) magnetic resonance imaging scans demonstrating a nonenhancing lesion involving the right medial parietal lobe.

	Hugues Duffau, MD, PhD, University Hospital of Montpellier, Montpellier, France	Shawn L. Hervey-Jumper, MD, University of California at San Francisco, San Francisco, CA, United States	Randy L. Jensen, MD, PhD, University of Utah, Salt Lake City, UT, United States	Stephen J. Price, MBBS, PhD, University of Cambridge, Cambridge, United Kingdom
Preoperative				
Additional tests requested	Neuropsychological assessment Repeat MRI for growth rate fMRI+DTI (research)	DTI MEG Neuropsychological assessment	Ophthalmology (visual field testing)	Ophthalmology (visual field testing) MRI perfusion with rCBV Steroid trial
Surgical approach selected	Right parietal awake craniotomy with cortical and subcortical mapping of precuneus, posterior cingulate, and splenium	Right parieto-occipital craniotomy with cortical and subcortical mapping	Right occipital craniotomy with interhemispheric	Right occipital craniotomy with 5-ALA if no response to steroids and rCBV greater than 3
Anatomic corridor	Right superior parietal lobule	Right parieto-occipital cortex	Right occipital interhemispheric	Right occipital interhemispheric
Goal of surgery	Extensive resection (GTR or NTR) with preservation of neurologic and cognitive functions	GTR with patient agreeing to accepting hemianopsia	GTR with expected visual field deficits	Resection of tumor with likely hemianopia
Perioperative				
Positioning	Lateral	Prone	Prone	Prone
Surgical equipment	Brain stimulator Dedicated team (anesthesia, neuropsychological, speech pathology) No neuronavigation, intraoperative MRI, microscope, or functional neuroimaging	Surgical navigation Surgical microscope Bipolar and monopolar brain stimulator Ultrasonic aspirator	Surgical navigation MEPs Ultrasonic aspirator Intraoperative MRI	Surgical navigation Surgical microscope with 5-ALA Ultrasound Ultrasonic aspirator Budde halo retractor
Medications	Steroids Antiepileptics	Antiepileptics Steroids Mannitol	Steroids	5-ALA Mannitol Steroids
Anatomic considerations	Postcentral sulcus anteriorly, intraparietal sulcus laterally, parieto-occipital sulcus posteriorly; somatosensory thalamocortical pathway anteriorly, SLF II laterally, optic tracts, cingulate	Superior sagittal sinus, callosomarginal and pericallosal arteries, cingulate gyrus	Visual cortex, visual fields	Venous sinuses and draining veins
Complications feared with approach chosen	Sensorimotor deficit, movement control, visual fields, spatial cognition, executive function, mentalizing, conscious awareness	Visual field defects, stroke	Visual field deficit	Hemianopia, central visual defect
Intraoperative				
Anesthesia	Asleep-awake-asleep	General	General	General
Skin incision	Arciform mark	U-shaped	Linear	Linear paramedian
Bone opening	Right parietal	Right occipital	Right parietal	Right occipital
Brain exposure	Right central and parietal	Right occipital	Right parietal	Right occipital

(continued on next page)

	Hugues Duffau, MD, PhD, University Hospital of Montpellier, Montpellier, France	Shawn L. Hervey-Jumper, MD, University of California at San Francisco, San Francisco, CA, United States	Randy L. Jensen, MD, PhD, University of Utah, Salt Lake City, UT, United States	Stephen J. Price, MBBS, PhD, University of Cambridge, Cambridge, United Kingdom
Method of resection	Opening under general anesthesia with laryngeal mask airway, bone flap exposing parietal lobe and perirolandic area, patient awoken prior to dural opening after dural anesthesia, cortical mapping at low intensity (1.5–3 mA) with counting/left upper and lower extremities/line bisection task/monitoring visual fields/conscious awareness, subpial dissection concurrent with mapping and functional testing, resection up to functional boundaries of somatosensory tracts/SLF/cingulate/optic tracts, general anesthesia for closure	Right parieto-occipital craniotomy ipsilateral to sagittal sinus, cortical bipolar motor mapping to identify somatosensory cortex, transparietal approach, focus on anterior and medial margins first, subpial dissection down to U-fibers, expose falx/cingulate sulcus/callosomarginal arteries, subcortical monopolar mapping along anterior and lateral margins finish with cingulate resection working medially within cingulate gyrus until corpus callosum is identified, cortical bipolar motor mapping to identify somatosensory cortex, transparietal approach focus on anterior and medial margins first, subpial dissection down to U fibers, expose falx/cingulate sulcus/callosomarginal arteries, subcortical monopolar mapping along anterior and lateral margins, finish with cingulate resection working medially within cingulate gyrus until corpus callosum is identified.	Right occipital craniotomy, interhemispheric approach, subpial dissection, identify tumor and corticectomy and debulk tumor, continuous MEP monitoring, intraoperative MRI for potential further resection	Right occipital craniotomy with burr holes on midline and spanning contralateral side above transverse sinus, cruciate dural opening and monitor for draining veins, mobilize occipital lobe, CSF drainage, retraction away from visual cortex, mobilize along falx to free end and visualize corpus callosum, blue light with fluorescence (unlikely), ultrasound to visualize best trajectory, continue corticectomy of posterior margin avoiding primary visual cortex, debulk tumor on deeper margin on medial side, rotate right side to get better view of lateral surface and debulk laterally, posterolateral corner may be difficult to visualize, watertight dural closure
Complication avoidance	Cortical and subcortical mapping with counting, left upper and lower extremity movement, line bisection, visual field monitoring, conscious awareness	Subpial resection, cortical and subcortical mapping, cingulate portion last	Interhemispheric approach, continuous MEP recording, intraoperative MRI for further resection	Craniotomy spans to contralateral side, monitor for bridging veins, avoid primary visual cortex, debulk medial side first
Postoperative				
Admission	ICU	Intermediate care	ICU	Floor
Postoperative complications feared	Movement, executive functions, spatial cognition, visual field, high-level mentalizing	Stroke, visual field defect (expected)	Visual field deficit	Visual field deficit
Follow-up testing	MRI within 24 hours after surgery Neuropsychological testing 2 days after surgery	MRI within 48 hours after surgery Neuropsychological testing at 1 and 3 months after surgery Cognitive rehab as needed	MRI within 48 hours after surgery Visual field testing 3 months	MRI within 72 hours after surgery Visual field testing 1 month after surgery
Follow-up visits	Cognitive rehabilitation, MRI 3 months and then every 3–6 months throughout lifetime	14 days after surgery, 1 and 3 months neuropsychological assessments	4–6 weeks after surgery	7 days after surgery

	Hugues Duffau, MD, PhD, University Hospital of Montpellier, Montpellier, France	Shawn L. Hervey-Jumper, MD, University of California at San Francisco, San Francisco, CA, United States	Randy L. Jensen, MD, PhD, University of Utah, Salt Lake City, UT, United States	Stephen J. Price, MBBS, PhD, University of Cambridge, Cambridge, United Kingdom
Adjuvant therapies recommended				
Diffuse astrocytoma (IDH mutant, retain 1p19q)	STR–observation for growth rate GTR–observation for growth rate	STR–radiation/temozolomide GTR–observation	STR–radiation/ temozolomide GTR–radiation/ temozolomide	STR–radiation/ temozolomide GTR–observation
Oligodendroglioma (IDH mutant, 1p19q LOH)	STR–growth rate observation GTR–growth rate observation	STR–tumor board discussion, likely chemoradiation GTR–observation	STR–radiation/ temozolomide GTR–observation	STR–radiation/PCV GTR–observation
Anaplastic astrocytoma (IDH wild type)	Homogenous AA-temozolomide AA foci removal with GTR of FLAIR abnormality–treatment as for diffuse astrocytoma	STR–radiation/temozolomide GTR–radiation/temozolomide	STR–radiation/ temozolomide GTR–radiation/ temozolomide	STR–radiation/ temozolomide GTR–radiation/ temozolomide

5-ALA, 5-aminolevulinic acid; *AA*, anaplastic astrocytoma; *CSF*, cerebrospinal fluid; *DTI*, diffusion tensor imaging; *FLAIR*, fluid attenuated inversion recovery; *fMRI*, functional magnetic resonance imaging; *GTR*, gross total resection; *ICU*, intensive care unit; *LOH*, loss of heterozygosity; *MEG*, magnetoencephalogram; *MEP*, motor evoked potential; *MRI*, magnetic resonance imaging; *NTR*, near total resection; *PCV*, procarbazine, lomustine, vincristine; *rCBV*, relative cerebral volume; *SLF*, superior longitudinal fasciculus; *STR*, subtotal resection.

Differential diagnosis and actual diagnosis

- LGG (astrocytoma, oligodendroglioma)
- High-grade glioma
- Demyelinating disease (i.e., multiple sclerosis)

Important anatomic and preoperative considerations

The parietal lobe is formed by the superior and inferior parietal lobules on the lateral surface and by the precuneus on the medial surface.[2,3] On the lateral surface, the parietal lobe is limited anteriorly by the postcentral sulcus, posteriorly by an imaginary line from the preoccipital notch to the parieto-occipital sulcus, and inferiorly by an imaging line from the end of the Sylvian fissure until it intersects the lateral parieto-occipital line at a right angle.[2,3] The parietal lobe is divided by the intraparietal sulcus that runs posteriorly from the postcentral sulcus in the direction of the occipital lobe, and divides the parietal lobe into the superior and inferior parietal lobules.[2,3] The inferior parietal lobule is formed by the supramarginal gyrus and the angular gyrus, in which the supramarginal gyrus is the gyrus that turns around the posterior end of the Sylvian fissure, and the angular gyrus is the gyrus that turns around the posterior end of the superior temporal sulcus.[2,3] The parietal lobe on the medial surface is called the precuneus, and is limited anteriorly by the marginal ramus of the cingulate gyrus, inferiorly by the cingulate gyrus, and posteriorly by the parieto-occipital sulcus. The subparietal sulcus separates the precuneus from the corpus callosum.[2,3]

Approaches to this lesion

As stated in Chapter 1, Fig. 1.2, the general approaches for these intrinsic lesions can be divided into asleep versus awake surgery.[4–9] As stated in Chapter 3, Fig. 3.2, the methods of identifying eloquent cortical and subcortical structures can be divided into direct and indirect methods.[7,10,11] Asleep surgery can be done with or without monitoring, in which monitoring involves somatosensory evoked potentials, motor evoked potentials, and/or electroencephalography.[8,9] Somatosensory evoked potentials can be used to identify the central sulcus with phase reversals, and cortical and subcortical mapping can be used to help identify motor and somatosensory cortex, as well as the corticospinal tract.[8,9] However, these monitoring and mapping techniques are sensitive to anesthetic regimen, prone to false positives and false negatives, exhibit changes in a delayed fashion, and cannot assess nonmotor/sensory functions.[8,9] Awake brain mapping can be used to identify and avoid eloquent cortical and subcortical regions to minimize surgical morbidity, but is associated with patient discomfort, longer surgical times, and risk of intraoperative seizures.[4,6–8] In this lesion location, awake mapping provides the opportunity to map language, visual, visuospatial, and lexical functions.

In terms of directionality of approach, accessing the lesion can be done directly perpendicular, anterior, or posterior to the lesion. Directly perpendicular to the lesion involves accessing the superior parietal lobule. The advantages of this approach are that it is the shortest distance to the lesion, the lesion extends near the pial surface over the lobule, and avoids the more eloquent anterior and posterior lobes, whereas the disadvantages include potential injury to

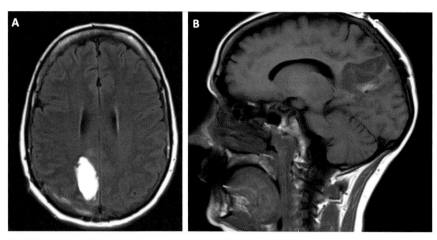

Fig. 9.2 Postoperative magnetic resonance imaging. (A) T2 axial fluid attenuation inversion recovery image; **(B)** T1 sagittal magnetic resonance imaging scans demonstrating gross total resection of the right parietal nonenhancing lesion.

the superior parietal lobule that is involved with sensation, three-dimensional orientation, mental constructional, dressing, and facial recognition. Anterior to the lesion involves potential damage to the postcentral gyrus and sensation, whereas posterior to the lesion involves potential damage to the superior occipital lobe and visual fields. A more lateral approach may endanger white matter tracts, including the superior longitudinal fasciculus.

What was actually done

The patient underwent a neuropsychological evaluation that showed mild disorders in visuospatial processing. The patient was taken to surgery for a right parieto-occipital craniotomy with awake motor, language, and visual mapping for resection of the lesion. The patient was intubated with a laryngeal mask airway. The scalp was blocked bilaterally with local anesthetic, and the head was fixed in pins, with two pins centered over the left external meatus and one pin over the right external meatus. The head was kept neutral, and the head was slightly flexed to minimize patient discomfort. A linear incision was planned in the coronal plane that centered over the lesion based on preoperative magnetic resonance imaging (MRI) navigation. The patient was draped in the usual standard fashion and given dexamethasone, levetiracetam, and cefazolin. A linear incision was made, and the skin was retracted with self-retaining retractors. A right parieto-occipital craniotomy was done to encompass the lesion plus approximately one gyrus in the anterior, lateral, and posterior dimension. Ultrasound and surgical navigation were used to confirm lesion boundaries, and the boundaries were designated with letter tags once the dura was opened. The dura was anesthetized with local anesthetics between the leaflets adjacent to the middle meningeal vessels. The patient was awakened, and the dura was opened once the patient followed commands consistently. Strip electrodes were placed in the subdural space for after-discharge monitoring. The cortex was initially stimulated at 2mA, and paresthesias occurred with stimulation of the somatosensory cortex at 5 mA with an Ojemann stimulator (Integra, Princeton, NJ). The rest of the cortical and subcortical mapping took place

at 5 mA. The patient participated in continuous motor, visuospatial, and visual field testing with right arm/face/leg movement, visuospatial picture identification, and visual field analyses. Positive mapping sites were designated with number tags. Negative mapping occurred over the surface of the lesion, and a corticectomy was done over this area that was between the postcentral sulcus and the parieto-occipital sulcus. Positive cortical mapping occurred anteriorly over the postcentral sulcus with leg paresthesias, and posteriorly over the occipital lobe with phosphenes. At the tumor depth, positive subcortical mapping occurred with visuospatial disorientation in close proximity to the splenium of the corpus callosum. Surgical resection was stopped at this depth. The dura, bone, and skin were closed in standard fashion.

The patient awoke at their neurologic baseline with intact speech, full strength bilaterally, and full visual fields, and was taken to the intensive care unit for recovery. Postoperative MRI done within 48 hours after surgery showed gross total resection of the lesion (Fig. 9.2). The patient participated with physical and occupational therapy and was discharged to home on postoperative day 2 with an intact neurologic examination. The patient was prescribed 3 months of levetiracetam, and dexamethasone was tapered to off over 5 days after surgery. The patient was seen at 2 weeks postoperatively for staple removal and was full strength. Pathology was a World Health Organization grade II astrocytoma (IDH mutant, 1p/19q wild type). The lesion was observed with serial MRI examinations at 3 months, followed by 6-month intervals, and has been without recurrence for 18 months. The patient had a repeat neuropsychological evaluation at 3 months postoperatively that showed no change from preoperative evaluation. The patient returned to work at 4 weeks postoperatively and remains without neurologic deficits.

Commonalities among the experts

For this lesion, the surgeons preferred to obtain formal visual field testing prior to surgery. The approach to the lesion varied from occipital interhemispheric in two, trans-occipital in one, and superior parietal lobule in one, with one surgeon preferring an awake mapping approach. The general goal was typically to achieve maximal and gross total resection. The most feared complication was a visual field deficit, which was expected by most surgeons. The anatomic considerations were varied, but the majority of surgeons were cognizant of visual cortex, draining veins, and sagittal sinus. Surgery was generally pursued with surgical navigation, brain stimulation, surgical microscope, and ultrasonic aspirator, with perioperative steroids and/or antiepileptics. The most common surgical techniques that most surgeons employed to avoid complications was subpial dissection and continuous neuro monitoring, either with mapping or intraoperative monitoring. Following surgery, most patients were admitted to the intensive care unit (others included intermediate care and floor), and MRIs were obtained within 72 hours after surgery. If the diagnosis was a diffuse astrocytoma, observation was typically chosen after gross total resection, and radiation and chemotherapy for subtotal resection. If the diagnosis was an oligodendroglioma, all surgeons opted for observation if gross total resection was achieved, and radiation and chemotherapy for subtotal resection. If the diagnosis was an anaplastic astrocytoma, radiation and temozolomide were chosen by all surgeons.

SUMMARY OF QUALITY OF EVIDENCE TO GUIDE SPECIFIC INTERVENTIONS FOR THIS CASE

- Surgery as opposed to biopsy or observation for LGGs—Class II-1.
- Increasing extent of resection associated with improved outcomes—Class II-2.
- Awake mapping versus asleep surgery for LGGs—Class II-2.

REFERENCES

1. Sanai N, Martino J, Berger MS. Morbidity profile following aggressive resection of parietal lobe gliomas. *J Neurosurg.* 2012;116:1182–1186.
2. Fernandez-Miranda JC, Rhoton AL Jr., Alvarez-Linera J, Kakizawa Y, Choi C, de Oliveira EP. Three-dimensional microsurgical and tractographic anatomy of the white matter of the human brain. *Neurosurgery.* 2008;62:989–1026; discussion 1026–1028.
3. Rhoton AL Jr. The cerebrum. Anatomy. *Neurosurgery.* 2007;61:37–118; discussion 118–119.
4. Duffau H. The reliability of asleep-awake-asleep protocol for intraoperative functional mapping and cognitive monitoring in glioma surgery. *Acta Neurochir (Wien).* 2013;155:1803–1804.
5. Eseonu CI, Eguia F, Garcia O, Kaplan PW, Quinones-Hinojosa A. Comparative analysis of monotherapy versus duotherapy antiseizure drug management for postoperative seizure control in patients undergoing an awake craniotomy. *J Neurosurg.* 2018;128:1661–1667.
6. Eseonu CI, Eguia F, ReFaey K, et al. Comparative volumetric analysis of the extent of resection of molecularly and histologically distinct low grade gliomas and its role on survival. *J Neurooncol.* 2017;134:65–74.
7. Eseonu CI, Rincon-Torroella J, ReFaey K, et al. Awake craniotomy vs craniotomy under general anesthesia for perirolandic gliomas: evaluating perioperative complications and extent of resection. *Neurosurgery.* 2017;81:481–489.
8. Bertani G, Fava E, Casaceli G, et al. Intraoperative mapping and monitoring of brain functions for the resection of low-grade gliomas: technical considerations. *Neurosurg Focus.* 2009;27:E4.
9. Nossek E, Korn A, Shahar T, et al. Intraoperative mapping and monitoring of the corticospinal tracts with neurophysiological assessment and 3-dimensional ultrasonography-based navigation. Clinical article. *J Neurosurg.* 2011;114:738–746.
10. Mandelli ML, Berger MS, Bucci M, Berman JI, Amirbekian B, Henry RG. Quantifying accuracy and precision of diffusion MR tractography of the corticospinal tract in brain tumors. *J Neurosurg.* 2014;121:349–358.
11. Pak RW, Hadjiabadi DH, Senarathna J, et al. Implications of neurovascular uncoupling in functional magnetic resonance imaging (fMRI) of brain tumors. *J Cereb Blood Flow Metab.* 2017;37:3475–3487.

10

Left temporal low-grade glioma

Case reviewed by Jeffrey N. Bruce, Victor Garcia-Navarro, John S. Kuo, Pierre A. Robe

Introduction

A common location of low-grade gliomas (LGGs) is the temporal lobe. In most series, this number ranges from 15% to 25%.[1-4] Patients with temporal lobe LGGs typically have subtle deficits, in which patients with left temporal lobe lesions typically have more deficits in attention, object naming, and language as compared with right temporal lesions.[5] Moreover, patients with left temporal glioma function poorer on neurocognitive tests than patients with right temporal gliomas.[5] In this chapter, we present a case of a left temporal lobe LGG.

Example case

Chief complaint: seizures
History of present illness
A 26-year-old, right-handed woman with no significant past medical history presented with confusion and possible seizures.

Over the past several months, her family has noted that she has several episodes in which she stares for several seconds and has several minutes of confusion following these events. They deny any loss of consciousness, tongue biting, and/or bowel/bladder incontinence. In addition, she has intermittent episodes in which she has trouble speaking. She saw her primary care physician who ordered brain imaging, which revealed a brain tumor (Fig. 10.1). She was referred for further evaluation and management.

Medications: None.
Allergies: No known drug allergies.
Past medical and surgical history: None.
Family history: No history of intracranial malignancies.
Social history: Nursing student. No smoking or alcohol.
Physical examination: Awake, alert, oriented to person, place, and time; Language: intact naming and repetition; Cranial nerves II to XII intact; No drift, moves all extremities with full strength.

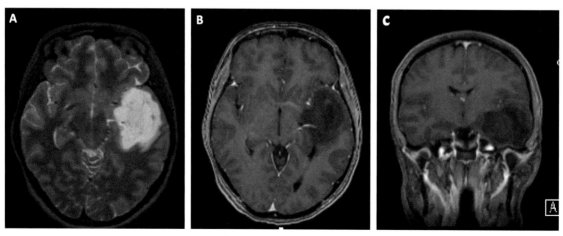

Fig. 10.1 Preoperative magnetic resonance imaging. (A) T2 axial fluid attenuation inversion recovery image; **(B)** T1 axial image with gadolinium contrast; **(C)** T1 coronal image with gadolinium contrast magnetic resonance imaging scan demonstrating a nonenhancing lesion involving the left temporal lobe and the inferior limiting sulcus of the insula.

	Jeffrey N. Bruce, MD, Columbia University, New York, NY, United States	Victor Garcia-Navarro, MD, Tec de Monterrey Institute, Campus Guadalajara, Mexico	John S. Kuo, MD, PhD University of Texas at Austin, Austin, TX, United States	Pierre A. Robe, MD, PhD, University Medical Center of Utrecht, The Netherlands
Preoperative				
Additional tests requested	DTI fMRI Neuropsychological assessment	fMRI, DTI, MRS Perfusion MRI (CBF/CBV) Neuropsychological assessment and language evaluation	fMRI Wada (sodium amytal) test Neuropsychological assessment	Neuropsychological assessment
Surgical approach selected	Left fronto-temporal awake craniotomy with speech and motor mapping	Left fronto-temporal awake craniotomy with speech and motor mapping	Left fronto-temporal craniotomy	Left temporal awake craniotomy with ECoG and cortical and subcortical mapping
Anatomic corridor	Left fronto-temporal	Left temporal	Left fronto-temporal	Left temporal
Goal of Surgery	Extensive resection with functional preservation	Diagnosis, maximal safe resection, seizure control	Diagnosis, maximal safe resection	Tumor removal to limits of neurocognitive function
Perioperative				
Positioning	Left supine with right rotation	Left semilateral	Left supine with right head rotation	Left park bench
Surgical equipment	Surgical navigation IOM (ECoG) Brain stimulator Ultrasound Ultrasonic aspirator Surgical microscope	Surgical navigation Ultrasound Brain stimulator IOM (ECoG) Ultrasonic aspirator	Surgical navigation Surgical microscope Ultrasound	Surgical navigation Ultrasound Neuropsychological testing IOM (EcoG) Surgical microscope
Medications	Steroids Antiepileptics	Steroids Antiepileptics Hypertonic saline	Steroids Antiepileptics Mannitol, furosemide	Steroids Mannitol
Anatomic considerations	Sylvian fissure, speech and motor areas	MCA perforators, cortical and bridging veins, motor and language tracts	Sylvian fissure, MCA and branches, anterior choroidal artery, temporal ventricular horns, perimesencephalic cisterns	Temporal cortex, optic radiations, IFOF
Complications feared with approach chosen	Language dysfunction, motor deficit, memory loss	Transient or permanent motor deficit, language or memory deficit, stroke	Speech deficit	Speech deficit, prosopagnosia, working memory deficit, quadrantopsia (upper right)
Intraoperative				
Anesthesia	Asleep-awake-asleep	Asleep-awake-asleep with bispectral index	General	Awake-awake-awake
Skin incision	Curvilinear/pterional	C-shaped	Pterional	Question mark
Bone opening	Left fronto-temporal	Left fronto-temporal		Left fronto-temporal
Brain exposure	Left fronto-temporal	Left fronto-temporal	Left fronto-temporal	Left temporal

(continued on next page)

	Jeffrey N. Bruce, MD, Columbia University, New York, NY, United States	Victor Garcia-Navarro, MD, Tec de Monterrey Institute, Campus Guadalajara, Mexico	John S. Kuo, MD, PhD University of Texas at Austin, Austin, TX, United States	Pierre A. Robe, MD, PhD, University Medical Center of Utrecht, The Netherlands
Method of resection	Monitored anesthesia care for opening, large fronto-temporal craniotomy and removal of lesser sphenoid wing, U-shaped dural opening based on sphenoid wing, ECoG grid, patient awoken, speech and motor mapping, identify margins based on navigation, resection starting at STG and dissecting from Sylvian fissure based on negative mapping of speech and motor, debulk tumor with ultrasonic aspirator, dissection from speech and motor fibers, ultrasound to guide further resection, watertight dural closure	Patient awakened, C-shaped dural incision and motor mapping to confirm a positive response, stimulation intensity determined by progressively increasing amplitude, language (counting, picture-naming tasks) mapping, eloquent areas marked by sterile number, ultrasound performed, transcortical subpial temporal lobectomy with lesionectomy, hippocampus and amygdala are identified in the temporal horn and tumor resected, functional structures determined by cortical and subcortical stimulation and represent the limits of surgery, goal is supramarginal resection, final ECoG and ultrasound to assess resection	Myocutaneous flap, left fronto-temporal craniotomy based on navigation, confirm location of Sylvian fissure, dural opening with copious antibiotic-impregnated irrigation, left anterior temporal lobectomy 4 cm from temporal tip, remove en bloc if possible under microscopic visualization, remove posterior and deep margins based on navigation, identify deep vasculature (MCA, anterior choroidal), use ultrasound to identify temporal ventricular horns and basal cisterns, protect with gelfoam, watertight dural closure	Local field block, myocutaneous opening, left temporal/pterional bone flap, ultrasound to delineate tumor margins, opening dura, ECoG, cortical stimulation for positive sites (1–3 mA), tumor resection with repetitive cortical and subcortical stimulation, decrease simulation to 2 and 1 mA near eloquent area, ultrasound to evaluate extent of resection and hematoma
Complication avoidance	Cortical and subcortical brain mapping, ultrasound	Preservation of bridging veins, motor and language mapping, resection to functional boundaries, ultrasound, ECoG	Limit temporal lobectomy to 4 cm from anterior edge of temporal lobe, en bloc resection, navigation-guided additional resection, ultrasound	ECoG, cortical and subcortical stimulation, ultrasound
Postoperative				
Admission	ICU	ICU	ICU	Floor
Postoperative complications feared	Language dysfunction, short-term memory loss, motor deficit, seizures	Seizures, stroke	Seizures, speech deficit	Vasospasm, seizures, CSF leak
Follow-up testing	MRI within 48 hours after surgery	CTA within 24 hours after surgery MRI within 72 hours after surgery	MRI within 24 hours after surgery	MRI within 72 hours after surgery
Follow-up visits	7 days after surgery	7 days after surgery	2 weeks after surgery	As needed
Adjuvant therapies recommended				
Diffuse astrocytoma (IDH mutant, retain 1p19q)	GTR–radiation/ temozolomide STR–radiation/ temozolomide	GTR–observation STR–temozolomide, possible radiation or repeat resection with recurrence	GTR–observation STR–second look surgery if resectable, neuro-oncology and radiation oncology evaluation if not resectable	GTR–radiation/ temozolomide STR–radiation/ temozolomide
Oligodendroglioma (IDH mutant, 1p19q LOH)	GTR–observation STR–radiation/ temozolomide or observation	GTR–observation STR–PCV or temozolomide, possible radiation or repeat resection for recurrence	GTR–observation STR–second look surgery if resectable, neuro-oncology and radiation oncology evaluation if not resectable	GTR–observation/ discussion STR–radiation/PCV

	Jeffrey N. Bruce, MD, Columbia University, New York, NY, United States	Victor Garcia-Navarro, MD, Tec de Monterrey Institute, Campus Guadalajara, Mexico	John S. Kuo, MD, PhD University of Texas at Austin, Austin, TX, United States	Pierre A. Robe, MD, PhD, University Medical Center of Utrecht, The Netherlands
Anaplastic astrocytoma (IDH wild type)	GTR–radiation/ temozolomide STR–radiation/ temozolomide	GTR–radiation/temozolomide STR–radiation/temozolomide	STR–second look surgery if resectable, radiation/ chemotherapy GTR–radiation/ chemotherapy	GTR–radiation/ temozolomide STR–radiation/ temozolomide

CBF, cerebral blood flow; *CBV*, cerebral blood volume; *CSF*, cerebrospinal fluid; *CTA*, computed tomography angiography; *DTI*, diffusion tensor imaging; *ECoG*, electrocorticography; *fMRI*, functional magnetic resonance imaging; *GTR*, gross total resection; *ICU*, intensive care unit; *IFOF*, inferior frontal occipital fasciculus; *IOM*, intraoperative monitoring; *LOH*, loss of heterozygosity; *MCA*, middle cerebral artery; *MRI*, magnetic resonance imaging; *MRS*, magnetic resonance spectroscopy; *PCV*, procarbazine, lomustine, vincristine; *STG*, superior temporal gyrus; *STR*, subtotal resection.

Differential diagnosis and actual diagnosis

- LGG (astrocytoma, oligodendroglioma)
- High-grade glioma
- Demyelinating disease (i.e., multiple sclerosis)

Important anatomic and preoperative considerations

The temporal lobe is separated from the frontal and parietal lobe by the Sylvian fissure and the occipital lobe by an imaginary line between the preoccipital notch and the parieto-occipital sulcus on the medial aspect of the hemisphere.[6,7] The temporal lobe has a lateral, inferior, medial, and anterior surface.[6,7] On the lateral surface, the superior and inferior temporal sulci divide the temporal lobe into superior, middle, and inferior temporal gyri.[6,7] The inferior surface of the temporal lobe consists of the inferior temporal, fusiform, and parahippocampal gyri, in which the occipito-temporal sulcus separates the inferior temporal from the fusiform gyrus, and the collateral sulcus separates the fusiform from the parahippocampal gyrus.[6,7] More anteriorly, the collateral sulcus becomes the rhinal sulcus that divides the uncus from the temporal pole.[6,7] The medial surface is formed by the uncus anteriorly and the parahippocampal gyrus posteriorly, and the anterior surface is the temporal pole laterally and the uncus medially.[6,7] For a full description of the mesial temporal lobe see Chapter 11.

Approaches to this lesion

As stated in Chapter 1, Fig. 1.2, the general approaches for these intrinsic lesions can be divided into asleep versus awake surgery.[8-13] As stated in Chapter 3, Fig. 3.2, the general ways of identifying eloquent cortical and subcortical structures can be divided into direct and indirect methods.[11,14,15] Asleep surgery can be done with or without monitoring, in which monitoring involves somatosensory evoked potentials, motor evoked potentials, and/or electroencephalography that are all indirect methods of identifying and monitoring elqoeunce.[12,13] For temporal lobe lesions, the use of these monitoring modalities are limited, as they provide extratemporal monitoring that may not provide sufficient neurologic feedback from surgery in the temporal lobe.[12,13] Awake brain mapping can be used to directly identify and avoid eloquent cortical and subcortical regions to minimize surgical morbidity, and can be used to identify the cortical and subcortical areas responsible for language and visual field functions, including the Wernicke area, Heschl gyrus, inferior longitudinal fasciculus, and inferior frontal occipital fasciculus (IFOF), as well as visual fields.

In terms of directionality, the most common approach is lateral as the lesion comes to the pial surface on the lateral side of the temporal lobe. Because this lesion is in the dominant hemisphere, accessing the inferior and middle temporal gyrus is typically done first before the superior temporal gyrus because they are more distal to the Broca area. As the lesion is resected more medially, the IFOF and uncinate fasciculus will come into play. Posteriorly in the lesion in close juxtaposition to the temporal horn of the lateral ventricle are the visual field tracts.

What was actually done

The patient underwent a neuropsychological evaluation that showed mild disorders in attention, object naming, and language. The patient was taken to surgery for a left temporal craniotomy with language and motor mapping for resection of the lesion. The patient was intubated with a laryngeal mask airway. The scalp was blocked bilaterally with local anesthetic, and the head was fixed in pins, with two pins centered over the inion and one pin over the right forehead in the midpupillary line. The head was turned 45 degrees to the right, and a bump was placed under the left shoulder and hip to facilitate turning and to minimize patient discomfort. A pterional incision was planned that spanned from the root of the zygoma to the vertex. The patient was draped in the usual standard fashion and given dexamethasone, levetiracetam, and cefazolin. A myocutaneous flap was raised and held in place with fishhooks attached to a retractor arm. A left pterional craniotomy was done that encompassed the lesion plus the inferior frontal gyrus and ventral premotor cortex based on preoperative magnetic resonance imaging (MRI) surgical navigation. Ultrasound and surgical navigation were used to confirm

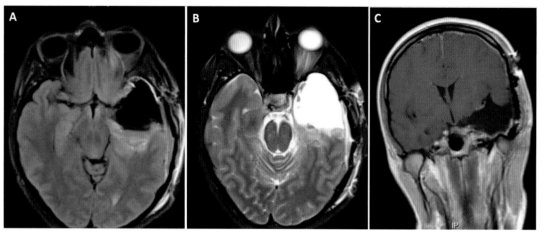

Fig. 10.2 Postoperative magnetic resonance imaging. (A) T2 axial fluid attenuation inversion recovery image; **(B)** T2 axial image; **(C)** T1 coronal image with gadolinium contrast magnetic resonance imaging scan demonstrating gross total resection of the left temporal nonenhancing lesion.

lesion boundaries, and the boundaries were designated with letter tags once the dura was opened. The dura was anesthetized with local anesthetics between the leaflets adjacent to the middle meningeal vessels. The patient was awakened, and the dura was opened once the patient followed commands consistently. Strip electrodes were placed in the subdural space for after-discharge monitoring. The cortex was initially stimulated at 2 mA, and speech arrest occurred with stimulation of the ventral premotor cortex at 3 mA with an Ojemann stimulator (Integra, Princeton, NJ). The rest of the cortical and subcortical mapping took place at 3 mA. The patient participated in continuous motor and language testing with right arm/face/leg movement and picture naming, as well as observing for phosphenes. Positive mapping sites were designated with number tags. Negative mapping occurred over the surface of the lesion, and a cortisectomy was done over the tumor. The order of resection was the inferior temporal, middle temporal, and then the superior temporal gyri, followed by the posterior aspects of these gyri until positive cortical and/or subcortical mapping occurred. After this was done, the resection proceeded to the inferior portion of the insula through the temporal operculum until positive mapping occurred with IFOF stimulation and semantic paraphasias. The positive cortical mapping site was the ventral premotor cortex (speech arrest), and positive subcortical mapping sites were the inferior longitudinal fasciculus medial to the lesion (prosopagnosia) and IFOF medial and superior to the lesion (semantic paraphasias). After the lesion was resected, the patient was put back to sleep, reintubated, and an intraoperative MRI was done to evaluate the extent of resection; no residual lesion was identified (Fig. 10.2). The dura, bone, and skin were closed in standard fashion.

The patient awoke at their neurologic baseline with intact speech, full strength bilaterally, and full visual fields, and was taken to the intensive care unit for recovery. The patient participated with physical, occupational, and speech therapy and was discharged to home on postoperative day 2 with an intact neurologic examination. The patient was prescribed 3 months of levetiracetam, and dexamethasone was tapered to off over 5 days after surgery. The patient was seen at 2 weeks postoperatively for staple removal and remained neurologically intact. Pathology was a World Health Organization grade II astrocytoma (IDH mutant, 1p/19q wild type). The lesion was observed with serial MRI examinations at 3 months, followed by 6-month intervals, and has been without recurrence for 12 months. The patient had a repeat neuropsychological evaluation at 3 months postoperatively that showed no change from preoperative evaluation except mild decrease in attention. The patient returned to work at 4 weeks postoperatively and remains without neurologic deficits.

Commonalities among the experts

For this lesion, the majority of surgeons preferred to have functional MRI prior to surgery for eloquent cortical localization, and all surgeons favored to obtain neuropsychiatry evaluation to obtain baseline neurocognitive function. The approach to the lesion was through an awake mapping procedure in the majority through an asleep-awake-asleep anesthetic algorithm. The general goal was typically to achieve maximal safe resection. The most feared complication was speech dysfunction, and most surgeons were cognizant of the Sylvian fissure, as well as the middle cerebral artery and perforating arterial branches. Surgery was generally pursued with surgical navigation, brain stimulation, surgical microscope, and ultrasonic aspirator, with perioperative steroids and/or antiepileptics. Most surgeons employed cortical and subcortical mapping to avoid iatrogenic injury. Following surgery, most patients were admitted to the intensive care unit (one to the floor), and MRIs were obtained within 72 hours after surgery. If the diagnosis was a diffuse astrocytoma, observation was chosen after gross total resection in half and radiation and temozolomide in the other half, whereas radiation and chemotherapy for the majority when subtotal resection was achieved. If the diagnosis was an oligodendroglioma, all surgeons opted for observation if gross total resection was achieved, and radiation and/or chemotherapy for subtotal resection. If the diagnosis was an anaplastic astrocytoma, radiation and temozolomide were chosen by all surgeons.

SUMMARY OF QUALITY OF EVIDENCE TO GUIDE SPECIFIC INTERVENTIONS FOR THIS CASE

- Surgery as opposed to biopsy or observation for LGGs—Class II-1.
- Increasing extent of resection associated with improved outcomes—Class II-2.
- Awake mapping versus asleep surgery for LGGs—Class II-2.
- Intraoperative MRI to assess for further resection—Class II-1.
- Neuropsychological evaluation for gliomas—Class III.

REFERENCES

1. Chaichana KL, McGirt MJ, Laterra J, Olivi A, Quinones-Hinojosa A. Recurrence and malignant degeneration after resection of adult hemispheric low-grade gliomas. *J Neurosurg.* 2010;112:10–17.
2. Chaichana KL, McGirt MJ, Niranjan A, Olivi A, Burger PC, Quinones-Hinojosa A. Prognostic significance of contrast-enhancing low-grade gliomas in adults and a review of the literature. *Neurol Res.* 2009;31:931–939.
3. McGirt MJ, Chaichana KL, Attenello FJ, et al. Extent of surgical resection is independently associated with survival in patients with hemispheric infiltrating low-grade gliomas. *Neurosurgery.* 2008;63:700–707; author reply 707–708.
4. Forst DA, Nahed BV, Loeffler JS, Batchelor TT. Low-grade gliomas. *Oncologist.* 2014;19:403–413.
5. Noll KR, Bradshaw ME, Weinberg JS, Wefel JS. Neurocognitive functioning is associated with functional independence in newly diagnosed patients with temporal lobe glioma. *Neurooncol Pract.* 2018;5:184–193.
6. Fernandez-Miranda JC, Rhoton AL Jr., Alvarez-Linera J, Kakizawa Y, Choi C, de Oliveira EP. Three-dimensional microsurgical and tractographic anatomy of the white matter of the human brain. *Neurosurgery.* 2008;62:989–1026; discussion 1026–1028.
7. Rhoton AL Jr. The cerebrum. Anatomy. *Neurosurgery.* 2007;61:37–118; discussion 118–119.
8. Duffau H. The reliability of asleep-awake-asleep protocol for intraoperative functional mapping and cognitive monitoring in glioma surgery. *Acta Neurochir (Wien).* 2013;155:1803–1804.
9. Eseonu CI, Eguia F, Garcia O, Kaplan PW, Quinones-Hinojosa A. Comparative analysis of monotherapy versus duotherapy antiseizure drug management for postoperative seizure control in patients undergoing an awake craniotomy. *J Neurosurg.* 2018;128:1661–1667.
10. Eseonu CI, Eguia F, ReFaey K, et al. Comparative volumetric analysis of the extent of resection of molecularly and histologically distinct low grade gliomas and its role on survival. *J Neurooncol.* 2017;134:65–74.
11. Eseonu CI, Rincon-Torroella J, ReFaey K, et al. Awake craniotomy vs craniotomy under general anesthesia for perirolandic gliomas: evaluating perioperative complications and extent of resection. *Neurosurgery.* 2017;81:481–489.
12. Bertani G, Fava E, Casaceli G, et al. Intraoperative mapping and monitoring of brain functions for the resection of low-grade gliomas: technical considerations. *Neurosurg Focus.* 2009;27:E4.
13. Nossek E, Korn A, Shahar T, et al. Intraoperative mapping and monitoring of the corticospinal tracts with neurophysiological assessment and 3-dimensional ultrasonography-based navigation. Clinical article. *J Neurosurg.* 2011;114:738–746.
14. Mandelli ML, Berger MS, Bucci M, Berman JI, Amirbekian B, Henry RG. Quantifying accuracy and precision of diffusion MR tractography of the corticospinal tract in brain tumors. *J Neurosurg.* 2014;121:349–358.
15. Pak RW, Hadjiabadi DH, Senarathna J, et al. Implications of neurovascular uncoupling in functional magnetic resonance imaging (fMRI) of brain tumors. *J Cereb Blood Flow Metab.* 2017;37:3475–3487.

Right temporal low-grade glioma

Case reviewed by Omar Arnaout, Santiago Gil-Robles, Manabu Natsumeda, Maryam Rahman

Introduction

A common location of low-grade gliomas (LGGs) is the temporal lobe, in which the number ranges from 15% to 25% in several series.[1–4] Patients with temporal lobe LGGs typically present with seizures in addition to deficits in neurocognitive function, namely attention, object naming, and language.[5,6] Surgery for left and right temporal lobe LGGs has different risk profiles and potentially different approaches.[5,6] Although nondominant-hemisphere lesions are considered to have lower risk profiles than their counterpart on the dominant hemisphere, surgery can be associated with significant morbidity.[5,6] In this chapter, we presents a case of a right temporal lobe LGG.

Example case

Chief complaint: seizures
History of present illness

An 18-year-old, right-handed man with no significant past medical history presented with seizures. He has complained of recurrent episodes of staring spells and abnormal smells. He saw his primary care physician who ordered brain imaging, which revealed a brain tumor (Fig. 11.1). He was started on levetiracetam. He was referred for further evaluation and management.

Medications: Levetiracetam.
Allergies: No known drug allergies.
Past medical and surgical history: None.
Family history: No history of intracranial malignancies.
Social history: Senior high school student. No smoking or alcohol.
Physical examination: Awake, alert, oriented to person, place, and time; Language: intact naming and repetition; Cranial nerves II to XII intact; No drift, moves all extremities with full strength.

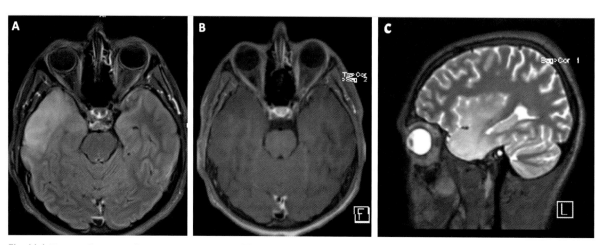

Fig. 11.1 Preoperative magnetic resonance imaging. (A) T2 axial fluid attenuation inversion recovery image; **(B)** T1 axial image with gadolinium contrast; **(C)** T2 sagittal magnetic resonance imaging scan demonstrating a nonenhancing lesion involving the right temporal lobe.

	Omar Arnaout, MD, Brigham and Women's Hospital, Boston, MA, United States	Santiago Gil-Robles, MD, PhD, Universidad Europea de Madrid, Madrid, Spain	Manabu Natsumeda, MD, PhD, Niigata University, Niigata, Japan	Maryam Rahman, MD, University of Florida, Gainesville, FL, United States
Preoperative				
Additional tests requested	None	DTI MR perfusion/MRS Neuropsychological assessment	Cerebral angiogram with Wada MRS with 2-HG analysis DTI 3D-CTA/V	DTI
Surgical approach selected	Right temporal craniotomy	Right pterional craniotomy with anterior temporal lobectomy with amygdalohippocampectomy and inferior insular resection with awake cortical and subcortical mapping	Right temporal craniotomy for temporal lobectomy with intraoperative CT	Right fronto-temporal craniotomy with intraoperative MRI
Anatomic corridor	Right temporal lobe	Right temporal lobe, opening of ventricle, amygdalohippocampectomy and inferior insular resection	Right temporal lobe	Right temporal lobe
Goal of surgery	Maximal safe resection, seizure control	Extensive resection with functional preservation	Gross total resection	Gross total resection
Perioperative				
Positioning	Right supine with left head rotation	Right lateral	Right supine 70-degree head rotation	Right supine
Surgical equipment	Surgical navigation Surgical microscope	Brain stimulator Ultrasonic aspirator Surgical navigation Speech therapist/ Neuropsychological assessment	Intraoperative CT/MRI Surgical navigation Ectrocorticography	Intraoperative MRI Surgical navigation Surgical microscope with fluorescent filter
Medications	Steroids Antiepileptics	Steroids Antiepileptics	Steroids Mannitol Antiepileptics	Steroids Mannitol Antiepileptics Fluorescein
Anatomic considerations	Sylvian fissure and vessels, temporal stem	Anterior choroidal artery, MCA M1 perforators IFOF	Right temporal gyri and sulci, temporal horn of lateral ventricle, temporobasal vein, SMCV, vein of Labbe, amygdala, hippocampus, uncus, anterior choroidal artery choroidal point	Sylvian fissure Meyer loop
Complications feared with approach chosen	Stroke	Subpial dissection to avoid vascular injury Awake cortical and subcortical mapping	Sylvian vascular injury Visual field deficit	Sylvian vascular injury Visual field deficit
Intraoperative				
Anesthesia	General	Awake-asleep-awake	General	General
Skin incision	Curvilinear	Pterional	Reverse question mark	Reverse question mark
Bone opening	Temporal	Frontal-temporal	Temporal	Frontal-temporal

(continued on next page)

	Omar Arnaout, MD, Brigham and Women's Hospital, Boston, MA, United States	Santiago Gil-Robles, MD, PhD, Universidad Europea de Madrid, Madrid, Spain	Manabu Natsumeda, MD, PhD, Niigata University, Niigata, Japan	Maryam Rahman, MD, University of Florida, Gainesville, FL, United States
Brain exposure	Temporal	Frontal-temporal	Temporal	Frontal-temporal
Method of resection	Skin opened separate from temporalis along different curve than incision, split temporalis, subperiosteal dissection to expose temporal squamosa, temporal craniotomy with single burr hole exposing STG/MTG/ITG, cruciate dural opening, lateral temporal lobe debulked with bipolar and suction, identify temporal horn and use as medial extent of resection, subpial resection up to Sylvian fissure as superior margin, temporal tip identified and folded in for resection, posterior margin confirmed by ultrasound and navigation, temporal stem identified and resected from insula respecting lenticulostriate vessels as medial border	Subfascial temporal muscle dissection, fronto-temporal craniotomy with posterior extension, intradural and muscle local anesthesia, dural opening, standard anterior temporal lobectomy with opening of ventricle, awaken patient, calibration of stimulation parameters (1.5–3 mA) based on anarthria over ventral premotor cortex, speech therapist for semantic association tasks to detect temporal stem and IFOF with stimulation, mark limits based on functional mapping, patient put to sleep, subpial resection of inferior insula and amygdalohippocampectomy, intraoperative scan to determine if additional nonfunctional tissue can be resected	Two layer skin flap, right fronto-temporal craniotomy, removal of temporal base and sphenoid ridge, determination of inferior horn and posterior aspect of tumor based on navigation, en bloc tumor resection through MTG as superior margin and posterior aspect of tumor and along base of tumor after opening inferior horn, keep temporobasal vein intact, and subpial removal of remaining tumor around inferior horn, intraoperative CT/MRI to assess resection, watertight dural closure, subgaleal drain	Myocutaneous flap, frontotemporal craniotomy maximizing exposure anteriorly and inferiorly, navigation to confirm posterior aspect of tumor and Meyer loops based on fMRI, identify Sylvian fissure, cortisectomy through superior and MTG at posterior aspect of tumor and resect everything anteriorly to this, leave arachnoid/pia intact to avoid cranial nerve III and PCA intact with microscopic visualization, avoid insula, intraoperative MRI and fluorescein to assess resection
Complication avoidance	Two-layered opening, anatomic boundaries	Subpial Awake cortical and subcortical mapping, mapping of IFOF	Subpial Intraoperative CT/MRI	Subpial Intraoperative MRI
Postoperative				
Admission	ICU	ICU	ICU	ICU
Postoperative complications feared	Stroke	Anterior choroidal artery, motor deficit, visual field deficit	Visual field impairment, cognitive dysfunction	MCA injury/stroke, visual field deficit
Follow-up testing	MRI within 48 hours after surgery	MRI within 48 hours after surgery Neuropsychological assessment	CT immediately postoperative MRI within 24 hours after surgery Neuropsychological assessment 1 week after surgery	MRI within 48 hours after surgery
Follow-up visits	7–10 days after surgery	7–10 days after surgery MRI 3–4 months	2–3 weeks after surgery	2 weeks after surgery with neuro-oncology 6 weeks after surgery

	Omar Arnaout, MD, Brigham and Women's Hospital, Boston, MA, United States	Santiago Gil-Robles, MD, PhD, Universidad Europea de Madrid, Madrid, Spain	Manabu Natsumeda, MD, PhD, Niigata University, Niigata, Japan	Maryam Rahman, MD, University of Florida, Gainesville, FL, United States
Adjuvant therapies recommended				
Diffuse astrocytoma (IDH mutant, retain 1p19q)	STR–radiation/ temozolomide GTR–radiation/ temozolomide	<4 mm/year growth rate– observation >4 mm/year growth rate– radiation/temozolomide	STR–radiation/ temozolomide GTR–observation	Screened for clinical trial STR–radiation/ temozolomide GTR–radiation/ temozolomide
Oligodendroglioma (IDH mutant, 1p19q LOH)	STR–second look surgery or radiation/ temozolomide GTR–observation	STR: <4 mm/year growth rate– observation; >4 mm/year growth rate–PCV GTR–observation	STR–radiation/PAV or temozolomide GTR–observation	Screened for clinical trial STR–radiation/ temozolomide or radiation/PCV GTR–radiation/ temozolomide or radiation/PCV
Anaplastic astrocytoma (IDH wild type)	STR–radiation/ temozolomide GTR–radiation/ temozolomide	Homogenous AA–radiation/ temozolomide AA foci removal–treatment as for diffuse astrocytoma	STR–radiation/ temozolomide GTR–radiation/ temozolomide	Screened for clinical trial STR–radiation/ temozolomide GTR–radiation/ temozolomide

2-HG, 2-hydroxyglutarate; *3D-CTA*, three-dimensional computed tomography angiography; *AA*, anaplastic astrocytoma; *CT*, computed tomography; *DTI*, diffusion tensor imaging; *fMRI*, functional magnetic resonance imaging; *GTR*, gross total resection; *ICU*, intensive care unit; *IFOF*, inferior frontal occipital fasciculus; *ITG*, inferior temporal gyrus; *LOH*, loss of heterozygosity; *MCA*, middle cerebral artery; *MR*, magnetic resonance; *MRI*, magnetic resonance imaging; *MRS*, magnetic resonance spectroscopy; *MTG*, middle temporal gyrus; *PAV*, procarbazine, *ACNU*, vincristine; *PCA*, posterior cerebral artery; *PCV*, procarbazine, lomustine, vincristine; *SMCV*, superficial middle cerebral vein; *STG*, superior temporal gyrus; *STR*, subtotal resection.

Differential diagnosis and actual diagnosis

- LGG (astrocytoma, oligodendroglioma)
- High-grade glioma
- Demyelinating disease (i.e., multiple sclerosis)

Important anatomic and preoperative considerations

For a full description of the surface anatomy of the temporal lobe, see Chapter 10. The medial temporal lobe is formed by the uncus, parahippocampal gyrus, dentate gyrus, and fimbria. The uncus is the anterior portion of the parahippocampal gyrus and separated from the parahippocampal gyrus by the uncal sulcus. The anterior part of the uncus is related to the amygdala and is separated from the temporal pole by the rhinal sulcus.

The portion of the uncus above the uncal sulcus is divided into three gyri from anterior to posterior: uncinate gyrus, band of Giacomini, and intralimbic gyrus, which collectively constitute the extraventricular portion of the head of the hippocampus. The ventricular component of the head of the hippocampus is seen when opening the temporal horn of the lateral ventricle. Posterior to the head of the hippocampus is the inferior choroidal point, which is the most inferior part of the choroidal fissure that divides the fornix from the thalamus. The structures below the choroidal fissure (hippocampus, subiculum, parahippocampal gyrus) may be removed in a medial temporal lobe resection, whereas the thalamus that resides above and medial to the choroidal fissure should not be removed. The optic tract is at the upper limit of the uncus, and above the optic tract is the basal ganglia.

Approaches to this lesion

As stated in Chapter 1, Fig. 1.2, the general approaches for these intrinsic lesions can be divided into asleep versus awake surgery, in which the methods of identifying eloquent cortical and subcortical structures can be divided into direct versus indirect methods (Chapter 3, Fig. 3.2).[7-12] For lesions isolated to the temporal lobe, monitoring during asleep surgery is not as useful until the motor and/or sensory cortex and corticospinal tracts are encountered.[11,12] This typically occurs in the vicinity of the thalamus and posterior limb of the internal capsule.[11,12] Awake brain mapping can be used to identify and avoid eloquent cortical and subcortical regions to minimize surgical morbidity, and can be used to identify the cortical and subcortical areas responsible for language, memory, and visual field functions, including the Wernicke area, Heschl gyrus, inferior longitudinal fasciculus, and inferior frontal-occipital fasciculus, as well as visual fields.[7-12] However, patients must be able to tolerate awake surgery, as this requires patient cooperation.[7-12]

In regard to directionality, the lesion involves the temporal lobe and extends upward to the frontal lobe via the uncinate fasciculus. The majority of the lesion is in the temporal lobe, therefore a lateral approach over the temporal lobe is typically done first and following the lesion into the uncinate fasciculus into the frontal lobe. An alternative is to approach the lesion through the frontal operculum first, but this would involve traversing uninvolved cortical and subcortical tissue.

What was actually done

The patient underwent a neuropsychological evaluation that showed mild disorders in processing speed and executive function. The patient was taken to surgery for an asleep right temporal craniotomy with general anesthesia. The patient was induced and intubated per routine. The head was fixed in pins, with two pins centered over the inion and one pin over the left forehead in the midpupillary line. The head was turned 90 degrees to the left, and a bump was placed under the right shoulder to facilitate turning. A pterional incision was planned that spanned from the root of the zygoma to the vertex. The patient was draped in the usual standard fashion and given dexamethasone, levetiracetam, and cefazolin. A myocutaneous flap was raised, and the flap was held in place with fishhooks attached to a retractor arm. A right pterional craniotomy was done that encompassed the lesion based on preoperative magnetic resonance imaging (MRI) surgical navigation. Ultrasound and surgical navigation were used to confirm lesion boundaries. The dura was then opened with the base along the sphenoid wing. The order of resection was the inferior temporal, middle temporal, and then the superior temporal gyri, followed by the uncinate fasciculus. After the lesion was resected, an intraoperative MRI was done to evaluate the extent of resection and no residual lesion was identified (Fig. 11.2). The dura, bone, and skin were closed in standard fashion.

The patient awoke at their neurologic baseline with intact speech, full strength bilaterally, and full visual fields, and was taken to the intensive care unit for recovery. The patient participated with physical and occupational therapy and was discharged to home on postoperative day 2 with an intact neurologic examination. The patient was prescribed 3 months of levetiracetam, and dexamethasone was tapered to off over 5 days after surgery. The patient was seen at 2 weeks postoperatively for staple removal and remained neurologically intact. Pathology was a World Health Organization grade II oligodendroglioma (IDH mutant, 1p/19q loss of heterozygosity). The lesion was observed with serial MRI examinations at 3 months, followed by 6-month intervals, and has been without recurrence for 12 months. The patient had a repeat neuropsychological evaluation at 3 months postoperatively that showed no change from preoperative evaluation. The patient returned to school at 2 weeks postoperatively and remains without neurologic deficits.

Commonalities among the experts

For this lesion, some of surgeons preferred to have diffusion tensor imaging prior to surgery to identify white matter tracts. The approach to the lesion was through the right temporal lobe with general anesthesia, except one surgeon favored an asleep-awake-asleep approach. The general goal was typically to achieve gross total resection, in which half of the surgeons favored the use of intraoperative imaging to guide possible further resection. The most feared complication was visual field deficit, and most surgeons were cognizant of the Sylvian fissure. Surgery was generally pursued with surgical navigation, surgical microscope, and ultrasonic aspirator, with perioperative steroids and/or antiepileptics. The key surgical technique was a subpial dissection to avoid vascular injury. The majority of surgeons favored a subpial dissection to avoid iatrogenic injury. Following surgery, all patients were admitted to the intensive care unit, and MRIs were obtained within 48 hours after surgery to assess the extent of resection and potential surgical complications. If the diagnosis was a diffuse astrocytoma, observation was chosen after gross total resection in one and radiation and temozolomide in two, whereas radiation and chemotherapy for the majority when subtotal resection was achieved. If the diagnosis was an oligodendroglioma, the majority of surgeons opted for observation if gross total resection was achieved, and radiation and/or chemotherapy

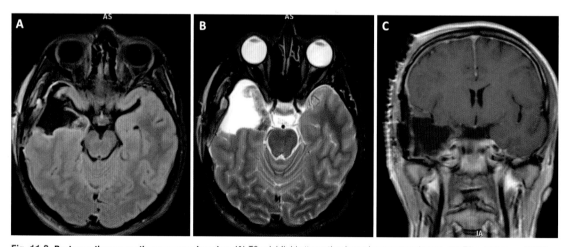

Fig. 11.2 Postoperative magnetic resonance imaging. (A) T2 axial fluid attenuation inversion recovery image; **(B)** T2 axial image; **(C)** T1 coronal image with gadolinium contrast magnetic resonance imaging scan demonstrating gross total resection of the right temporal nonenhancing lesion.

for subtotal resection. If the diagnosis was an anaplastic astrocytoma, radiation and temozolomide were chosen by all surgeons.

SUMMARY OF QUALITY OF EVIDENCE TO GUIDE SPECIFIC INTERVENTIONS FOR THIS CASE

- Surgery as opposed to biopsy or observation for LGGs—Class II-1.
- Increasing extent of resection associated with improved outcomes—Class II-2.
- Intraoperative MRI to assess for further resection—Class II-1.
- Neuropsychological evaluation for gliomas—Class III.

REFERENCES

1. Chaichana KL, McGirt MJ, Laterra J, Olivi A, Quinones-Hinojosa A. Recurrence and malignant degeneration after resection of adult hemispheric low-grade gliomas. *J Neurosurg.* 2010;112:10–17.
2. Chaichana KL, McGirt MJ, Niranjan A, Olivi A, Burger PC, Quinones-Hinojosa A. Prognostic significance of contrast-enhancing low-grade gliomas in adults and a review of the literature. *Neurol Res.* 2009;31:931–939.
3. McGirt MJ, Chaichana KL, Attenello FJ, et al. Extent of surgical resection is independently associated with survival in patients with hemispheric infiltrating low-grade gliomas. *Neurosurgery.* 2008;63:700–707; author reply 707–708.
4. Forst DA, Nahed BV, Loeffler JS, Batchelor TT. Low-grade gliomas. *Oncologist.* 2014;19:403–413.
5. Noll KR, Bradshaw ME, Weinberg JS, Wefel JS. Neurocognitive functioning is associated with functional independence in newly diagnosed patients with temporal lobe glioma. *Neurooncol Pract.* 2018;5:184–193.
6. Kemerdere R, Yuksel O, Kacira T, et al. Low-grade temporal gliomas: surgical strategy and long-term seizure outcome. *Clin Neurol Neurosurg.* 2014;126:196–200.
7. Duffau H. The reliability of asleep-awake-asleep protocol for intraoperative functional mapping and cognitive monitoring in glioma surgery. *Acta Neurochir (Wien).* 2013;155:1803–1804.
8. Eseonu CI, Eguia F, Garcia O, Kaplan PW, Quinones-Hinojosa A. Comparative analysis of monotherapy versus duotherapy antiseizure drug management for postoperative seizure control in patients undergoing an awake craniotomy. *J Neurosurg.* 2018;128:1661–1667.
9. Eseonu CI, Eguia F, ReFaey K, et al. Comparative volumetric analysis of the extent of resection of molecularly and histologically distinct low grade gliomas and its role on survival. *J Neurooncol.* 2017;134:65–74.
10. Eseonu CI, Rincon-Torroella J, ReFaey K, et al. Awake craniotomy vs craniotomy under general anesthesia for perirolandic gliomas: evaluating perioperative complications and extent of resection. *Neurosurgery.* 2017;81:481–489.
11. Bertani G, Fava E, Casaceli G, et al. Intraoperative mapping and monitoring of brain functions for the resection of low-grade gliomas: technical considerations. *Neurosurg Focus.* 2009;27:E4.
12. Nossek E, Korn A, Shahar T, et al. Intraoperative mapping and monitoring of the corticospinal tracts with neurophysiological assessment and 3-dimensional ultrasonography-based navigation. Clinical article. *J Neurosurg.* 2011;114:738–746.

12

Gliomatosis cerebri

Case reviewed by Gordon Li, Nader Sanai, Shota Tanaka, Graeme F. Woodworth

Introduction

Gliomatosis cerebri is characterized by widespread infiltration of the brain in three or more lobes with bilateral involvement.[1] Gliomatosis cerebri type 1 is when there is no obvious mass, but there is a widespread tumor pattern, whereas gliomatosis cerebri type 2 shows a widespread tumor pattern with a tumor mass.[1] The symptoms of gliomatosis cerebri depend on the tumor location.[1] The management of these lesions is typically limited to surgical biopsy, as there usually is no mass lesion to remove.[1] The tissue obtained through the biopsy will be used to guide possible adjuvant therapy.[1] In this chapter, we present a case with bilateral multifocal disease characteristic of gliomatosis cerebri.

Example case

Chief complaint: seizures
History of present illness
A 57-year-old, right-handed woman with no significant past medical history presented with seizures. She was driving when she had a witnessed acute onset of right facial and arm twitching followed by loss of consciousness with resulting motor vehicle collision. She was brought to the emergency room where imaging revealed multifocal brain lesions (Fig. 12.1).
Medications: None.
Allergies: No known drug allergies.
Past medical and surgical history: None.
Family history: No history of intracranial malignancies.
Social history: Elementary school teacher. No smoking or alcohol.
Physical examination: Awake, alert, oriented to person, place, and time; Language: intact naming and repetition; Cranial nerves II to XII intact; No drift, moves all extremities with full strength.

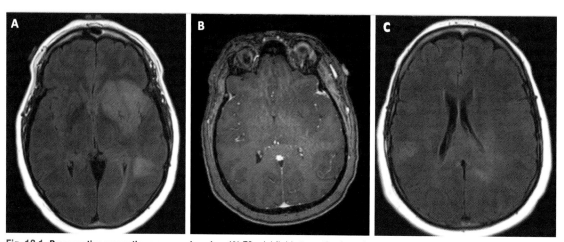

Fig. 12.1 Preoperative magnetic resonance imaging. (A) T2 axial fluid attenuation inversion recovery image; **(B)** T1 axial image with gadolinium contrast; **(C)** T2 axial fluid attenuation inversion recovery image at a higher level demonstrating a multifocal, nonenhancing lesion involving the left frontal, left insular, left temporal, and right parietal lobes.

	Gordon Li, MD, Stanford University, Palo Alto, CA, United States	Nader Sanai, MD, Barrow Neurological Institute, Phoenix, AZ, United States	Shota Tanaka, MD, PhD, The University of Tokyo, Tokyo, Japan	Graeme F. Woodworth, MD, University of Maryland School of Medicine, Baltimore, MD, United States
Preoperative				
Additional tests requested	CSF analysis	DTI fMRI	DTI fMRI PET methionine	Neurology evaluation
Surgical approach selected	Left posterior temporal stereotactic needle biopsy	Left frontal stereotactic needle biopsy	Left fronto-temporal craniotomy for temporal lobectomy and partial insular resection	Left temporal craniotomy for open excisional biopsy
Anatomic corridor	Left posterior MTG/ITG	Left frontal	Left temporal	Left anterior ITG
Goal of surgery	Diagnosis	Diagnosis	Diagnosis, debulking of highest-grade potion of lesion based on PET	Diagnosis, molecular testing
Perioperative				
Positioning	Left supine	Left supine	Left supine with right rotation	Left supine with rotation
Surgical equipment	Needle biopsy kit Surgical navigation	Needle biopsy kit Surgical navigation	Surgical navigation IOM (MEP) Surgical microscope with 5-ALA Doppler ultrasound	Surgical navigation Surgical microscope
Medications	Antiepileptics	None	Steroids Antiepileptics	Steroids after biopsy Antiepileptics Mannitol
Anatomic considerations	Wernicke area	Sylvian vessels Internal capsule	MCA, lenticulostriate artery	Eloquent language regions
Complications feared with approach chosen	Language deficit with Wernicke superiorly, left insula, and right perirolandic	Aphasia Motor deficit	Motor deficit, semantic paraphasias	Speech dysfunction, nondiagnostic tissue
Intraoperative				
Anesthesia	General	General	General	General
Skin incision	Linear	Linear	Curvilinear	Curvilinear
Bone opening	Left temporal burr hole	Left frontal burr hole	Left fronto-temporal	Left anterior temporal
Brain exposure	Left MTG/ITG	Left SFG/MFG (Kocher point)	Left fronto-temporal	Left anterior temporal
Method of resection	Preplan entry point for left MTG/ITG, twist drill burr hole, puncture dura with k-wire, navigation biopsy kit, take four biopsies at the same depth with one biopsy in each quadrant, frozen diagnosis, incision closed if pathology is lesional	Left frontal linear incision, Kocher point identified, and burr hole made, stereotactic needle biopsy passed into left basal ganglia, biopsies taken, frozen pathology, incision closed if pathology is lesional	Left fronto-temporal craniotomy, dural opening, left temporal lobectomy up to 4 cm with microscope, identify and preserve Sylvian fissure vessels including MCA, debulk insular portion through resection cavity	Preplan entry point based on navigation, craniotomy over inferior anterior temporal region, cruciate dural opening, enter temporal region low and anterior based on navigation, open biopsy, microscope as needed for visualization
Complication avoidance	Avoid Wernicke area	Avoid Sylvian vessels and internal capsule	IOM, awareness of Sylvian vessels, debulk insular portion through resection cavity	Low and anterior trajectory, open biopsy with direct visualization

(continued on next page)

	Gordon Li, MD, Stanford University, Palo Alto, CA, United States	Nader Sanai, MD, Barrow Neurological Institute, Phoenix, AZ, United States	Shota Tanaka, MD, PhD, The University of Tokyo, Tokyo, Japan	Graeme F. Woodworth, MD, University of Maryland School of Medicine, Baltimore, MD, United States
Postoperative				
Admission	Floor	ICU	ICU	ICU
Postoperative complications feared	Hemorrhage, language deficit	Hemorrhage	Vessel spasm/stroke	Speech loss, seizures, hemorrhage, cerebral edema
Follow-up testing	None	Head CT immediately after surgery	MRI within 48 hours after surgery	Head CT immediately after surgery
Follow-up visits	10 days after surgery	14 days after surgery	12–31 days after surgery	14 days after surgery Radiation Oncology and Neuro Oncology pending pathology results
Adjuvant therapies recommended				
Diffuse astrocytoma (IDH mutant, retain 1p19q)	Radiation/temozolomide	Radiation/temozolomide	Radiation/temozolomide	Radiation, possible chemotherapy
Oligodendroglioma (IDH mutant, 1p19q LOH)	Radiation/PCV or radiation/ temozolomide	Radiation/temozolomide	Radiation/PAV	Radiation/PCV
Anaplastic astrocytoma (IDH wild type)	Radiation/temozolomide	Radiation/temozolomide	Radiation/temozolomide	Radiation/temozolomide

5-ALA, 5-aminolevulinic acid; *CSF*, cerebrospinal fluid; *CT*, computed tomography; *DTI*, diffusion tensor imaging; *fMRI*, functional magnetic resonance imaging; *ICU*, intensive care unit; *IOM*, intraoperative monitoring; *ITG*, inferior temporal gyrus; *LOH*, loss of heterozygosity; *MCA*, middle cerebral artery; *MEP*, motor evoked potential; *MFG*, middle frontal gyrus; *MRI*, magnetic resonance imaging; *MTG*, middle temporal gyrus; *PAV*, procarbazine, ACNU, vincristine; *PCV*, procarbazine, lomustine, vincristine; *PET*, positron emission tomography; *SFG*, superior frontal gyrus.

Differential diagnosis and actual diagnosis

- Multifocal low-grade glioma (astrocytoma, oligodendroglioma)
- Multifocal high-grade glioma
- Demyelinating disease (i.e., multiple sclerosis)

Important anatomic and preoperative considerations

In cases in which tissue is needed for multifocal lesions, the goal of lesion selection is to obtain the highest-yield tissue in the area with the least risk of neurologic deficit. The highest-yield tissue is typically considered contrast-enhancing tissue and lesion sizes that are larger. The regions that are the least risk of neurologic deficits are those that are more superficially located and avoid eloquent cortical and subcortical areas. The critical eloquent cortical areas include language cortices (ventral premotor, Broca, Wernicke), motor/sensory cortex, and visual cortex, whereas the eloquent subcortical regions include corticospinal tract, superior longitudinal fasciculus, arcuate fasciculus, inferior frontal occipital fasciculus, and inferior longitudinal fasciculus. The typical order of white matter tract preservation is projection fibers, association fibers, and then commissural fibers.

Approaches to this lesion

There is currently no role for extensive surgical resection for cases of true gliomatosis cerebri.[1] The goal of surgery is to obtain tissue for diagnosis and to guide adjuvant therapy.[1] Tissue can be obtained via needle biopsy or excisional biopsy.[2] The advantages of needle biopsy is that it is minimally invasive, high diagnostic yield (96%–99%), can be applied to eloquent cortical and subcortical areas, minimal morbidity, and decreased hospital stay.[2] The disadvantages of the needle biopsy is that there is minimal tissue obtained, risk of intraparenchymal hemorrhage, and sampling error.[2] An excisional biopsy typically involves a small craniotomy with direct visualization of the tissue that is biopsied, without the goal of extensive resection.[2] The advantages of an excisional biopsy are that it provides more tissue for pathology and tissue banking and is less prone to sampling error, whereas the disadvantages are that it is more invasive, potentially more morbidity, and difficulty with applying it to eloquent regions.[2]

In terms of directionality of approach, there are generally three lesions to target: the left insular, left posterior superior temporal, and right parietal. The left insular lesion is the largest of the lesions but is associated with the most eloquence, as it involves the dominant hemisphere, close proximity to middle cerebral artery (MCA) vessels, and eloquent subcortical structures (caudate, basal ganglia, superior longitudinal fasciculus [SLF], arcuate fasciculus [AF]). This area can be accessed through a lateral or anterior approach, in which the lateral approach involves potentially traversing the Broca area, Sylvian fissure with MCA vessels, SLF, and AF, whereas an anterior approach from the Kocher point is the longest distance to the insula but avoids these structures. The left posterior superior temporal is the shortest distance from the cortical surface, but potentially involves the Wernicke area and the temporal-parietal component of the SLF and AF. The right parietal has the least dense fluid attenuation inversion recovery hyperintensity area but is the least eloquent area of the three.

What was actually done

The patient was taken to surgery for an asleep right parietal needle biopsy with general anesthesia. The patient was induced and intubated per routine. The head was fixed in pins, with two pins centered over the left external auditory meatus and one pine over the right external auditory meatus. The head was kept in a neutral position. A linear incision was planned over the right parietal region based on preoperative surgical navigation. The right parietal lesion was chosen because of its lesser degree of eloquence as compared with the left fronto-insular and left temporal lesion. The right parietal trajectory was chosen to be posterior to the postcentral gyrus based on anatomic landmarks. The patient was draped in the usual standard fashion and given cefazolin and levetiracetam. A 2-cm linear incision was made, and the skin was retracted with a self-retaining retractor. A burr hole was made, and the dura was opened in a cruciate fashion. Under navigation guidance, a stereotactic needle was passed into the white matter, and samples were taken. Preliminary pathology was consistent with infiltrating glioma. The dura, bone, and skin were closed in standard fashion.

The patient awoke at their neurologic baseline with an intact neurologic examination and was taken to the postanesthesia care unit. The patient was discharged to home on postoperative day 1 with an intact neurologic examination without imaging. The patient was prescribed 3 months of levetiracetam. The patient returned to work 3 days after surgery. The patient was seen at 2 weeks postoperatively for staple removal and remained neurologically intact. Pathology was a World Health Organization grade II astrocytoma (IDH mutant, 1p/19q wild type). The patient underwent temozolomide chemotherapy with radiation therapy. The patient unfortunately had progression at 6 months and was administered bevacizumab.

Commonalities among the experts

For this lesion, most of the surgeons preferred to have functional magnetic resonance imaging and diffusion tensor imaging prior to surgery to identify white eloquent cortical areas and white matter tracts. A needle biopsy for diagnosis was chosen by most surgeons because of the multifocal nature of the lesion, but the biopsied area varied from frontal to temporal. The general goal was to obtain tissue for diagnosis. Most surgeons were cognizant of cortical language areas and MCA and its vessels, and the most feared complication was language and motor deficits. Surgery was generally pursued with surgical navigation and standard needle biopsy kits, in which most surgeons did not give perioperative steroids and/or antiepileptics. The key surgical technique was to avoid eloquent cortical areas, as well as MCA and its vessels. Following surgery, most patients were admitted to the intensive care unit, and imaging (computed tomography or magnetic resonance imaging) was obtained within 48 hours after surgery to assess for potential surgical complications. For all low- and high-grade diagnoses, all surgeons favored the use of radiation and chemotherapy because of expected subtotal resection.

SUMMARY OF QUALITY OF EVIDENCE TO GUIDE SPECIFIC INTERVENTIONS FOR THIS CASE

- Surgical resection versus biopsy for gliomatosis cerebri— Class III.

REFERENCES

1. Herrlinger U, Jones DTW, Glas M, et al. Gliomatosis cerebri: no evidence for a separate brain tumor entity. *Acta Neuropathol.* 2016;131:309–319.
2. Jackson C, Gallia GL, Chaichana KL. Minimally invasive biopsies of deep-seated brain lesions using tubular retractors under exoscopic visualization. *J Neurol Surg A Cent Eur Neurosurg.* 2017;78:588–594.

Pontine brainstem low-grade glioma

Case reviewed by Clark C. Chen, Shlomi Constantini, Danil A. Kozyrev, George I. Jallo, Vicent Quilis-Quesada

Introduction

Surgery in the brainstem can be associated with significant morbidity and mortality.[1,2] This is because the brainstem has a high density of eloquent gray and white matter structures, including cranial nerve (CN) nuclei, CN tracts, and craniospinal tracts, among others.[1,2] With a better understanding of brainstem anatomy, improved neuroimaging, and advances in surgical techniques and monitoring, surgery within the brainstem can occur with reduced morbidity.[1,2] In this chapter, we present a case of dorsal pontine brainstem lesion.

Example case

Chief complaint: left facial weakness

History of present illness

A 19-year-old, right-handed woman with no significant past medical history presented with prolonged facial weakness. Six months prior she developed left-sided facial weakness with inability to close her eye. She was treated for Bell palsy with steroids with no improvement after 6 months. Imaging was done and revealed a brain lesion (Fig. 13.1).

Medications: None.

Allergies: No known drug allergies.

Past medical and surgical history: None.

Family history: No history of intracranial malignancies.

Social history: College student. No smoking or alcohol.

Physical examination: Awake, alert, oriented to person, place, and time; Language: intact naming and repetition; CNs II to XII intact except left House-Brackmann 5/6; No drift, moves all extremities with full strength.

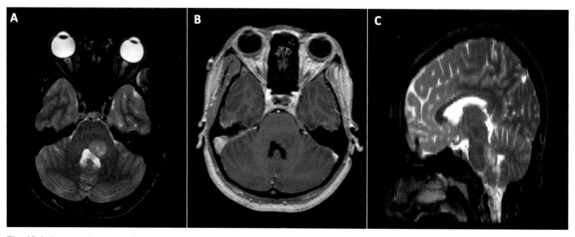

Fig. 13.1 Preoperative magnetic resonance imaging. (A) T2 axial image; **(B)** T1 axial image with gadolinium contrast; **(C)** T2 sagittal magnetic resonance imaging scan demonstrating a nonenhancing lesion involving the left pontine region.

	Clark C. Chen, MD, PhD, University of Minnesota, Minneapolis, MN, United States	Shlomi Constantini, MD, Danil A. Kozyrev, MD, Tel Aviv Sourasky Medical Center, Tel Aviv, Israel	George I. Jallo, MD, Johns Hopkins All Children's Hospital, St. Petersburg, FL, United States	Vicent Quilis-Quesada, MD, PhD, University of Valencia, Valencia, Spain
Preoperative				
Additional tests requested	Spine MRI Neuroophthalmology evaluation ENT evaluation Speech and swallow evaluation Intraoperative MRI	Diffusion MRI Spine MRI	Spine MRI	Spine MRI Lumbar puncture/CSF analysis DTI Echocardiogram
Surgical approach selected	Midline suboccipital craniotomy with intraoperative MRI	Midline suboccipital craniotomy for open biopsy	Midline suboccipital craniotomy	Midline suboccipital craniotomy
Anatomic corridor	Telovelar	Target inferior medullary aspect	Left telovelar	Left telovelar
Goal of surgery	Diagnosis, maximal resection	Diagnosis	Maximal resection without neurological deficit	GTR
Perioperative				
Positioning	Prone	Prone	Prone	Semisitting
Surgical equipment	Surgical navigation IOM (MEP, SSEP, BAERs, facial nerve EMG) Intraoperative MRI with 5-ALA	Ultrasound IOM Surgical microscope Electrified ultrasonic aspirator	Surgical navigation IOM (SSEP, MEPs, BAERs, cranial nerve EMG) Ultrasound Surgical microscope Nerve stimulator	IOM (SSEP, MEPs, BAERs, cranial nerve EMG) Surgical microscope Ultrasonic aspirator
Medications	Steroids Mannitol	Steroids	Steroids	None
Anatomic considerations	Inion, foramen magnum, C1, torcula, transverse sinus, sulcus arteriosus	Cerebellar tonsils	Cerebellar tonsils, PICA, floor of fourth ventricle	Floor of the fourth ventricle, PICA, dentate nuclei
Complications feared with approach chosen	Venous sinus and vertebral artery injury, brainstem/spinal cord injury	Injury to cranial nerves VI–VII, paramedian pontine reticular formation	Injury to cranial nerves at fourth ventricular floor, PICA stroke	Venous air embolism
Intraoperative				
Anesthesia	General	General	General	General
Skin incision	Midline linear from 1–2 cm above inion to C1	Midline linear from under inion to C2	Midline linear from under inion to C2	Midline from inion to C2
Bone opening	Midline occipital bone below transverse sinus, including foramen magnum	Midline occipital bone below transverse sinus, including foramen magnum	Midline occipital bone below transverse sinus, including foramen magnum	Midline occipital bone 1 cm below superior nuchal line, including foramen magnum
Brain exposure	Cerebellum, tonsils	Cerebellum	Cerebellum, tonsils	Cerebellum, tonsils

(continued on next page)

	Clark C. Chen, MD, PhD, University of Minnesota, Minneapolis, MN, United States	Shlomi Constantini, MD, Danil A. Kozyrev, MD, Tel Aviv Sourasky Medical Center, Tel Aviv, Israel	George I. Jallo, MD, Johns Hopkins All Children's Hospital, St. Petersburg, FL, United States	Vicent Quilis-Quesada, MD, PhD, University of Valencia, Valencia, Spain
Method of resection	Mark Frazier burr hole, incision with preservation of the pericranium, midline muscle dissection with exposure of C1, midline craniotomy, Y-shaped dural opening, open cerebellomedullary fissure, dissect up to rostral half of fourth ventricle, identify abnormal region and confirm with navigation, establish new baseline IOM, biopsy lesion, repeat IOM, debulk lesion and attempt to identify plane, intraoperative MRI to assess need for further resection, watertight closure with pericranium, bone flap fixation	Midline muscle dissection, stripping muscle from C1 and atlanto-axial membrane, midline craniotomy below transverse sinus, opening of foramen magnum, midline Y-shaped dural opening, separate tonsils to visualize the fourth ventricle, biopsy of exophytic medullary component leaving floor of fourth ventricle intact	Midline muscle dissection, exposing C1 lamina, midline occipital craniectomy below sinus incorporating foramen magnum, midline Y-shaped dural openings, section arachnoid between tonsils, identifying and incising tela choroidea +/− inferior medullary velum on left, ultrasound probe and navigation to confirm lesion location if not readily apparent on fourth ventricular floor, stimulate with nerve stimulator to confirm no facial nerve activity, intralesional debulking with suction, stop if lesion is fibrous or neuromonitoring changes, watertight dural closure with synthetic graft, bone flap fixation	Midline muscle dissection, suboccipital craniotomy, Y-shaped dural openings, cerebellomedullary fissure dissection, left tonsil dissection and left PICA protection, open vallecula to expose fourth ventricle, division of inferior medullary velum and tela choroidea, removal of inferior part of the lesion, expose left MCP and SCP and remove remainder, reconstruct cisterna magna with 9-0 suture, watertight dural closure, bone flap fixation
Complication avoidance	Frazier burr hole preparation, pericranium for closure, opening foramen magnum, telovelar approach, repeated IOM, intraoperative MRI	Separate muscle from atlanto-occipital membrane, opening foramen magnum, working between cerebellar tonsils, biopsy only exophytic medullary component, leave floor of fourth ventricle intact	Opening foramen magnum, left-sided telovelar opening, ultrasound and navigation to confirm lesion, nerve stimulator to identify safe entry zone, intralesional debulking	IOM, left PICA identification and protection, telovelar tonsillar opening, removal of inferior or exophytic portion first
Postoperative				
Admission	ICU	ICU	ICU	ICU
Postoperative complications feared	Facial nerve injury, cerebellar retraction injury, CSF leak	Loss of cough and gag reflexes, posterior fossa syndrome, eye movement issues	Facial nerve weakness, diplopia, dysphagia, aspiration, CSF leak	Cranial neuropathies, motor deficit, respiratory insufficiency
Follow-up testing	MRI within 48 hours after surgery Swallow evaluation Physical and occupational therapy	MRI within 48 hours after surgery	MRI within 48 hours after surgery Swallow evaluation	MRI within 24 hours after surgery
Follow-up visits	2 weeks after surgery Initiation of radiation/ chemotherapy pending diagnosis	14 days after surgery MRI 3 months after surgery	14–21 days after surgery MRI 3 months after surgery	14 days after surgery

	Clark C. Chen, MD, PhD, University of Minnesota, Minneapolis, MN, United States	Shlomi Constantini, MD, Danil A. Kozyrev, MD, Tel Aviv Sourasky Medical Center, Tel Aviv, Israel	George I. Jallo, MD, Johns Hopkins All Children's Hospital, St. Petersburg, FL, United States	Vicent Quilis-Quesada, MD, PhD, University of Valencia, Valencia, Spain
Adjuvant therapies recommended				
Diffuse astrocytoma (IDH mutant, retain 1p19q)	STR–chemotherapy, delayed radiation for recurrence GTR–observation	STR–radiation/ chemotherapy GTR–observation	STR–observation GTR–observation	STR–radiation/PCV GTR–radiation/PCV
Oligodendroglioma (IDH mutant, 1p19q LOH)	STR–radiation/PCV GTR–observation	STR–chemotherapy GTR–observation	STR–observation GTR–observation	STR–radiation/PCV GTR–radiation/PCV
Anaplastic astrocytoma (IDH wild type)	STR–radiation/ temozolomide GTR–radiation/ temozolomide	STR–radiation +/– chemotherapy GTR–radiation +/– chemotherapy	STR–radiation/ temozolomide GTR–radiation/ temozolomide	STR–radiation/ temozolomide GTR–radiation/ temozolomide

5-ALA, 5-aminolevulinic acid; *BAERs*, brainstem auditory evoked responses; *CSF*, cerebrospinal fluid; *DTI*, diffusion tensor imaging; *EMG*, electromyogram; *ENT*, ear, nose, and throat; *ICU*, intensive care unit; *IOM*, intraoperative monitoring; *GTR*, gross total resection; *LOH*, loss of heterozygosity; *MCP*, middle cerebellar peduncle; *MEP*, motor evoked potential; *MRI*, magnetic resonance imaging; *PCV*, procarbazine, lomustine, vincristine; *PICA*, posterior inferior cerebellar artery; *SCP*, superior cerebellar peduncle; *SSEP*, somatosensory evoked potential; *STR*, subtotal resection.

Differential diagnosis and actual diagnosis

- Low-grade glioma (astrocytoma, oligodendroglioma)
- High-grade glioma
- Demyelinating disease (i.e., multiple sclerosis)

Important anatomic and preoperative considerations

The pons has four surfaces: anterior, two posterior-lateral, and posterior, and is separated from the midbrain by the ponto-mesencephalic sulcus and the medulla by the pontine-bulbar sulcus that are both well defined on the anterior and lateral surfaces.[3] The two posterolateral faces continue with the cerebellar peduncles, in which anteriorly is the middle cerebellar peduncle (MCP), superior is the superior cerebellar peduncle, and inferior is the inferior cerebellar peduncle. The posterior face corresponds to the floor of the fourth ventricle.[3] The CN nuclei that are located at the level of the pons are the nuclei of CN V, VI, VII, and VIII.[3] From ventral to dorsal at the level of the pons at the level of the sensory and motor nucleus of CN V resides the superficial pontine fibers, corticospinal tract, medial and deep transverse fibers, medial lemniscus (immediately dorsal to the crossed cerebellopontine fibers), central tegmental tract, nucleus ceruleus, and the mesencephalic nucleus of CN V.[3] Medial to the central tegmental tract is the tectospinal tract that is ventral to the middle longitudinal fasciculus.[3]

The floor of the fourth ventricle that is located over the dorsal surface of the brainstem has a rhomboidal shape that is longer in the cranio-caudal than transverse dimension and extends from the distal portion of the cerebral aqueduct to the obex, which is immediately anterior to the foramen of Magendie.[3] The floor can be divided into three triangles: superior (pontine) (between the cerebral aqueduct and the line connecting the lateral recesses), intermediate (between the superior and inferior boundaries of the lateral recesses), and

inferior or medullary (inferolateral margin of the floor of the fourth ventricle or obex).[3] The medial sulcus divides the floor of the ventricle in the midline, and lateral to the medial sulcus is the sulcus limitans that further divides the floor of the fourth ventricle.[3] The area in-between the medial sulcus and the sulcus limitans is the median eminence, which is the site where the facial colliculus resides and is the prominence on the floor of the ventricle over CN X and XII nuclei and the area postrema.[3] The superior limit of the facial colliculus is the superior intrapontine segment of the facial nerve, and the inferior limit is formed by the intrapontine portion of the facial nerves that curve beneath the nucleus of CN VI.[3] The sulcus limitans itself has two depressions or fovea along the ventricular floor.[3] The superior fovea lies laterally to the facial colliculus, whereas the inferior fovea lies lateral to the hypoglossal triangle in the medullary portion of the ventricular floor and between the vestibular area superiorly and the superior border of the vagal triangle inferiorly.[3] Over the median eminence, caudal to the facial colliculus, lies the hypoglossal trigone medially and the vagal trigone laterally.[3]

Approaches to this lesion

There are generally three different approaches for lesions located dorsally in the pons at the junction of the pons and MCP, and include posterior, posterolateral, and lateral approaches. The direct posterior approach is done by accessing the floor of the fourth ventricle through a telovelar approach. The use of bilateral telovelar openings can provide a wider access to the floor of the fourth ventricle. The advantage of this approach is that it minimizes potential injury to the brain parenchyma but exposes the posterior inferior cerebellar artery (PICA) to potential injury. The posterolateral approach involves accessing the MCP through the cerebellar hemisphere or the cerebellopontine angle. This minimizes exposure of critical vessels but exposes the parenchyma at risk for injury, especially the MCP. This, however, can be done with tubular retractors to minimize potential parenchymal

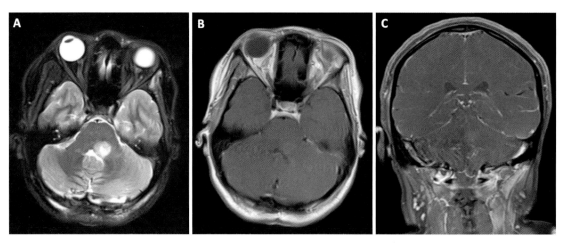

Fig. 13.2 Postoperative magnetic resonance imaging. (A) T2 axial image; **(B)** T1 axial image with gadolinium contrast; **(C)** T1 coronal image with gadolinium contrast magnetic resonance imaging scan demonstrating subtotal resection of the pontine lesion.

injury.[4–6] The lateral face of the pons can also be exposed, and accessed via the peritrigeminal zones, where the lateral limits are defined by the cranial, motor, and sensory trigeminal roots. This area can be accessed by transcavernous, anterior transpetrosal, or presigmoid approaches.

What was actually done

The patient underwent spinal imaging prior to rule out the presence of drop and/or concomitant lesions. The patient was taken to surgery for midline suboccipital craniotomy with right telovelar approach for pontine glioma with general anesthesia. The patient was induced and intubated per routine. Intraoperative monitoring was used to monitor somatosensory evoked potentials, as well as CN V, VII, IX, X, and XII. The head was fixed in neutral position with two pins centered over the left external auditory meatus and one pin over the right external auditory meatus. The patient was then placed prone onto chest rolls with the neck flexed and reduced. A midline incision was planned that spanned from just above the inion to the C2 spinous process. The patient was draped in the usual standard fashion and given dexamethasone and cefazolin. A midline incision was made, and dissection took place in the avascular plane between the suboccipital muscles. The skin and muscles were retracted with a cerebellar retractor, and the C1 spinous process and occipital bone with foramen magnum were identified. A suboccipital craniotomy was made below the transverse sinus and incorporated the foramen magnum. The dura was then opened in a Y-shaped fashion, and the surgical microscope was brought in for the remainder of the case. The arachnoid between the tonsils and the cerebellar hemispheres were opened with sharp dissection, making sure to identify and protect the bilateral PICAs. The tonsils were then retracted laterally with dynamic retraction without fixed retractors to expose the tela choroidea and inferior medullary velum on the right side. This exposed the floor of the fourth ventricle, and the posterior aspect of the pons was stimulated with a bipolar electrode looking for firing of the facial colliculi, as well as CNs IX and X. The tumor was then entered and debulked until facial nerve firing was elicited medially in the tumor cavity. At this point, the tumor resection was stopped. The dura, bone, and skin were closed in standard fashion.

The patient awoke at their neurologic baseline with intact speech, full strength bilaterally, and baseline left facial nerve weakness, and was taken to the intensive care unit for recovery. A magnetic resonance imaging (MRI) scan was done within 48 hours after surgery and showed expected subtotal resection with residual medially in the tumor cavity (Fig. 13.2). The patient participated with physical and occupational therapy and was discharged to home on postoperative day 3 with an intact neurologic examination. The patient was prescribed dexamethasone that was tapered to off over 10 days after surgery. The patient was seen at 2 weeks postoperatively for suture removal and remained neurologically intact with stable left facial weakness. Pathology was a World Health Organization grade II astrocytoma (IDH mutant, 1p/19q wild type). The lesion was observed with serial MRI examinations at 3 months, followed by 6-month intervals, and has been without recurrence for 24 months. The patient returned to school at 4 weeks postoperatively and remained at their neurological baseline but with improved facial nerve function (left House-Brackmann 2/6).

Commonalities among the experts

For this lesion, all surgeons would have patients undergo spine imaging to evaluate for drop lesions. A midline suboccipital approach was used for all, in which most surgeons preferred a left telovelar approach to the lesion. The general goal was typically to achieve maximal safe resection, and one surgeon favored the use of intraoperative imaging to guide potential further resection. Most surgeons were cognizant of the cerebellar tonsils, PICA, and floor of the fourth ventricle, in which the most feared complication was PICA vascular injury and cranial neuropathy owing to injury to the floor of the fourth ventricle. Surgery was generally pursued with surgical navigation, surgical microscope, and ultrasonic aspirator, with perioperative steroids. The key surgical technique was to open the foramen magnum, identify and protect the PICA, and focus primarily on the exophytic portion of the tumor to avoid iatrogenic injury. Following surgery, all patients were admitted to the intensive care unit, and MRIs were obtained within 48 hours after surgery to assess extent of resection and potential surgical complications, and most patients would undergo swallow evaluation postoperatively prior to advancing their diet. If the diagnosis was a diffuse astrocytoma, observation was chosen after gross total resection in the majority, whereas radiation and/or chemotherapy for the majority when subtotal resection was achieved. If the diagnosis was an oligodendroglioma, half of the surgeons chose observation and the other half chose radiation and PCV (procarbazine, lomustine, vincristine) chemotherapy for gross total resection, and radiation and/or chemotherapy for subtotal resection. If the diagnosis was an anaplastic astrocytoma, radiation and temozolomide were chosen by all surgeons.

SUMMARY OF QUALITY OF EVIDENCE TO GUIDE SPECIFIC INTERVENTIONS FOR THIS CASE

- Surgery as opposed to biopsy or observation for brainstem low-grade gliomas—Class III.
- Monitoring and brainstem mapping for brainstem surgery—Class III.

REFERENCES

1. Cavalheiro S, Yagmurlu K, da Costa MD, et al. Surgical approaches for brainstem tumors in pediatric patients. *Childs Nerv Syst.* 2015;31:1815–1840.
2. Jallo GI, Shiminski-Maher T, Velazquez L, Abbott R, Wisoff J, Epstein F. Recovery of lower cranial nerve function after surgery for medullary brainstem tumors. *Neurosurgery.* 2005;56:74–77; discussion 78.
3. Ribas EC. Yagmurlu K, de Oliveira E, Ribas GC, Rhoton A Jr. Microsurgical anatomy of the central core of the brain. *J Neurosurg.* 2018;129:752–769.
4. Gassie K, Wijesekera O, Chaichana KL. Minimally invasive tubular retractor-assisted biopsy and resection of subcortical intra-axial gliomas and other neoplasms. *J Neurosurg Sci.* 2018;62:682–689.
5. Iyer R, Chaichana KL. Minimally invasive resection of deep-seated high-grade gliomas using tubular retractors and exoscopic visualization. *J Neurol Surg A Cent Eur Neurosurg.* 2018;79:330–336.
6. Jackson C, Gallia GL, Chaichana KL. Minimally invasive biopsies of deep-seated brain lesions using tubular retractors under exoscopic visualization. *J Neurol Surg A Cent Eur Neurosurg.* 2017;78:588–594.

14

Medullary brainstem low-grade glioma

Case reviewed by Victor Garcia-Navarro, George I. Jallo, Maciej S. Lesniak, Andreas Raabe

Introduction

Brainstem tumors are a rare subset of intrinsic tumors that occur in adults that account for less than 1% of the primary brain tumors in adults.[1,2] These tumors typically occur in children and younger adults.[1,2] Surgery for these lesions can be associated with significant morbidity and include significant cranial nerve (CN) dysfunction and motor deficits.[1,2] Therefore because of the high risk of neurologic deficits, the optimal treatment of intrinsic brainstem lesions remains controversial.[1,2] In this chapter, we present a case of a medullary brainstem tumor.

Example case

Chief complaint: headaches and progressive imbalance
History of present illness
A 31-year-old, right-handed woman with no significant past medical history presented with headaches, facial pressure, and progressive imbalance. For the past 3 months, she has had progressive sensation of facial pressure and worsened headaches. She was treated with antibiotics for sinusitis, without improvement. More recently, over the past 2 weeks, she has had progressive imbalance with frequent falls. Imaging was done and revealed a brain lesion (Fig. 14.1).
Medications: None.
Allergies: No known drug allergies.
Past medical and surgical history: None.
Family history: No history of intracranial malignancies.
Social history: Accountant. No smoking or alcohol.
Physical examination: Awake, alert, oriented to person, place, and time; CNs II to XII intact; No drift, moves all extremities with full strength; right greater than left finger-to-nose dysmetria.

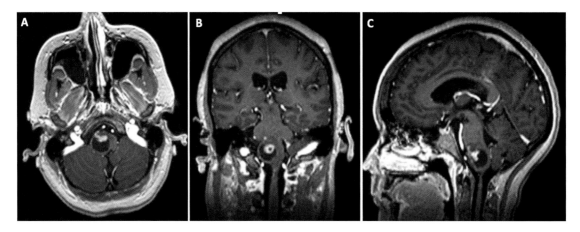

Figure 14.1 Preoperative magnetic resonance imaging. (A) T1 axial image with gadolinium contrast; **(B)** T1 coronal image with gadolinium contrast; **(C)** T1 sagittal image with gadolinium contrast magnetic resonance imaging scan demonstrating a heterogeneously enhancing lesion within the medullary brainstem region.

	Victor Garcia-Navarro, MD, Tec de Monterrey Institute, Campus Guadalajara, Mexico	George I. Jallo, MD, Johns Hopkins All Children's Hospital, St. Petersburg, FL, United States	Maciej S. Lesniak, MD, Northwestern University, Chicago, IL, United States	Andreas Raabe, MD, University Hospital at Inselspital, Bern, Switzerland
Preoperative				
Additional tests requested	MR perfusion Genetic/evaluation evaluation for VHL	Spinal MRI MR angiography	None	DTI Cerebral angiogram
Surgical approach selected	Right far lateral craniotomy	Midline suboccipital craniotomy with cortical and subcortical mapping	Right suboccipital craniectomy	Midline suboccipital craniotomy with cortical and subcortical mapping
Anatomic corridor	Right lateral medullary	Right telovelar	Right lateral medullary	Right telovelar
Goal of surgery	Diagnosis, resect enhancing portion	Extensive resection with cyst decompression and avoiding neurologic deficit	Diagnosis, resect enhancing portion	Diagnosis, resection of enhancing portion and cyst
Perioperative				
Positioning	Right park bench	Prone	Right park bench	Prone
Surgical equipment	Surgical navigation IOM (SSEP, MEP, BAERs, cranial nerve 7, 10–12 EMG)	Surgical navigation IOM (SSEP, MEPs, BAERs, cranial nerve EMG) Ultrasound Surgical microscope Nerve stimulator	Surgical navigation IOM Brain stimulator	Surgical navigation Ultrasound IOM (SSEP, MEP, cranial nerve EMG) Brain stimulator
Medications	Steroids Hypertonic saline solution	Steroids	Mannitol Steroids	None
Anatomic considerations	Sigmoid sinus, PCA, cranial nerves 7–12, brainstem, white matter tracts	Cerebellar tonsils, PICA, floor of fourth ventricle	Cranial nerve nuclei and tracts	Cranial nerves 9–12, CST, sensory tracts
Complications feared with approach chosen	Vascular injury, brainstem and cerebellar retraction injury	Lower cranial nerve dysfunction, motor or sensory deficit	Hemiparesis	Lower cranial nerve dysfunction, motor or sensory deficit
Intraoperative				
Anesthesia	General	General	General	General
Skin incision	Inverted hockey stick	Midline	Right paramedian	Midline
Bone opening	Extended retrosigmoid suboccipital craniotomy and posterior third of the occipital condyle	Suboccipital craniotomy with foramen magnum and C1 laminectomy	Suboccipital craniectomy	Suboccipital craniotomy with foramen magnum and C1 laminectomy
Brain exposure	Inferior cerebellum, right lateral medulla	Cerebellum and cervicomedullary junction	Inferior cerebellum, right lateral medulla	Cerebellum and cervicomedullary junction

(continued on next page)

	Victor Garcia-Navarro, MD, Tec de Monterrey Institute, Campus Guadalajara, Mexico	George I. Jallo, MD, Johns Hopkins All Children's Hospital, St. Petersburg, FL, United States	Maciej S. Lesniak, MD, Northwestern University, Chicago, IL, United States	Andreas Raabe, MD, University Hospital at Inselspital, Bern, Switzerland
Method of resection	Myocutaneous flap, retrosigmoid suboccipital craniotomy 3–4 cm posterior to sigmoid sinus, skeletonizing of transverse/sigmoid sinus, posterior third of the occipital condyle drilled away, L-shaped dural opening paralleling sinuses, drain CSF from cisterns, identification of neurovascular structures, stimulation to identify safe entry zone, lesion resection at tumor margin with decompression of cyst and removal of enhancing lesion, watertight dural closure with dural substitutes, titanium mesh or bone flap fixation	Midline suboccipital with slight right eccentricity with C1 laminectomy, Y-shaped dural opening, section arachnoid between tonsils, identifying and sectioning tela choroidea +/− inferior medullary velum on right, ultrasound probe and navigation to confirm lesion location if not readily apparent, stimulate with nerve stimulator to confirm no lower cranial nerve activity, intralesional debulking with suction, stop if lesion is fibrous or neuromonitoring changes, watertight dural closure with dural substitute if necessary, bone flap fixation	Right suboccipital craniectomy, identify right lateral medullary area anatomically, stimulate brainstem to find entry point with negative stimulation, resect as much lesion based on continuous monitoring and stimulating of CSTs, watertight dural closure, titanium mesh	Midline suboccipital craniotomy with opening of foramen magnum, +/− C1 laminectomy based on navigation, dural opening, opening of right tela choroidea and inferior medullary velum, expose part of cyst that reaches surface, map dorsal wall using cranial nerve/dorsal column/motor mapping, enter the cyst and spread tissue with fine forceps, release cyst fluid, map again, remove solid enhancing tumor, expected/planned subtotal resection, dural closure, bone fixation
Complication avoidance	Large bony opening, nerve stimulation for safe entry zone, decompress cyst	Opening foramen magnum, right-sided telovelar opening, ultrasound and navigation to confirm lesion, nerve stimulator to identify safe entry zone, intralesional debulking	IOM to guide entry and resection	Motor, dorsal column, and cranial nerve mapping; IOM; resecting only enhancing portion
Postoperative				
Admission	ICU	ICU	ICU	ICU
Postoperative complications feared	Hydrocephalus, lower cranial nerve dysfunction	Lower cranial nerve dysfunction, motor or sensory deficit, CSF leak	Hemiparesis, infarct	Lower cranial nerve dysfunction, motor or sensory deficit
Follow-up testing	CT/CTA within 24 hours after surgery ENT evaluation within 24 hours after surgery MRI within 72 hours of surgery	MRI within 48 hours after surgery Swallow evaluation	MRI within 48 hours after surgery	MRI within 48 hours after surgery
Follow-up visits	10–12 days after surgery	14–21 days after surgery	14 days after surgery	4 weeks after surgery
Adjuvant therapies recommended				
Diffuse astrocytoma (IDH mutant, retain 1p19q)	STR–radiation/ temozolomide GTR–temozolomide	STR–observation GTR–observation	STR–observation GTR–observation	STR–radiation/ temozolomide GTR–radiation/ temozolomide

	Victor Garcia-Navarro, MD, Tec de Monterrey Institute, Campus Guadalajara, Mexico	George I. Jallo, MD, Johns Hopkins All Children's Hospital, St. Petersburg, FL, United States	Maciej S. Lesniak, MD, Northwestern University, Chicago, IL, United States	Andreas Raabe, MD, University Hospital at Inselspital, Bern, Switzerland
Oligodendroglioma (IDH mutant, 1p19q LOH)	STR–radiation/PCV (if available) or temozolomide GTR–observation	STR–observation GTR–observation	STR–chemotherapy GTR–chemotherapy	STR–PCV GTR–not possible
Anaplastic astrocytoma (IDH wild type)	STR–radiation/ temozolomide GTR–radiation/ temozolomide	STR–radiation/ temozolomide GTR–radiation/ temozolomide	STR–radiation/ temozolomide GTR–radiation/ temozolomide	STR–radiation/ temozolomide GTR–radiation/ temozolomide

BAERs, brainstem auditory evoked responses; *CSF*, cerebrospinal fluid; *CST*, corticospinal tract; *CT*, computed tomography; *CTA*, computed tomography angiography; *DTI*, diffusion tensor imaging; *EMG*, electromyography; *ENT*, ear, nose, and throat; *GTR*, gross total resection; *ICU*, intensive care unit; *IOM*, intraoperative monitoring; *LOH*, loss of heterozygosity; *MEP*, motor evoked potentials; *MR*, magnetic resonance; *MRI*, magnetic resonance imaging; *MRS*, magnetic resonance spectroscopy; *PCA*, posterior cerebral artery; *PCV*, procarbazine, lomustine, vincristine; *PICA*, posterior inferior cerebellar artery; *SSEP*, somatosensory evoked potentials; *STR*, subtotal resection; *VHL*, von Hippel-Lindau.

Differential diagnosis and actual diagnosis

- Low-grade glioma (pilocytic astrocytoma, astrocytoma, oligodendroglioma)
- High-grade glioma
- Demyelinating disease (i.e., multiple sclerosis)

Important anatomic and preoperative considerations

The medulla and bulbar regions have posterior, anterior, and lateral faces.[3] The posterior face of the medulla can be divided into superior and inferior halves, in which the superior posterior surface corresponds to the inferior half of the floor of the fourth ventricle, and the inferior half takes on the morphological features of the spinal medulla.[3] The delineation between the superior and inferior halves is the imaginary line that is projected posteriorly from the bulbar-protuberantial sulcus along the anterior face of the medulla.[3] Lateral to the floor of the fourth ventricle is the inferior cerebellar peduncles (ICPs).[3] The inferior half of the bulbar region is divided in the midline by the posterior medial sulcus, which extends upward ending in the obex.[3] On each side of the posterior medial sulcus lies the gracile fasciculus medially and the cuneate fasciculus laterally, which themselves are separated by the intermediate sulcus that continues toward the spinal medulla as the posterior intermediate sulcus. On the anterior face of the bulbar region is the anterior sulcus that is interrupted by the pyramidal decussations.[3] The bulbar pyramids are comprised of corticospinal tracts (behind which are the medial lemniscus and olivary-olivary fibers) and reside on both sides of the sulcus, and superior to the bulbar pyramids is the origin of CN VI and lateral are the bulbar olives.[3] Over the bulbar olives lies the supraolivary fossa, where CN VII to VIII run.[3] The lateral face of the medullary bulbar region is comprised mainly of the bulbar olive.[3] Anterior to the bulbar olive is the preolivary sulcus that lies between the bulbar pyramid and bulbar olive and is the origin of CN XII, whereas posterior to the bulbar olive is the retro-olivary sulcus where the CN IX, X, and XI nerves run.[3] The transverse olive-olivary

fibers cross the medial sulcus and follow a dorsal direction to enter the cerebellum through the ICP.[3] The dorsolateral sulcus lies behind the retro-olivary sulcus and continues downward with the posterior collateral sulcus of the medulla.[3] The nucleus ambiguous lies dorsal to the olive.[3] The roots of CN IX, X, and XI run laterally to the nucleus ambiguous and pass through the spinal nucleus of the trigeminal nerve and the spinal trigeminal tract.[3]

Approaches to this lesion

There are generally three different approaches for lesions at the medullary bulb: anterior, lateral, and posterior. The anterior face can be exposed by a transclival approach through an endoscopic endonasal approach, in which it provides adequate access to lesions located in the anterior midline, and the medial sulcus can be used to access lesions in the midline and anterior half of the bulb. A lateral or, more specifically, an antero- and dorsolateral approach can be achieved with a far lateral approach, which provides access to the ICP. A vertical corticectomy below the cochlear nucleus and posterior to the origin of the lower CNs, which provides access through the inferior olivary nucleus and through the post-olivary sulcus, can be used to access the ICP. The posterior approach to the superior half of the bulb, as well as the dorsal aspect of the pons, is done through a telovelar approach (as described in Chapter 13). The safe entry zone through the posterior aspect of the medulla is through the posterior medial sulcus, which gives access to lesions on the posterior half of the medulla near the midline. For more dorsolateral lesions, the intermediate sulcus and the posterior collateral sulcus can also be used.

What was actually done

The patient was taken to surgery for a midline suboccipital craniotomy with right far lateral transcondylar extension for a telovelar approach for medullary glioma resection with general anesthesia. The patient was induced and intubated per routine. Intraoperative monitoring was used to monitor somatosensory evoked potentials, as well as CN V, VII, IX, X, XI, and XII. The head was fixed in neutral position with two pins centered over the left external auditory meatus and one pin over the right external auditory meatus. The patient was then placed prone onto chest rolls with the neck flexed and reduced. A midline incision was planned that spanned from just above the inion to the C2 spinous process. The patient was draped in the usual standard fashion and given dexamethasone and cefazolin. A midline incision was made, and dissection took place in the avascular plane between the suboccipital muscles. The skin and muscles were retracted with a cerebellar retractor, and the C1 spinous process and occipital bone with foramen magnum were identified. A suboccipital craniotomy was made below the transverse sinus and incorporated the foramen magnum, and a right C1 laminectomy was done to facilitate dural opening. The dura was then opened in a semicircular shape with the base of the concavity at the level of the foramen magnum and tacked up to the surrounding muscles. The arachnoid between the tonsils and the cerebellar hemispheres were opened with sharp dissection, making sure to identify and protect the posterior inferior cerebellar arteries. The right cerebellar tonsil was retracted laterally with dynamic retraction without fixed retractors to expose the tela choroidea and inferior medullary velum on the right side. The tela choroidea was opened on the right side to expose the superior aspect of the medulla, whereas the inferior medullary velum was left intact. The dorsal aspect of the lesion was stimulated with a bipolar electrode looking for response from CN IX to XII. The intermediate sulcus was identified, and a small corticectomy was made over the sulcus. The lesion was entered, and the cystic component was drained. The tumor continued to be debulked, but the patient had intermittent episodes of hypertension and tachycardia. As expected, there was a slight decline in the contralateral somatosensory evoked potential. At this point, the tumor resection was stopped. The dura, bone, and skin were closed in standard fashion.

The patient awoke at their neurologic baseline with intact speech, full strength bilaterally, and intact CNs, and was taken to the intensive care unit for recovery. A magnetic resonance imaging (MRI) scan was done within 48 hours after surgery and showed expected subtotal resection with residual anteriorly in the tumor cavity (Fig. 14.2). The patient participated with physical and occupational therapy

and was discharged to home on postoperative day 3 with an intact neurologic examination, including proprioception. The patient was prescribed dexamethasone that was tapered to off over 10 days after surgery. The patient was seen at 2 weeks postoperatively for suture removal and remained neurologically intact with improved balance. Pathology was a World Health Organization grade I pilocytic astrocytoma. The lesion was observed with serial MRI examinations at 3 months, followed by 6-month intervals, and has been without recurrence for 12 months. The patient returned to work at 6 weeks postoperatively and remains without neurologic deficits with improved balance.

Commonalities among the experts

For this lesion, the majority of surgeons favored having vascular imaging to better characterize the lesion. A midline suboccipital combined with a telovelar approach was used by half of the surgeons, whereas the other half favored a right suboccipital retrosigmoid with a lateral medullary approach to the lesion. The majority of surgeons also opted to supplement their surgery with brainstem mapping. The general goal was to achieve diagnosis and resect only the enhancing nodule. Most surgeons were cognizant of the cerebellar tonsils, posterior inferior cerebellar arteries, CNs, and floor of the fourth ventricle, in which the most feared complication was lower cranial neuropathy. Surgery was generally pursued with surgical navigation, surgical microscope, and intraoperative monitoring, with perioperative steroids. The key surgical technique was to open the foramen magnum, brainstem mapping to guide entry and resection, intralesional debulking, and focusing on resecting only the enhancing nodule. Following surgery, all patients were admitted to the intensive care unit, and MRIs were typically obtained within 48 hours after surgery to assess extent of resection and potential surgical complications. If the diagnosis was a diffuse astrocytoma, half of the surgeons favored observation, and the other half elected for radiation and/or temozolomide whether gross or subtotal resection was achieved. If the diagnosis was an oligodendroglioma, observation was chosen if gross total resection was achieved, whereas half of the surgeons chose observation, and the other half chose

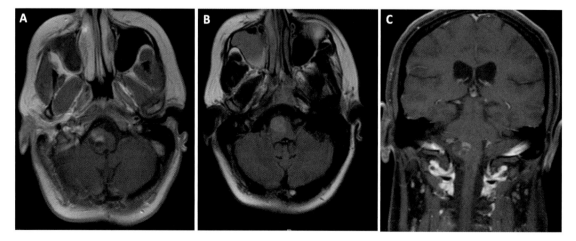

Figure 14.2 Postoperative magnetic resonance imaging. (A) T1 axial image with gadolinium contrast; **(B)** T2 axial fluid attenuation inversion recovery image; **(C)** T1 coronal image with gadolinium contrast magnetic resonance imaging scan demonstrating subtotal resection of the medullary brainstem lesion.

radiation and/or chemotherapy for subtotal resection. If the diagnosis was an anaplastic astrocytoma, radiation and temozolomide were chosen by all surgeons.

SUMMARY OF QUALITY OF EVIDENCE TO GUIDE SPECIFIC INTERVENTIONS FOR THIS CASE

- Surgery as opposed to biopsy or observation for brainstem low-grade gliomas—Class III.
- Monitoring and brainstem mapping for brainstem surgery—Class III.

REFERENCES

1. Cavalheiro S, Yagmurlu K, da Costa MD, et al. Surgical approaches for brainstem tumors in pediatric patients. *Childs Nerv Syst.* 2015;31:1815–1840.
2. Jallo GI, Shiminski-Maher T, Velazquez L, Abbott R, Wisoff J, Epstein F. Recovery of lower cranial nerve function after surgery for medullary brainstem tumors. *Neurosurgery.* 2005;56:74–77; discussion 78.
3. Ribas EC. Yagmurlu K, de Oliveira E, Ribas GC, Rhoton A Jr. Microsurgical anatomy of the central core of the brain. *J Neurosurg.* 2018;129:752–769.

15

Right frontal high-grade glioma

Case reviewed by Chetan Bettegowda, Orin Bloch, Guilherme C. Ribas, Walter Stummer

Introduction

The factors associated with worse outcomes for patients with high-grade gliomas include older patients, poorer neurologic function, tumors in close proximity to the subventricular zone, and decreasing extent of resection.[1–8] In several studies, increasing extent of resection is associated with prolonged survival and delayed recurrence; however, the development of neurologic deficits reverses the benefits of extent of resection.[2,4,6–9] In general, lesions in the right frontal lobe are amenable to extensive resection, as they are more remote from eloquent brain regions.[2] In this chapter, we present a case of a right frontal likely high-grade glioma.

Example case

Chief complaint: seizures

History of present illness

A 73-year-old, right-handed woman with a history of aneurysmal subarachnoid hemorrhage s/p coil embolization presented with seizures. She was with her family when she developed acute onset of left twisting of her body, left-sided head turn, and unresponsiveness. She was brought to the emergency room, where imaging revealed a brain lesion (Fig. 15.1).

Medications: None.

Allergies: No known drug allergies.

Past medical and surgical history: right paraophthalmic aneurysm coil 7 years prior.

Family history: No history of intracranial malignancies.

Social history: Retired school teacher, remote smoking history, occasional alcohol.

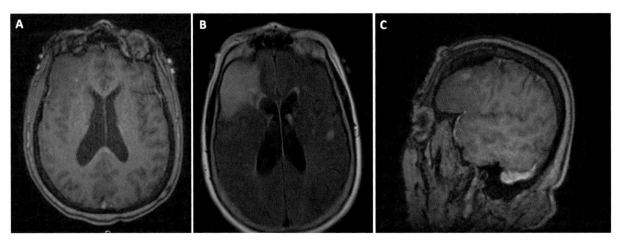

Fig. 15.1 Preoperative magnetic resonance imaging. (A) T1 axial image with gadolinium contrast; **(B)** T2 axial fluid attenuation inversion recovery image; **(C)** T1 sagittal image with gadolinium contrast magnetic resonance imaging scan demonstrating a right frontal glioma with small areas of enhancement that involves the right middle and inferior frontal gyri.

Physical examination: Awake, alert, oriented to person, place, and time; Cranial nerves II to XII intact; No drift, moves all extremities with full strength.

Imaging: Chest/abdomen/pelvis computed tomography negative for primary malignancy.

	Chetan Bettegowda, MD, PhD, Johns Hopkins University, Baltimore, MD, United States	Orin Bloch, MD, University of California-Davis, Sacramento, CA, United States	Guilherme C. Ribas, MD, PhD, Hospital Israelita Albert Einstein, São Paulo, Brazil	Walter Stummer, MD, PhD, University of Munster, Munster, NRW, Germany
Preoperative				
Additional tests requested	CT angiogram MRS	MRS Neurooncology evaluation	MRS MR perfusion	FET PET fMRI
Surgical approach selected	Right frontal craniotomy	Right pterional craniotomy with asleep cortical and subcortical motor mapping	Right frontal temporal craniotomy	Right frontal craniotomy with 5-ALA and asleep cortical and subcortical motor mapping
Anatomic corridor	Right frontal	Right frontal	Right frontal	Right frontal SFG, MFG, STG
Goal of surgery	Gross total resection	Attempted supratotal resection	Maximal resection	Maximal safe resection, biopsy fluorescent areas for representative histology
Perioperative				
Positioning	Right supine	Right supine left head rotation	Right supine with left head rotation	Right supine left 60-degree head rotation
Surgical equipment	Surgical navigation IOM (SSEP, EEG) Surgical microscope	Surgical navigation IOM (MEP) Ultrasonic aspirator	Surgical navigation Ultrasound Ultrasonic aspirator	Surgical navigation IOM (MEP) Ultrasound Surgical microscope with 5-ALA Ultrasonic aspirator
Medications	Steroids Antiepileptics Mannitol	Steroids Antiepileptics Mannitol	Antiepileptics	Steroids
Anatomic considerations	Frontal sinus, aneurysm	Primary motor cortex (face), SMA, subcortical CST, lateral ventricle, MCA and lenticulostriates	Sylvian fissure, inferior frontal gyrus convolutions	Primary motor cortex
Complications feared with approach chosen	Inadvertent aneurysm injury	Motor deficit, stroke	Typical postoperative complications	Tongue weakness, dysarthria, vascular injury
Intraoperative				
Anesthesia	General	General	General	General
Skin incision	Pterional	Right linear coronal	Pterional	Pterional
Bone opening	Right frontal	Right fronto-temporal	Right fronto-temporal	Right fronto-temporal
Brain exposure	Right frontal	Right fronto-temporal	Right fronto-temporal	Right fronto-temporal

(continued on next page)

	Chetan Bettegowda, MD, PhD, Johns Hopkins University, Baltimore, MD, United States	Orin Bloch, MD, University of California-Davis, Sacramento, CA, United States	Guilherme C. Ribas, MD, PhD, Hospital Israelita Albert Einstein, São Paulo, Brazil	Walter Stummer, MD, PhD, University of Munster, Munster, NRW, Germany
Method of resection	Right frontal craniotomy guided by navigation, C-shaped dural opening, navigation-guided sampling of contrast enhancing areas, resection of FLAIR abnormality, ultrasound to evaluate for extent of resection and need for additional resection	Separate dissection of temporalis muscle, fronto-temporal craniotomy, dural opening, identify boundaries based on navigation, asleep mapping of face and upper extremity to find primary motor cortex, sample tumor in center, perform corticectomy and subcortical dissection beyond tumor margin if possible, subpial resection posteriorly adjacent to primary motor cortex, debulk tumor with ultrasonic aspirator, open into ventricle for anatomic localization, remove tumor en bloc, place EVD at posterior aspect of tumor margin, subgaleal drain	Wide right fronto-temporal craniotomy with large exposure of the frontal lobe especially its antero-lateral basal aspect, drill outer aspect of the sphenoid wing, wide dural opening with exposure of frontal and temporal operculi, anatomic identification of the exposed sulci and gyri especially including inferior frontal and lateral orbital gyri with aid of neuronavigation and ultrasound, open Sylvian fissure especially of stem, dissect tumor from superior and posterior margins, removal of tumor with dissection and suction with aid of ultrasonic aspirator, outer to inner debulking	Tailored craniotomy to lesion boundaries based on navigation, MEP mapping of cortex (<10 mA) and subcortical space (<20 mA) with monopolar stimulator, biopsy hot spots based of FET PET and fluorescence, subpial dissection at Sylvian fissure and SFS with subcortical mapping, resect posterior portion of tumor with constant monopolar subcortical simulation to identify CST, ultrasound and microscope for deep portion of the tumor
Complication avoidance	IOM	IOM, cortical and subcortical mapping, subpial dissection at posterior aspect of tumor, en bloc resection, EVD	Wide bony opening, anatomic landmark identification, outer to inner debulking	Cortical and subcortical mapping, subpial dissection, ultrasound and fluorescence to guide resection

Postoperative

Admission	ICU	ICU	ICU	ICU or intermediate care
Postoperative complications feared	Abulia, motor deficit, CSF leak	Motor deficit, stroke, hydrocephalus	General postoperative complications	Motor deficit including tongue and face
Follow-up testing	MRI within 24 hours after surgery Physical and occupational therapy	MRI within 48 hours after surgery	MRI within 48 hours after surgery	MRI within 48 hours after surgery
Follow-up visits	14 days after surgery	14 days after surgery	2–3 months after surgery	3 months after surgery

Adjuvant therapies recommended

IDH status	Mutant–radiation/temozolomide Wild type–radiation/temozolomide	Mutant–radiation/temozolomide Wild type–radiation/temozolomide	Mutant–radiation/temozolomide Wild type–radiation/temozolomide	Mutant–radiation/temozolomide +/– TTF Wild type–radiation/temozolomide +/– TTF
MGMT status	Methylated–radiation/temozolomide Unmethylated–radiation/temozolomide	Methylated–radiation/temozolomide Unmethylated–radiation/temozolomide	Methylated–radiation/temozolomide Unmethylated–radiation/temozolomide	Methylated–radiation/temozolomide +/– TTF Unmethylated–radiation/temozolomide +/– TTF

5-ALA, 5-aminolevulinic acid; *CSF*, cerebrospinal fluid; *CST*, corticospinal tract; *CT*, computed tomography; *EEG*, electroencephalogram; *EVD*, external ventricular drain; *FET*, fluoro-O-(2) fluoroethyl-l-tyrosine; *ICU*, intensive care unit; *IOM*, intraoperative monitoring; *FLAIR*, fluid attenuation inversion recovery image; *fMRI*, functional magnetic resonance imaging; *MCA*, middle cerebral artery; *MEP*, motor evoked potential; *MFG*, middle frontal gyrus; *MGMT*, O6-methylguanine-DNA methyl-transferase; *MR*, magnetic resonance; *MRI*, magnetic resonance imaging; *MRS*, magnetic resonance spectroscopy; *PET*, positron emission tomography; *SFG*, superior frontal gyrus; *SFS*, superior frontal sulcus; *SMA*, supplementary motor area; *SSEP*, somatosensory evoked potential; *STG*, superior temporal gyrus; *TTF*, tumor treatment fields.

Differential diagnosis

- High-grade glioma
- Low-grade glioma (astrocytoma, oligodendroglioma)
- Demyelinating disease (i.e., multiple sclerosis)
- Lymphoma

Important anatomic considerations

For a full discussion on frontal lobe anatomy see Chapters 1 and 2. The right frontal lobe is often considered a safe site for extensive surgical resection, especially in right-handed patients, because language areas, such as Broca and Wernicke, are thought of as only residing in the left hemisphere.[10,11] However, the right hemisphere can also possess language functions even in right hand–dominant patients, as well as other critical functions, including executive function, memory, and proprioception, among others.[12,13] Therefore it is important to understand and identify the same eloquent locations present in the left frontal lobe as in the right frontal lobe, which can possess critical language and motor functions.[12,13] Based on the description of the frontal lobe in Chapters 1 and 2, this lesion involves the middle and inferior frontal gyrus, in which the inferior frontal gyrus involvement is the pars orbitalis and triangularis. Posterior to the lesion should reside the ventral premotor cortex (speech initiation), and superior should be the supplementary motor area (motor coordination). Deep to the lesion are the superior longitudinal fasciculus (SLF; phonetics) and inferior frontal occipital fasciculus (semantics), and the deepest part of the lesion involves the head of the caudate (articulation and fluency).

Approaches to this lesion

The methods of identifying eloquent cortical and subcortical structures can be divided into direct or indirect methods (Chapter 3, Fig. 3.2), and the primary surgical approaches for right frontal gliomas can be divided into either asleep or awake surgery (Chapter 1, Fig. 1.2).[14–19] The conventional approach for noneloquent, intrinsic tumors is asleep surgery with general anesthesia.[14–19] The definition of eloquence is different for individual surgeons; however, the conventional definition is involvement of the language, motor, and/or somatosensory cortex with or without cortical spinal involvement.[2] However, there are other neurologic functions that can be assessed and tested intraoperatively and include phonetics, semantics, executive function, orientation, proprioception, and visual fields, among others.[14–19] These functions are present in historically noneloquent regions and in both hemispheres, but require awake surgery with brain mapping and intricate testing to identify and avoid.[14–19] Besides brain mapping, there are a variety of imaging modalities that have been used to attempt to identify these eloquent regions, and include functional magnetic resonance imaging (MRI) and diffusion tensor imaging. The difficulties with these modalities are they are prone to false positive and false negatives, are not accurate in tumor infiltrated regions, lack sensitivity with peritumoral edema, and are unable to identify thresholds of resection, among others.[20,21] These limitations can preclude extensive resection with avoidance of iatrogenic deficits.[20,21]

In terms of directionality, the options include anterior and lateral. This lesion comes to the surface at the anterolateral portion of the frontal lobe, and therefore both directions can be incorporated simultaneously. The primary advantage of a solely anterior approach is that the lesion comes to the cortical surface on the anterior side, as well as keeping potentially a nondominant Broca area and the SLF lateral to the surgical approach. A solely lateral approach potentially exposes the nondominant Broca area and the SLF but is less of an issue as long as the trajectory is anterior to these eloquent structures.

What was actually done

The patient underwent a neuropsychological evaluation that showed no deficits. The patient was taken to surgery for a right frontal craniotomy with awake language and motor mapping for resection of the lesion. The patient was intubated with a laryngeal mask airway. The scalp was blocked bilaterally with local anesthetic, and the head was fixed in pins, with two pins straddling the inion and one pin on the left forehead in the midpupillary line. The head was turned 30 degrees to the left. A pterional incision posterior to the lesion that extended from the root of the zygoma to the vertex was planned with the aid of preoperative MRI navigation. The patient was draped in the usual standard fashion and given dexamethasone, levetiracetam, and cefazolin. A myocutaneous flap was made, and the flap was held in place with fishhooks attached to the drapes. A standard pterional craniotomy was done to encompass the lesion plus one gyrus in each dimension. Ultrasound and surgical navigation were used to confirm lesion boundaries, and the boundaries were designated with letter tags once the dura was opened. The dura was anesthetized with local anesthetics between the leaflets adjacent to the middle meningeal vessels. The patient was awakened, and the dura was opened once the patient followed commands consistently. Strip electrodes were placed in the subdural space for after discharge monitoring. The cortex was stimulated with an Ojemann stimulator (Integra, Princeton, NJ) starting at 2 mA while the patient underwent a battery of motor tests involving the left face, arm, and leg concurrently with picture naming and counting. The patient had speech motor arrest at 4 mA near the ventral premotor area with number counting, and the rest of the cortical and subcortical mapping took place at 4 mA. Positive mapping sites were designated with number tags. Negative mapping occurred over the tumor and the cortical boundaries that were identified were the ventral premotor (speech arrest) and motor cortex posteriorly (decreased strength), as well as the supplementary motor cortex medially. The subcortical boundaries that were identified were the SLF (phonetic paraphasias) deep and medial to the lesion, and the head of the caudate (speech perseveration). Resection was limited over the head of the caudate because of speech perseveration. Preliminary diagnosis was infiltrating glioma. Once the resection was complete, the patient was put back to sleep with deep sedation without a laryngeal mask airway. The dura, bone, and skin were closed in standard fashion.

The patient awoke at their neurologic baseline with intact speech and full strength bilaterally and was taken to the intensive care unit for recovery. An MRI scan was done within 48 hours that showed near total resection of the lesion with expected residual near the caudate head

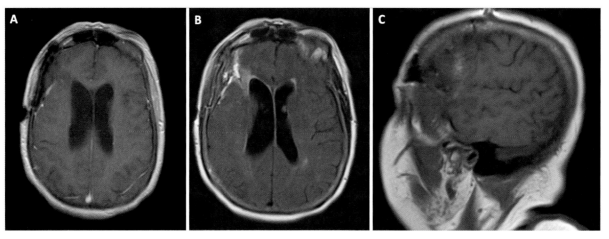

Fig. 15.2 **Postoperative magnetic resonance imaging. (A)** T1 axial with gadolinium contrast; **(B)** T2 axial fluid attenuation inversion recovery image; **(C)** T1 sagittal image with gadolinium contrast magnetic resonance imaging scan demonstrating near total resection of the lesion with small residual at the caudate head.

(Fig. 15.2). The patient participated with physical and occupational therapy and was discharged to home on post-operative day 2. The patient was discharged on 3 months of levetiracetam, and the dexamethasone was tapered to off over 5 days. The patient was seen at 2 weeks postoperatively for staple removal. Pathology was a World Health Organization grade III anaplastic astrocytoma (IDH wild type, 1p/19q wild type). The patient underwent concurrent temozolomide and radiation therapy for 6 weeks followed by six adjuvant cycles. The lesion was observed with serial MRI examinations at 3 months, followed by 6-month intervals, and has been without recurrence for 18 months. The patient had a repeat neuropsychological evaluation at 3 months postoperatively that showed no change from preoperative evaluation. The patient returned to work 4 weeks postoperatively and remains without neurologic deficits.

Commonalities among the experts

The majority of the surgeons preferred to obtain magnetic resonance spectroscopy for lesion characterization prior to surgery. The majority of the surgeons elected to perform the surgery with cortical and subcortical mapping, in which half chose to perform cortical and subcortical mapping with general anesthesia. The general goal was typically to achieve maximal resection, in which one surgeon aimed for supratotal resection and one based it on fluorescence. Most surgeons were cognizant of the primary motor cortex at the posterior aspect of the lesion. The most feared complication was motor deficit. Surgery was pursued with surgical navigation, intraoperative monitoring (motor evoked potential), ultrasonic aspirator, and surgical microscope, with perioperative steroids and antiepileptics. The majority of surgeons favored a large craniotomy, navigation-guided resection, and subpial resection to avoid iatrogenic injuries. Following surgery, patients were admitted to the intensive care unit, and MRIs were obtained within 48 hours after surgery. For a diagnosis of a high-grade glioma, regardless of O6-methylguanine-DNA methyl-transferase and IDH status, radiation and temozolomide were selected by all surgeons, in which one considered the use of tumor treatment fields.

SUMMARY OF QUALITY OF EVIDENCE TO GUIDE SPECIFIC INTERVENTIONS FOR THIS CASE

- Surgery as opposed to biopsy or observation for high-grade gliomas—Class II-1.
- Increasing extent of resection associated with improved outcomes for high-grade gliomas—Class II-2.
- Awake mapping versus asleep surgery for noneloquent gliomas—Class II-3.
- Neuropsychological testing for gliomas—Class III.

REFERENCES

1. Chaichana K, Parker S, Olivi A, Quinones-Hinojosa A. A proposed classification system that projects outcomes based on preoperative variables for adult patients with glioblastoma multiforme. *J Neurosurg.* 2010;112:997–1004.
2. Chaichana KL, Cabrera-Aldana EE, Jusue-Torres I, et al. When gross total resection of a glioblastoma is possible, how much resection should be achieved. *World Neurosurg.* 2014;82:e257–e265.
3. Chaichana KL, Garzon-Muvdi T, Parker S, et al. Supratentorial glioblastoma multiforme: the role of surgical resection versus biopsy among older patients. *Ann Surg Oncol.* 2011;18:239–245.
4. Chaichana KL, Jusue-Torres I, Navarro-Ramirez R, et al. Establishing percent resection and residual volume thresholds affecting survival and recurrence for patients with newly diagnosed intracranial glioblastoma. *Neuro Oncol.* 2014;16:113–122.
5. Chaichana KL, McGirt MJ, Frazier J, Attenello F, Guerrero-Cazares H, Quinones-Hinojosa A. Relationship of glioblastoma multiforme to the lateral ventricles predicts survival following tumor resection. *J Neurooncol.* 2008;89:219–224.
6. McGirt MJ, Chaichana KL, Attenello FJ, et al. Extent of surgical resection is independently associated with survival in patients with hemispheric infiltrating low-grade gliomas. *Neurosurgery.* 2008;63:700–707; author reply 707–708.
7. McGirt MJ, Chaichana KL, Gathinji M, et al. Independent association of extent of resection with survival in patients with malignant brain astrocytoma. *J Neurosurg.* 2009;110:156–162.
8. McGirt MJ, Mukherjee D, Chaichana KL, Than KD, Weingart JD, Quinones-Hinojosa A. Association of surgically acquired motor and language deficits on overall survival after resection of glioblastoma multiforme. *Neurosurgery.* 2009;65:463–469; discussion 469–470.
9. Rahman M, Abbatematteo J, De Leo EK, et al. The effects of new or worsened postoperative neurological deifcts on survival of patients with glioblastoma. *J Neurosurg.* 2017;127:123–131.

10. Rhoton AL Jr. The cerebrum. Anatomy. *Neurosurgery.* 2007;61:37–118; discussion 118–119.
11. Fernandez-Miranda JC, Rhoton AL Jr., Alvarez-Linera J, Kakizawa Y, Choi C, de Oliveira EP. Three-dimensional microsurgical and tractographic anatomy of the white matter of the human brain. *Neurosurgery.* 2008;62:989–1026; discussion 1026–1028.
12. Duffau H, Mandonnet E. The "onco-functional balance" in surgery for diffuse low-grade glioma: integrating the extent of resection with quality of life. *Acta Neurochir (Wien).* 2013;155:951–957.
13. Vilasboas T, Herbet G, Duffau H. Challenging the myth of right nondominant hemisphere: lessons from corticosubcortical stimulation mapping in awake surgery and surgical implications. *World Neurosurg.* 2017;103:449–456.
14. Duffau H. The reliability of asleep-awake-asleep protocol for intraoperative functional mapping and cognitive monitoring in glioma surgery. *Acta Neurochir (Wien).* 2013;155:1803–1804.
15. Eseonu CI, Eguia F, Garcia O, Kaplan PW, Quinones-Hinojosa A. Comparative analysis of monotherapy versus duotherapy antiseizure drug management for postoperative seizure control in patients undergoing an awake craniotomy. *J Neurosurg.* 2018;128:1661–1667.
16. Eseonu CI, Eguia F, ReFaey K, et al. Comparative volumetric analysis of the extent of resection of molecularly and histologically distinct low grade gliomas and its role on survival. *J Neurooncol.* 2017;134:65–74.
17. Eseonu CI, Rincon-Torroella J, ReFaey K, et al. Awake craniotomy vs craniotomy under general anesthesia for perirolandic gliomas: evaluating perioperative complications and extent of resection. *Neurosurgery.* 2017;81:481–489.
18. Bertani G, Fava E, Casaceli G, et al. Intraoperative mapping and monitoring of brain functions for the resection of low-grade gliomas: technical considerations. *Neurosurg Focus.* 2009;27:E4.
19. Nossek E, Korn A, Shahar T, et al. Intraoperative mapping and monitoring of the corticospinal tracts with neurophysiological assessment and 3-dimensional ultrasonography-based navigation. Clinical article. *J Neurosurg.* 2011;114:738–746.
20. Duffau H. The dangers of magnetic resonance imaging diffusion tensor tractography in brain surgery. *World Neurosurg.* 2014;81:56–58.
21. Sternberg EJ, Lipton ML, Burns J. Utility of diffusion tensor imaging in evaluation of the peritumoral region in patients with primary and metastatic brain tumors. *AJNR Am J Neuroradiol.* 2014;35:439–444.

16

Left frontal high-grade glioma

Case reviewed by Miguel A. Arraez, Juan A. Barcia, Linda M. Liau, Ian F. Parney

Introduction

The primary modifiable risk factor for patients with high-grade gliomas is extent of resection.[1–7] For patients with primary glioblastoma, the maximum residual volume threshold is 5 cm³, in which patients with higher residual volume had a median survival of 11.6 months as compared with 15.3 months for patients with lesser residual volume.[3] In regard to percent resection, patients with less than 70% resection had a median survival of 10.5 months as compared with 14.4 months for patients with more than 70% resection.[3] In patients in which gross total resection can be achieved, at least 95% resection needs to be achieved.[1] These studies are based on resection of the contrast-enhancing regions.[1–7] For tumors involving the frontal pole, these lesions are typically more amenable to extensive resection.[1] In this chapter, we present a case of a left frontal pole high-grade glioma.

Example case

Chief complaint: headaches
History of present illness
A 28-year-old, right-handed man with no significant past medical history presented with headaches. He complained of progressive headaches not responsive to over-the-counter pain medications for 3 weeks, and most recently developed nausea and vomiting. He was taken to the emergency room where imaging revealed a brain lesion (Fig. 16.1).
Medications: Aspirin, acetaminophen.
Allergies: No known drug allergies.
Past medical and surgical history: None.
Family history: No history of intracranial malignancies.
Social history: Waiter, no smoking or alcohol.
Physical examination: Awake, alert, oriented to person, place, and time; Cranial nerves II to XII intact; No drift, moves all extremities with full strength.
Imaging: Chest / abdomen / pelvis computed tomography negative for primary malignancy.

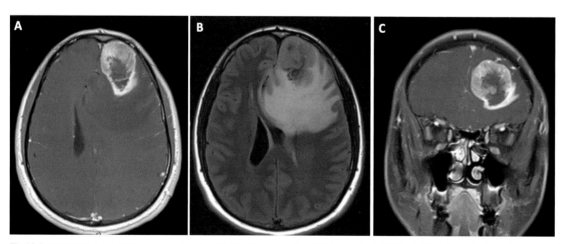

Fig 16.1 Preoperative magnetic resonance imaging. (A) T1 axial image with gadolinium contrast; **(B)** T2 axial fluid attenuation inversion recovery image; **(C)** T1 coronal image with gadolinium contrast magnetic resonance imaging scan demonstrating a left frontal heterogeneously enhancing lesion that involves the left anterior superior and middle frontal gyri.

	Miguel A. Arraez, MD, PhD, Carlos Haya University Hospital, Malaga, Spain	Juan A. Barcia, MD, PhD, Hospital Clínico San Carlos, Complutense University, Madrid, Spain	Linda M. Liau, MD, PhD, University of California-Los Angeles, Los Angeles, CA, United States	Ian F. Parney, MD, PhD, Mayo Clinic, Rochester, MN, United States
Preoperative				
Additional tests requested	Neuropsychological	DTI fMRI Neuropsychological assessment	DTI fMRI Neuropsychological assessment and language evaluation	None
Surgical approach selected	Left frontal craniotomy	Left frontal craniotomy with 5-ALA	Left frontal craniotomy with awake language and motor mapping	Left frontal craniotomy with possible fluorescence
Anatomic corridor	Left frontal	Left frontal	Left SFG and MFG and interhemispheric	Left frontal
Goal of surgery	Maximal resection of contrast enhancing lesion	Gross total removal of 5-ALA strong and weak fluorescent tissue	Maximal safe resection of contrast enhancing and FLAIR	Gross total resection of contrast enhancing (second look surgery for FLAIR if IDH mutant)
Perioperative				
Positioning	Supine neutral	Supine neutral	Left supine with slight right rotation	Supine neutral
Surgical equipment	Surgical navigation Surgical microscope with 5-ALA Ultrasonic aspirator Intraoperative MRI if available	Surgical navigation Surgical microscope with 5-ALA Ultrasonic aspirator	Surgical navigation Surgical microscope IOM (MEP/SSEP/ECoG) Brain stimulator	Surgical navigation Ultrasonic aspirator Surgical microscope +/− fluorescence
Medications	Steroids Antiepileptics	Steroids Antiepileptics	Steroids Antiepileptics	Mannitol Steroids Antiepileptics
Anatomic considerations	Frontal lobe sulci and gyri	Sagittal suture, superior sagittal sinus, falx, ACA, frontopolar arteries, anterior parasagittal draining veins	Broca area inferolaterally, ACA medially, SMA and motor cortex/CST posteriorly	Frontal sinus, ACA medially, Broca area laterally
Complications feared with approach chosen	Motor deficit, aphasia	Left frontal lobe syndrome	Expressive aphasia, motor deficit	Expressive aphasia, motor deficit
Intraoperative				
Anesthesia	General	General	Asleep-awake-asleep	General
Skin incision	Wide fronto-parietal-temporal	Pterional	Pterional	Pterional or bicoronal
Bone opening	Left frontal	Left frontal	Left frontal	Left frontal
Brain exposure	Left frontal	Left frontal	Left frontal	Left frontal

(continued on next page)

	Miguel A. Arraez, MD, PhD, Carlos Haya University Hospital, Malaga, Spain	Juan A. Barcia, MD, PhD, Hospital Clínico San Carlos, Complutense University, Madrid, Spain	Linda M. Liau, MD, PhD, University of California-Los Angeles, Los Angeles, CA, United States	Ian F. Parney, MD, PhD, Mayo Clinic, Rochester, MN, United States
Method of resection	Left frontal craniotomy, dura opened and reflected toward midline, corticectomy at most superficial aspect of tumor to cortical surface, microsurgical resection with 5-ALA, inspection of cavity with fluorescence, intraoperative MRI to guide further resection if available, subgaleal drain to low suction pressure	Left frontal craniotomy, dural opening, subpial resection of tumor inside SFG and MFG based on 5-ALA fluorescence, resect until no strong or weak fluorescence remains	Left frontal craniotomy, peripheral tack up sutures, U-shaped dural opening with base along sagittal sinus observing for draining veins, motor strip mapping to identify primary motor cortex, awaken patient for language mapping with cortical stimulation to identify the Broca and other eloquent language areas, protect positive mapping sites, dissect around tumor with continuous cortical and subcortical mapping, remove tumor en bloc if possible, use microscope if necessary around ACA and eloquent white matter tracts, put back to sleep for remainder of case, watertight dural closure	Left frontal craniotomy ipsilateral to sagittal sinus based on navigation, dural opening, resection of tumor en bloc under microscopic visualization +/– fluorescence, further resection of any remaining lesion
Complication avoidance	Shortest trajectory	Subpial resection, resection of strong and weak fluorescence	Observe for cortical veins, language and motor mapping, en bloc resection	En bloc resection, possible use of fluorescence
Postoperative				
Admission	ICU	ICU	Floor if no deficits	ICU
Postoperative complications feared	Cognitive dysfunction	CSF leak, left frontal lobe syndrome	SMA syndrome, expressive aphasia	Expressive aphasia, motor deficit
Follow-up testing	MRI within 72 hours after surgery	MRI within 48 hours after surgery	MRI within 24 hours after surgery	MRI within 24 hours after surgery
Follow-up visits	7 days after surgery	7 days after surgery 1 month after surgery	14 days after surgery	3 months after surgery 7 days after surgery with radiation and neurooncology
Adjuvant therapies recommended				
IDH status	Mutant–radiation/ temozolomide Wild type–radiation/ temozolomide	Mutant–radiation/ temozolomide Wild type–radiation/ temozolomide	Mutant–radiation/temozolomide Wild type–radiation/ temozolomide	Mutant–possible second look surgery of FLAIR Wild type–radiation/ temozolomide +/– TTF
MGMT status	Methylated–radiation/ temozolomide Unmethylated–radiation/ temozolomide	Methylated–radiation/ temozolomide Unmethylated– radiation/ temozolomide	Methylated–radiation/ temozolomide Unmethylated–radiation/ temozolomide	Methylated–radiation/ temozolomide +/– TTF Unmethylated– radiation/ temozolomide +/– TTF

5-ALA, 5-aminolevulinic acid; *ACA*, anterior cerebral artery; *CSF*, cerebrospinal fluid; *CST*, corticospinal tracts; *DTI*, diffusion tensor imaging; *ECoG*, electrocorticography; *FLAIR*, fluid attenuation inversion recovery image; *fMRI*, functional magnetic resonance imaging; *ICU*, intensive care unit; *IOM*, intraoperative monitoring; *MEP*, motor evoked potential; *MFG*, middle frontal gyrus; *MGMT*, O6-methylguanine-DNA methyl-transferase; *MRI*, magnetic resonance imaging; *SFG*, superior frontal gyrus; *SMA*, supplementary motor area; *SSEP*, somatosensory evoked potentials; *TTF*, tumor treatment fields.

Differential diagnosis

- High-grade glioma
- Metastatic tumor
- Lymphoma
- Demyelinating disease (i.e., multiple sclerosis)

Important anatomic considerations

Based on the description of the frontal lobe in Chapters 1 and 2, this lesion involves the anterior portion of the superior and middle frontal gyrus. Directly posterior to the lesion is the pre-supplementary area (pre-SMA), and posterior to that is the SMA. Lateral and posterior to the lesion is the ventral premotor cortex and the Broca area within the inferior frontal gyrus. Deep to the lesion is the default mode network (DFN), lateral to the DFN is the frontal aslant tract (FAT), and lateral to that is the superior longitudinal fasciculus (SLF). The DFN plays a role in executive function and attention, the FAT in speech initiation, and the SLF in phonetics. The lesion itself also abuts the superior sagittal sinus.

Approaches to this lesion

The primary methods of identifying eloquent structures can be divided into direct and indirect methods (Chapter 3, Fig. 3.2), and the primary surgical approaches for frontal anterior pole gliomas can be divided into either asleep or awake surgery Chapter 1, Fig. 1.2).[8–13] The conventional approach for non-eloquent, intrinsic tumors is asleep surgery with general anesthesia.[8–13] This lesion, by conventional neuroanatomy, does not appear to involve eloquent function, as the SMA, ventral premotor cortex, and the Broca area are posterior, posterolateral, and posterolateral to the lesion, respectively. Asleep surgery can be supplemented with intraoperative monitoring of motor and somatosensory pathways, but these pathways are posterior to the lesion. Besides asleep surgery with general anesthesia, the surgery can be done awake with brain mapping. The advantage of this method is that pathways including the DFN, FAT, and SMA involvement of the corticospinal, and the language pathways can be mapped and potentially facilitate supratotal resection, as has been described for low grade gliomas.[14] However, recent studies have shown that extensive resection of fluid attenuation inversion recovery does not correspond with improved outcomes for high-grade gliomas.[15]

In terms of directionality, the options include anterior and lateral. The primary advantage of the anterior approach is that the lesion comes to the cortical surface on the anterior side, as well as keeping the Broca area and the SLF lateral to the surgical approach. If the craniotomy of the anterior approach is too low, a breach of the frontal sinus may occur. The lateral approach requires transgression of cortex and subcortical white matter to resect the lesion and also potentially incorporates the Broca area and the SLF. This is less of an issue as long as the trajectory is anterior to these eloquent structures.

What was actually done

The patient was taken to surgery for a left frontal craniotomy with general anesthesia. The patient was induced and intubated by anesthesia per routine. The head was fixed in pins, with two pins straddling the right external auditory meatus in the superior temporal line and one pin posterior to the left external auditory meatus below the superior temporal line. The head was kept neutral and slightly extended to make the lesion perpendicular with the ground. A left pterional incision posterior to the lesion that extended from just below the superior temporal line to the vertex was planned with the aid of preoperative magnetic resonance imaging (MRI) navigation. The patient was draped in the usual standard fashion and given dexamethasone, levetiracetam, and cefazolin. A skin flap was made staying above the temporalis muscle, and the flap was held in place with fishhooks attached to a retractor arm. A left frontal craniotomy that remained just ipsilateral to the sagittal sinus and spanned the lesion and was superior to the frontal sinus was done. Ultrasound and surgical navigation were used to confirm lesion boundaries, and the boundaries were designated with letter tags once the dura was opened. The dura was opened in a semicircular fashion with the base along the sagittal sinus and tacked up with sutures. A corticectomy was done over the anterior portion of the superior frontal gyrus and middle frontal gyrus, and the tumor was removed until white matter was seen on all the edges. The fluid attenuation inversion recovery or edematous white matter was not resected. The dura, bone, and skin were closed in standard fashion.

The patient awoke at their neurologic baseline with intact speech and full strength bilaterally, and was taken to the intensive care unit for recovery. An MRI scan was done within 48 hours that showed gross total resection of the enhancing portion of the lesion (Fig. 16.2). The patient participated with physical and occupational therapy and was discharged to home on postoperative day 2. The patient was discharged on 3 months of levetiracetam, and the dexamethasone was tapered to off over 10 days. The patient was seen at 2 weeks postoperatively for staple removal. Pathology was a World Health Organization grade IV glioblastoma (IDH wild type, 1p/19q wild type, O6-methylguanine-DNA methyl-transferase unmethylated). The patient returned to work 4 weeks postoperatively and underwent concurrent temozolomide and radiation therapy for 6 weeks followed by six adjuvant cycles. The lesion was observed with serial MRI examinations at 3 months but had recurrence at 9 months and underwent repeat resection. The patient died 18 months after the initial surgery.

Commonalities among the experts

The majority of the surgeons preferred to obtain functional MRI and diffusion tensor imaging prior to surgery to identify functional cortical areas and white matter tracts, as well as neuropsychiatry evaluation to obtain baseline neurocognitive function. All surgeons performed a left frontal craniotomy for the lesion, in which two supplemented their approach with awake language and motor mapping, and three used adjuvant modalities to facilitate extensive resection (fluorescence in two and intraoperative MRI in one). The general goal was typically to achieve gross total resection of enhancing or fluorescing portions. Most surgeons were cognizant of the Broca area inferolaterally to the lesion, as well as anterior cerebral artery vessels medially. The most feared complication was language and motor deficits with injury to the language

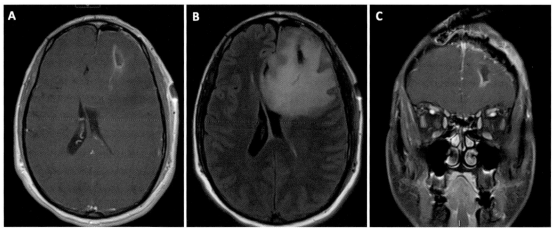

Fig. 16.2 Postoperative magnetic resonance imaging. (A) T1 axial image with gadolinium contrast; **(B)** T2 axial fluid attenuation inversion recovery image; **(C)** T1 coronal image with gadolinium contrast magnetic resonance imaging scan demonstrating gross total resection of the enhancing portion of the tumor.

areas and the motor cortex, respectively. Surgery was pursued with surgical navigation, surgical microscope, and ultrasonic aspirator with perioperative steroids and antiepileptics. The majority of surgeons favored en bloc resection, resection of fluorescence, subpial dissection, and preservation of veins to avoid iatrogenic injuries. Following surgery, patients were typically admitted to the intensive care unit (one to the floor), and MRIs were obtained within 72 hours after surgery. For a diagnosis of a high-grade glioma, regardless of O6-methylguanine-DNA methyl-transferase and IDH status, radiation and temozolomide were selected by all surgeons, in which one considered the use of tumor treatment fields.

SUMMARY OF QUALITY OF EVIDENCE TO GUIDE SPECIFIC INTERVENTIONS FOR THIS CASE

- Surgery as opposed to biopsy or observation for high-grade gliomas—Class II-1.
- Increasing extent of resection associated with improved outcomes for high-grade gliomas—Class II-2.
- Repeat resection for recurrent high-grade glioma—Class II-2.
- Supratotal resection of high-grade gliomas—Class III.

REFERENCES

1. Chaichana KL, Cabrera-Aldana EE, Jusue-Torres I, et al. When gross total resection of a glioblastoma is possible, how much resection should be achieved? *World Neurosurg.* 2014;82:e257–e265.
2. Chaichana KL, Garzon-Muvdi T, Parker S, et al. Supratentorial glioblastoma multiforme: the role of surgical resection versus biopsy among older patients. *Ann Surg Oncol.* 2011;18:239–245.
3. Chaichana KL, Jusue-Torres I, Navarro-Ramirez R, et al. Establishing percent resection and residual volume thresholds

affecting survival and recurrence for patients with newly diagnosed intracranial glioblastoma. *Neuro Oncol.* 2014;16:113–122.
4. Chaichana KL, Parker SL, Mukherjee D, Cheng JS, Gokaslan ZL, McGirt MJ. Assessment of the extent of surgical resection as a predictor of survival in patients with primary osseous spinal neoplasms. *Clin Neurosurg.* 2011;58:117–121.
5. Chaichana KL, Zadnik P, Weingart JD, et al. Multiple resections for patients with glioblastoma: prolonging survival. *J Neurosurg.* 2013;118:812–820.
6. Lacroix M, Abi-Said D, Fourney DR, et al. A multivariate analysis of 416 patients with glioblastoma multiforme: prognosis, extent of resection, and survival. *J Neurosurg.* 2001;95:190–198.
7. Sanai N, Polley MY, McDermott MW, Parsa AT, Berger MS. An extent of resection threshold for newly diagnosed glioblastomas. *J Neurosurg.* 2011;115:3–8.
8. Duffau H. The reliability of asleep-awake-asleep protocol for intraoperative functional mapping and cognitive monitoring in glioma surgery. *Acta Neurochir (Wien).* 2013;155:1803–1804.
9. Eseonu CI, Eguia F, Garcia O, Kaplan PW, Quinones-Hinojosa A. Comparative analysis of monotherapy versus duotherapy antiseizure drug management for postoperative seizure control in patients undergoing an awake craniotomy. *J Neurosurg.* 2018;128:1661–1667.
10. Eseonu CI, Eguia F, ReFaey K, et al. Comparative volumetric analysis of the extent of resection of molecularly and histologically distinct low grade gliomas and its role on survival. *J Neurooncol.* 2017;134:65–74.
11. Eseonu CI, Rincon-Torroella J, ReFaey K, et al. Awake craniotomy vs craniotomy under general anesthesia for perirolandic gliomas: evaluating perioperative complications and extent of resection. *Neurosurgery.* 2017;81:481–489.
12. Bertani G, Fava E, Casaceli G, et al. Intraoperative mapping and monitoring of brain functions for the resection of low-grade gliomas: technical considerations. *Neurosurg Focus.* 2009;27:E4.
13. Nossek E, Korn A, Shahar T, et al. Intraoperative mapping and monitoring of the corticospinal tracts with neurophysiological assessment and 3-dimensional ultrasonography-based navigation. Clinical article. *J Neurosurg.* 2011;114:738–746.
14. Duffau H. Long-term outcomes after supratotal resection of diffuse low-grade gliomas: a consecutive series with 11-year follow-up. *Acta Neurochir (Wien).* 2016;158:51–58.
15. Mampre D, Ehresman J, Pinilla-Monsalve G, et al. Extending the resection beyond the contrast-enhancement for glioblastoma: feasibility, efficacy, and outcomes. *Br J Neurosurg.* 2018;32:528–535.

17

Right perirolandic high-grade glioma

Case reviewed by Mark Bernstein, Chetan Bettegowda, Randy L. Jensen, Eslam Mohsen Mahmoud Hussein

Introduction

The surgery of brain tumors, namely gliomas, requires a delicate balance between extensive resection and avoidance of neurologic deficits.[1–8] The risk of neurologic deficits is highest in those tumors that involve eloquent motor and/or language cortical and subcortical regions.[9–12] There are a variety of methods for monitoring these pathways, which include passive monitoring, including motor evoked potentials (MEP) and somatosensory evoked potentials (SSEP), as well as direct monitoring, including cortical stimulation.[9–12] These methods are most utilized for lesions involving motor pathways.[9–12] In this chapter, we present a high-grade glioma that is in close proximity and possibly involves the perirolandic region and corticospinal tracts in the nondominant hemisphere.

Example case

Chief complaint: left-sided weakness
History of present illness
A 41-year-old, right-handed man with no significant past medical history presented with progressive left-sided weakness. Over the past 3 weeks, he developed progressive left arm and leg weakness to the point in which he could not button his shirt and was dragging his leg while he was walking. He was seen by his primary care physician who ordered brain imaging that revealed a brain lesion (Fig. 17.1). He was referred for evaluation and management.
Medications: None.
Allergies: No known drug allergies.
Past medical and surgical history: None.
Family history: Father died of glioblastoma within the last couple of months.
Social history: Works as an engineer. No smoking history or alcohol.

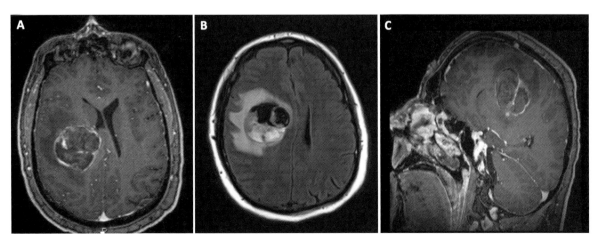

Fig. 17.1 Preoperative magnetic resonance imaging. (A) T1 axial image with gadolinium contrast; **(B)** T2 axial fluid attenuation inversion recovery image; **(C)** T1 sagittal image with gadolinium contrast magnetic resonance imaging scan demonstrating a right frontal and perirolandic heterogeneously enhancing lesion involving the supplementary motor and perirolandic areas, as well as corticospinal tracts.

Physical examination: Awake, alert, oriented to person, place, and time; Cranial nerves II to XII intact; Left drift, left upper extremity 4/5, left lower extremity 4+/5, right upper extremity/right lower extremity 5/5.

Imaging: Chest/abdomen/pelvis computed tomography negative for primary malignancy.

	Mark Bernstein, MD, University of Toronto, Toronto, Canada	Chetan Bettegowda, MD, PhD, Johns Hopkins University, Baltimore, MD, United States	Randy L. Jensen, MD, PhD, University of Utah, Salt Lake City, UT, United States	Eslam Mohsen Mahmoud Hussein, MBBS, MSc, Ain Shams University, Cairo, Egypt
Preoperative				
Additional tests requested	DTI fMRI	DTI	DTI	DTI fMRI Neuropsychological assessment
Surgical approach selected	Right frontal awake craniotomy for tumor for motor and sensory mapping	Right frontal craniotomy with tubular retractor and asleep motor mapping	Right frontal-parietal craniotomy for tumor with asleep cortical mapping and intraoperative MRI	Right posterior frontal or parieto-occipital craniotomy
Anatomic corridor	Right frontal	Right frontal lateral and anterior to motor cortex	Right frontal	Right posterior frontal
Goal of surgery	Maximal safe resection of enhancing portion of the tumor	Gross total resection of enhancing component	Gross total resection of enhancing component	Gross total resection of enhancing component
Perioperative				
Positioning	Right supine with left rotation	Right supine	Right supine 30-degree rotation	Right supine with left rotation
Surgical equipment	Surgical navigation Surgical microscope Brain stimulator	Surgical navigation IOM (MEP, SSEP, EEG) Brain stimulator Surgical microscope Tubular retractors	Surgical navigation Ultrasonic aspirator Brain stimulator IOM (SSEP/MEP/phase reversal) Intraoperative MRI	Surgical navigation Ultrasonic aspirator Surgical microscope
Medications	Steroids	Steroids Antiepileptics Mannitol	Steroids	Steroids Antiepileptics Mannitol Diuretics
Anatomic considerations	Precentral gyrus	Precentral gyrus, SMA, internal capsule	Central sulcus, precentral gyrus	Precentral gyrus
Complications feared with approach chosen	Motor deficit	Motor deficit	Motor deficit	Motor deficit
Intraoperative				
Anesthesia	Asleep	General	General	General
Skin incision	Linear	Linear	Linear/curvilinear	Linear
Bone opening	Right frontal	Right frontal	Right frontal-parietal	Right posterior frontal or parieto-occipital
Brain exposure	Right frontal	Right frontal	Right frontal-parietal	Right posterior frontal or parieto-occipital

	Mark Bernstein, MD, University of Toronto, Toronto, Canada	Chetan Bettegowda, MD, PhD, Johns Hopkins University, Baltimore, MD, United States	Randy L. Jensen, MD, PhD, University of Utah, Salt Lake City, UT, United States	Eslam Mohsen Mahmoud Hussein, MBBS, MSc, Ain Shams University, Cairo, Egypt
Method of resection	Regional field block with local anesthetic, craniotomy based on navigation over lesion, cruciate dural opening, motor and speech mapping with electrocortical stimulation, find pseudoplane between tumor and normal parenchyma, stay 1 cm away from positive mapping sites, periodic confirmation with navigation, close when satisfied with maximal resection	Craniotomy to encompass lesion based on navigation, cruciate dural opening, placement of strip electrode and phase reversal to identify motor cortex, stimulate cortex to confirm absence of motor cortex, small corticectomy over negative motor mapping site, place tubular retractor into hematoma, debulk hematoma to reduce mass effect, debulk remaining tumor with continuous subcortical mapping	Craniotomy based on navigation, dural opening, placement of strip electrode, and phase reversal assessment, identify tumor volume based on navigation, cortical mapping to confirm absence of motor cortex, corticectomy over negative mapping sites, microscopic guided resection with continuous MEP, subcortical mapping as needed for deep portion of tumor, intraoperative MRI when maximal resection anticipated, further resection with recalibrated navigation if necessary	Larger craniotomy to avoid postoperative edema, monitor for increased intracranial pressure based on dural pulsation, cruciate dural opening if not tense, trajectory based on DTI and navigation, small corticectomy over nonfunctional areas, attempt to find a cleavage plane, debulk tumor without violating neural structures, expansile duraplasty if brain swelling, closure with subgaleal drain
Complication avoidance	Awake motor and speech mapping, staying 1 cm away from positive mapping sites	IOM, cortical and subcortical mapping	IOM, cortical and subcortical mapping, intraoperative MRI	DTI, finding cleavage plane around tumor
Postoperative				
Admission	Outpatient	ICU	ICU	ICU
Postop complications feared	Motor deficit	Seizures, motor deficit, hydrocephalus, intraventricular hemorrhage	Motor deficit	Motor deficit, seizure, altered mental status
Follow-up testing	CT within 4 hours after surgery MRI prior to radiation	CT immediately after surgery MRI within 24 hours after surgery Physical and occupational therapy	MRI within 48 hours after surgery	CT with and without contrast within 48 hours after surgery MRI before radiation therapy
Follow-up visits	10–14 days after surgery and follow-up with radiation and neurooncology	14 days after surgery	2–4 weeks with neurooncology 4–6 weeks after surgery	10 days after surgery
Adjuvant therapies recommended				
IDH status	Mutant–radiation/ temozolomide Wild type–radiation/ temozolomide	Mutant–radiation/ temozolomide Wild type–radiation/ temozolomide	Mutant–radiation/ temozolomide Wild type–radiation/ temozolomide	Mutant–whole brain radiation/ temozolomide or bevacizumab Wild type–whole brain radiation therapy, neurooncology evaluation
MGMT status	Methylated–radiation/ temozolomide Unmethylated–radiation/ temozolomide	Methylated–radiation/ temozolomide Unmethylated–radiation/ temozolomide	Methylated–radiation/ temozolomide Unmethylated–radiation/ temozolomide	Methylated–whole brain radiation/ temozolomide or bevacizumab Unmethylated–whole brain radiation therapy, neurooncology evaluation

CST, corticospinal tracts; CT, computed tomography; DTI, diffusion tensor imaging; EEG, electroencephalogram; fMRI, functional magnetic resonance imaging; ICU, intensive care unit; IOM, intraoperative monitoring; MEP, motor evoked potentials; MGMT, O6-methylguanine-DNA methyl-transferase; MRI, magnetic resonance imaging; SMA, supplementary motor area; SSEP, somatosensory evoked potentials.

Differential diagnosis and actual diagnosis

- High-grade glioma
- Metastatic tumors
- Lymphoma
- Low-grade glioma (astrocytoma, oligodendroglioma)
- Demyelinating disease (i.e., multiple sclerosis)

Important anatomic and preoperative considerations

For a full description of the anatomic considerations of the frontal and central lobes, see Chapters 1 and 2 and Chapters 3 and 4, respectively. The central lobe can typically be located by following the superior frontal sulcus posteriorly to where it communicates with the precentral gyrus, but can also be located by the omega shape of the precentral gyrus or the location of the marginal ramus of the cingulate gyrus along the interhemispheric fissure.[13,14] The central sulcus extends from the medial aspect of the interhemispheric region and runs on the lateral surface of the brain from a posterior to anterior direction toward the Sylvian fissure, where it makes contact via the subcentral gyrus that connects the pre- and postcentral gyri.[13,14] At the level of the middle frontal gyrus anterior to the precentral gyrus is the premotor cortex, and at the level of the superior frontal gyrus is the supplementary motor area (SMA).[13,14] The corticospinal tract itself has neurons that originate not only in the primary motor cortex but also premotor, SMA, and somatosensory cortices, and travel through the posterior limb of the internal capsule to enter the cerebral crus within the midbrain before entering the brainstem and terminating on the neurons within the spinal cord.[13,14] This lesion lies below the cortical surface of the SMA and precentral gyrus at the level of the superior frontal gyrus, and involves the corticospinal tracts.

Approaches to this lesion

As discussed in Chapter 1, Fig. 1.2, the approaches to this lesion can be divided into asleep and awake procedures. As discussed in Chapter 3, Fig. 3.2, the methods for identifying eloquent cortical and subcortical structures can be divided into direct and indirect methods. Asleep procedures can be done with or without monitoring, and asleep monitoring can be done with or without mapping. The advantages of asleep procedures are that they are the conventional approach, do not require patient participation, which is especially critical for anxious patients, and decrease surgical time, whereas its disadvantages include lack of real-time neurologic monitoring, lack of sensitivity and specificity in identifying motor pathways, and inability to monitor nonmotor/sensory functions.[9,15] Some of these disadvantages can be decreased with monitoring for motor (MEP) and sensory (SSEP) tracts during the surgery, and can be augmented with asleep brain mapping whereby the cortex and subcortical regions are stimulated to identify electrical activity in distal muscles groups.[9,15] However, these modalities for asleep surgery lack the advantages of awake brain mapping whereby the surgeon has real-time feedback of neurologic function, ability to identify critical thresholds of resection before deficits occur,

and ability to monitor nonmotor/sensory functions, including language.[9–12] The disadvantages of awake brain mapping include necessity of patient cooperation and resulting potential discomfort, critical understanding of cortical and subcortical structures, and potentially increased risk of intraoperative seizures.[9–12]

In terms of trajectory, there are several options with different potential morbidity. The lesion is in the subcortical space, and therefore requires transgression of the cortex and superficial white matter. The lesion therefore can be accessed via a transgyral or transsulcal approach. The transgyral approach involves performing a corticectomy over the gyrus and dissecting through the white matter to enter the lesion. The advantage of this approach is that it does not engage the transsulcal arteries and veins, but the disadvantages include increased working distance and distance of parenchyma involved and engaging projection and association fibers. The transsulcal approach involves opening the sulcus and dissecting through the white matter at the bottom of the sulcus to enter the lesion. The advantages of this approach are that it decreases working distance and distance of parenchyma involved and engages less critical subcortical U-fibers, whereas the disadvantages include potential injury to sulcal vessels. Moreover, this lesion most likely is below the motor and sensory cortex and the proximal portion of the corticospinal tract. An anterior approach could endanger the motor cortex and corresponding motor component of the corticospinal tract, whereas a posterior approach could endanger the sensory cortex and corresponding sensory portion of the corticospinal tract.

What was actually done

The patient declined an awake surgery because of anxiety. The patient was taken to surgery for a right frontal craniotomy with general anesthesia with intraoperative SSEP, MEP, and electroencephalogram with motor mapping. The patient was induced and intubated per routine. The head was pinned, with two pins centered on the inion and one pin over the left forehead in the midpupillary line. A right pterional incision was planned based on preoperative magnetic resonance imaging (MRI) navigation that spanned from just above the root of the zygoma to the vertex and was posterior to the lesion. The patient was draped in the usual standard fashion and given dexamethasone, levetiracetam, and cefazolin. The flap was made and held in place with fishhooks attached to a retractor arm, making sure to stay above the temporalis fascia. A right frontal-parietal craniotomy was done to encompass the lesion, as well as extend at least one gyrus anterior, posterior, and lateral to the lesion. Ultrasound and surgical navigation were used to confirm lesion boundaries, and the boundaries were designated with letter tags once the dura was opened. A strip electrode was placed in the subdural space perpendicular to the central sulcus, and a phase reversal was done to identify the rolandic fissure, which was posterior to the lesion and the precentral gyrus involved the posterior aspect of the lesion. In addition, the cortex was stimulated with an Ojemann stimulator (Integra, Princeton, NJ) over the precentral gyrus to confirm this was the motor cortex with response in the distal muscle groups within the contralateral arm and leg. The exoscope was brought in, and the precentral sulcus was opened sharply

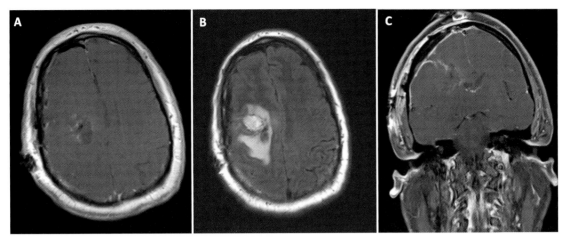

Fig. 17.2 Postoperative magnetic resonance imaging. (A) T1 axial image with gadolinium contrast; **(B)** T2 axial fluid attenuation inversion recovery image; **(C)** T1 coronal image with gadolinium contrast demonstrating gross total resection of the enhancing portion of the tumor.

with microdissection. A 50-mm tubular retractor was placed in the precentral sulcus to dilate the sulcus and provide a protected corridor for access and resection. The lesion was removed piecemeal from internally to externally until white matter was seen on all the edges. The retractor was removed, and no obvious tumor was identified. The ultrasound was also used to confirm extent of resection. Preliminary diagnosis was high-grade glioma. The dura, bone, and skin were closed in standard fashion.

The patient awoke at their neurologic baseline with stable left-sided weakness and was taken to the intensive care unit for recovery. On postoperative day 1, patient's strength improved to nearly full strength in the left lower extremity, but the left upper extremity remained 4/5. Postoperative MRI done within 48 hours after surgery showed gross total resection of the contrast-enhancing portion of the tumor (Fig. 17.2). The patient participated with physical and occupational therapy and had near full strength in the left upper extremity on postoperative day 3 and was discharged to home. The patient was prescribed 3 months of levetiracetam, and dexamethasone was tapered to off over 10 days after surgery. The patient was seen at 2 weeks postoperatively for staple removal and was full strength with continued physical therapy. Pathology was a World Health Organization grade IV glioblastoma (IDH wild type, O6-methylguanine-DNA methyl-transferase unmethylated). The patient underwent 6 weeks of radiation and temozolomide chemotherapy followed by six adjuvant cycles. He had recurrence at 10 months and underwent bevacizumab chemotherapy for concern of recurrence. He died 16 months after surgery.

Commonalities among the experts

All surgeons preferred to obtain diffusion tensor imaging prior to surgery to identify white matter tracts, half opted for functional MRI to identify eloquent cortical areas, and half chose to have their patient undergo neuropsychiatry evaluation to obtain baseline neurocognitive function. All surgeons performed a right frontal craniotomy for the lesion, in which the majority supplemented their approach with motor mapping (one awake and two asleep), and one opted for surgery through a tubular retractor. The general goal

was typically to achieve gross total resection of the enhancing portion. Most surgeons were cognizant of the precentral gyrus, and all feared motor deficit with this surgery. Surgery was pursued with surgical navigation, surgical microscope, ultrasonic aspirator, and brain stimulator with perioperative steroids and antiepileptics. The majority of surgeons favored cortical and subcortical mapping to avoid iatrogenic injuries. Following surgery, patients were typically admitted to the intensive care unit (one as an outpatient), and MRIs were obtained within 48 hours after surgery or prior to radiation therapy. For a diagnosis of a high-grade glioma, regardless of O6-methylguanine-DNA methyl-transferase and IDH status, radiation and temozolomide were selected by most surgeons.

SUMMARY OF QUALITY OF EVIDENCE TO GUIDE SPECIFIC INTERVENTIONS FOR THIS CASE

- Surgery as opposed to biopsy or observation for high-grade gliomas—Class II-1.
- Increasing extent of resection associated with improved outcomes for high-grade gliomas—Class II-2.
- Awake versus asleep surgery for eloquent high-grade gliomas—Class II-2.
- Asleep brain mapping for eloquent gliomas—Class III.
- Use of tubular retractors for deep-seated gliomas—Class III.
- Use of diffusion tensor imaging to guide glioma resection within white matter—Class III.

REFERENCES

1. Chaichana KL, Cabrera-Aldana EE, Jusue-Torres I, et al. When gross total resection of a glioblastoma is possible, how much resection should be achieved? *World Neurosurg.* 2014;82:e257–e265.
2. Chaichana KL, Garzon-Muvdi T, Parker S, et al. Supratentorial glioblastoma multiforme: the role of surgical resection versus biopsy among older patients. *Ann Surg Oncol.* 2011;18:239–245.
3. Chaichana KL, Jusue-Torres I, Navarro-Ramirez R, et al. Establishing percent resection and residual volume thresholds affecting survival and recurrence for patients with newly diagnosed intracranial glioblastoma. *Neuro Oncol.* 2014;16:113–122.

4. Chaichana KL, Parker SL, Mukherjee D, Cheng JS, Gokaslan ZL, McGirt MJ. Assessment of the extent of surgical resection as a predictor of survival in patients with primary osseous spinal neoplasms. *Clin Neurosurg.* 2011;58:117–121.

5. Chaichana KL, Zadnik P, Weingart JD, et al. Multiple resections for patients with glioblastoma: prolonging survival. *J Neurosurg.* 2013;118:812–820.

6. Lacroix M, Abi-Said D, Fourney DR, et al. A multivariate analysis of 416 patients with glioblastoma multiforme: prognosis, extent of resection, and survival. *J Neurosurg.* 2001;95:190–198.

7. Sanai N, Polley MY, McDermott MW, Parsa AT, Berger MS. An extent of resection threshold for newly diagnosed glioblastomas. *J Neurosurg.* 2011;115:3–8.

8. De Witt Hamer PC, Robles SG, Zwinderman AH, Duffau H, Berger MS. Impact of intraoperative stimulation brain mapping on glioma surgery outcome: a meta-analysis. *J Clin Oncol.* 2012;30:2559–2565.

9. Bertani G, Fava E, Casaceli G, et al. Intraoperative mapping and monitoring of brain functions for the resection of low-grade gliomas: technical considerations. *Neurosurg Focus.* 2009;27:E4.

10. Duffau H. The reliability of asleep-awake-asleep protocol for intraoperative functional mapping and cognitive monitoring in glioma surgery. *Acta Neurochir (Wien).* 2013;155:1803–1804.

11. Eseonu CI, Eguia F, ReFaey K, et al. Comparative volumetric analysis of the extent of resection of molecularly and histologically distinct low grade gliomas and its role on survival. *J Neurooncol.* 2017;134:65–74.

12. Eseonu CI, Rincon-Torroella J, ReFaey K, et al. Awake craniotomy vs craniotomy under general anesthesia for perirolandic gliomas: evaluating perioperative complications and extent of resection. *Neurosurgery.* 2017;81:481–489.

13. Fernandez-Miranda JC, Rhoton AL Jr., Alvarez-Linera J, Kakizawa Y, Choi C, de Oliveira EP. Three-dimensional microsurgical and tractographic anatomy of the white matter of the human brain. *Neurosurgery.* 2008;62:989–1026; discussion 1026–1028.

14. Rhoton AL Jr. The cerebrum. Anatomy. *Neurosurgery.* 2007;61:37–118; discussion 118–119.

15. Nossek E, Korn A, Shahar T, et al. Intraoperative mapping and monitoring of the corticospinal tracts with neurophysiological assessment and 3-dimensional ultrasonography-based navigation. Clinical article. *J Neurosurg.* 2011;114:738–746.

18

Left perirolandic high-grade glioma

Case reviewed by Linda M. Liau, Ian F. Parney, Zvi Ram, Pierre A. Robe

Introduction

In general, the most critical eloquent locations are the language and motor areas. In a meta-analysis on intraoperative stimulation brain mapping for glioma surgery, De Witt Hammer and colleagues found that late severe neurologic deficits were seen in 8.2% of patients without brain mapping and in 3.4% of patients with brain mapping.[1] In addition, the percent of radiographically confirmed gross total resection was 58% in cases without brain mapping as compared with 75% with brain mapping, in which eloquent involvement was seen in 95.8% of nonbrain mapping cases, and 99.9% of brain mapping cases.[1] In this chapter, we present a case that involves the left perirolandic region in close proximity to the corticospinal and superior longitudinal white matter tracts.

Example case

Chief complaint: right-sided weakness and double vision
History of present illness
A 53-year-old, right-handed man with a history of liver disease presented with progressive right-sided weakness and diplopia. Over the past 3 weeks, he developed progressive right arm and leg weakness to the point in which he had difficulty with coordination. He was seen by his primary care physician who ordered brain imaging that revealed a brain lesion (Fig. 18.1). He was referred for evaluation and management.
Medications: None.
Allergies: No known drug allergies.
Past medical and surgical history: Liver disease.
Family history: No history of intracranial malignancies.
Social history: Engineer, no smoking or alcohol.

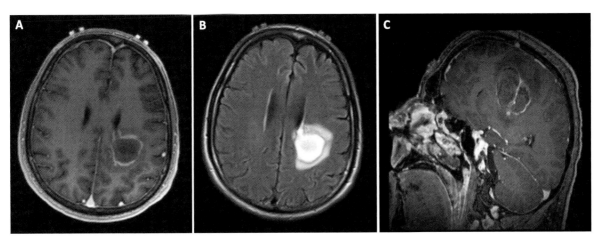

Fig. 18.1 Preoperative magnetic resonance imaging. (A) T1 axial image with gadolinium contrast; **(B)** T2 axial fluid attenuation inversion recovery image; **(C)** T1 sagittal image with gadolinium contrast magnetic resonance imaging scan demonstrating a left perirolandic heterogeneously enhancing lesion that likely involves the corticospinal and superior longitudinal white matter tracts in the dominant hemisphere.

Physical examination: Awake, alert, oriented to person, place, and time; Cranial nerves II to XII intact; Right drift, right upper extremity 4/5, right lower extremity 4+/5.

Imaging: Chest/abdomen/pelvis computed tomography negative for primary malignancy.

	Linda M. Liau, MD, PhD, University of California-Los Angeles, Los Angeles, CA, United States	Ian F. Parney, MD, PhD, Mayo Clinic, Rochester, MN, United States	Zvi Ram, MD, Tel Aviv Medical Center, Tel Aviv, Israel	Pierre A. Robe, MD, PhD, University Medical Center of Utrecht, The Netherlands
Preoperative				
Additional tests requested	DTI fMRI Neuropsychological assessment Possible Wada (sodium amytal) test	DWI ESR/CRP	Neuropsychological assessment	DWI Surgery if biopsy confirms glioma
Surgical approach selected	Left fronto-parietal craniotomy with awake language and motor mapping	Left parietal stereotactic needle biopsy	Left frontal stereotactic needle biopsy	Left awake parietal craniotomy with cortical and subcortical mapping with 5-ALA
Anatomic corridor	Left fronto-parietal transsulcal based on DTI and mapping	Left superior parietal lobule	Left anterior frontal	Left parietal
Goal of surgery	Extensive resection of contrast-enhancing portion	Diagnosis	Diagnosis	Extensive resection and preservation of neurologic function
Perioperative				
Positioning	Left lateral	Left lateral	Supine neutral	Left park bench
Surgical equipment	IOM (MEP, SSEP, ECoG), Surgical navigation Brain stimulator Surgical microscope	Surgical navigation Biopsy kit	Surgical navigation Biopsy kit	Surgical navigation Ultrasound Neuropsychological testing Surgical microscope 5-ALA
Medications	Mannitol Steroids Antiepileptics	Steroids	Steroids	Steroids Mannitol
Anatomic considerations	Primary motor and sensory cortex, CST	Primary motor and sensory cortex, CST	Motor cortex	Motor cortex, language pathways
Complications feared with approach chosen	Motor deficit	Motor deficit, hemisensory loss	Motor deficit	Motor, cognitive, proprioception, and speech deficits
Intraoperative				
Anesthesia	Awake-asleep-awake	General	General	Awake
Skin incision	Inverted U	Linear	Linear	Linear
Bone opening	Left frontal-parietal	Left parietal	Left frontal burr hole	Left parietal
Brain exposure	Left frontal-parietal	Left superior parietal	Kocher point (SFG)	Left parietal

	Linda M. Liau, MD, PhD, University of California-Los Angeles, Los Angeles, CA, United States	Ian F. Parney, MD, PhD, Mayo Clinic, Rochester, MN, United States	Zvi Ram, MD, Tel Aviv Medical Center, Tel Aviv, Israel	Pierre A. Robe, MD, PhD, University Medical Center of Utrecht, The Netherlands
Method of resection	Left frontal-parietal bone flap, U-shaped dural opening based on sagittal sinus protecting draining veins, phase reversal to identify central sulcus, if unclear perform cortical mapping, open sulcus closest to tumor under microscopic visualization, resect tumor circumferentially if plane exists and guided by DTI, debulk inside-out if no plane or in close proximity to eloquent white matter tracts on DTI, watertight dural closure, tack up sutures	Left parietal incision, burr hole, open dura, insert needle under navigation guidance, four circumferential core biopsies, leave introducer in place while awaiting pathology review, 5 mm deeper biopsies if nondiagnostic, remove needle and introducer	Left frontal incision, burr hole, navigation-guided needle biopsy, await intraoperative path review prior to closure	Titrate sedation with intravenous anesthetics, scalp field block with local anesthetics, left parietal bone flap based on navigation, ultrasound to delineate tumor margins, open dura, cortical stimulation for positive language and motor sites with neuropsychologists, tumor resection with 5-ALA fluorescence, debulk tumor with ultrasonic aspirator, repetitive cortical and subcortical stimulation, ultrasound to evaluate extent of resection and hematoma
Complication avoidance	Phase reversal, cortical mapping, resection strategy based on planes	Needle biopsy through superior parietal lobule	Needle biopsy anterior to motor cortex	Cortical and subcortical stimulation, ultrasound
Postoperative				
Admission	ICU	ICU	ICU	Floor
Postoperative complications feared	Right motor weakness or sensory deficit	Hemorrhage	Hemorrhage, motor deficit	Motor, cognitive, proprioception, and speech deficits
Follow-up testing	MRI brain with DTI within 24 hours after surgery	CT within 24 hours after surgery	Immediate postoperative head CT MRI within 48 hours after surgery	MRI within 72 hours after surgery
Follow-up visits	2 weeks after surgery	3 months after surgery 7 days after surgery with radiation and neurooncology	On obtaining pathology	As needed
Adjuvant therapies recommended				
IDH status	Mutant–radiation/ temozolomide Wild type–radiation/ temozolomide	If GBM, surgical resection through superior parietal lobule Mutant–radiation/ temozolomide +/– TTF Wild type– radiation/ temozolomide +/– TTF	Mutant–radiation/ temozolomide Wild type–radiation/ temozolomide	Mutant: radiation/ temozolomide Wild type: radiation/ temozolomide

(continued on next page)

	Linda M. Liau, MD, PhD, University of California-Los Angeles, Los Angeles, CA, United States	Ian F. Parney, MD, PhD, Mayo Clinic, Rochester, MN, United States	Zvi Ram, MD, Tel Aviv Medical Center, Tel Aviv, Israel	Pierre A. Robe, MD, PhD, University Medical Center of Utrecht, The Netherlands
MGMT status	Methylated–radiation/ temozolomide Unmethylated–radiation/ temozolomide	If GBM, surgical resection through superior parietal lobule Methylated–radiation/ temozolomide +/– TTF Unmethylated–radiation/ temozolomide +/– TTF	Methylated–radiation/ temozolomide Unmethylated–radiation/ temozolomido	Methylated: radiation/ temozolomide Unmethylated: radiation/ temozolomide

5-ALA, 5-aminolevulinic acid; *CRP*, C-reactive protein; *CST*, corticospinal tract; *CT*, computed tomography; *DTI*, diffusion tensor imaging; *DWI*, diffusion-weighted imaging; *ECoG*, electrocorticography; *ESR*, erythrocyte sedimentation rate; *fMRI*, functional magnetic resonance imaging; *GBM*, glioblastoma multiforme; *ICU*, intensive care unit; *IOM*, intraoperative monitoring; *MEP*, motor evoked potentials; *MGMT*, O6-methylguanine-DNA methyl-transferase; *MRI*, magnetic resonance imaging; *SFG*, superior frontal gyrus; *SSEP*, somatosensory evoked potentials; *TTF*, tumor treatment fields.

Differential diagnosis

- High-grade glioma
- Metastatic tumor
- Lymphoma
- Demyelinating disease (i.e., multiple sclerosis)

Important anatomic considerations

For a full description of the anatomic considerations of the frontal and central lobes, see Chapters 1 and 2 and Chapters 3 and 4, respectively. The frontal lobe is separated from the central lobe by the precentral sulcus. The superior frontal sulcus that is oriented in an anterior-posterior dimension usually connects to the precentral gyrus.[2,3] The superior frontal sulcus typically points to the omega-shaped portion of the precentral gyrus, which corresponds to the hand portion of the precentral gyrus.[2,3] Posterior to the postcentral sulcus is the parietal lobe.[2,3] In the dominant hemisphere, the parietal lobe can have several different associated functions, including language, calculation, reading, coordination, object recognition, and visual fields.[2,3] The white matter tracts that extend from the supplementary motor, motor, sensory, and parietal cortices form the corticospinal tract.[2,3] This lesion lies below the cortical surface of the supplementary motor area (coordination) and precentral gyrus (contralateral strength) at the level of the superior frontal gyrus, and involves the corticospinal tracts (contralateral strength). In addition, this lesion abuts the lateral ventricle, and therefore it is also in close juxtaposition to the superior longitudinal fasciculus (phonetics) and arcuate fasciculus (phonetics, repetition).

Approaches to this lesion

The primary surgical approaches for eloquent intrinsic tumors can be divided into either asleep or awake surgery (Chapter 1, Fig. 1.2), and the primary methods of eloquent identification can be divided into either direct or indirect methods (Chapter 3, Fig. 3.2).[4–9] Surgery in perirolandic regions can be done via both asleep or awake surgery.[4–9] The goals in either approach is to maximize resection while avoiding eloquent cortical and subcortical tissue.[4–9] In asleep surgery, intraoperative monitoring can be done to monitor motor (motor evoked potentials) and sensory (somatosensory evoked potentials) pathways.[1] In motor evoked potentials, the motor pathways are stimulated transcranially and observed in the distal muscles, in which reductions in amplitudes by 50% or increase in stimulus thresholds greater than 100 V typically corresponds with neurologic injury.[1] In somatosensory evoked potentials, the distal nerves are stimulated and observed over the somatosensory cortex, in which more than 50% decrease in amplitude and 10% increase in latency corresponds with neurologic injury.[1] The problem with these monitoring pathways is that they are sensitive to anesthetics, associated with false positive and false negatives, and provide delayed information after neurologic injury has occurred.[1] The alternative is awake surgery in which the patient participates in motor and other neurologic tests in real time.[4–9] The brain is stimulated with bipolar electrodes to prevent normal neurologic firing, and therefore mimics neurologic injury.[4–9] This allows one to gauge whether or not the tissue is eloquent and can be resected.[4–9] This, however, requires patient participation, potential patient discomfort and anxiety, surgical experience, and potentially increased risk of seizures, among others.[4–9]

For a full description of approaches to this perirolandic high-grade glioma, see Chapter 17. This lesion most likely is below the motor and sensory cortex and the proximal portion of the corticospinal tract. The cortical-based approaches for this subcortical lesion include transgyral and transsulcal approaches. In terms of directionality of approach, this includes anterior, perpendicular, or posterior. An anterior approach could endanger the motor cortex and corresponding motor component of the corticospinal tract, whereas a posterior approach could endanger the sensory cortex and corresponding sensory portion of the corticospinal tract. A direct perpendicular approach could potentially endanger both motor and sensory cortices and their corresponding corticospinal tracts.

What was actually done

The patient was taken to surgery for a left frontal-parietal craniotomy with awake language and motor mapping for resection of the lesion. The patient was intubated with a laryngeal mask airway. The scalp was blocked bilaterally with local anesthetic, and the head was fixed in pins, with two pins centered on the inion and one pin over the right forehead in the midpupillary line. The head was turned 45 degrees to the right, and a bump was placed under the left shoulder and hip to facilitate turning. A pterional incision was planned that spanned from just below the superior temporal line on the left to the vertex and was posterior to the lesion based on preoperative magnetic resonance imaging navigation. The patient was draped in the usual standard fashion and given dexamethasone, levetiracetam, and cefazolin. The flap was made and held in place with fishhooks attached to a retractor arm. A left frontal-parietal craniotomy was done to encompass the lesion, as well as extend at least one gyrus anterior, posterior, and lateral to the lesion. Ultrasound and surgical navigation were used to confirm lesion boundaries, and the boundaries were designated with letter tags once the dura was opened. The dura was anesthetized with local anesthetics between the leaflets adjacent to the middle meningeal vessels. The patient was awakened, and the dura was opened once the patient followed commands consistently. Strip electrodes were placed in the subdural space for after-discharge monitoring. The cortex was initially stimulated at 2 mA, and hand dysfunction was achieved at 3 mA with an Ojemann stimulator (Integra, Princeton, NJ) over the precentral gyrus. The rest of the cortical and subcortical mapping took place at 3 mA. The patient participated in continuous motor movement of the right face, arm, and leg with concurrent picture naming. Positive mapping sites were designated with number tags, which included the precentral gyrus with hand weakness and postcentral gyrus with hand paresthesias. It was determined at this point to access the lesion via the precentral sulcus. The microscope was brought in for the remainder of the case. The sulcus was opened sharply, and a 50-mm tubular retractor was placed through the sulcus into the lesion. The lesion was resected continuously while the patient participated in continual

right face, arm, and leg movement with picture naming to monitor for phonetics and, more specifically, the superior longitudinal fasciculus. Once white matter was seen on all the edges, the retractor was withdrawn. The patient continued to be at their baseline strength and speech. Preliminary diagnosis was infiltrating glioma. The dura, bone, and skin were closed in standard fashion.

The patient remained awake at their neurologic baseline with right-sided weakness and was taken to the intensive care unit for recovery. Postoperative magnetic resonance imaging done within 48 hours after surgery showed gross total resection (Fig. 18.2). The patient participated with physical and occupational therapy and was discharged to home on postoperative day 2 with an improved neurologic examination with 5/5 in the right lower extremity but remained 4/5 in the right upper extremity, but with intact speech. The patient was prescribed 3 months of levetiracetam, and dexamethasone was tapered to off over 7 days after surgery. The patient was seen at 2 weeks postoperatively for staple removal and was full strength with continued physical therapy. Pathology was a World Health Organization grade IV glioblastoma (IDH wild type, O6-methylguanine-DNA methyl-transferase unmethylated). The patient returned to work 4 weeks after surgery with an intact neurologic examination. The patient underwent temozolomide with concurrent radiation therapy for 6 weeks followed by three adjuvant temozolomide cycles, in which the adjuvant cycles had to be stopped because of thrombocytopenia. The patient had recurrence at 7 months after surgery and was given bevacizumab. The patient died 12 months after surgery.

Commonalities among the experts

Half of the surgeons wanted to rule out abscess with diffusion imaging, and half chose to have their patient undergo neuropsychiatry evaluation to obtain baseline neurocognitive function. The approach involved an awake motor mapping with the goal of extensive resection in half of surgeons, whereas the other half of surgeons preferred to perform a needle biopsy for diagnosis. Two surgeons favored an anterior frontal approach to the lesion, whereas the other

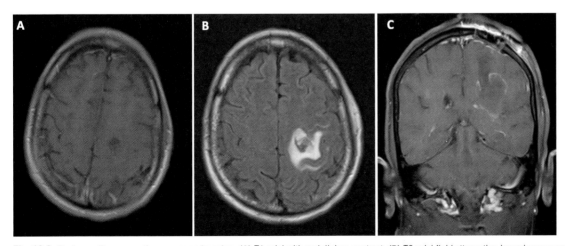

Fig. 18.2 Postoperative magnetic resonance imaging. (A) T1 axial with gadolinium contrast; **(B)** T2 axial fluid attenuation inversion recovery image; **(C)** T1 coronal image with gadolinium contrast magnetic resonance imaging scan demonstrating gross total resection of the enhancing portion of the tumor through a transsulcal approach.

two favored a posterior parietal approach to the lesion. All surgeons were cognizant of the primary motor cortex and corticospinal tracts, and all feared motor deficit with this surgery. For those surgeons pursing surgical resections, surgery was pursued with surgical navigation, surgical microscope, ultrasonic aspirator, and brain stimulator with perioperative steroids and antiepileptics, in which one surgeon also favored 5-aminolevulinic acid (5-ALA). The majority of surgeons favored cortical and subcortical mapping to avoid iatrogenic injuries in the resection cases and needle biopsies to avoid deficits in the nonresection cases. Following surgery, patients were typically admitted to the intensive care unit (one to the floor), and imaging was obtained within 72 hours after surgery to assess extent of resection and/or potential complications. For a diagnosis of a high grade-glioma, regardless of O6-methylguanine-DNA methyl-transferase and IDH status, radiation and temozolomide were selected by all surgeons, and one provided an additional option of tumor treatment fields.

SUMMARY OF QUALITY OF EVIDENCE TO GUIDE SPECIFIC INTERVENTIONS FOR THIS CASE

- Surgery as opposed to biopsy or observation for high-grade gliomas—Class II-1.
- Increasing extent of resection associated with improved outcomes for high-grade gliomas—Class II-2.
- Awake versus asleep surgery for eloquent high-grade gliomas—Class II-2.
- Use of tubular retractors for deep-seated gliomas—Class III.
- Transsulcal approach for deep-seated brain lesions—Class III.

REFERENCES

1. De Witt Hammer PC. Robles SG, Zwinderman AH, Duffau H, Berger MS. Impact of intraoperative stimulation brain mapping on glioma surgery outcome: a meta-analysis. *J Clin Oncol.* 2012;10:302559–302565.
2. Stecker MM. A review of intraoperative monitoring for spinal surgery. *Surg Neurol Int.* 2012;3:S174–S187.
3. Fernandez-Miranda JC, Rhoton AL Jr. Alvarez-Linera J, Kakizawa Y, Choi C, de Oliveira EP. Three-dimensional microsurgical and tractographic anatomy of the white matter of the human brain. *Neurosurgery.* 2008;62:989–1026; discussion 1026–1028.
4. Rhoton AL Jr. The cerebrum. Anatomy. *Neurosurgery.* 2007;61:37–118; discussion 118–119.
5. Duffau H. The reliability of asleep-awake-asleep protocol for intraoperative functional mapping and cognitive monitoring in glioma surgery. *Acta Neurochir (Wien).* 2013;155:1803–1804.
6. Eseonu CI, Eguia F, Garcia O, Kaplan PW, Quinones-Hinojosa A. Comparative analysis of monotherapy versus duotherapy antiseizure drug management for postoperative seizure control in patients undergoing an awake craniotomy. *J Neurosurg.* 2018;128:1661–1667.
7. Eseonu CI, Eguia F, ReFaey K, et al. Comparative volumetric analysis of the extent of resection of molecularly and histologically distinct low grade gliomas and its role on survival. *J Neurooncol.* 2017;134:65–74.
8. Eseonu CI, Rincon-Torroella J, ReFaey K, et al. Awake craniotomy vs craniotomy under general anesthesia for perirolandic gliomas: evaluating perioperative complications and extent of resection. *Neurosurgery.* 2017;81:481–489.
9. Bertani G, Fava E, Casaceli G, et al. Intraoperative mapping and monitoring of brain functions for the resection of low-grade gliomas: technical considerations. *Neurosurg Focus.* 2009;27:E4.
10. Nossek E, Korn A, Shahar T, et al. Intraoperative mapping and monitoring of the corticospinal tracts with neurophysiological assessment and 3-dimensional ultrasonography-based navigation. Clinical article. *J Neurosurg.* 2011;114:738–746.

19

Broca area high-grade glioma

Case reviewed by Jeffrey N. Bruce, Chae-Yong Kim, Ganesh Rao, Jinsong Wu

Introduction

Historically, the Broca area has been defined as residing primarily within the pars triangularis of the inferior frontal gyrus or frontal operculum on the dominant hemisphere.[1,2] The methods of identifying this area radiographically primarily involves functional magnetic resonance imaging (fMRI), in which neurovascular coupling allows the identification of flow changes in conjunction with neuronal activity.[3] The difficulty with fMRI is that it is prone to false positives and false negatives, does not identify critical threshold of functions, and can be less sensitive and/or specific in tumor-infiltrated and/or edematous areas that is common for gliomas.[3] The direct method of identifying these areas is awake brain mapping with direct electrical stimulation, whereby electrical stimulation impairs normal neurologic firing to identify functional processes.[4] In this chapter, we present a case of a high-grade glioma in close proximity to the inferior frontal gyrus, which has historically been identified as the Broca area.

Example case

Chief complaint: speaking problems and confusion
History of present illness
A 59-year-old, right-handed woman with a history of hypertension, hyperlipidemia, and anxiety presented with confusion and speaking problems. Her family states that over the past couple of months they have noted that she has become increasingly confused and with difficulty getting her words out. She was seen by a neurologist who ordered imaging that showed a large brain lesion (Fig. 19.1).
Medications: Lisinopril, atorvastatin, sertraline.
Allergies: No known drug allergies.
Past medical and surgical history: Hypertension, hyperlipidemia, anxiety.
Family history: No history of intracranial malignancies.

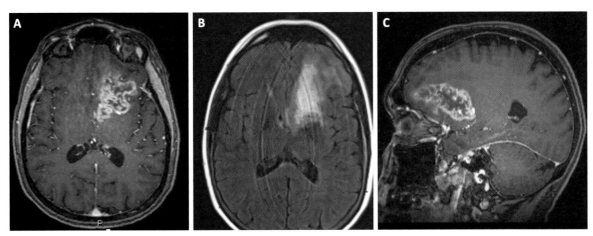

Fig. 19.1 Preoperative magnetic resonance imaging. (A) T1 axial image with gadolinium contrast; **(B)** T2 axial fluid attenuation inversion recovery image; **(C)** T1 sagittal image with gadolinium contrast scan demonstrating an enhancing lesion involving the left inferior frontal gyrus or Broca region.

Social history: Homemaker, no smoking or alcohol history.
Physical examination: Awake, alert, oriented to person, place, and time; Language: slowness in speech, dysarthria, intact naming and repetition; Cranial nerves II to

XII intact; Right drift, moves all extremities with full strength.
Imaging: Chest/abdomen/pelvis imaging negative for primary malignancy.

	Jeffrey N. Bruce, MD, Columbia University, New York City, NY, United States	Chae-Yong Kim, MD, PhD, Seoul National University, Bundang Hospital, Seoul, South Korea	Ganesh Rao, MD, Baylor College of Medicine, Houston, TX, United States	Jinsong Wu, MD, PhD, Fudan University, Huashan Hospital, Shanghai, China
Preoperative				
Additional tests requested	DTI fMRI Neuropsychological assessment	DTI Perfusion and diffusion MRI +/– fMRI PET	fMRI Neuropsychological assessment	DTI Task-based BOLD fMRI MRS Neuropsychological assessment
Surgical approach selected	Left frontal craniotomy with awake language and motor mapping	Left frontal craniotomy with 5-ALA	Left frontal craniotomy	Left frontal craniotomy with awake language and motor mapping with intraoperative MRI
Anatomic corridor	Left frontal over tumor	Left frontal	Left frontal above frontal sinus	Left frontal
Goal of surgery	Extensive resection of contrast and FLAIR with functional preservation	Attempted gross total resection	Diagnosis because of insula involvement and maximal safe resection	Maximal safe resection of enhancing component
Perioperative				
Positioning	Left supine with slight right rotation	Left supine with 5-degree right rotation	Left supine	Left supine with 30-degree right rotation
Surgical equipment	Surgical navigation IOM (ECoG) Brain stimulator Ultrasound Ultrasonic aspirator Surgical microscope	Surgical navigation IOM Ultrasound Surgical microscope with 5-ALA Ultrasonic aspirator	Surgical navigation Ultrasound	Surgical navigation IOM Brain stimulator Ultrasonic aspirator Intraoperative MRI
Medications	Steroids Antiepileptics 5-ALA or Fluorescein	Antiepileptics	Steroids	Steroids Antiepileptics
Anatomic considerations	Sylvian fissure, speech and motor areas, lateral ventricle	Corpus callosum, MCA	Sphenoid wing, frontal sinus, sagittal sinus, Broca area, lateral ventricles, ACA	Coronal suture, IFG, orbital gyrus, frontal horn lateral ventricle, caudate head, fornix, ventral striatal pallidum, anterior perforated substance, mesial basal frontal cortex, genu of corpus callosum, prefrontal veins and arteries
Complications feared with approach chosen	Language dysfunction, motor deficit	Language dysfunction	Language dysfunction, ACA injury	Language dysfunction, motor deficit, cognitive dysfunction
Intraoperative				
Anesthesia	Asleep-awake-asleep	General	General	Awake (MAC)
Skin incision	Bicoronal	Bicoronal	Modified bicoronal	Bicoronal linear
Bone opening	Left frontal near sagittal sinus	Left frontal	Left frontal above frontal sinus	Left frontal
Brain exposure	Left SFG, MFG, IFG	Left frontal	Left frontal pole	Left SFG, MFG, IFG

	Jeffrey N. Bruce, MD, Columbia University, New York City, NY, United States	Chae-Yong Kim, MD, PhD, Seoul National University, Bundang Hospital, Seoul, South Korea	Ganesh Rao, MD, Baylor College of Medicine, Houston, TX, United States	Jinsong Wu, MD, PhD, Fudan University, Huashan Hospital, Shanghai, China
Method of resection	Local anesthetic application, craniotomy planning based on navigation, large left frontal craniotomy to encompass lesion and Sylvian fissure, cruciate dural opening over lesion, patient awoken, ECoG grids, awake speech and motor mapping, outline tumor with navigation, corticectomy in negative mapping areas starting lateral to tumor, dissect posteriorly and leave medial portion for last, extend resection to skull base and into frontal horn of lateral ventricle, debulk tumor with ultrasonic aspirator, dissect from critical white matter tracts identified during mapping, ultrasound to guide further resection, resect fluorescing tissue, watertight dural closure	Craniotomy based on navigation, open dura, delineate tumor margins with navigation and ultrasound, attempt en bloc, inspect cavity with 5-ALA and ultrasound	Semibicoronal incision taken down to just temporalis fascia, craniotomy ipsilateral to sagittal sinus, ultrasound to locate hyperechoic component, intralesional resection, remove as much of the suckable portion of tumor as possible, no attempt at en bloc or supratotal resection	Craniotomy based on navigation, dural opening, identify and protect the Broca area, resection from lateral fissure to intercerebral fissure to 2 cm in front of coronal suture and close to the frontal horn of the lateral ventricle, attempt to avoid opening lateral ventricle, removal of the prefrontal lobe en bloc with ultrasonic aspirator, removal of deep portion of residual tumor guided by navigation, continuous MEP, intraoperative MRI to guide further resection, watertight dural closure
Complication avoidance	Cortical and subcortical mapping, leave medial portion for last, fluorescence, ultrasound	Attempt en bloc, 5-ALA and ultrasound to guide resection	Ultrasound, limiting resection to suckable component	Cortical and subcortical mapping, continuous MEP, obey anatomic boundaries, intraoperative MRI
Postoperative				
Admission	ICU	ICU	Intermediate care	ICU
Postoperative complications feared	Language dysfunction, motor deficit, seizures	Language dysfunction	Language dysfunction, vascular injury	Language dysfunction, cognitive disorder
Follow-up testing	MRI within 48 hours after surgery	MRI within 48 hours after surgery	MRI within 24 hours after surgery Neuropsychological and speech assessment 3 days after surgery	Intraoperative MRI on completion of surgery or MRI within 72 hours after surgery
Follow-up visits	7 days after surgery	3–4 weeks after adjuvant therapy	7 days after surgery 1 month after surgery with MRI	1 month after surgery
Adjuvant therapies recommended				
IDH status	Mutant–radiation/temozolomide Wild type–radiation/temozolomide	Mutant–radiation/ temozolomide Wild type–radiation/ temozolomide	Mutant–radiation/ temozolomide Wild type–radiation/ temozolomide	Mutant–radiation/ temozolomide Wild type–radiation/ temozolomide
MGMT status	Methylated–radiation/ temozolomide Unmethylated–radiation/ temozolomide	Methylated– radiation/ temozolomide Unmethylated– radiation/ temozolomide	Methylated–radiation/ temozolomide Unmethylated–radiation/ temozolomide	Methylated–radiation/ temozolomide Unmethylated–radiation/ temozolomide

5-ALA, 5-aminolevulinic acid; ACA, anterior cerebral artery; BOLD, blood-oxygen-level-dependent; DTI, diffusion tensor imaging; ECoG, electrocorticography; FLAIR, fluid attenuation inversion recovery; fMRI, functional magnetic resonance imaging; ICU, intensive care unit; IFG, inferior frontal gyrus; IOM, intraoperative monitoring; MAC, monitored anesthesia care; MCA, middle cerebral artery; MEP, motor evoked potential; MFG, middle frontal gyrus; MGMT, O6-methylguanine-DNA methyl-transferase; MRI, magnetic resonance imaging; MRS, magnetic resonance spectroscopy; PET, positron emission tomography; SFG, superior frontal gyrus.

Differential diagnosis and actual diagnosis

- High-grade glioma
- Lymphoma
- Demyelinating disease (i.e., tumefactive multiple sclerosis)

Important anatomic and preoperative considerations

For a full description of the frontal lobe and its relevant anatomy, see Chapters 1 and 2. The lateral surface of the frontal lobe is limited posteriorly by the precentral sulcus and inferiorly by the Sylvian fissure, and is divided by two longitudinal sulci (superior and inferior frontal sulci) into three gyri (superior, middle, and inferior frontal gyri).[5,6] The inferior frontal gyrus is divided by the horizontal and ascending rami of the Sylvian fissure into the pars orbitalis, pars triangularis, and pars opercularis, in which the latter is frequently divided by the diagonal sulcus.[5,6] The inferior surface of the frontal lobe lies over the orbit and is divided by the olfactory sulcus into the gyrus rectus medially and orbital gyrus laterally.[5,6] The orbital sulcus forms the letter H, and divides the orbital gyrus into four gyri: anterior, posterior, medial, and lateral, in which the lateral and posterior orbital gyri are continuous on the lateral surface with the pars orbitalis of the inferior frontal gyrus.[5,6] The Broca area, by convention, typically consists of the pars triangularis and pars opercularis on the dominant hemisphere.[5,6] Superior to the Broca area is the ventral premotor cortex that plays a role in speech initiation and functions in both hemispheres.[7,8] Posterior to Broca is the precental gyrus that controls contralateral motor movement primarily of the face.[5,6] There are several white matter tracts that terminate in the vicinity of the Broca area, and include the superior longitudinal fasciculus (SLF, phonetics), arcuate fasciculus (AF, phonetics and repetition), frontal aslant tract (FAT, speech initiation), and inferior frontal occipital fasciculus (IFOF, semantics).[5,6] This lesion involves the gyrus rectus, orbital gyrus, and inferior frontal gyrus, with subcortical involvement of the SLF and AF, IFOF, FAT, head of the caudate, and anterior limb of the internal capsule.

Approaches to this lesion

The general approaches to this lesion can be divided into biopsy or extensive surgical resection, and the methods of doing this can be further divided into asleep or awake surgery (Chapter 1, Fig. 1.2). The goal in this surgery would be to avoid eloquent structures that can be identified with direct or indirect methods both in and outside of the operating room (Chapter 3, Fig. 3.2). This lesion primarily involves the gyrus rectus, orbital gyrus, and inferior frontal gyrus in the dominant hemisphere, with subcortical involvement of the SLF and AF, IFOF, FAT, head of the caudate, and anterior limb of the internal capsule. The best trajectory into this lesion would likely be an anterior frontal approach in the midpupillary line into the gyrus rectus, thus avoiding the laterally positioned Broca area and cortex of the inferior frontal gyrus, as well as the SLF, AF, and IFOF. The deepest part of the lesion is important to avoid as this would involve the head of the caudate and the FAT. Another structure to keep in mind medially and posteriorly is the default mode network that is adjuvant to the anterior genus of the corpus callosum. An alternative approach is laterally but this would engage the Broca area, SLF, AF, and IFOF.

What was actually done

The patient was taken to surgery for a left pterional craniotomy with awake motor and language mapping for resection of the lesion. The patient was intubated with a laryngeal mask airway. The scalp was blocked bilaterally with local anesthetic, and the head was fixed in pins, with two pins centered on the external auditory meatus on the right and one pin posterior to the external auditory meatus below the superior temporal line on the left. The head was kept neutral to minimize patient discomfort. A pterional incision was then planned that spanned from above the root of the zygoma to the vertex. The patient was draped in the usual standard fashion and given dexamethasone, levetiracetam, and cefazolin. A pterional flap was formed staying above the temporalis fascia and held in place with fishhooks attached to a retracting arm. A left frontal craniotomy was done to encompass the anterior pole of the lesion and staying above the frontal sinus. Ultrasound and surgical navigation were used to confirm lesion boundaries, and the boundaries were designated with letter tags once the dura was opened. The dura was anesthetized with local anesthetics between the leaflets adjacent to the middle meningeal vessels. The patient was awakened, and the dura was opened once the patient followed commands consistently. Strip electrodes were placed in the subdural space for after discharge monitoring. The cortex was initially stimulated at 2 mA, and no speech arrest occurred over the cortical surface at 6 mA with an Ojemann stimulator (Integra, Princeton, NJ). The rest of the cortical and subcortical mapping took place at 6 mA. The patient participated in continuous language testing with picture naming, phonetic tests, and repetition, with concurrent motor movement of the right face and arm. Positive mapping sites were designated with number tags. Negative mapping occurred initially over the cortical surface of the anterior pole of the tumor; however, at the tumor depths, positive subcortical mapping sites were elicited, and included the head of the caudate (speech perseveration) at the posterior margin of the lesion, FAT (difficulty with speech initiation) at the posterolateral margin, and SLF (phonetic paraphasias) lateral to the FAT. When these areas were encountered, resection stopped at these boundaries, and the patient was put back to sleep. Preliminary diagnosis was infiltrating glioma. The dura, bone, and skin were closed in standard fashion.

The patient awoke at their neurologic baseline with intact speech and full strength bilaterally and was taken to the intensive care unit for recovery. On postoperative day 1, they developed some mild dysarthria. Postoperative MRI done within 48 hours after surgery showed near total resection with expected residual posteriorly near the caudate head (Fig. 19.2). The patient participated with physical, occupational, and speech therapy and was discharged to home on postoperative day 2 with an intact neurologic examination. The patient was prescribed 3 months of levetiracetam, and dexamethasone was tapered to off over 7 days after surgery.

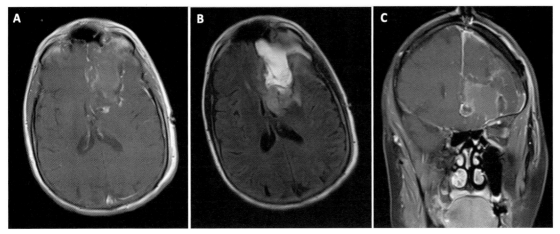

Fig. 19.2 Postoperative magnetic resonance imaging. (A) T1 axial imaging with gadolinium contrast; **(B)** T2 axial fluid attenuation inversion recovery image; **(C)** T1 coronal image with gadolinium contrast magnetic resonance imaging scan demonstrating near total resection of the tumor involving the Broca region with residual posteriorly along the resection cavity.

The patient was seen at 2 weeks postoperatively for staple removal and was full strength with intact speech. Pathology was a World Health Organization grade IV glioblastoma (IDH wild type, methylguanine-DNA methyl-transferase methylated). The patient underwent adjuvant temozolomide chemotherapy with concurrent radiation therapy for 6 weeks followed by five adjuvant temozolomide cycles. The patient unfortunately had recurrence at 12 months and underwent repeat resection. The patient remains alive at 18 months after the initial surgery.

Commonalities among the experts

All surgeons opted for patients having fMRI and diffusion tensor imaging to help identify areas of eloquent and white matter tracts, respectively. The majority of surgeons also requested neuropsychiatry evaluation to obtain baseline neurocognitive function. The approach involved an awake language and motor mapping in half, and one surgeons each elected for using intraoperative MRI and 5-aminolevulinic acid (5-ALA) to guide more extensive resection. All surgeons favored an anterior frontal approach to the lesion, and the goal was typically maximal safe resection of the enhancing portion. Most surgeons identified the importance of awareness of the Sylvian fissure and Broca area, and most feared language and motor dysfunction. For those surgeons pursing surgical resections, surgery was pursued with surgical navigation, surgical microscope, ultrasonic aspirator, ultrasound, and brain stimulator with perioperative steroids and antiepileptics. The use of cortical and subcortical mapping was used in half, whereas the majority of surgeons favored ultrasound to guide resection to avoid iatrogenic injuries. Following surgery, patients were typically admitted to the intensive care unit (one to intermediate care), and imaging was obtained within 72 hours after surgery to assess extent of resection and/or potential complications. For a diagnosis of a high-grade glioma, regardless of methylguanine-DNA methyl-transferase and IDH status, all surgeons favored the use of postoperative radiation and temozolomide.

SUMMARY OF QUALITY OF EVIDENCE TO GUIDE SPECIFIC INTERVENTIONS FOR THIS CASE

- Surgery as opposed to biopsy or observation for high-grade gliomas—Class II-1.
- Increasing extent of resection associated with improved outcomes for high-grade gliomas—Class II-2.
- Awake versus asleep surgery for eloquent high-grade gliomas—Class II-2.
- Repeat resection for recurrent glioblastoma—Class II-2.

REFERENCES

1. Picart T, Duffau H. Awake resection of a left operculo-insular low-grade glioma guided by cortico-subcortical mapping. *Neurosurg Focus.* 2018;45:V1.
2. Saito T, Muragaki Y, Maruyama T, et al. Difficulty in identification of the frontal language area in patients with dominant frontal gliomas that involve the pars triangularis. *J Neurosurg.* 2016;125:803–811.
3. Hua J, Miao X, Agarwal S, et al. Language mapping using T2-prepared BOLD functional MRI in the presence of large susceptibility artifacts-initial results in patients with brain tumor and epilepsy. *Tomography.* 2017;3:105–113.
4. Eseonu CI, Rincon-Torroella J, ReFaey K, et al. awake craniotomy vs craniotomy under general anesthesia for perirolandic gliomas: evaluating perioperative complications and extent of resection. *Neurosurgery.* 2017;81:481–489.
5. Rhoton AL Jr. The cerebrum. Anatomy. *Neurosurgery.* 2007;61:37–118; discussion 118–119.
6. Fernandez-Miranda JC, Rhoton AL Jr., Alvarez-Linera J, Kakizawa Y, Choi C, de Oliveira EP. Three-dimensional microsurgical and tractographic anatomy of the white matter of the human brain. *Neurosurgery.* 2008;62:989–1026; discussion 1026–1028.
7. Duffau H. Long-term outcomes after supratotal resection of diffuse low-grade gliomas: a consecutive series with 11-year follow-up. *Acta Neurochir (Wien).* 2016;158:51–58.
8. Duffau H, Mandonnet E. The "onco-functional balance" in surgery for diffuse low-grade glioma: integrating the extent of resection with quality of life. *Acta Neurochir (Wien).* 2013;155:951–957.

20

Wernicke area high-grade glioma

Case reviewed by Mitchel S. Berger, Shawn L. Hervey-Jumper, Manabu Natsumeda, Pierre A. Robe

Introduction

Historically, the Wernicke area has been defined as residing primarily within the posterior superior temporal lobe in the dominant hemisphere.[1,2] However, there is great individual variability.[1,2] The methods of identifying this area radiographically primarily involve functional magnetic resonance imaging (MRI), in which neurovascular coupling allows the identification of flow changes in conjunction with neuronal activity.[3] The difficulty with functional MRI is that it is prone to false positives and false negatives, does not identify critical functional thresholds, and can be less sensitive and/or specific in tumor-infiltrated and/or edematous areas that are common for gliomas, especially high-grade gliomas.[3] The direct method of identifying these areas is awake brain mapping with direct electrical stimulation, whereby electrical stimulation impairs normal neurologic firing to identify functional processes.[4] In this chapter, we present a case of a high-grade glioma in close proximity to the superior temporal gyrus, which has historically been identified as the Wernicke area.

Example case

Chief complaint: speaking difficulties

History of present illness

A 51-year-old, right-handed man with a history of hypertension presented with difficulty speaking. Over the past 2 months, he has noticed an increased difficulty getting the right words out, especially during business meetings. He has also had several instances in which his words did not sound right. He underwent brain imaging that revealed a brain lesion (Fig. 20.1).

Medications: Hydrochlorothiazide.

Allergies: No known drug allergies.

Past medical and surgical history: Hypertension.

Family history: No history of intracranial malignancies.

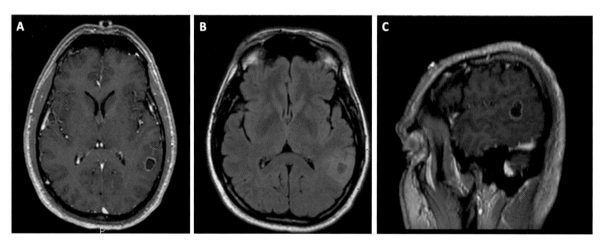

Fig. 20.1 Preoperative magnetic resonance imaging. (A) T1 axial image with gadolinium contrast; **(B)** T2 axial fluid attenuation inversion recovery image; **(C)** T1 sagittal image with gadolinium contrast magnetic resonance imaging scan demonstrating a heterogeneously enhancing lesion involving the left posterior superior temporal gyrus or Wernicke area.

Social history: Business executive, no smoking or alcohol history.

Physical examination: Awake, alert, oriented to person, place, and time; Language: slowness in speech, dysarthria, intact naming and repetition; Cranial nerves II to XII intact; No drift, moves all extremities with full strength.

Imaging: Chest/abdomen/pelvis imaging negative for primary malignancy.

	Mitchel S. Berger, MD, University of California at San Francisco, San Francisco, CA, United States	Shawn L. Hervey-Jumper, MD, University of California at San Francisco, San Francisco, CA, United States	Manabu Natsumeda, MD, PhD, Niigata University, Niigata, Japan	Pierre A. Robe, MD, PhD, University Medical Center of Utrecht, The Netherlands
Preoperative				
Additional tests requested	DTI MEG	DTI MEG Neuropsychological assessment	fMRI DTI Neuropsychological assessment Angiography and Wada test 3D-CTA/CTV	Neuropsychological assessment
Surgical approach selected	Left temporal-parietal craniotomy with awake language and motor cortical and subcortical mapping with 5-ALA	Left temporal craniotomy with awake language mapping with 5-ALA	Left parietal awake craniotomy with cortical and subcortical mapping	Left temporo-parietal awake craniotomy with cortical and subcortical mapping with 5-ALA
Anatomic corridor	Left temporal-parietal with awake cortical and subcortical mapping	Left STG	Left parietal	Left posterior temporal
Goal of surgery	Complete resection of the enhancing and as much FLAIR as possible	Maximal resection of enhancing core and FLAIR with minimal language morbidity	Complete resection of the enhancing and as much FLAIR as possible	Maximal resection of FLAIR according to functional boundaries
Perioperative				
Positioning	Left supine	Left semilateral	Right lateral (left side up)	Left park bench
Surgical equipment	Surgical navigation Surgical microscope with 5-ALA Brain stimulator	Surgical navigation IOM (ECoG) Surgical microscope with 5-ALA Brain stimulator Ultrasonic aspirator	Surgical navigation IOM (MEP/SSEP) Brain stimulator Surgical microscope with 5-ALA Intraoperative CT	Surgical navigation Ultrasound Neuropsychological testing Surgical microscope
Medications	Mannitol Steroids Antiepileptics	Mannitol Steroids Antiepileptics	Mannitol Steroids Antiepileptics	Steroids Mannitol
Anatomic considerations	Language cortical and subcortical areas	STG, MTG, SLF, AF, IFOF, uncinate, ILF, MdLF	Angular artery, temporal occipital artery, SMG, AG, STG, AF, IFOF, MdLF, Sylvian fissure, vein of Labbe	Temporal cortex, optic radiations, IFOF
Complications feared with approach chosen	Language deficits	Long-term language deficits	Language dysfunction, Gerstmann syndrome, visual field deficit	Speech deficit, prosopagnosia, working memory deficit, quadrantopsia
Intraoperative				
Anesthesia	Asleep-awake-asleep	Asleep-awake-asleep	Asleep-awake-asleep	Awake
Skin incision	Inverted U	Inverted U	Horseshoe	Semicircular, supraauricular

(continued on next page)

	Mitchel S. Berger, MD, University of California at San Francisco, San Francisco, CA, United States	Shawn L. Hervey-Jumper, MD, University of California at San Francisco, San Francisco, CA, United States	Manabu Natsumeda, MD, PhD, Niigata University, Niigata, Japan	Pierre A. Robe, MD, PhD, University Medical Center of Utrecht, The Netherlands
Bone opening	Left temporal-parietal with 2-cm margin	Left temporal	Left temporal-parietal	Left temporal-parietal
Brain exposure	Left temporal-parietal	Left temporal	Left temporal-parietal	Left temporal-parietal
Method of resection	Skin anesthetized, craniotomy overlying lesion with 2-cm margin based on navigation, dural opening, awake language cortical mapping, corticectomy based on negative mapping areas, continue resection with continuous subcortical language mapping, aim to resect all enhancement as well as FLAIR pending mapping results, resection until positive cortical and subcortical mapping, 5-ALA fluorescence assessemnts for residual, watertight dural closure, subgaleal drain insertion	Local anesthetic into pins sites, wide scalp block, myocutaneous flap extended inferiorly, confirm body temperature and optimal mapping conditions, mapping team present including neurology and speech pathology, language mapping over STG and MTG to determine positive mapping threshold, mapping over tumor site with 1-cm margin around FLAIR, entry into functional free zones with ultrasonic aspirator, resection first along anterior and medial FLAIR margins subpially and then lateral margin down to subcortical U-fibers, mass truncated at bottom of sulcus, subcortical stimulation until medial margin reached	Scalp bloc, LMA, craniotomy based on navigation, awaken patient and removal of LMA, language mapping, corticectomy based on negative mapping results, resection of enhancing portion with ultrasonic aspirator and suction, check for 5-ALA staining, removal of FLAIR portion until positive mapping areas reached, patient put back to sleep with LMA, continuous monitoring, intraoperative CT to guide further resection, watertight dural closure, insertion of subgaleal drain	Local field block, myocutaneous opening, left temporal/pterional bone flap, ultrasound to delineate tumor margins, opening dura, ECoG, cortical stimulation for positive sites (1–3 mA), tumor resection with repetitive cortical and subcortical stimulation, decrease simulation to 2 and 1 mA near eloquent area, ultrasound to evaluate extent of resection and hematoma
Complication avoidance	Language mapping, continuous monitoring	Language mapping, subcortical mapping once sulcus level reached	Language mapping, continuous monitoring, intraoperative CT	Cortical and subcortical stimulation, ultrasound
Postoperative				
Admission	ICU	ICU	ICU	Floor
Postoperative complications feared	Language dysfunction, seizures	Language dysfunction, venous infarct	Language dysfunction, Gerstmann syndrome, visual field deficit	Language dysfunction, vasospasm, seizure
Follow-up testing	MRI within 24 hours after surgery with DWI and DTI	MRI within 48 hours after surgery Speech evaluation 24 hours after surgery	CT immediate postoperative MRI within 24 hours after surgery Neuropsychological assessment 7 days after surgery	MRI within 72 hours after surgery Postoperative neuropsychological assessment and 3 months after surgery
Follow-up visits	10 days after surgery with neurooncology	14 days after surgery	On pathology diagnosis	As needed with neurosurgery Speech therapy

	Mitchel S. Berger, MD, University of California at San Francisco, San Francisco, CA, United States	Shawn L. Hervey-Jumper, MD, University of California at San Francisco, San Francisco, CA, United States	Manabu Natsumeda, MD, PhD, Niigata University, Niigata, Japan	Pierre A. Robe, MD, PhD, University Medical Center of Utrecht, The Netherlands
Adjuvant therapies recommended				
IDH status	Mutant–radiation/ temozolomide +/– lomustine Wild type–radiation/ temozolomide +/– lomustine	Mutant–radiation/ temozolomide Wild type–radiation/ temozolomide	Mutant–radiation/ temozolomide with TTF Wild type–radiation/ temozolomide with TTF	Mutant–radiation/ temozolomide Wild type–radiation/ temozolomide
MGMT status	Methylated–radiation/ temozolomide Unmethylated–radiation/ temozolomide under 65 years of age	Methylated–radiation/ temozolomide Unmethylated–radiation/ temozolomide	Methylated–radiation/ temozolomide +/– TTF Unmethylated–radiation/ temozolomide +/– TTF	Methylated–radiation/ temozolomide Unmethylated–radiation/ temozolomide

3D-CTA, three-dimensional computed tomography angiography; *5-ALA*, 5-aminolevulinic acid; *AF*, arcuate fasciculus; *AG*, angular gyrus; lomustine; *CT*, computed tomography; *CTV*, CT venography; *DTI*, diffusion tensor imaging; *DWI*, diffusion-weighted imaging; *ECoG*, electrocorticography; *FLAIR*, fluid attenuation inversion recovery; *fMRI*, functional magnetic resonance imaging; *ICU*, intensive care unit; *IFOF*, inferior occipital fasciculus; *ILF*, inferior longitudinal fasciculus; *IOM*, intraoperative monitoring; *LMA*, laryngeal mask airway; *MEG*, magnetoencephalogram; *MdLF*, middle longitudinal fasciculus; *MEP*, motor evoked potential; MGMT, O6-methylguanine-DNA methyltransferase; MRI, magnetic resonance imaging; *MTG*, middle temporal gyrus; *SLF*, superior longitudinal fasciculus; *SMG*, supramarginal gyrus; *SSEP*, somatosensory evoked potential; *STG*, superior temporal gyrus; *TTF*, tumor treatment fields.

Differential diagnosis and actual diagnosis

- High-grace glioma
- Metastatic brain tumor
- Cerebral abscess
- Low-grade glioma (oligodendroglioma)

Important anatomic and preoperative considerations

This lesion is in close proximity to the language networks and, more specifically, the Wernicke area.[5,6] The Wernicke area is classically described as involving the posterior superior temporal gyrus.[1,2] The transverse temporal gyrus or Heschl gyrus is the primary auditory cortex that extends anterolaterally from the posterior end of the insula, and can be identified on sagittal images as a protuberance between the posterior insula and superior temporal gyrus.[5,6] The planum temporale, which is involved in language processing, is the area in-between the posterior end of the Sylvian fissure and Heschl gyrus.[5,6] The initial cortical processing of speech takes place along the Heschl gyrus, where it then projects to the posterior half of the superior temporal sulcus for phonological processing or the Wernicke area. From here, language processing is distributed along the dorsal-phonetic (superior longitudinal fasciculus [SLF] and arcuate fasciculus [AF]) and the ventral-semantic stream (inferior frontal occipital fasciculus).[7] For this lesion, it is located in close proximity to the Wernicke area, and on the medial surface is the temporal-parietal component of the SLF and AF.

Approaches to this lesion

The general approaches to this lesion can be divided into asleep or awake surgery (Chapter 1, Fig. 1.2). The goal in this surgery would be to avoid eloquent structures that can be identified with direct or indirect methods both in and outside of the operating room (Chapter 3, Fig. 3.2). This lesion primarily involves the Wernicke area, as well as the SLF and AF on its medial surfaces. The best trajectory to this lesion would be lateral, as this is the shortest distance to the lesion, however, the eloquent function of the superficial cortex must be understood, as this correlates to the Wernicke area anatomically. There is no overlying sulcus to allow a transsulcal approach to the lesion. At the medial aspect of the tumor, especially if the fluid attenuation inversion recovery image (FLAIR) changes are targeted, it is important to understand if eloquent white matter tracts are involved, namely SLF and AF.

What was actually done

The patient was taken to surgery for a left temporal-parietal craniotomy with awake motor and language mapping for resection of the lesion. The patient was intubated with a laryngeal mask airway. The scalp was blocked bilaterally with local anesthetic, and the head was fixed in pins, with two pins centered on the inion and one pin on the right forehead in the midpupillary line. The head was turned 60 degrees to the right, and a bump was placed under the shoulder and hip to facilitate turning and minimize patient discomfort. A trap-door incision was then planned that spanned from the mastoid process to the superior temporal line, and anteriorly to a line connecting the zygoma with the superior temporal line. The patient was draped in the usual standard fashion and given dexamethasone, levetiracetam, and cefazolin. A myocutaneous flap was made, reflected inferiorly, and held in place with fishhooks attached to a retractor arm. A left temporal-parietal craniotomy was done to encompass the lesion, and at least one gyrus in each direction to facilitate positive mapping. Ultrasound and surgical navigation were used to confirm lesion boundaries, and the boundaries were designated with letter tags once the dura was opened. The dura was anesthetized with local anesthetics between the leaflets adjacent to the middle meningeal vessels. The patient was awakened, and the dura was opened once the patient followed commands consistently. Strip electrodes were placed in the subdural space for after discharge monitoring. The cortex was initially stimulated at 2 mA, and facial paresthesias were elicited over the sensory cortex superiorly to the lesion at 4 mA with an Ojemann stimulator (Integra, Princeton, NJ), as well as adjacent to the lesion with dysarthria. The rest of the cortical and subcortical mapping took place at 4 mA. The patient participated in continuous language testing with picture naming, phonetic tests, and repetition, with concurrent motor movement of the right face and arm. Positive mapping sites were designated with number tags. Negative mapping occurred initially over the cortical surface of the tumor, but dysarthria occurred anteriorly and posteriorly to the lesion (Wernicke). The corticectomy was done between the positive mapping sites, and the lesion was resected until the SLF and AF (phonetic paraphasias) medial to the lesion were encountered. When these areas were identified with positive stimulation, the resection stopped at these boundaries, and the patient was put back to sleep. Preliminary diagnosis was infiltrating glioma. The dura, bone, and skin were closed in standard fashion.

The patient awoke at their neurologic baseline with intact speech and full strength bilaterally and was taken to the intensive care unit for recovery. Postoperative MRI done within 48 hours after surgery showed gross total resection of the contrast-enhancing portion but expected FLAIR residual medial within the resection cavity (Fig. 20.2). The patient participated with physical, occupational, and speech therapy and was discharged to home on postoperative day 2 with an intact neurologic examination. The patient was prescribed 3 months of levetiracetam, and dexamethasone was tapered to off over 5 days after surgery. The patient was seen at 2 weeks postoperatively for staple removal and was full strength with intact speech. Pathology was a World Health Organization grade IV glioblastoma (IDH wild type, O6-methylguanine-DNA methyl-transferase unmethylated). The patient returned to work 3 weeks after surgery. The patient underwent adjuvant temozolomide chemotherapy with concurrent radiation therapy for 6 weeks followed by six adjuvant temozolomide cycles. The patient remains recurrence-free at 12 months after the initial surgery.

Commonalities among the experts

Most surgeons opted for patients having diffusion tensor imaging to help identify white matter tracts, and neuropsychiatry evaluation to obtain baseline neurocognitive function, and two surgeons favored the use of magnetoencephalogram to help identify eloquent cortical areas. All surgeons opted for an awake surgery with language cortical and subcortical mapping, with the majority using 5-aminolevulinic acid, and the goal was maximal resection of the enhancing and FLAIR components. Most surgeons identified the importance of awareness of language cortical areas and underlying language white matter tracts, namely the inferior frontal occipital fasciculus, and all were concerned about speech dysfunction and half were concerned about a visual field deficit. The majority of surgeons used an asleep-awake-asleep anesthetic regimen, and the remaining surgeon used an entirely awake approach. Surgery was pursued with surgical navigation, surgical microscope, ultrasonic aspirator, and brain stimulator with perioperative steroids and antiepileptics. One surgeon used intraoperative computed tomography. All surgeons used language cortical and subcortical mapping to avoid iatrogenic injuries. Following surgery, patients were typically admitted to the intensive care unit (one to the floor), and imaging was obtained within 72 hours after surgery to assess extent of resection and/or potential complications. For a diagnosis of a high-grade glioma, regardless of O6-methylguanine-DNA methyl-transferase and IDH status, all surgeons favored the use of postoperative radiation and temozolomide.

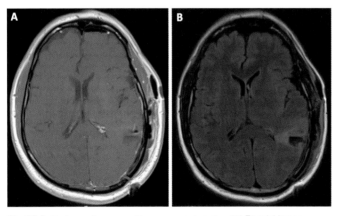

Fig. 20.2 Postoperative magnetic resonance imaging. (A) T1 axial image with gadolinium contrast; **(B)** T2 axial FLAIR magnetic resonance imaging scan demonstrating gross total resection of the contrast-enhancing portion of the tumor, but with residual fluid attenuation inversion recovery image abnormality medial to the lesion involving the Wernicke region.

SUMMARY OF QUALITY OF EVIDENCE TO GUIDE SPECIFIC INTERVENTIONS FOR THIS CASE

- Surgery as opposed to biopsy or observation for high-grade gliomas—Class II-1.
- Increasing extent of resection associated with improved outcomes for high-grade gliomas—Class II-2.
- Awake versus asleep surgery for eloquent high-grade gliomas—Class II-2.

REFERENCES

1. Sarubbo S, Latini F, Sette E, et al. Is the resection of gliomas in Wernicke's area reliable? Wernicke's area resection. *Acta Neurochir (Wien)*. 2012;154:1653–1662.
2. Wang J, Fan L, Wang Y, et al. Determination of the posterior boundary of Wernicke's area based on multimodal connectivity profiles. *Hum Brain Mapp*. 2015;36:1908–1924.
3. Hua J, Miao X, Agarwal S, et al. Language mapping using T2-prepared BOLD functional MRI in the presence of large susceptibility artifacts-initial results in patients with brain tumor and epilepsy. *Tomography*. 2017;3:105–113.
4. Eseonu CI, Rincon-Torroella J, ReFaey K, et al. Awake craniotomy vs craniotomy under general anesthesia for perirolandic gliomas: evaluating perioperative complications and extent of resection. *Neurosurgery*. 2017;81:481–489.
5. Fernandez-Miranda JC, Rhoton AL Jr., Alvarez-Linera J, Kakizawa Y, Choi C, de Oliveira EP. Three-dimensional microsurgical and tractographic anatomy of the white matter of the human brain. *Neurosurgery*. 2008;62:989–1026; discussion 1026–1028.
6. Rhoton AL Jr. The cerebrum. Anatomy. *Neurosurgery*. 2007;61:37–118; discussion 118–119.
7. Hickok G, Poeppel D. Dorsal and ventral streams: a framework for understanding aspects of the functional anatomy of language. *Cognition*. 2004;92:67–99.

21

Right insular high-grade glioma

Case reviewed by Mitchel S. Berger, Jorge Navarro-Bonnet, Ganesh Rao, George Samandouras, Matthew A. Kirkman

Introduction

The insula is a complex structure both anatomically and functionally.[1–3] Functionally, the insula plays critical roles in memory, executive function, motor integration, and motor planning, among others.[1–4] Although the majority of insular gliomas are low grade, a significant portion of high-grade gliomas can also involve the insula.[5–7] Surgery in this region is challenging because of its complex anatomic location with several adjacent critical cortical and subcortical structures, in which morbidity rates are as high as 60%, and subtotal resections rates range from 62% to 100% in several series.[4–7] In this chapter, we present a case of a nondominant insular high-grade glioma.

Example case

Chief complaint: seizures

History of present illness

A 47-year-old, right-handed woman with a history of hypertension presented with a seizure. She was working and developed generalized tonic-clonic movement with loss of consciousness. She was seen locally where an excisional biopsy was done 2 weeks prior and revealed a grade II astrocytoma, but tissue from the enhancing portion was not obtained. She is being referred for further evaluation and management (Fig. 21.1).

Medications: Lisinopril, levetiracetam.

Allergies: No known drug allergies.

Past medical and surgical history: Hypertension, right temporal biopsy 2 weeks prior.

Family history: No history of intracranial malignancies.

Social history: Nurse, smokes 1 pack per day for 20 years, social alcohol.

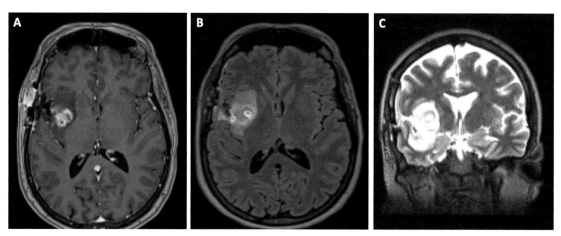

Fig. 21.1 Preoperative magnetic resonance imaging. (A) T1 axial image with gadolinium contrast; **(B)** T2 axial fluid attenuation inversion recovery image; **(C)** T2 coronal magnetic resonance imaging scan demonstrating a partially enhancing lesion involving the right insular region.

Physical examination: Awake, alert, oriented to person, place, and time; Language: intact naming and repetition; Cranial nerves II to XII intact; No drift, moves all extremities with full strength.

Imaging: Chest/abdomen/pelvis imaging negative for primary disease.

	Mitchel S. Berger, MD, University of California at San Francisco, San Francisco, CA, United States	Jorge Navarro-Bonnet, MD, Oncologic Neurosurgery, Medica Sur, Tlalpan, Mexico	Ganesh Rao, MD, Baylor College of Medicine, Houston, TX, United States	George Samandouras, MD, Matthew A. Kirkman, MEd, National Hospital for Neurology and Neurosurgery, Queen Square, London, United Kingdom
Preoperative				
Additional tests requested	DTI MEG	DTI Neuropsychological assessment EEG	DTI fMRI Neuropsychological assessment	DTI fMRI Perfusion MRI, MRS CT angiogram Neuropsychological assessment Neurooncology multidisciplinary meeting
Surgical approach selected	Right fronto-temporal craniotomy with awake motor mapping with 5-ALA	Right fronto-temporal awake craniotomy with awake cortical and subcortical mapping with 5-ALA	Right fronto-insular craniotomy with awake motor cortical and subcortical mapping	Right fronto-temporal craniotomy with intraoperative MRI and 5-ALA
Anatomic corridor	Right fronto-temporal with awake motor mapping	Right fronto-temporal trans-Sylvian	Right frontal and temporal opercula	Right trans-Sylvian, and frontal and temporal opercula
Goal of surgery	Gross total resection of enhancing and FLAIR components	Maximal safe resection	Maximal safe resection including FLAIR	Maximal safe resection including FLAIR
Perioperative				
Positioning	Right supine with left rotation	Right lateral decubitus	Right supine with left rotation	Right supine with left rotation
Surgical equipment	Surgical navigation Surgical microscope with 5-ALA Brain stimulator	Surgical navigation Ultrasound Surgical microscope with 5-ALA Brain stimulator Ultrasonic aspirator	Surgical navigation Ultrasound Surgical microscope	Surgical navigation Surgical microscope with 5-ALA Ultrasonic aspirator Intraoperative MRI
Medications	Steroids Antiepileptics	Steroids Antiepileptics	Steroids Antiepileptics	Steroids
Anatomic considerations	Insular anatomy MCA and its branches	MCA, head of the caudate and putamen	Lenticulostriate arteries medial and deep, internal capsule, Sylvian veins, primary motor cortex	M2 and M3 segments of MCA, CST at level of superior limiting insular sulcus, globus pallidus, head of caudate
Complications feared with approach chosen	Injury to MCA branches or lenticulostriate branches, as well as CST	MCA stroke, injury to internal capsule and basal ganglia	MCA and Sylvian vein injury, retraction on frontal and temporal lobes	M2 or M3 injury, motor deficit, injury to lateral lenticulostriate arteries, facial weakness
Intraoperative				
Anesthesia	Asleep-awake-asleep	Awake	Asleep-awake-asleep	General
Skin incision	Pterional	Dandy incision	Pterional	Pterional
Bone opening	Right fronto-temporal	Right fronto-temporal	Right fronto-temporal	Right fronto-temporal

(continued on next page)

	Mitchel S. Berger, MD, University of California at San Francisco, San Francisco, CA, United States	Jorge Navarro-Bonnet, MD, Oncologic Neurosurgery, Medica Sur, Tlalpan, Mexico	Ganesh Rao, MD, Baylor College of Medicine, Houston, TX, United States	George Samandouras, MD, Matthew A. Kirkman, MEd, National Hospital for Neurology and Neurosurgery, Queen Square, London, United Kingdom
Brain exposure	Right fronto-temporal	Right fronto-temporal	Right fronto-temporal	Right fronto-temporal
Method of resection	Local anesthetic in scalp, craniotomy, awaken patient, cortical mapping of frontal operculum and posteriorly until identification of face motor cortex, corticectomy based on negative mapping sites, resection of STG and frontal operculum, resection of insular component with subcortical mapping and navigation, tack up sutures, insertion of subgaleal drain	Keep patient awake from beginning to monitor for patient comfort, infiltrate skin with local anesthetic, right fronto-temporal craniotomy anterior to projection of Sylvian fissure with one-half frontal and one-half temporal, anesthetize dura, open dura monitoring for MCA vessels, Sylvian fissure opening, mapping of adjacent cortex, entry based on negative mapping areas, avoid coagulation unless necessary, safe maximal resection between vascular branches that are silent based on mapping and navigation, resection aided by navigation, ultrasound, and 5-ALA, stop resection at internal capsule	LMA placement and regional scalp block, myocutaneous flap, right fronto-temporal craniotomy, large dural opening, ultrasound to identify hyperechoic areas, awaken patient and perform motor function testing, resection of frontal and temporal opercula based on negative motor mapping, open pia of insula, periodic motor mapping, resection until all of hyperechoic area removed, place patient back under anesthesia for closure	Right fronto temporal craniotomy, dural openings, split Sylvian fissure, visualize/understand MCA anatomy, including lateral lenticulostriate arteries, open two cortical windows in the frontal and temporal opercula, join surgical cavities behind the M2 and M3 branches, obtain intraoperative MRI to confirm resection/avoid CST damage at level of superior limiting insular sulcus and globus pallidus if not infiltrated by tumor, use 5-ALA to help target enhancing components, debulk tumor with ultrasonic aspirator on low settings (tissue select medium or high and 40% amplitude), avoid bipolar cautery if possible
Complication avoidance	Cortical and subcortical mapping	Cortical and subcortical mapping, minimal bipolar cautery, stop resection at internal capsule	Resection of frontal and temporal opercula based on motor mapping, continuous motor mapping through resection	Sylvian fissure split to understand MCA anatomy, transopercular to resect insular lesion, intraoperative MRI to guide extent of resection and avoidance of critical areas, avoid bipolar coagulation
Postoperative				
Admission	ICU	Floor	ICU	Floor
Postoperative complications feared	MCA and lenticulostriate ischemia, motor deficit	MCA and Sylvian vessel ischemia, injury to internal capsule and basal ganglia	Vascular injury, damage to descending white matter tracts, motor deficit	Motor deficit, vascular injury to M2 or M3 segments as well as lenticulostriate vessels
Follow-up testing	MRI within 24 hours after surgery Full molecular panel	CT immediately after surgery MRI within 48 hours after surgery	MRI within 24 hours after surgery	MRI within 24 hours after surgery
Follow-up visits	10 days after surgery with neurooncology	10 days after surgery	7–10 days after surgery 1 month after surgery with MRI	7 days after surgery with neurooncology multidisciplinary clinic

	Mitchel S. Berger, MD, University of California at San Francisco, San Francisco, CA, United States	Jorge Navarro-Bonnet, MD, Oncologic Neurosurgery, Medica Sur, Tlalpan, Mexico	Ganesh Rao, MD, Baylor College of Medicine, Houston, TX, United States	George Samandouras, MD, Matthew A. Kirkman, MEd, National Hospital for Neurology and Neurosurgery, Queen Square, London, United Kingdom
Adjuvant therapies recommended				
IDH status	Mutant–radiation/ temozolomide +/– lomustine Wild type–radiation/ temozolomide +/– lomustine	Mutant–temozolomide Wild type–radiation/ temozolomide	Mutant–temozolomide Wild type–radiation/ temozolomide	Mutant–radiation/ temozolomide Wild type–radiation/ temozolomide
MGMT status	Methylated–radiation/ temozolomide Unmethylated– radiation/ temozolomide under 65 and radiation only over 65 years of age	Methylated– temozolomide Unmethylated–radiation/ temozolomide	Methylated– temozolomide Unmethylated–radiation/ temozolomide	Methylated–radiation/ temozolomide Unmethylated–radiation/ temozolomide

5-ALA, 5-aminolevulinic acid; lomustine; *CST*, corticospinal tract; *CT*, computed tomography; *DTI*, diffusion tensor imaging; *EEG*, electroencephalogram; *FLAIR*, fluid attenuation inversion recovery; *fMRI*, functional magnetic resonance imaging; *ICU*, intensive care unit; *LMA*, laryngeal mask airway; *MCA*, middle cerebral artery; *MEG*, magentoencepahlography; *MGMT*, O6-methylguanine-DNA methyl-transferase; *MRI*, magnetic resonance imaging; *MRS*, magnetic resonance spectroscopy; *STG*, superior temporal gyrus.

Differential diagnosis and actual diagnosis

- High-grade glioma
- Low-grade glioma (astrocytoma, oligodendroglioma)
- Demyelinating disease (i.e., multiple sclerosis)

Important anatomic and preoperative considerations

For a full description of anatomic delineations and classification schemes of insular tumors, see Chapters 7 and 8. The insula is a pyramidal-shaped structure that lies deep to the Sylvian fissure and is covered by the frontal, parietal, and temporal opercula.[1-3] The insula is separated from the adjoining cortical structures by the circular sulcus of Reil at anterior, superior, and inferior interfaces.[1-3] The insular cortex can be divided into the larger anterior insula and smaller posterior insula by the central insular sulcus.[1-3] The anterior insula is covered by the orbito-frontal operculum, whereas the posterior insula is covered superiorly by the fronto-parietal operculum and inferiorly by the temporal operculum.[1-3] The base of the insular pyramid and central portion of the insula lies lateral to the extreme capsule, claustrum, external capsule, putamen, globus pallidus, internal capsule, and thalamus in that order from lateral to medial.[1-3] Critical white matter tracts lie deep to the insula and include the arcuate (AF) and superior longitudinal fasciculi (SLF) of the dorsal language stream that lie deep, anterior and superior to the insula; inferior frontal occipital (IFOF) and uncinate fasciculi of the ventral language stream lie deep, inferior, and anterior to the insula; posterior limb of the internal capsule is medial and posterior to the insula; and the corticospinal tract within the centrum semiovale that lies medial and superior to the insula.[1-3] There are several classification schemes for tumors involving the insula.[8-10] For the full description scheme, see Chapter 8.

Approaches to this lesion

As with any intrinsic brain tumor, the surgical approaches can be divided into awake and asleep procedures (Chapter 1, Fig. 1.2). In terms of directionality, the approach is typically lateral to the insula based on the anatomy and superficial extension when nonbiopsy surgical resection is pursued. The case presented in this chapter is a Yasargil type 3A, Berger zone 1–4, Duffau AF and IFOF insular glioma. This lesion is different from other insular lesions because it does not extend to the opercula surface. This lack of extension makes the approach to this lesion somewhat less clear-cut. A nonbiopsy surgical approach can be either through a trans-Sylvian or a transopercular route.[4] In the trans-Sylvian approach, the Sylvian fissure is split widely, and resection proceeds between the perforating vessels from M2 of the middle cerebral artery (MCA).[10] The advantages of the trans-Sylvian approach are direct access to the insula without having to directly compromise the overlying frontal, parietal, and/or temporal opercula, as well as direct identification of MCA perforating vessels.[10] The disadvantage of the trans-Sylvian approach is the risk of vascular damage to these perforating vessels either from direct injury or vasospasm, and small working corridors between each of these vessels.[10] The transcortical or transopercular approach involves accessing the insula through the overlying opercula followed by entering the cortex of the insula.[5] The advantage of this approach is that it minimizes injury to and potential vasospasm of the MCA and its branches by preserving the pia around these vessels, avoids the use of retractors to hold the Sylvian fissure open, and allows easier access to lesions below the parietal opercula.[5] The disadvantage of the transopercular is that it involves transgressing the overlying opercula, which can have functional and epileptic consequences.[5] When needle biopsy is pursued, a superior frontal approach through the Kocher point is typically preferred because it avoids the MCA arteries within the Sylvian fissure, as well as the MCA perforators. This point should be anterior to the motor cortex, lateral to the sagittal stratum, and medial to the SLF/AF.

What was actually done

The patient underwent a neuropsychological evaluation that showed no deficits. The patient was taken to surgery for a right pterional craniotomy with awake motor and language mapping for resection of the lesion. The patient was intubated with a laryngeal mask airway. The scalp was blocked bilaterally with local anesthetic, and the head was fixed in pins, with two pins centered on the inion and one on the left forehead in the midpupillary line. The head was turned 45 degrees to the left, and a bump was placed under the right shoulder and hip to facilitate turning. The old linear incision over the temporal lobe was identified and extended inferiorly toward the zygoma and superiorly above the superior temporal line. The patient was draped in the usual standard fashion and given dexamethasone, levetiracetam, and cefazolin. A myocutaneous flap was formed and held in place with cerebellar retractors. The previous right pterional craniotomy was used and extended posteriorly to encompass the lesion based on preoperative magnetic resonance imaging (MRI) navigation. Ultrasound and surgical navigation were used to confirm lesion boundaries, and the boundaries were designated with letter tags once the dura was opened. The dura was anesthetized with local anesthetics between the leaflets adjacent to the middle meningeal vessels. The patient was awakened, and the dura was opened once the patient followed commands consistently. Strip electrodes were placed in the subdural space for after-discharge monitoring. The cortex was initially stimulated at 2 mA, and speech arrest occurred

with stimulating the ventral premotor cortex at 4 mA with an Ojemann stimulator (Integra, Princeton, NJ). The rest of the cortical and subcortical mapping took place at 4 mA. The patient participated in continuous language testing with picture naming with concurrent motor movement of the left face, arm, and leg. Positive mapping sites were designated with number tags. Negative mapping occurred over the frontal operculum in the region of the pars opercularis and pars triangularis, as well as the temporal operculum, and a corticectomy was done over both of these areas to access the insula. Resection took place in the insula with continuous mapping until the lateral lenticulostriates were identified anteromedially, and numbness and tingling in the leg designating the posterior limb of the internal capsule posteromedially. At the tumor depth, positive subcortical mapping occurred with stimulation of the SLF and AF that resulted in phonetic paraphasias anteromedial and superior to the tumor, and IFOF anteromedial and inferior to the tumor. Preliminary diagnosis was infiltrating glioma. Once the tumor was disconnected from the deep tracts, the patient was placed back asleep and reintubated with a laryngeal mask airway. The dura, bone, and skin were closed in standard fashion.

The patient awoke at their neurologic baseline with intact speech and full strength bilaterally and was taken to the intensive care unit for recovery. Postoperative MRI done within 48 hours after surgery showed gross total resection of the lesion but with some edema of the caudate head likely from vasospasm (Fig. 21.2). The patient participated with physical and occupational therapy and was discharged to home on postoperative day 3 with an intact neurologic examination. The patient was prescribed 3 months of levetiracetam, and dexamethasone was tapered to off over 5 days after surgery. The patient was seen at 2 weeks postoperatively for staple removal and was full strength. Pathology was a World Health Organization grade III anaplastic astrocytoma (IDH wild type, 1p/19q wild type, and O6-methylguanine-DNA methyltransferase unmethylated). The patient underwent 6 weeks of temozolomide and radiation therapy, as well as six adjuvant temozolomide cycles. The patient remains without recurrence

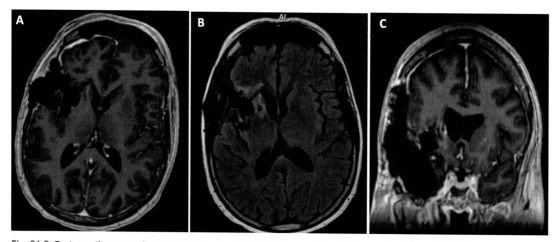

Fig. 21.2 Postoperative magnetic resonance imaging. (A) T1 axial image with gadolinium contrast; **(B)** T2 axial fluid attenuation inversion recovery image; **(C)** T1 coronal image with gadolinium contrast magnetic resonance imaging scan demonstrating gross total resection of the insular tumor including the fluid attenuation inversion recovery portion of the tumor.

at 18 months after surgery, in which the patient is being monitored with serial MRI examinations at 3-month intervals. The patient had a repeat neuropsychological evaluation at 3 months postoperatively that showed no change from preoperative evaluation. The patient returned to work at 4 weeks postoperatively and remains without neurologic deficits.

Commonalities among the experts

All surgeons opted for patients having diffusion tensor imaging to help identify white matter tracts, most requested neuropsychiatry evaluation to obtain baseline neurocognitive function, and half favored having functional MRI to help identify eloquent cortical areas. The majority of surgeons opted for an awake surgery primarily with motor cortical and subcortical mapping (two surgeons through an asleep-awake-asleep and the other an awake), with the majority using 5-aminolevulinic acid, and the goal was maximal safe resection of the enhancing and fluid attenuation inversion recovery components. The majority of surgeons opted for a transopercular approach with likely the frontal operculum, and one opted for a trans-Sylvian approach. Most surgeons identified the importance of using insular anatomy to guide resection, as well as preserving MCA lenticulostriate vessels, and all were concerned about motor deficits from injury to the MCA perforating vessels. Surgery was generally pursued with surgical navigation, surgical microscope with 5-aminolevulinic acid filter, ultrasonic aspirator, and brain stimulator with perioperative steroids and antiepileptics. One surgeon used intraoperative MRI. The majority of surgeons relied on cortical and subcortical mapping, as well as using the lenticulostriate vessels as the medial boundary to avoid iatrogenic injury. Following surgery, half of the surgeons admitted their patients to the intensive care unit and the other half to the floor, and imaging was obtained within 48 hours after surgery to assess extent of resection and/or potential complications. For a diagnosis of a high-grade glioma, regardless of O6-methylguanine-DNA methyl-transferase and IDH status, all surgeons favored the use of postoperative radiation and temozolomide.

SUMMARY OF QUALITY OF EVIDENCE TO GUIDE SPECIFIC INTERVENTIONS FOR THIS CASE

- Surgery as opposed to biopsy or observation for high-grade gliomas—Class II-1.
- Surgery as opposed for biopsy for insular high-grade gliomas—Class II-3.
- Increasing extent of resection associated with improved outcomes—Class II-2.
- Awake mapping versus asleep surgery for high-grade gliomas—Class II-2.
- Transopercular versus trans-Sylvian access for insular gliomas—Class III.

REFERENCES

1. Ribas EC, Yagmurlu K, de Oliveira E, Ribas GC, Rhoton A Jr. Microsurgical anatomy of the central core of the brain. *J Neurosurg*. 2018;129:752–769.
2. Ture U, Yasargil DC, Al-Mefty O, Yasargil MG. Topographic anatomy of the insular region. *J Neurosurg*. 1999;90:720–733.
3. Ture U, Yasargil MG, Al-Mefty O, Yasargil DC. Arteries of the insula. *J Neurosurg*. 2000;92:676–687.
4. Lu VM, Goyal A, Quinones-Hinojosa A, Chaichana KL. Updated incidence of neurological deficits following insular glioma resection: a systematic review and meta-analysis. *Clin Neurol Neurosurg*. 2018;177:20–26.
5. Duffau H. Surgery of insular gliomas. *Prog Neurol Surg*. 2018;30:173–185.
6. Eseonu CI, ReFaey K, Garcia O, Raghuraman G, Quinones-Hinojosa A. Volumetric analysis of extent of resection, survival, and surgical outcomes for insular gliomas. *World Neurosurg*. 2017;103:265–274.
7. Kim YH, Kim CY. Current surgical management of insular gliomas. *Neurosurg Clin N Am*. 2012;23:199–206. vii.
8. Mandonnet E, Capelle L, Duffau H. Extension of paralimbic low grade gliomas: toward an anatomical classification based on white matter invasion patterns. *J Neurooncol*. 2006;78:179–185.
9. Sanai N, Polley MY, Berger MS. Insular glioma resection: assessment of patient morbidity, survival, and tumor progression. *J Neurosurg*. 2010;112:1–9.
10. Yasargil MG, von Ammon K, Cavazos E, Doczi T, Reeves JD, Roth P. Tumours of the limbic and paralimbic systems. *Acta Neurochir (Wien)*. 1992;118:40–52.

22

Left insular high-grade glioma

Case reviewed by Frederick F. Lang, Linda M. Liau, Stephen J. Price, Jinsong Wu

Introduction

Surgery within the insula is associated with significant morbidity because it is adjacent to and involves critical cortical structures, white matter tracts, and cerebral vasculature.[1] The incidence of subtotal resections for insular gliomas ranges from 62% to 100% in several series.[1–4] Despite this high rate of subtotal resection, the risk of temporary and permanent deficits are 11% and 4%, respectively, in a recent meta-analysis.[1] Insular tumors, however, are far from uniform, as some extend to the opercular surface and involve eloquent cortical and subcortical structures.[1–4] In this chapter, we present a case of a large, dominant-hemisphere high-grade glioma that involves the insula and extends to the opercular surfaces.

Example case

Chief complaint: headaches and lethargy
History of present illness
A 41-year-old, right-handed, Spanish-speaking man with a history of previous biopsy of a left temporal/insular World Health Organization (WHO) grade II fibrillary astrocytoma presented with increasing headaches and lethargy. He had undergone an excisional biopsy 6 years prior of the left temporal tip with a diagnosis of a WHO grade II fibrillary astrocytoma and was lost to follow-up. Over the past 3 to 4 months, he complained of increasing headaches, lethargy, and brain imaging was concerning for disease progression (Fig. 22.1).
Medications: None.
Allergies: No known drug allergies.
Past medical and surgical history: Left temporal biopsy 6 years prior for fibrillary astrocytoma.
Family history: No history of intracranial malignancies.

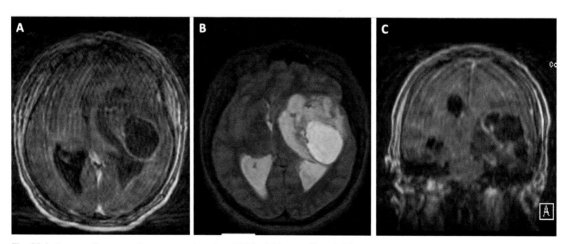

Fig. 22.1 Preoperative magnetic resonance imaging. (A) T1 axial image with gadolinium contrast; **(B)** T2 axial image; **(C)** T1 coronal image with gadolinium contrast magnetic resonance imaging scan demonstrating a large left singular contrast-enhancing tumor that extends to the frontal and temporal opercula.

Social history: Landscaper, no smoking, social alcohol.
Physical examination: Awake, alert, oriented to person, place, and time; Language: intact naming and repetition in Spanish; Cranial nerves II to XII intact; No drift, moves all extremities with full strength.

	Frederick F. Lang, MD, MD Anderson Cancer Center, Houston, TX, United States	Linda M. Liau, MD, PhD, University of California-Los Angeles, Los Angeles, CA, United States	Stephen J. Price, MBBS, PhD, University of Cambridge, Cambridge, United Kingdom	Jinsong Wu, MD, PhD, Fudan University, Huashan Hospital, Shanghai, China
Preoperative				
Additional tests requested	MRA fMRI Neuropsychological assessment	fMRI DTI Neuropsychological assessment DOPA-PET Possible Wada (sodium amytal) test	DTI Neuropsychological assessment	fMRI task-based BOLD DTI MRS Neuropsychological assessment
Surgical approach selected	Left fronto-temporal craniotomy with awake language mapping if possible after debulking	Left fronto-temporal craniotomy with awake language and motor mapping	Left pterional craniotomy with awake language and motor mapping and 5-ALA	Left modified pterional with asleep motor mapping and intraoperative MRI
Anatomic corridor	Temporal, temporal-opercular and possible trans-Sylvian	Temporal, temporal-opercular	Temporal, temporal-opercular	Left temporal-insular
Goal of surgery	Maximal safe resection of contrast-enhancing and FLAIR components	Maximal safe resection of contrast-enhancing and FLAIR components	Maximal safe resection of fluorescent tumor while preserving speech and motor	Maximal safe resection of contrast-enhancing and FLAIR components
Perioperative				
Positioning	Left supine with 45-degree right rotations	Left supine with right rotation	Left semilateral	Left supine with 45-degree right rotations
Surgical equipment	Surgical navigation Brain stimulator Ultrasonic aspirator	Surgical navigation IOM (MEP/SSEP/ECoG) Brain stimulator Surgical microscope Weck clips	Surgical navigation Brain stimulator–bipolar and monopolar IOM (SSEP, MEP) Surgical microscope with 5-ALA Ultrasonic aspirator	Surgical navigation IOM (MEP, SSEP, phase reversal) Brain stimulator Ultrasonic aspirator Intraoperative MRI
Medications	Steroids Antiepileptics Milrinone for vasospasm	Mannitol Steroids Antiepileptics	Mannitol Steroids 5-ALA	Steroids Antiepileptics
Anatomic considerations	Sylvian fissure, vein of Labbe, MCA (M1 and M2), lateral ventricle, uncus, AF, Wernicke area, CST	MCA, lenticulostriates, Broca area, internal capsule	Language areas, AF, MCA and branches	Temporal pole, STG, MTG, mesial temporal lobe, temporal stem, striatum, IFOF, ILF, optic radiation, MCA, PCA, oculomotor nerve, choroidal fissure
Complications feared with approach chosen	Language dysfunction, motor deficit	Language dysfunction, motor deficit	Language dysfunction, motor deficit	Language dysfunction, motor deficit, hemianopia
Intraoperative				
Anesthesia	Asleep-awake-asleep (if mass effect can be reduced)	Asleep-awake-asleep	Asleep-awake-asleep	General (because of mass effect)
Skin incision	Left question mark	Left curvilinear	Left question mark	Left pterional

(continued on next page)

	Frederick F. Lang, MD, MD Anderson Cancer Center, Houston, TX, United States	Linda M. Liau, MD, PhD, University of California-Los Angeles, Los Angeles, CA, United States	Stephen J. Price, MBBS, PhD, University of Cambridge, Cambridge, United Kingdom	Jinsong Wu, MD, PhD, Fudan University, Huashan Hospital, Shanghai, China
Bone opening	Left fronto-temporal	Left fronto-temporal	Left fronto-temporal	Left fronto-temporal
Brain exposure	Left fronto-temporal	Left fronto-temporal	Left fronto-temporal	Left fronto-temporal
Method of resection	Left craniotomy with navigation guidance, open dura, assess fullness of brain, drain cyst early to provide decompression if necessary, as well as hyperventilation and head elevation, if brain relaxed then wake patient up, if brain is not relaxed then safe anterior temporal lobectomy, map temporal lobe for speech to define posterior edge of temporal lobectomy, temporal lobectomy then insular resection, dissect M2 vessels from tumor, identify superior periinsular sulcus, dissect perforators off the back of M2, remove tumor based on insular anatomy	Left craniotomy, dural tack up sutures, C-shaped dural opening based anteroinferiorly, motor strip mapping to identify primary motor cortex, awaken patient to perform language mapping to identify the Broca area and other eloquent language areas, right temporal lobectomy, enter insula from temporal operculum, decompress cyst and resect insular portions of tumor, continuous language and motor mapping, watertight dural closure	Myocutaneous flap, left craniotomy, reduce bone overlying temporal fossa, temporal lobectomy while patient asleep, superior aspect through MTG and posteriorly within tumor, subpial dissection in both planes, map for motor function with strip electrode on cortical surface and phase reversal, stimulate cortex to obtain continuous MEP, wake patient up, map language namely with picture naming with neuropsychologist in English and Spanish, complete lobectomy once language areas identified, subpial dissection to expose MCA and branches in Sylvian fissure, resect posterior margin with fluorescence and mapping, medial resection using subpial dissection for fluorescent tumor, open cyst superiorly, resect fluorescent wall of cyst, language mapping over insular cortex, once language mapping complete patient is put back asleep, careful resection between insular vessels, motor mapping of deep margins using sucker with monopolar stimulator starting at 8 mA and can lower based on depth, inspect for residual fluorescence	Surgical navigation with MRS/DTI/fMRI, left fronto-temporal craniotomy based on navigation, dural tack up sutures, dural opening, strip electrode placed for phase reversal to identify central sulcus, cortical and subcortical motor mapping, outline border of tumor with navigation, cortical incisions based on negative mapping area, subpial dissection, near the Sylvian fissure the ultrasonic aspirator is changed to tissue selection, resection along periinsular sulcus and temporal lobectomy with resection of uncus and opening into ventricle, papaverine to MCA vessels, monopolar stimulation in the subcortical space, intraoperative MRI to guide further resection
Complication avoidance	Debulk tumor prior to waking up patient, language mapping, define insular sulci, dissect M2 and its perforators from tumor, identify lenticulostriate vessels	Motor strip mapping, awake language mapping, temporal lobectomy first, temporal opercular approach to insula	Asleep motor mapping, awake language mapping, temporal lobectomy first, subpial dissection, temporal opercular approach to insula, 5-ALA	Surgical navigation with DTI/fMRI, phase reversal, cortical and subcortical asleep motor mapping, continuous MEP, papaverine to vessels, intraoperative MRI
Postoperative				
Admission	ICU	ICU	Floor	ICU
Postoperative complications feared	Motor deficit, language dysfunction, visual field cut	Vasospasm of MCA vessels, language dysfunction, motor deficit	Language dysfunction, motor deficit	Motor deficit, hemianopia, aphasia, ptosis, working memory loss, emotional disorder

	Frederick F. Lang, MD, MD Anderson Cancer Center, Houston, TX, United States	Linda M. Liau, MD, PhD, University of California-Los Angeles, Los Angeles, CA, United States	Stephen J. Price, MBBS, PhD, University of Cambridge, Cambridge, United Kingdom	Jinsong Wu, MD, PhD, Fudan University, Huashan Hospital, Shanghai, China
Follow-up testing	MRI within 24 hours after surgery	MRI within 24 hours after surgery	MRI within 72 hours after surgery	Intraoperative MRI on completion of surgery or MRI within 72 hours after surgery
Follow-up visits	10 days after surgery with neurosurgery, radiation oncology, neurooncology	2 weeks after surgery	7 days after surgery	1 month after surgery
Adjuvant therapies recommended				
IDH status	Mutant–radiation/ temozolomide Wild type–radiation/ temozolomide	Mutant–radiation/ temozolomide Wild type–radiation/ temozolomide	Mutant–radiation/ temozolomide Wild type–radiation/ temozolomide	Mutant–radiation/ temozolomide Wild type–radiation/ temozolomide
MGMT status	Methylated–radiation/ temozolomide Unmethylated–radiation/ temozolomide	Methylated–radiation/ temozolomide Unmethylated–radiation/ temozolomide	Methylated–radiation/ temozolomide Unmethylated–radiation/ temozolomide	Methylated–radiation/ temozolomide Unmethylated–radiation/ temozolomide

5-ALA, 5-aminolevulinic acid; *AF*, arcuate fasciculus; *BOLD*, blood-oxygen-level-dependent; *CST*, corticospinal tract; *DOPA*, [8] F-dihydroxyphenylalanine; *DTI*, diffusion tensor imaging; *ECoG*, electrocorticography; *FLAIR*, fluid attenuation inversion recovery; *fMRI*, functional magnetic resonance imaging; *ICU*, intensive care unit; *IFOF*, inferior frontal occipital fasciculus; *ILF*, inferior longitudinal fasciculus; *IOM*, intraoperative monitoring; *MCA*, middle cerebral artery; *MEP*, motor evoked potential; *MGMT*, O6-methylguanine-DNA methyl-transferase; *MRA*, magnetic resonance angiography; *MRI*, magnetic resonance imaging; *MRS*, magnetic resonance spectroscopy; *MTG*, middle temporal gyrus; *PCA*, posterior cerebral artery; *PET*, positron emission tomography; *SSEP*, somatosensory evoked potential; *STG*, superior temporal gyrus.

Differential diagnosis and actual diagnosis

- High-grade glioma
- Low-grade glioma (astrocytoma, oligodendroglioma)

Important anatomic and preoperative considerations

For a full description of anatomic delineations and classification schemes of insular tumors, see Chapters 7 and 8. The insula is considered the fifth lobe in some nomenclature, in which the other lobes are the frontal, parietal, temporal, and occipital lobes.[5–7] The insula lies deep to the Sylvian fissure and is covered by the frontal, parietal, and temporal opercula, where it is separated from these structures by the anterior, superior, and inferior insular sulci.[5–7] On its medial surface, the insula is lateral to the extreme capsule, and in close juxtaposition to the arcuate (AF) and superior longitudinal fasciculi on its medial, anterior, and superior border; the inferior frontal occipital (IFOF) and uncinate fasciculi (UF) on its medial, anterior, and inferior border; posterior limb of the internal capsule on its medial and posterior border; and the corticospinal tract within the centrum semiovale on its medial and superior border.[5–7] Gliomas that involve the insula rarely involve just the insula, but more commonly involve the overlying opercula and the more medial white matter tracts.[5–7] There are several classification schemes for tumors involving the insula (see Chapter 8).[8–10] Yasargil et al.[10] classified gliomas limited to the insula as

type 3A, opercular involvement as type 3B, orbito-frontal and temporal-polar structures as type 5A, and mesial temporal structures as type 5B. Berger classified insular tumors into four zones by the bisection of a line through the foramen of Monro and the Sylvian fissure, in which zone 1 is the anterior-superior quadrant, zone 2 is the posterior-superior quadrant, zone 3 is the inferior-posterior quadrant, and zone 4 is the anterior-inferior quadrant.[9] Duffau classified based on white matter tract involvement (AF, IFOF, and/or UF).[8] This lesion is a Yasargil 5B, Berger zone 1–4, and Duffau AF/IFOF/UF.

Approaches to this lesion

As with any intrinsic brain tumor, the surgical approaches can be divided into awake and asleep procedures (Chapter 1, Fig. 1.2). Eloquent cortical and subcortical structures can be identified directly or indirectly (Chapter 3, Fig. 3.2). In terms of directionality, the approach to insular tumors is typically lateral (trans-Sylvian or transopercular) when nonbiopsy surgical resection is pursued. For lesions that extend to the opercular surface, an opercular approach is typically preferred because a trans-Sylvian approach would bypass the superficial portion of the tumor. In terms of opercular approaches, this can be through the frontal, temporal, and/or parietal opercula depending on the direction of opercular extension from the insula and eloquence of the overlying opercula. In the dominant hemisphere, the temporal operculum is usually safer as compared with the frontal and parietal opercula, which typically possess the Broca and Wernicke

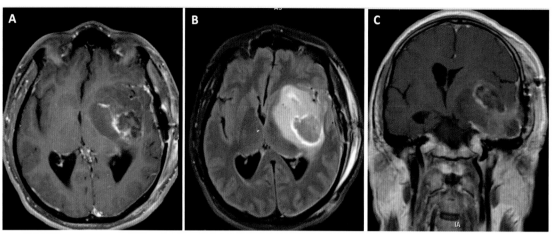

Fig. 22.2 Postoperative magnetic resonance imaging. (A) T1 axial image with gadolinium contrast; **(B)** T2 axial fluid attenuation inversion recovery image; **(C)** T1 coronal image with gadolinium contrast magnetic resonance imaging scan demonstrating subtotal resection of the insular tumor with residual within the insula.

areas, respectively. However, for larger tumors, several transopercular approaches are often required to access the lesion. In addition to a lateral approach, an anterior approach is typically what is preferred for biopsies. This approach is typically through the Kocher point, which places the superior longitudinal fasciculus and AF laterally and the cingulum medially. Because of the long working distance, this is typically only used for needle biopsies.

What was actually done

Because of the significant edema and mass effect, it was elected to perform the surgery asleep with intraoperative monitoring. The patient was taken to surgery for a left pterional craniotomy with somatosensory evoked potential and electroencephalogram for resection of the lesion. The patient was induced and intubated per routine. The head was fixed in pins, with two pins centered on the inion and one on the right forehead in the midpupillary line. The head was turned 90 degrees to the right, and a bump was placed under the left shoulder to facilitate turning. The old linear incision over the temporal lobe was identified and extended inferiorly toward the zygoma and superiorly and anteriorly to the vertex. The patient was draped in the usual standard fashion and given dexamethasone, levetiracetam, and cefazolin. A myocutaneous flap was formed and held in place with fishhooks attached to the retractor arm. The previous left pterional craniotomy was used. Ultrasound and surgical navigation were used to confirm lesion boundaries, and the boundaries were designated with letter tags once the dura was opened. The dura was opened in a semicircular fashion with the base along the sphenoid wing. A temporal lobectomy was done first spanning 4.5 cm from the temporal tip. After the this was done, the microscope was brought in for the remainder of the case. After performing the temporal lobectomy, the lesion was followed into the insula by staying within the lesion. The tumor continued to be debulked until no more grossly obvious necrotic tumor was present. Because of the wildly infiltrative lesion, it was not determined safe to resect into the frontal portion of the insula and deep

white matter tracts. Preliminary diagnosis was infiltrating glioma. The dura, bone, and skin were closed in standard fashion.

The patient awoke at their neurologic baseline with intact speech and full strength bilaterally and was taken to the intensive care unit for recovery. Postoperative magnetic resonance imaging (MRI) done within 48 hours after surgery showed subtotal resection with residual within the insula (Fig. 22.2). The patient participated with physical and occupational therapy and was discharged to home on postoperative day 3 with an intact neurologic examination. The patient was prescribed 3 months of levetiracetam, and dexamethasone was tapered to off over 7 days after surgery. The patient was seen at 2 weeks postoperatively for staple removal and was full strength. Pathology was a WHO grade IV glioblastoma (IDH mutant, O6-methylguanine-DNA methyl-transferase unmethylated). The patient underwent 6 weeks of temozolomide and radiation therapy, as well as three adjuvant temozolomide cycles. The patient had recurrence at 6 months after surgery and was started on bevacizumab. The patient died 11 months after surgery.

Commonalities among the experts

The majority of surgeons opted for having patients undergo functional MRI to identify eloquent cortical regions, diffusion tensor imaging to help identify white matter tracts, and neuropsychiatry evaluation to obtain baseline neurocognitive function prior to surgery. All surgeons elected for cortical and subcortical brain mapping (three awake through an asleep-awake-asleep anesthetic protocol, one under general). The approach was through the temporal lobe to the insula, in which the goal was maximal safe resection, in which one surgeon supplemented their surgery with 5-aminolevulinic acid, and another with intraoperative MRI. Most surgeons emphasized the importance of protecting the middle cerebral artery and its perforating arteries, avoiding eloquent language cortex and the AF, and preserving the internal capsule, in which the most feared complications were language dysfunction and motor deficits. Surgery was generally pursued with surgical navigation, surgical microscope, ultrasonic aspirator, and brain stimulator with perioperative steroids and antiepileptics. The majority of surgeons relied on cortical and subcortical mapping and addressing the temporal lobe component first to minimize risk of iatrogenic injury. Following surgery, the majority of patients were admitted to the intensive care unit (one to the floor), and imaging was obtained within 72 hours after surgery to assess extent of resection and/or potential complications. For a diagnosis of a high-grade glioma, regardless of O6-methylguanine-DNA methyl-transferase and IDH status, all surgeons favored the use of postoperative radiation and temozolomide.

SUMMARY OF QUALITY OF EVIDENCE TO GUIDE SPECIFIC INTERVENTIONS FOR THIS CASE

- Surgery as opposed to biopsy or observation for high-grade gliomas—Class II-1.
- Surgery as opposed for biopsy for insular high-grade gliomas—Class II-3.
- Increasing extent of resection associated with improved outcomes—Class II-2.
- Awake mapping versus asleep surgery for high-grade gliomas—Class II-2.
- Transopercular versus trans-Sylvian access for insular gliomas—Class III.

REFERENCES

1. Lu VM, Goyal A, Quinones-Hinojosa A, Chaichana KL. Updated incidence of neurological deficits following insular glioma resection: a systematic review and meta-analysis. *Clin Neurol Neurosurg.* 2018;177:20–26.
2. Duffau H. Surgery of insular gliomas. *Prog Neurol Surg.* 2018;30:173–185.
3. Eseonu CI, ReFaey K, Garcia O, Raghuraman G, Quinones-Hinojosa A. Volumetric analysis of extent of resection, survival, and surgical outcomes for insular gliomas. *World Neurosurg.* 2017;103:265–274.
4. Kim YH, Kim CY. Current surgical management of insular gliomas. *Neurosurg Clin N Am.* 2012;23:199–206. vii.
5. Ribas EC, Yagmurlu K, de Oliveira E, Ribas GC, Rhoton A Jr. Microsurgical anatomy of the central core of the brain. *J Neurosurg.* 2018;129:752–769.
6. Ture U, Yasargil DC, Al-Mefty O, Yasargil MG. Topographic anatomy of the insular region. *J Neurosurg.* 1999;90:720–733.
7. Ture U, Yasargil MG, Al-Mefty O, Yasargil DC. Arteries of the insula. *J Neurosurg.* 2000;92:676–687.
8. Mandonnet E, Capelle L, Duffau H. Extension of paralimbic low grade gliomas: toward an anatomical classification based on white matter invasion patterns. *J Neurooncol.* 2006;78:179–185.
9. Sanai N, Polley MY, Berger MS. Insular glioma resection: assessment of patient morbidity, survival, and tumor progression. *J Neurosurg.* 2010;112:1–9.
10. Yasargil MG, von Ammon K, Cavazos E, Doczi T, Reeves JD, Roth P. Tumours of the limbic and paralimbic systems. *Acta Neurochir (Wien).* 1992;118:40–52.

23

Left temporal high-grade glioma

Case reviewed by Hossam El-Husseiny, Gordon Li, Walter Stummer, Robert E. Wharen

Introduction

A common location for high-grade gliomas is the temporal lobe.[1-4] In most series, this number ranges from 15% to 25%.[1-4] Patients with dominant-hemisphere temporal lobe gliomas most commonly present with seizures, but those that do not typically have subtle deficits in attention, object naming, and language as compared with right temporal lobe lesions.[1-4] In this chapter, we present a case of a dominant-hemisphere temporal lobe high-grade glioma.

Example case

Chief complaint: confusion
History of present illness
A 44-year-old, right-handed man with a history of traumatic brain injury (TBI) with left-sided ventriculoperitoneal shunt (VPS) 20 years prior presented with confusion. He had sustained a TBI after a motor vehicle accident (MVA) and developed hydrocephalus requiring a left frontal VPS (nonprogrammable) 20 years prior. Over the past 3 weeks, his parents noted that he has become increasingly confused with the time of day and where he is. He denies any loss of consciousness, staring episodes, or arm/leg shaking. Imaging was done and revealed a brain lesion (Fig. 23.1).
Medications: None.
Allergies: No known drug allergies.
Past medical and surgical history: Right VPS after MVA and TBI.
Family history: No history of intracranial malignancies.
Social history: Dependent on his parents for activities of daily living after MVA. No smoking or alcohol.
Physical examination: Awake, alert, oriented to person, place, and time; Language: intact naming and repetition; Cranial nerves II to XII intact; No drift, moves all extremities with full strength.
Imaging: Chest/abdomen/pelvis with no evidence of primary disease.

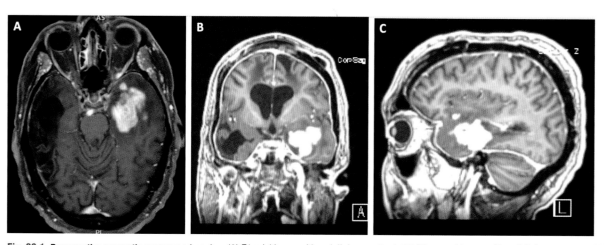

Fig. 23.1 Preoperative magnetic resonance imaging. (A) T1 axial image with gadolinium contrast; **(B)** T1 coronal image with gadolinium contrast; **(C)** T1 sagittal with gadolinium contrast magnetic resonance imaging scan demonstrating a contrast-enhancing lesion involving the left temporal lobe.

	Hossam El-Husseiny, MBBS, Ain Shams University, Cairo, Egypt	Gordon Li, MD, Stanford University, Palo Alto, CA, United States	Walter Stummer, MD, PhD, University of Munster, Munster, NRW, Germany	Robert E. Wharen, MD, Mayo Clinic, Jacksonville, FL, United States
Preoperative				
Additional tests requested	fMRI MRI flowmetry MRS EEG Neuroophthalmology evaluation	None	fMRI DTI Language evaluation	fMRI Wada test Neuropsychological assessment Neurooncology evaluation
Surgical approach selected	Left temporal awake craniotomy with speech and motor mapping	Left temporal craniotomy	Left temporal awake craniotomy with 5-ALA and language mapping	Left temporal awake craniotomy with language mapping (after determining patency of shunt)
Anatomic corridor	Left temporal	Left temporal	Left temporal	Left temporal
Goal of surgery	Decompression, diagnosis	Complete resection of enhancing portion and as much FLAIR as possible	Complete safe resection of fluorescent components that typically extend past enhancement	Extensive resection of enhancing portion without neurologic compromise
Perioperative				
Positioning	Left supine with 60 degree right rotation	Left supine	Left supine	Left supine
Surgical equipment	Ultrasound Brain stimulator	Surgical navigation Surgical microscope Ultrasonic aspirator	Surgical navigation Ultrasound Brain stimulator Surgical microscope with 5-ALA Ultrasonic aspirator	Surgical navigation Brain stimulator Surgical microscope
Medications	Steroids Antiepileptics	Steroids	Steroids	Steroids Antiepileptics
Anatomic considerations	Speech centers	Sylvian fissure, Wernicke, pial boundary	Wernicke, Ludders temporobasal language, IFOF, AF, choroidal fissure, internal capsule, cranial nerve 3	Speech and memory centers
Complications feared with approach chosen	Language dysfunction, upper quadrantopsia	Language dysfunction	Language dysfunction, quadrantopsia, cranial 3 palsy	Language dysfunction, memory issues
Intraoperative				
Anesthesia	Asleep-awake-asleep	General	Awake-awake-awake (asleep)	Asleep-awake-asleep
Skin incision	Pterional	Question mark	Pterional	Question mark
Bone opening	Left temporal	Left temporal	Left fronto-temporal	Left temporal
Brain exposure	Left temporal	Left temporal	Left fronto-temporal	Left temporal

(continued on next page)

	Hossam El-Husseiny, MBBS, Ain Shams University, Cairo, Egypt	Gordon Li, MD, Stanford University, Palo Alto, CA, United States	Walter Stummer, MD, PhD, University of Munster, Munster, NRW, Germany	Robert E. Wharen, MD, Mayo Clinic, Jacksonville, FL, United States
Method of resection	Left temporal myocutaneous flap, left temporal craniotomy with drilling down toward skull base, dural tack up sutures, awaken patient after dural opening, ultrasound to localize lesion, speech and motor mapping with cortical and subcortical stimulation, subpial anterior lobectomy, put patient back to asleep for closure	Myocutaneous flap, craniotomy based on navigation, dural opening, corticectomy anterior and low to the lesion, attempt to dissect planes, internally debulk with ultrasonic aspirator if margins are not apparent, debulk to margins, subpial dissection medially to ensure medial borders, extend resection to anterior middle fossa dura, go to floor for inferior margin, confirm posterior margin with navigation	Scalp block, position while responsive, deepen sedation for craniotomy, left temporal craniotomy, reduce sedation, dural opening, language mapping in exposed temporal cortex and find positive mapping over the Broca area, map temporal lobe, resect posterior margin based on fluorescence, then cranial and then medial and along Sylvian fissure/parahippocampal gyrus/hippocampus, subpial dissection into choroidal fissure to border of fluorescence	Preoperative scalp block, myocutaneous flap, right temporal craniotomy, cortical language mapping, enter tumor anterior ITG, resect contrast-enhancement with continuous language and memory testing
Complication avoidance	Awake motor and speech mapping, anterior temporal lobectomy, ultrasound to localize, subpial dissection	Subpial dissection, anatomic boundaries, attempted en bloc resection	Language mapping, fluorescence, subpial dissection	Language and memory mapping, enter anterior ITG
Postoperative				
Admission	ICU	ICU	ICU or intermediate care	ICU
Postoperative complications feared	Language dysfunction, visual field deficit	Seizures, stroke	Language dysfunction, visual field deficit	Language dysfunction, memory loss
Follow-up testing	MRI within 48 hours after surgery	MRI within 24 hours after surgery	MRI within 48 hours after surgery	MRI within 48 hours after surgery
Follow-up visits	2 months after surgery Neuropsychological assessment 2 months after surgery	10 days after surgery with radiation and neurooncology	3 months after surgery	2 weeks after surgery with neuro and radiation oncology
Adjuvant therapies recommended				
IDH status	Referral to neurooncology and radiation oncology	Mutant–radiation/temozolomide Wild type–radiation/temozolomide Consideration of TTF	Mutant–radiation/temozolomide +/– TTF Wild type–radiation/temozolomide +/– TTF	Mutant–determined by neuro and radiation oncology Wild type–determined by neuro and radiation oncology
MGMT status	Referral to neurooncology and radiation oncology	Methylated–radiation/temozolomide Unmethylated–radiation/temozolomide Consideration of TTF	Methylated– radiation/temozolomide +/– TTF Unmethylated–radiation/temozolomide +/– TTF	Methylated–determined by neuro and radiation oncology Unmethylated–determined by neuro and radiation oncology

5-ALA, 5-aminolevulinic acid; AF, arcuate fasciculus; DTI, diffusion tensor imaging; EEG, electroencephalogram; FLAIR, fluid attenuation inversion recovery; fMRI, functional magnetic resonance imaging; ICU, intensive care unit; IFOF, inferior frontal occipital fasciculus; ITG, inferior temporal gyrus; MGMT, O6-methylguanine-DNA methyl-transferase; MRI, magnetic resonance imaging; MRS, magnetic resonance spectroscopy; TTF, tumor treatment fields.

Differential diagnosis and actual diagnosis

- High-grade glioma
- Metastatic brain tumor
- Lymphoma
- Low-grade glioma (pilocytic astrocytoma, oligodendroglioma)

Important anatomic and preoperative considerations

For a full description of the temporal lobe anatomy, see Chapters 10 and 11. The temporal lobe is separated from the frontal and parietal lobe by the Sylvian fissure and the occipital lobe by an imaginary line between the preoccipital notch and the parieto-occipital sulcus on the medial aspect of the hemisphere.[5,6] On the lateral surface or the temporal lobe is the superior temporal gyrus (STG), middle temporal gyrus (MTG), and inferior temporal gyrus (ITG) that are separated by the superior temporal sulcus between the STG and MTG, and the inferior temporal sulcus between the MTG and the ITG.[5,6] The inferior surface of the temporal lobe consists of the inferior temporal, fusiform, and parahippocampal gyri, in which the occipitotemporal sulcus separates the inferior temporal from the fusiform gyrus, and the collateral sulcus separates the fusiform from the parahippocampal gyrus.[5,6] More anteriorly, the collateral sulcus becomes the rhinal sulcus that divides the uncus from the temporal pole.[5,6] The Wernicke area is typically along the posterior STG and superior temporal sulcus, but there is individual variability.[7,8] To minimize damage to the Wernicke area, most advocate for lobectomies in the dominant hemisphere that are no greater than 5.5 cm from the temporal tip.[7,8]

Approaches to this lesion

As stated in Chapter 1, Fig. 1.2, the general approaches for these intrinsic lesions can be divided into asleep versus awake surgery.[9–14] Asleep surgery can be done with or without monitoring, in which monitoring involves somatosensory evoked potentials, motor evoked potentials, and/or electroencephalography that are all indirect methods of identifying and monitoring elqoeunce.[13,14] For temporal lobe lesions, the use of these monitoring modalities are limited, as they provide extratemporal monitoring that may not provide sufficient neurologic feedback from surgery in the temporal lobe.[13,14] Awake brain mapping, however, can be used to directly identify and avoid eloquent cortical and subcortical regions to minimize surgical morbidity. This, however, requires a cooperative patient.

In terms of directionality, the most common approach is lateral, in which the lateral entry can be through some combination of STG, MTG, and/or ITG, as the lesion is below the cortical surface. The access through more inferior gyri exposes less of the Sylvian fissure and potentially the Broca area to risk. As the lesion is resected more medially, the inferior frontal occipital fasciculus and uncinate fasciculus will come into play on the medial surface.

What was actually done

The patient was taken to surgery for a left temporal craniotomy without monitoring for resection of the lesion because of his depressed cognitive state from his TBI. The patient was induced and intubated per routine. The head was fixed in pins, with two pins centered on the inion and one on the right forehead in the midpupillary line, making sure to identify and avoid the shunt catheter. The head was turned 90 degrees to the right, and a bump was placed under the left shoulder to facilitate turning. A linear incision was made that extended from the zygoma to just above the superior temporal line. The patient was draped in the usual standard fashion and given dexamethasone, levetiracetam, and cefazolin. A myocutaneous flap was formed and held in place with cerebellar retractors. A left temporal craniotomy was done that encompassed the lesion based on surgical navigation. Ultrasound and surgical navigation were used to confirm lesion boundaries, and the boundaries were designated with letter tags once the dura was opened. The dura was opened in a semicircular fashion with the base along the sphenoid wing. A temporal lobectomy was done by entering the lesion through the middle temporal gyri at the posterior aspect of the lesion based on navigation and ultrasound. The tumor was removed piecemeal until white matter was seen on all the edges. Preliminary diagnosis was infiltrating glioma. The dura, bone, and skin were closed in standard fashion.

The patient awoke at their neurologic baseline with intact speech and full strength bilaterally and was taken to the intensive care unit for recovery. Postoperative magnetic resonance imaging done within 48 hours after surgery showed gross resection of the contrast-enhancing portion of the tumor (Fig. 23.2). The patient participated with physical and occupational therapy and was discharged to home on postoperative day 2 with an intact neurologic examination. The patient was prescribed 3 months of levetiracetam, and dexamethasone was tapered to off over 5 days after surgery. The patient was seen at 2 weeks postoperatively for staple removal and was neurologically intact. Pathology was a World Health Organization grade IV glioblastoma (IDH mutant, O6-methylguanine-DNA methyl-transferase unmethylated). The patient underwent 6 weeks of temozolomide and radiation therapy, as well as six adjuvant temozolomide cycles. The patient has been without recurrence for 12 months after his surgery.

Commonalities among the experts

The majority of surgeons opted for patients having functional magnetic resonance imaging to identify eloquent cortical regions prior to surgery. In addition, the majority of surgeons elected for performing this surgery with awake language mapping through an asleep-awake-asleep anesthetic protocol, in which the trajectory in all was through the temporal lobe. One surgeon supplemented their surgery with 5-aminolevulinic acid. The goal of surgery was generally maximal resection of the enhancing tumor portion. Most surgeons identified the importance of protecting the language centers, as well as the Sylvian fissure, in which the most feared complications was language dysfunction. Surgery was generally pursued with surgical navigation, surgical microscope, and brain stimulator with perioperative

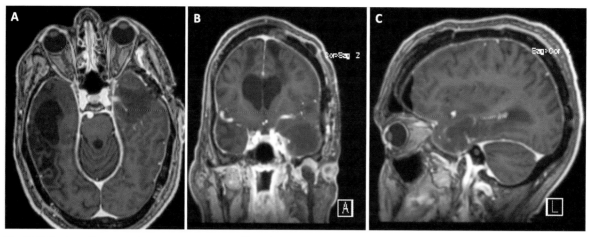

Fig. 23.2 Postoperative magnetic resonance imaging. (A) T1 axial image with gadolinium contrast; **(B)** T1 coronal image with gadolinium contrast; **(C)** T1 sagittal with gadolinium contrast magnetic resonance imaging scan demonstrating gross total resection of the contrast-enhancing portion of the lesion involving the left temporal lobe.

steroids and antiepileptics. The majority of surgeons relied on cortical and subcortical mapping, as well as subpial dissection to minimize risk of iatrogenic injury. Following surgery, all patients were admitted to the intensive care unit, and imaging was obtained within 48 hours after surgery to assess extent of resection and/or potential complications. For a diagnosis of a high-grade glioma, regardless of O6-methylguanine-DNA methyl-transferase and IDH status, all surgeons favored the use of postoperative radiation and temozolomide. One surgeon also suggested possible use of tumor treatment fields.

SUMMARY OF QUALITY OF EVIDENCE TO GUIDE SPECIFIC INTERVENTIONS FOR THIS CASE

- Surgery as opposed to biopsy or observation for high-grade gliomas—Class II-1.
- Increasing extent of resection associated with improved outcomes—Class II-2.
- Awake mapping versus asleep surgery for high-grade gliomas—Class II-2.

REFERENCES

1. Chaichana KL, Jusue-Torres I, Navarro-Ramirez R, et al. Establishing percent resection and residual volume thresholds affecting survival and recurrence for patients with newly diagnosed intracranial glioblastoma. *Neuro Oncol.* 2014;16:113–122.
2. Lacroix M, Abi-Said D, Fourney DR, et al. A multivariate analysis of 416 patients with glioblastoma multiforme: prognosis, extent of resection, and survival. *J Neurosurg.* 2001;95:190–198.
3. McGirt MJ, Chaichana KL, Gathinji M, et al. Independent association of extent of resection with survival in patients with malignant brain astrocytoma. *J Neurosurg.* 2009;110:156–162.
4. Sanai N, Polley MY, McDermott MW, Parsa AT, Berger MS. An extent of resection threshold for newly diagnosed glioblastomas. *J Neurosurg.* 2011;115:3–8.
5. Fernandez-Miranda JC, Rhoton AL Jr., Alvarez-Linera J, Kakizawa Y, Choi C, de Oliveira EP. Three-dimensional microsurgical and tractographic anatomy of the white matter of the human brain. *Neurosurgery.* 2008;62:989–1026; discussion 1026–1028.
6. Rhoton AL Jr. The cerebrum. Anatomy. *Neurosurgery.* 2007; 61:37–118; discussion 118–119.
7. Sarubbo S, Latini F, Sette E, et al. Is the resection of gliomas in Wernicke's area reliable?: Wernicke's area resection. *Acta Neurochir (Wien).* 2012;154:1653–1662.
8. Wang J, Fan L, Wang Y, et al. Determination of the posterior boundary of Wernicke's area based on multimodal connectivity profiles. *Hum Brain Mapp.* 2015;36:1908–1924.
9. Duffau H. The reliability of asleep-awake-asleep protocol for intraoperative functional mapping and cognitive monitoring in glioma surgery. *Acta Neurochir (Wien).* 2013;155:1803–1804.
10. Eseonu CI, Eguia F, Garcia O, Kaplan PW, Quinones-Hinojosa A. Comparative analysis of monotherapy versus duotherapy antiseizure drug management for postoperative seizure control in patients undergoing an awake craniotomy. *J Neurosurg.* 2018;128:1661–1667.
11. Eseonu CI, Eguia F, ReFaey K, et al. Comparative volumetric analysis of the extent of resection of molecularly and histologically distinct low grade gliomas and its role on survival. *J Neurooncol.* 2017;134:65–74.
12. Eseonu CI, Rincon-Torroella J, ReFaey K, et al. Awake craniotomy vs craniotomy under general anesthesia for perirolandic gliomas: evaluating perioperative complications and extent of resection. *Neurosurgery.* 2017;81:481–489.
13. Bertani G, Fava E, Casaceli G, et al. Intraoperative mapping and monitoring of brain functions for the resection of low-grade gliomas: technical considerations. *Neurosurg Focus.* 2009;27:E4.
14. Nossek E, Korn A, Shahar T, et al. Intraoperative mapping and monitoring of the corticospinal tracts with neurophysiological assessment and 3-dimensional ultrasonography-based navigation. Clinical article. *J Neurosurg.* 2011;114:738–746.

24

Right temporal high-grade glioma

Case reviewed by Ricardo Díez Valle, Peter Nakaji, Ian F. Parney, Shota Tanaka

Introduction

A relatively common location for high-grade gliomas is the temporal lobe, in which the incidence ranges from 15% to 25% in several series.[1–4] Patients with temporal lobe gliomas typically present with seizures but can have more subtle deficits in neurocognitive function, including attention, object naming, and language.[5,6] Although nondominant temporal lobe lesions are considered to have lower risk profiles than corresponding lesions in the dominant hemisphere, surgery can still be associated with significant morbidity.[5,6] In this chapter, we present a case of a right temporal lobe high-grade glioma.

Example case

Chief complaint: confusion

History of present illness

A 65-year-old, right-handed man with a history of coronary artery disease and hypertension presented with acute confusion. He was in his usual state of health until earlier this morning when he had an acute onset of confusion on awakening in which he did not know where he was or what time of day it was. This was witnessed by his wife. He was taken to the emergency room, where imaging revealed a brain lesion. He denies any loss of consciousness, arm/leg shaking, or urinary incontinence (Fig. 24.1).

Medications: Lisinopril, metoprolol, aspirin.

Allergies: No known drug allergies.

Past medical and surgical history: Coronary artery disease, hypertension, cholecystectomy, appendectomy.

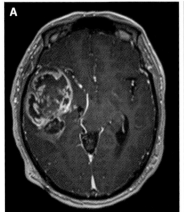
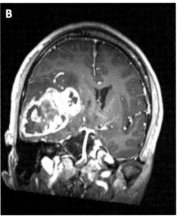
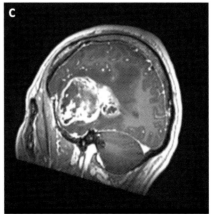

Fig. 24.1 Preoperative magnetic resonance imaging. (A) T1 axial image with gadolinium contrast; **(B)** T1 coronal image with gadolinium contrast; **(C)** T1 sagittal with gadolinium contrast magnetic resonance imaging scan demonstrating a contrast-enhancing lesion involving the right temporal lobe.

Family history: No history of intracranial malignancies.

Social history: Store owner, 0.5 pack/day for 30-year smoking history, social drinker.

Physical examination: Awake, alert, oriented to person, place, and time; Language: intact naming and repetition; Cranial nerves II to XII intact; No drift, moves all extremities with full strength.

Imaging: Chest/abdomen/pelvis with no evidence of primary disease.

	Ricardo Díez Valle, MD, PhD, Fundación Jiménez Díaz University Clinic, Madrid, Spain	Peter Nakaji, MD, Barrow Neurological Institute, Phoenix, AZ, United States	Ian F. Parney, MD, PhD, Mayo Clinic, Rochester, MN, United States	Shota Tanaka, MD, PhD, The University of Tokyo, Tokyo, Japan
Preoperative				
Additional tests requested	DTI Cardiology evaluation	DTI fMRI	None	DTI PET FDG Chest/abdomen/pelvis CT Cardiac ultrasound
Surgical approach selected	Right temporal craniotomy with 5-ALA and asleep motor mapping	Right temporal craniotomy with fluorescein	Right fronto-temporal craniotomy with possible fluorescence	Right fronto-temporal craniotomy with 5-ALA and asleep motor mapping
Anatomic corridor	Right temporal	Right ITG, MTG	Right temporal	Right temporal
Goal of surgery	Gross total resection of enhancing component guided by mapping	Maximal resection, decrease mass effect	Gross total resection of enhancing component	Gross total resection of enhancing component
Perioperative				
Positioning	Right supine with 90-degree left rotation	Right supine with left rotation	Right supine with left rotation	Right supine with left rotation
Surgical equipment	Surgical navigation Surgical microscope with 5-ALA IOM (MEP) Brain stimulator	Surgical navigation IOM (MEP, SSEP) Surgical microscope with fluorescein	Surgical navigation Ultrasonic aspirator Surgical microscope +/– fluorescence	Surgical navigation IOM (MEP) Brain stimulator Surgical microscope with 5-ALA Doppler
Medications	Steroids	Steroids	Steroids Antiepileptics Mannitol	Steroids Antiepileptics Mannitol
Anatomic considerations	Basal ganglia, internal capsule, temporal horn, PCA, MCA branches	Basal ganglia, internal capsule	MCA, lateral lenticulostriate arteries, basal ganglia	CST, internal capsule
Complications feared with approach chosen	Vascular injury, damage to internal capsule	Motor deficit	Stroke	Motor deficit
Intraoperative				
Anesthesia	General	General	General	General
Skin incision	Mini pterional	Linear	Pterional	Curved pterional
Bone opening	Right temporal	Right temporal	Right fronto-temporal	Right fronto-temporal
Brain exposure	Right temporal	Right temporal	Right temporal	Right fronto-temporal

	Ricardo Díez Valle, MD, PhD, Fundación Jiménez Díaz University Clinic, Madrid, Spain	Peter Nakaji, MD, Barrow Neurological Institute, Phoenix, AZ, United States	Ian F. Parney, MD, PhD, Mayo Clinic, Rochester, MN, United States	Shota Tanaka, MD, PhD, The University of Tokyo, Tokyo, Japan
Method of resection	Mini pterional incision, fascial and muscle opening in separate layers, craniotomy based on navigation, dural opening, cortical entry based on navigation and most superficial portion, debulk necrotic tumor first if brain is full, 5-ALA-guided resection, access to basal cistern to relax brain, continue debulking with forceps and bipolar, monopolar stimulation at deep and medial aspects of the tumor, resection of red fluorescence completely and pale fluorescence based on mapping, intraoperative MRI to assess for further resection	Small temporal craniotomy, intratumoral debulking, anterior temporal lobectomy, subpial removal along anterior Sylvian fissure, care along posterior and deep portions, leave residual if necessary, fluorescein to help guide additional resection	Right fronto-temporal craniotomy, dural openings, attempted en bloc resection under microscopic visualization +/– fluorescence, further resection of obvious residual +/– fluorescence	Navigation and transcranial MEP monitoring setup, right fronto-temporal craniotomy, dural opening, right temporal lobectomy with 5-ALA under microscopic visualization, further resection with subcortical stimulation at bottom of resection cavity to prevent pyramidal tract injury
Complication avoidance	Avoid ultrasonic aspirator, resection limited first to 5-ALA positive areas, cortical and subcortical asleep mapping	Anterior temporal lobectomy, subpial dissection along Sylvian fissure, caution along posterior and medial portions, fluorescein	En bloc resection, possible fluorescence-guided resection	Temporal lobectomy, 5-ALA, subcortical stimulation of CST

Postoperative

Admission	ICU	ICU	ICU	ICU
Postoperative complications feared	Motor deficit, hemianopsia	Motor deficit	Motor deficit	Stroke
Follow-up testing	MRI within 24 hours after surgery	MRI within 48 hours after surgery Physical, occupational, speech therapy	MRI within 24 hours after surgery	MRI within 48 hours after surgery
Follow-up visits	7 days after surgery	10–14 days after surgery	3 months after surgery 7 days after surgery with radiation and neurooncology	14–21 days after surgery

Adjuvant therapies recommended

IDH status	Mutant–radiation/ temozolomide Wild type–radiation/ temozolomide	Mutant–radiation/ temozolomide Wild type–radiation/ temozolomide	Mutant–possible second look surgery of FLAIR Wild type–radiation/ temozolomide +/– TTF	Mutant–radiation/ temozolomide Wild type–radiation/ temozolomide
MGMT status	Methylated–radiation/ temozolomide Unmethylated–radiation/ temozolomide	Methylated–radiation/ temozolomide Unmethylated–radiation/ temozolomide	Methylated–radiation/ temozolomide +/– TTF Unmethylated–radiation/ temozolomide +/– TTF	Methylated–radiation/ temozolomide Unmethylated–radiation/ temozolomide

5-ALA, 5-aminolevulinic acid; CST, corticospinal tract; CT, computed tomography; DTI, diffusion tensor imaging; FDG, fludeoxyglucose; FLAIR, fluid attenuation inversion recovery; fMRI, functional magnetic resonance imaging; ICU, intensive care unit; IOM, intraoperative monitoring; ITG, inferior temporal gyrus; MCA, middle cerebral artery; MEP, motor evoked potentials; MGMT, O6-methylguanine-DNA methyl-transferase; MRI, magnetic resonance imaging; MTG, middle temporal gyrus; PCA, posterior cerebral artery; PET, positron emission tomography; SSEP, somatosensory evoked potentials; TTG, tumor treatment fields.

Differential diagnosis and actual diagnosis

- High-grade glioma
- Metastatic brain tumor
- Lymphoma

Important anatomic and preoperative considerations

For a full description of the temporal lobe anatomy, see Chapters 10 and 11. The temporal lobe has lateral, inferior, medial, and anterior surfaces.[7,8] On the lateral surface, the superior and inferior temporal sulci divide the temporal lobe into the superior temporal gyrus, middle temporal gyrus, and inferior temporal gyrus (ITG)[7,8] The inferior surface of the temporal lobe consists of the ITG, fusiform, and parahippocampal gyri, in which the occipitotemporal sulcus separates the inferior temporal from the fusiform gyrus, and the collateral sulcus separates the fusiform from the parahippocampal gyrus.[7,8] More anteriorly, the collateral sulcus becomes the rhinal sulcus that divides the uncus from the temporal pole.[7,8] The medial surface is formed by the uncus anteriorly and the parahippocampal gyrus posteriorly, and the anterior surface is the temporal pole laterally and the uncus medially.[7,8] The important white matter tracts in the area of the anterior temporal lobe include the inferior longitudinal fasciculus (ILF), uncinate fasciculus (UF), inferior frontal occipital fasciculus (IFOF), and optic radiations. The ILF is an associative white matter tract that connects the occipital and occipital-temporal areas with the anterior temporal areas, in which injury typically results in neuropsychological impairments of visual cognition, including visual agnosia, prosopagnosia, and alexia.[7,8] Medial and dorsal to the ILF is the IFOF, which runs at the level of the external capsule medial to the corona radiata and connects the occipital lobe with the inferior frontal lobe.[7,8] Injury to the IFOF can lead to semantic paraphasias.[7,8] The UF connects the mesial portion of the temporal lobe and the limbic system with the orbitofrontal cortex, and plays a role in auditory-verbal and declarative memory.[7,8]

Approaches to this lesion

As stated in Chapter 1, Fig. 1.2, the general approaches for these intrinsic lesions can be divided into asleep versus awake surgery.[9–14] Asleep surgery can be done with or without monitoring, in which monitoring involves somatosensory evoked potentials and/or motor evoked potentials that are all indirect methods of primarily identifying and monitoring the motor and sensory pathways, which are not involved in temporal lobe surgery.[13,14] Awake brain mapping, however, can be used to directly identify and avoid eloquent cortical and subcortical regions to minimize surgical morbidity. This, however, requires a cooperative patient and is more challenging in larger tumors with more edema, as the ability to hyperventilate is obviated.[9,12]

In terms of directionality, the most common approach is lateral, in which the lateral entry can be through some combination of superior temporal gyrus, middle temporal gyrus, and/or ITG as the lesion is below the cortical surface. The access through more inferior gyri exposes less of the Sylvian fissure and potentially the Broca area to risk. As the lesion is resected more medially, the ILF, IFOF, and optic radiations can be injured, as well as the UF more anteriormedially.

What was actually done

The patient was taken to surgery for a right temporal craniotomy without monitoring for resection of the lesion without awake mapping because of the significant mass effect associated with the lesion. The patient was induced and intubated per routine. The head was fixed in pins, with two pins centered on the inion and one on the left forehead in the midpupillary line. The head was turned 90 degrees to the left, and a bump was placed under the right shoulder to facilitate turning. A pterional incision was planned from the root of the zygoma to the vertex, making sure to stay posterior to the lesion on surgical navigation. The patient was draped in the usual standard fashion and given dexamethasone, levetiracetam, and cefazolin. A myocutaneous flap was formed and held in place with fishhooks attached to a retractor arm. A right pterional craniotomy that was more temporally based was done that encompassed the lesion based on surgical navigation. Ultrasound and surgical navigation were used to confirm lesion boundaries, and the boundaries were designated with letter tags once the dura was opened. The dura was opened in a semicircular fashion with the base along the sphenoid wing. A temporal lobectomy was done by entering the lesion through the middle temporal gyri at the posterior aspect of the lesion based on navigation and ultrasound. Once the middle and inferior temporal components were removed, the superior temporal portion was removed making sure to preserve the pia over the Sylvian fissure. The insula was then entered, and the tumor was removed until white matter was seen on all the edges. Preliminary diagnosis was infiltrating glioma. The dura, bone, and skin were closed in standard fashion.

The patient awoke at their neurologic baseline with intact speech and full strength bilaterally and was taken to the intensive care unit for recovery. Postoperative magnetic resonance imaging done within 48 hours after surgery showed gross resection of the contrast-enhancing portion of the tumor (Fig. 24.2). The patient participated with physical and occupational therapy and was discharged to home on postoperative day 2 with an intact neurologic examination. The patient was prescribed 3 months of levetiracetam, and dexamethasone was tapered to off over 7 days after surgery. The patient was seen at 2 weeks postoperatively for staple removal and was neurologically intact. Pathology was a World Health Organization grade IV glioblastoma (IDH wild type, O6-methylguanine-DNA methyl-transferase unmethylated). The patient underwent 6 weeks of temozolomide and radiation therapy, as well as five adjuvant temozolomide cycles that were stopped because of thrombocytopenia. The patient had recurrence at 12 months after surgery and was started on bevacizumab. The patient died 16 months after surgery.

Commonalities among the experts

The majority of surgeons opted for patients having diffusion tensor imaging to identify white matter tracts prior to surgery. All surgeons elected for performing this surgery with

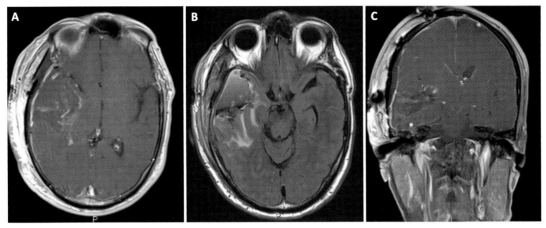

Fig. 24.2 Postoperative magnetic resonance imaging. (A) T1 axial image with gadolinium contrast; **(B)** T2 axial fluid attenuation inversion recovery image; **(C)** T1 coronal with gadolinium contrast magnetic resonance imaging scan demonstrating gross total resection of the contrast-enhancing portion of the lesion involving the right temporal lobe.

general anesthesia with fluorescence (half 5-aminolevulinic acid, half fluorescein), in which the trajectory in all was through the temporal lobe. Half of the surgeons also employed asleep motor mapping to identify the internal capsule. The goal of surgery in all surgeons was gross total resection of the enhancing portion. Most surgeons identified the importance of protecting the basal ganglia and internal capsule, in which the most feared complication was a motor deficit. Surgery was generally pursued with surgical navigation, surgical microscope with fluorescent filter, intraoperative monitoring, and brain stimulator with perioperative steroids and antiepileptics. The majority of surgeons relied on performing a temporal lobectomy and fluorescent-guided resection to minimize risk of iatrogenic injury. Following surgery, all patients were admitted to the intensive care unit, and imaging was obtained within 48 hours after surgery to assess extent of resection and/or potential complications. For a diagnosis of a high-grade glioma, regardless of O6-methylguanine-DNA methyl-transferase and IDH status, all surgeons favored the use of postoperative radiation and temozolomide.

SUMMARY OF QUALITY OF EVIDENCE TO GUIDE SPECIFIC INTERVENTIONS FOR THIS CASE

- Surgery as opposed to biopsy or observation for high-grade gliomas—Class II-1.
- Increasing extent of resection associated with improved outcomes—Class II-2.
- Awake mapping versus asleep surgery for high-grade gliomas—Class II-2.
- Bevacizumab for recurrent high-grade gliomas—Class I.

REFERENCES

1. Chaichana KL, McGirt MJ, Laterra J, Olivi A, Quinones-Hinojosa A. Recurrence and malignant degeneration after resection of adult hemispheric low-grade gliomas. *J Neurosurg.* 2010;112:10–17.
2. Chaichana KL, McGirt MJ, Niranjan A, Olivi A, Burger PC, Quinones-Hinojosa A. Prognostic significance of contrast-enhancing low-grade gliomas in adults and a review of the literature. *Neurol Res.* 2009;31:931–939.
3. McGirt MJ, Chaichana KL, Attenello FJ, et al. Extent of surgical resection is independently associated with survival in patients with hemispheric infiltrating low-grade gliomas. *Neurosurgery.* 2008;63:700–707; author reply 707–708.
4. Forst DA, Nahed BV, Loeffler JS, Batchelor TT. Low-grade gliomas. *Oncologist.* 2014;19:403–413.
5. Noll KR, Bradshaw ME, Weinberg JS, Wefel JS. Neurocognitive functioning is associated with functional independence in newly diagnosed patients with temporal lobe glioma. *Neurooncol Pract.* 2018;5:184–193.
6. Kemerdere R, Yuksel O, Kacira T, et al. Low-grade temporal gliomas: surgical strategy and long-term seizure outcome. *Clin Neurol Neurosurg.* 2014;126:196–200.
7. Fernandez-Miranda JC, Rhoton AL Jr., Alvarez-Linera J, Kakizawa Y, Choi C, de Oliveira EP. Three-dimensional microsurgical and tractographic anatomy of the white matter of the human brain. *Neurosurgery.* 2008;62:989–1026; discussion 1026–1028.
8. Rhoton AL Jr. The cerebrum. Anatomy. *Neurosurgery.* 2007;61:37–118; discussion 118–119.
9. Duffau H. The reliability of asleep-awake-asleep protocol for intraoperative functional mapping and cognitive monitoring in glioma surgery. *Acta Neurochir (Wien).* 2013;155:1803–1804.
10. Eseonu CI, Eguia F, Garcia O, Kaplan PW, Quinones-Hinojosa A. Comparative analysis of monotherapy versus duotherapy antiseizure drug management for postoperative seizure control in patients undergoing an awake craniotomy. *J Neurosurg.* 2018;128:1661–1667.
11. Eseonu CI, Eguia F, ReFaey K, et al. Comparative volumetric analysis of the extent of resection of molecularly and histologically distinct low grade gliomas and its role on survival. *J Neurooncol.* 2017;134:65–74.
12. Eseonu CI, Rincon-Torroella J, ReFaey K, et al. Awake craniotomy vs craniotomy under general anesthesia for perirolandic gliomas: evaluating perioperative complications and extent of resection. *Neurosurgery.* 2017;81:481–489.
13. Bertani G, Fava E, Casaceli G, et al. Intraoperative mapping and monitoring of brain functions for the resection of low-grade gliomas: technical considerations. *Neurosurg Focus.* 2009;27:E4.
14. Nossek E, Korn A, Shahar T, et al. Intraoperative mapping and monitoring of the corticospinal tracts with neurophysiological assessment and 3-dimensional ultrasonography-based navigation. Clinical article. *J Neurosurg.* 2011;114:738–746.

25

Left occipital high-grade glioma

Case reviewed by Bob S. Carter, Sunit Das, Maciej S. Lesniak, Jinsong Wu

Introduction

An uncommon location for gliomas is the occipital lobe, in which the incidence ranges from 5% to 10% in several series.[1–4] Patients with occipital lobe gliomas typically present with seizures but can have more subtle deficits in visual fields and neurocognitive function, including attention, proprioception, reading, and writing.[5,6] Moreover, dominant hemisphere lesions can be in close juxtaposition to language-associated white matter tracts, in which surgery can be associated with significant morbidity.[5,6] In this chapter, we present a case of a dominant hemisphere occipital high-grade glioma.

Example case

Chief complaint: right-sided vision loss and difficulty speaking
History of present illness
A 73-year-old, right-handed woman with a history of hypertension, hypercholesterolemia, and asthma presented with progressive right-sided vision loss and difficulty speaking. She was seen by her primary care physician when she stated she noticed having a blind spot on the right side when she was at a four-way intersection. In addition, she complains of difficulty with word pronunciation (Fig. 25.1).
Medications: Lisinopril, fluticasone, simvastatin.
Allergies: No known drug allergies.
Past medical and surgical history: Hypertension, hypercholesterolemia, asthma, right knee replacement.
Family history: No history of intracranial malignancies.
Social history: Retired teacher, no smoking, social alcohol.
Physical examination: Awake, alert, oriented to person, place, and time; Language: intact naming and repetition but with slight dysarthria; Cranial nerves II to XII intact except right homonymous hemianopsia; No drift, moves all extremities with full strength.
Imaging: Chest/abdomen/pelvis with no evidence of primary disease.

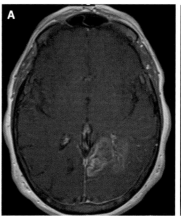 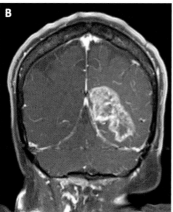 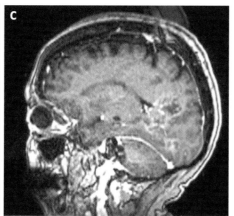

Fig 25.1 Preoperative magnetic resonance imaging. (A) T1 axial image with gadolinium contrast; **(B)** T1 coronal image with gadolinium contrast; **(C)** T1 sagittal with gadolinium contrast magnetic resonance imaging scan demonstrating a contrast-enhancing lesion involving the left occipital lobe.

	Bob S. Carter, MD, PhD, Massachusetts General Hospital, Boston, MA, United States	Sunit Das, MD, PhD, St. Michael's Hospital, University of Toronto, Toronto, Canada	Maciej S. Lesniak, MD, Northwestern University, Chicago, IL, United States	Jinsong Wu, MD, PhD, Fudan University, Huashan Hospital, Shanghai, China
Preoperative				
Additional tests requested	None	Visual field testing	Visual field testing	Tasked-based BOLD DTI MRS PWI Neuropsychological assessment
Surgical approach selected	Left occipital craniotomy with 5-ALA	Left temporo-occipital craniotomy	Left occipital craniotomy	Left parietal needle biopsy (because of age)
Anatomic corridor	Occipital-parietal	Occipital–lingual gyrus	Occipital	Angular gyrus, IPL
Goal of surgery	Diagnosis, debulking	Resection of contrast-enhancing portion	Resection of contrast-enhancing portion	Diagnosis
Perioperative				
Positioning	Left lateral	Left lateral	Left park bench	Prone with 30-degree left rotation
Surgical equipment	Surgical navigation Surgical microscope with 5-ALA Ultrasonic aspirator	Surgical navigation Ultrasound Surgical microscope Ultrasonic aspirator	Surgical navigation Surgical microscope	Surgical navigation Needle biopsy kit
Medications	5-ALA Mannitol, furosemide Antiepileptics	Steroids	Mannitol Steroids	Steroids Antiepileptics
Anatomic considerations	Posterior corpus callosum	Visual pathways, corpus callosum, ventricle	Motor and visual cortex, visual fields	Angular gyrus, STG/MTG, optic radiations, IFOF, splenium, major forceps of corpus callosum, precuneus, cuneus, parieto-occipital sulcus
Complications feared with approach chosen	Speech deficits	Visual deficit	Visual and motor deficit	Hemorrhage
Intraoperative				
Anesthesia	General	General	General	General
Skin incision	U-shaped	Horseshoe	Linear	Linear
Bone opening	Left parieto-occipital	Left temporo-occipital	Left occipital	Left parietal (burr hole)
Brain exposure	Left parieto-occipital	Left temporo-occipital	Left occipital	Angular gyrus
Method of resection	Craniotomy based on navigation, dural opening, trans parieto-occipital based on navigation using shortest distance, internal debulking, resect residual with 5-ALA, anticipate residual anteriorly near corpus callosum	Craniotomy based on navigation, flap designed based on axial planes, ultrasound to visualize most superficial portion of tumor to cortical surface, dural opening, corticectomy based on ultrasound, surgical microscope to dissect through white matter, internal debulking and working to the edges using ultrasound and microscope, dural tack up sutures	Craniotomy based on navigation, determine shortest distance based on navigation, internal debulking under microscopic visualization, minimize retraction, resection of enhancing portion	Trajectory based on navigation, burr hole, dural opening over angular gyrus, targeting three sites within lesion, four samples from each target point

(continued on next page)

	Bob S. Carter, MD, PhD, Massachusetts General Hospital, Boston, MA, United States	Sunit Das, MD, PhD, St. Michael's Hospital, University of Toronto, Toronto, Canada	Maciej S. Lesniak, MD, Northwestern University, Chicago, IL, United States	Jinsong Wu, MD, PhD, Fudan University, Huashan Hospital, Shanghai, China
Complication avoidance	Internal debulking, 5-ALA, anticipate anterior residual	Internal debulking	Internal debulking	Angular gyrus starting point, needle biopsy
Postoperative				
Admission	ICU	ICU	ICU	ICU
Postoperative complications feared	Expect visual deficit, speech deficit	Visual deficit, CSF leak	Visual deficit, seizure	Hemorrhage
Follow-up testing	MRI within 48 hours after surgery	MRI within 48 hours after surgery	CT within 12 hours after surgery MRI within 48 hours after surgery	CT head immediately after surgery
Follow-up visits	7–10 days after surgery	1 month after surgery	14 days after surgery	1 month after surgery
Adjuvant therapies recommended				
IDH status	Mutant–radiation/ temozolomide Wild type–radiation/ temozolomide	Mutant–radiation/ temozolomide Wild type–radiation/ temozolomide	Mutant–radiation/ temozolomide + TTF Wild type–radiation/ temozolomide + TTF	Mutant–radiation/ temozolomide Wild type–radiation/ temozolomide
MGMT status	Methylated–radiation/ temozolomide Unmethylated–radiation/ temozolomide	Methylated–radiation/ temozolomide Unmethylated–radiation/ temozolomide	Methylated–radiation/ temozolomide + TTF Unmethylated–radiation/ temozolomide + TTF	Methylated– temozolomide Unmethylated–radiation/ temozolomide

5-ALA, 5-aminolevulinic acid; BOLD, blood-oxygen-level-dependent; CSF, cerebrospinal fluid; CT, computed tomography; DTI, diffusion tensor imaging; ICU, intensive care unit; IFOF, inferior frontal occipital fasciculus; IPL, inferior parietal lobule; MGMT, O6-methylguanine-DNA methyl-transferase; MRI, magnetic resonance imaging; MRS, magnetic resonance spectroscopy; MTG, middle temporal gyrus; PWI, perfusion-weighted imaging; STG, superior temporal gyrus; TTF, tumor treatment fields.

Differential diagnosis and actual diagnosis

- High-grade glioma
- Metastatic brain tumor
- Lymphoma

Important anatomic and preoperative considerations

Similar to the other lobes, the occipital lobe has lateral, inferior, and medial surfaces.[7,8] On the lateral surface of the occipital lobe, there are three gyri: superior occipital gyrus (SOG), middle occipital gyrus (MOG), and inferior occipital gyrus (IOG).[7,8] The SOG is between the interhemispheric fissure and the intraoccipital sulcus, which is a continuation of the intraparietal sulcus.[7,8] The MOG is between the intraoccipital sulcus and the lateral occipital sulcus, which is a continuation of the superior temporal sulcus, and the IOG is below the lateral occipital sulcus.[7,8] The SOG is continuous on the medial surface with the cuneus, which is limited by the parietal-occipital sulcus superiorly and the calcarine sulcus inferiorly.[7,8] The parieto-occipital sulcus separates the calcarine into an anterior and posterior segment, and the calcarine sulcus extends laterally near the atrium and occipital horn where it forms the calcar avis on the medial side of the atrium.[7,8] The primary visual cortex resides on the upper and lower banks of the posterior part of the calcarine

sulcus.[7,8] The lingual gyrus, which is a continuation of the parahippocampal gyrus, is below the calcarine sulcus, as well as medial to the posterior end of the collateral sulcus.[7,8] The white matter tracts that connect the occipital lobe with other areas include the visual field tracts, superior longitudinal fasciculus (SLF), inferior longitudinal fasciculus, and inferior frontal occipital fasciculus.[7,8]

Approaches to this lesion

The general approaches for these intrinsic lesions can be divided into asleep versus awake surgery (Chapter 1, Fig. 1.2), and eloquent cortical and subcortical structures can be identified by direct and indirect methods (Chapter 3, Fig. 3.2).[9–14] Asleep surgery can be done with or without monitoring, in which monitoring involves somatosensory evoked potentials and/or motor evoked potentials that are all indirect methods of primarily identifying and monitoring the motor and sensory pathways that should be anterior to the lesion.[13,14] Awake brain mapping, however, can be used to directly identify and avoid eloquent cortical and subcortical regions to minimize surgical morbidity. It can be used to identify language, motor, and visual areas, among others.[9,12]

In terms of directionality, the approaches can be divided into superior, posterior, and lateral. The superior approach is approaching the lesion from either the parietal or SOG near the interhemispheric fissure, in which the advantages include avoiding the macula and the SLF but requires traversing the

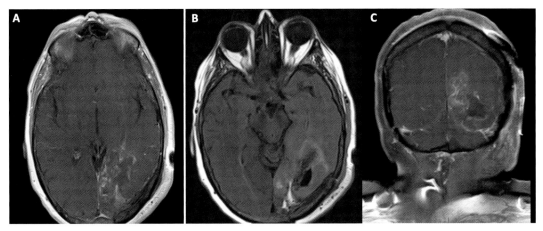

Fig. 25.2 Postoperative magnetic resonance imaging. (A) T1 axial image with gadolinium contrast; **(B)** T2 axial fluid attenuation inversion recovery image; **(C)** T1 coronal with gadolinium contrast magnetic resonance imaging scan demonstrating near total resection of the contrast-enhancing portion of the lesion involving the left occipital lobe, with expected residual anteromedially within the resection in close proximity to the splenium of the corpus callosum.

entire occipital lobe to reach the inferior portion of the lesion and potentially injuring the posterior corpus callosum on the dominant hemisphere that is responsible for reading and writing. A posterior approach involves going through the occipital pole, in which the primary advantage includes providing the shortest working distance, but traverses through the macula. A lateral approach involves coming in through the lateral surface of the occipital lobe through the SOG, MOG, and/or IOG, in which the advantages include short working distance and convenient access to the anterior and posterior portions of the tumor, but it requires crossing several critical white matter tracts, including the SLF, inferior longitudinal fasciculus, inferior frontal occipital fasciculus, and visual tracts.

What was actually done

The patient underwent formal visual fields and had a partial right homonymous hemianopsia. The patient was taken to surgery for a left occipital craniotomy with awake motor and language mapping for resection of the lesion. The patient was intubated with a laryngeal mask airway. The scalp was blocked bilaterally with local anesthetic, and the head was fixed in pins, with two pins over the right superior nuchal line and one pin over the left forehead in the midpupillary line. The patient was positioned lateral with their head turned to the right. A linear incision was then planned over the occipital lobe based on preoperative magnetic resonance imaging surgical navigation. The patient was draped in the usual standard fashion and given dexamethasone, levetiracetam, and cefazolin. A linear incision was made, and the skin incision was retracted with cerebellar retractors. A left occipital craniotomy was done to encompass the occipital pole of the lesion and staying above the transverse sinus. Ultrasound and surgical navigation were used to confirm lesion boundaries, and the boundaries were designated with letter tags once the dura was opened. The dura was anesthetized with local anesthetics between the leaflets adjacent to the middle meningeal vessels. The patient was awakened, and the dura was opened once the patient followed commands consistently. Strip electrodes were placed in the subdural space for after discharge monitoring. The cortex was initially stimulated at 2 mA, and no phosphenes were elicited at

6 mA with an Ojemann stimulator (Integra, Princeton, NJ). The rest of the cortical and subcortical mapping took place at 6 mA. The patient participated in continuous language testing with picture naming, reading, and writing, with concurrent motor movement of the right face and arm. Positive mapping sites were designated with number tags. Negative mapping occurred initially over the occipital surface; however, at the tumor depths, positive subcortical mapping sites were elicited and included splenium of the corpus callosum (alexia) at the anterior margin and SLF (phonetic paraphasias) at the lateral margin. When these areas were encountered, resection stopped at these boundaries and the patient was put back to sleep. Preliminary diagnosis was infiltrating glioma. The dura, bone, and skin were closed in standard fashion.

The patient awoke at their neurologic baseline with intact speech and full strength bilaterally with baseline right homonymous hemianopsia and was taken to the intensive care unit for recovery. Postoperative magnetic resonance imaging done within 48 hours after surgery showed near total resection with expected residual anterior to the lesion in close proximity to the corpus callosum (Fig. 25.2). The patient participated with physical, occupational, and speech therapy and was discharged to home on postoperative day 2 with baseline preoperative neurologic examination. The patient was prescribed 3 months of levetiracetam, and dexamethasone was tapered to off over 7 days after surgery. The patient was seen at 2 weeks postoperatively for staple removal and was full strength with intact speech. Pathology was a World Health Organization grade IV glioblastoma (IDH wild type, O6-methylguanine-DNA methyl-transferase methylated). The patient underwent adjuvant temozolomide chemotherapy with concurrent radiation therapy for 6 weeks followed by four adjuvant temozolomide cycles. The patient unfortunately had recurrence at 7 months and was transitioned to bevacizumab. The patient died 13 months after surgery.

Commonalities among the experts

In this case, half of the surgeons opted for patients having preoperative visual field testing to assess for visual field deficits. The majority of the surgeons elected for resection of the contrast-enhancing portion of the lesion through primarily an occipital approach. Most surgeons identified the importance of identifying the corpus callosum and optic radiations, in which the most feared complication was a visual field deficit. Surgery was generally pursued with surgical navigation, surgical microscope, and ultrasonic aspirator with perioperative steroids and antiepileptics. The majority of surgeons relied on internal debulking to minimize risk of iatrogenic injury. Following surgery, all patients were admitted to the intensive care unit, and imaging was obtained within 48 hours after surgery to assess extent of resection and/or potential complications. For a diagnosis of a high-grade glioma, regardless of O6-methylguanine-DNA methyl-transferase and IDH status, all surgeons favored the use of postoperative radiation and temozolomide.

SUMMARY OF QUALITY OF EVIDENCE TO GUIDE SPECIFIC INTERVENTIONS FOR THIS CASE

- Surgery as opposed to biopsy or observation for high-grade gliomas—Class II-1.
- Increasing extent of resection associated with improved outcomes—Class II-2.
- Awake mapping versus asleep surgery for high-grade gliomas—Class II-2.
- Bevacizumab for recurrent high-grade gliomas—Class I.
- Visual field mapping—Class III.

REFERENCES

1. Chaichana KL, McGirt MJ, Laterra J, Olivi A, Quinones-Hinojosa A. Recurrence and malignant degeneration after resection of adult hemispheric low-grade gliomas. *J Neurosurg*. 2010;112:10–17.
2. Chaichana KL, McGirt MJ, Niranjan A, Olivi A, Burger PC, Quinones-Hinojosa A. Prognostic significance of contrast-enhancing low-grade gliomas in adults and a review of the literature. *Neurol Res*. 2009;31:931–939.
3. McGirt MJ, Chaichana KL, Attenello FJ, et al. Extent of surgical resection is independently associated with survival in patients with hemispheric infiltrating low-grade gliomas. *Neurosurgery*. 2008;63:700–707; author reply 707–708.
4. Forst DA, Nahed BV, Loeffler JS, Batchelor TT. Low-grade gliomas. *Oncologist*. 2014;19:403–413.
5. Noll KR, Bradshaw ME, Weinberg JS, Wefel JS. Neurocognitive functioning is associated with functional independence in newly diagnosed patients with temporal lobe glioma. *Neurooncol Pract*. 2018;5:184–193.
6. Kemerdere R, Yuksel O, Kacira T, et al. Low-grade temporal gliomas: surgical strategy and long-term seizure outcome. *Clin Neurol Neurosurg*. 2014;126:196–200.
7. Fernandez-Miranda JC, Rhoton AL Jr., Alvarez-Linera J, Kakizawa Y, Choi C, de Oliveira EP. Three-dimensional microsurgical and tractographic anatomy of the white matter of the human brain. *Neurosurgery*. 2008;62:989–1026; discussion 1026–1028.
8. Rhoton AL Jr. The cerebrum. Anatomy. *Neurosurgery*. 2007;61:37–118; discussion 118–119.
9. Duffau H. The reliability of asleep-awake-asleep protocol for intraoperative functional mapping and cognitive monitoring in glioma surgery. *Acta Neurochir (Wien)*. 2013;155:1803–1804.
10. Eseonu CI, Eguia F, Garcia O, Kaplan PW, Quinones-Hinojosa A. Comparative analysis of monotherapy versus duotherapy antiseizure drug management for postoperative seizure control in patients undergoing an awake craniotomy. *J Neurosurg*. 2018;128:1661–1667.
11. Eseonu CI, Eguia F, ReFaey K, et al. Comparative volumetric analysis of the extent of resection of molecularly and histologically distinct low grade gliomas and its role on survival. *J Neurooncol*. 2017;134:65–74.
12. Eseonu CI, Rincon-Torroella J, ReFaey K, et al. Awake craniotomy vs craniotomy under general anesthesia for perirolandic gliomas: evaluating perioperative complications and extent of resection. *Neurosurgery*. 2017;81:481–489.
13. Bertani G, Fava E, Casaceli G, et al. Intraoperative mapping and monitoring of brain functions for the resection of low-grade gliomas: technical considerations. *Neurosurg Focus*. 2009;27:E4.
14. Nossek E, Korn A, Shahar T, et al. Intraoperative mapping and monitoring of the corticospinal tracts with neurophysiological assessment and 3-dimensional ultrasonography-based navigation. Clinical article. *J Neurosurg*. 2011;114:738–746.

26

Left thalamic high-grade glioma

Case reviewed by Frederick F. Lang, Fredric B. Meyer, Stephen J. Price, Andreas Raabe

Introduction

The general treatment paradigm for high-grade gliomas is maximal resection followed by adjuvant chemoradiation; however, patients who develop deficits have worsened survival independent of the extent of resection.[1] Deep-seated high-grade gliomas have arguably the highest surgical risk of developing neurologic deficits.[1–4] Therefore the management of deep-seated high-grade gliomas remains unclear.[4–6] Some practitioners perform stereotactic needle biopsies to minimize surgical morbidity, whereas others perform open resections with significant risk of iatrogenic deficits.[5,6] In this chapter, we present a case of a dominant-hemisphere thalamic high-grade glioma.

Example case

Chief complaint: right-sided arm and leg weakness

History of present illness

An 18-year-old, right-handed woman with no significant past medical history presented with progressive right arm and leg weakness. She stated that over the past 2 to 3 months her right arm has become weaker to the point where she has problems writing. In addition, her leg seems to drag more when she walks. She denies any speaking or vision problems (Fig. 26.1).

Medications: None.

Allergies: No known drug allergies.

Past medical and surgical history: None.

Family history: No history of intracranial malignancies.

Social history: College student, no smoking, no alcohol.

Physical examination: Awake, alert, oriented to person, place, and time; Language: intact naming and repetition; Cranial nerves

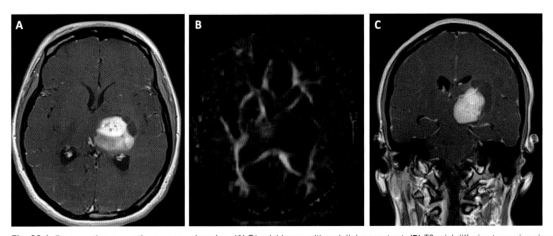

Fig. 26.1 Preoperative magnetic resonance imaging. (A) T1 axial image with gadolinium contrast; **(B)** T2 axial diffusion tensor imaging; **(C)** T1 coronal with gadolinium contrast magnetic resonance imaging scan demonstrating a contrast-enhancing lesion involving the left posterior thalamus with anterior displacement of the internal capsule.

II-XII intact except slight decreased right nasolabial fold, right drift, right upper extremity 4/5, right lower extremity 4+/5, left upper extremity/left lower extremity 5/5.

Imaging: Chest/abdomen/pelvis with no evidence of primary disease.

	Frederick F. Lang, MD, MD Anderson Cancer Center, Houston, TX, United States	Fredric B. Meyer, MD, Mayo Clinic, Rochester, MN, United States	Stephen J. Price, MBBS, PhD, University of Cambridge, Cambridge, United Kingdom	Andreas Raabe, MD, University Hospital at Inselspital Bern, Switzerland
Preoperative				
Additional tests requested	fMRI DTI MRV	+/− fMRI +/− DTI	DTI	DTI Neuropsychological assessment
Surgical approach selected	Left parietal craniotomy with intraoperative MRI and 5-ALA, if available	Left parietal craniotomy with asleep subcortical stimulation	Supracerebellar infratentorial	Left parietal craniotomy with tubular retractor with intraoperative MRI
Anatomic corridor	Left superior parietal lobule	Left superior parietal lobule, transsulcal, transventricular to pulvinar	Supracerebellar infratentorial	Left postcentral-intraparietal transsulcal
Goal of surgery	Complete resection of contrast-enhancing portion if possible	Extensive resection of enhancing portion of the tumor	Extensive resection of enhancing portion of the tumor	Extensive resection guided by mapping and intraoperative MRI
Perioperative				
Positioning	Left supine	Right lateral with head turned to the right	Prone	Left lateral with 20-degree head tilt and turn to the right
Surgical equipment	Surgical navigation IOM (SSEP, phase reversal) Brain retractor Surgical microscope with 5-ALA, if possible Ultrasonic aspirator Intraoperative MRI	Surgical navigation IOM (MEP) Surgical microscope Brain retractor Suction brain stimulator	Surgical navigation Surgical microscope Ultrasonic aspirator Ultrasound Budde halo retractor	Surgical navigation IOM (MEP, SSEP) Ultrasound Surgical microscope with augmented reality Ultrasonic aspirator Intraoperative MRI
Medications	Steroids Antiepileptics	Steroids Antiepileptics	Steroids Mannitol	Steroids Antiepileptics
Anatomic considerations	Motor cortex, AF, internal capsule/CST	Posterior limb of internal capsule	Avoiding optic tracts and CST	Sensory pathways, AF, optic tract, thalamus, internal capsule, crus cerebri, CST, perforating arteries
Complications feared with approach chosen	Motor deficit, sensory deficit, language dysfunction	Worsening motor deficit	Motor, visual deficit	Motor, language, or visual deficit
Intraoperative				
Anesthesia	General	General	General	General
Skin incision	Lateral-based U-shaped flap	Linear horizontal	Midline linear from occiput to C2 with option of hockey stick incision	Linear
Bone opening	Left parietal	Left parietal	Occipital craniotomy eccentric to the right	Left parietal
Brain exposure	Left superior parietal lobule	Left superior parietal lobule	Cerebellar hemispheres and transverse sinus	Left parietal

	Frederick F. Lang, MD, MD Anderson Cancer Center, Houston, TX, United States	Fredric B. Meyer, MD, Mayo Clinic, Rochester, MN, United States	Stephen J. Price, MBBS, PhD, University of Cambridge, Cambridge, United Kingdom	Andreas Raabe, MD, University Hospital at Inselspital Bern, Switzerland
Method of resection	Craniotomy centered over superior parietal lobule near midline, open dura medially, phase reversal to identify perirolandic area, confirm entry point behind sensory cortex in superior parietal lobule, preserve veins, 2 x 2 cm corticectomy, follow path down to lesion with navigation, advance retractors once tumor is reached, internally debulk, dissect tumor until completely removed, intraoperative MRI for possible further resection	Craniotomy centered on selected sulcus based on navigation, dural tack up sutures, dural opening, sulcus opened and retracted with brain retractor (circular or single blade), divide U-fibers vertically, enter ventricle under navigation, choroid plexus is swept away and cottonoid placed to prevent spillage of blood products and tumor, horizontal incision in pulvinar based on appearance and stereotaxis, debulk tumor with suction and bipolar, stimulate with suction tip to identify internal capsule at 3–4 mA, continuous MEP, debulk tumor from medial to lateral, protect small perforators, avoid aggressive cauterization, water tight dural closure	Midline dissection from occiput to C1, burr holes on each side of the keel, craniotomy going up to transverse sinus eccentric to the right, Y-shaped dural opening, care of draining veins, drain CSF, depress cerebellum from tentorium, enter pineal region, corticectomy over tumor (ultrasound and image guidance), internal debulking of tumor, aim for cyst laterally, aim for subtotal resection, watertight dural closure	Left parietal craniotomy based on navigation, identification of interparietal and postcentral sulci, placement of tubular retractor, resect tumor with ultrasonic aspirator under microscopic visualization with augmented reality and continuous motor mapping, resect tumor until 3–4 mA threshold reached, intraoperative MRI with DTI, further resection until 2 mA threshold reached, repeat intraoperative MRI with DTI as needed
Complication avoidance	Phase reversal to confirm superior parietal lobule, preserve veins, navigation for trajectory, brain retractor to hold corridor, intraoperative MRI for possible further resection	Transsulcal approach, corridor kept open with retractor, cottonoid pledge to protect spillage, use of stimulating suction to identify internal capsule, continuous MEP, medial to lateral resection, avoid aggressive cauterization	Supracerebellar approach to minimize cortical entry, internally debulking of tumor, target lateral cyst	Transsulcal approach, tubular retractor, augmented reality, continuous motor mapping, intraoperative MRI with DTI
Postoperative				
Admission	ICU	ICU	Floor	ICU
Postoperative complications feared	Motor weakness, language dysfunction	Progressive hemiparesis, thalamic pain syndrome	Difficulty accessing tumor, hemianopia, motor deficit, CSF leak	Motor of language deficit, seizures
Follow-up testing	MRI within 24 hours after surgery	MRI within 24 hours after surgery Physical and occupational therapy evaluation	MRI within 72 hours after surgery	MRI within 48 hours after surgery Neuropsychological assessment Visual field testing

(continued on next page)

	Frederick F. Lang, MD, MD Anderson Cancer Center, Houston, TX, United States	Fredric B. Meyer, MD, Mayo Clinic, Rochester, MN, United States	Stephen J. Price, MBBS, PhD, University of Cambridge, Cambridge, United Kingdom	Andreas Raabe, MD, University Hospital at Inselspital Bern, Switzerland
Follow-up visits	2 weeks after surgery with neurosurgery, neurooncology, radiation oncology	6 weeks after surgery with neurosurgery 2 weeks after surgery with neurooncology and radiation oncology	7 days after surgery	4 weeks after surgery
Adjuvant therapies recommended				
IDH status	Mutant–radiation followed by temozolomide Wild type–radiation/ temozolomide	Mutant–radiation/ temozolomide Wild type–radiation/ temozolomide	Mutant–radiation/ temozolomide Wild type–radiation/ temozolomide	Mutant–temozolomide (GTR), temozolomide/ radiation (STR) Wild type–radiation/ temozolomide
MGMT status	Methylated–radiation/ temozolomide Unmethylated–radiation/ temozolomide	Methylated–radiation/ temozolomide Unmethylated–radiation/ temozolomide	Methylated–radiation/ temozolomide Unmethylated–radiation/ temozolomide	Methylated–radiation/ temozolomide Unmethylated–radiation/ temozolomide

5-ALA, 5-aminolevulinic acid; *AF*, arcuate fasciculus; *CSF*, cerebrospinal fluid; *CST*, corticospinal tract; *DTI*, diffusion tensor imaging; *DWI*, diffusion-weighted imaging; *fMRI*, functional magnetic resonance imaging; *GTR*, gross total resection; *ICU*, intensive care unit; *IOM*, intraoperative monitoring; *MEP*, motor evoked potential; *MGMT*, O6-methylguanine-DNA methyl-transferase; *MRI*, magnetic resonance imaging; *MRV*, magnetic resonance venogram; *SSEP*, somatosensory evoked potential; *STR*, subtotal resection.

Differential diagnosis and actual diagnosis

- High-grade glioma
- Metastatic brain tumor
- Low-grade glioma (pilocytic astrocytoma)
- Lymphoma

Important anatomic and preoperative considerations

The thalamus is a critical deep-seated nuclear complex that is a relay center for motor and sensory signals, as well as other functions, including sleep and wakefulness.[7] It is covered by a thin layer of white matter on its superior surface by the stratum zonale, and on its lateral surface by the external medullary lamina. Within the gray matter of the thalamus is the internal medullary lamina that separates the thalamus into anterior, medial, and lateral parts.[7] The anterior thalamic nuclei primarily functions in conjunction with the limbic system (emotion and memory), and receives the mammillothalamic tract from the mammillary nuclei and has reciprocal connections with the cingulate gyrus and hypothalamus.[7] The medial part that forms the upper lateral walls of the third ventricle is primarily composed of the dorsomedial nucleus and functions in the integration of a large variety of sensory information and subjective emotions, and has reciprocal connections with the prefrontal cortex, hypothalamic nuclei, and other thalamic nuclei.[7] The lateral part is further subdivided into dorsal and ventral components.[7] The dorsal component of the lateral thalamic nuclei consists of the lateral dorsal nucleus, lateral posterior nucleus, and pulvinar, and has reciprocal connections with other thalamic nuclei, parietal lobe, cingulate gyrus, and temporal lobes.[7] The ventral component of the lateral thalamic nuclei consists of the ventral anterior nucleus, ventral lateral nucleus, and ventral posterior nucleus.[7] The ventral anterior nucleus influences the activity of the motor cortex and has connections with the reticular formation, substantia nigra, corpus striatum, and premotor cortex.[7] The ventral lateral nucleus also influences motor activity and has connections with the cerebellum, red nuclei, reticular formation, substantia nigra, corpus striatum, and premotor cortex.[7] The ventral posterior nucleus influences sensory activity and has inputs from the trigeminal and gustatory pathways, spinothalamic tracts, and dorsal column medial lemniscus pathways.[7]

Approaches to this lesion

The general approaches for intrinsic lesions can be divided into asleep versus awake surgery (Chapter 1, Fig. 1.2), and eloquent cortical and subcortical structures can be identified by direct and indirect methods (Chapter 3, Fig. 3.2).[8–13] Asleep surgery can be done with or without monitoring, in which monitoring involves somatosensory evoked potentials and/or motor evoked potentials that are all indirect methods of primarily identifying and monitoring the motor and sensory pathways.[12,13] These modalities, however, are limited in that changes occur in a delayed fashion after deficits occur.[12,13] Awake brain mapping, however, can be used to directly identify and avoid eloquent cortical and subcortical regions to minimize surgical morbidity.[8,11] Awake brain mapping, however, can be limited when working in deeps-seated locations because of the limited access, visualization, and corridor for subcortical stimulation.

In terms of directionality, the approaches can be divided into anterior, posterior, and lateral. The anterior approach involves accessing the lesion from a frontal or Kocher point, whereby the entry is anterior to the motor cortex, medial to superior longitudinal fasciculus and language tracts, and lateral to the cingulum. The anterior approach is best for anterior thalamic lesions. The posterior approach involves accessing the lesion from a superior parietal lobule approach, whereby the entry is posterior to the sensory cortex, anterior to the visual cortex, and medial to the language tracts. The posterior approach is best for posterior thalamic lesions. The lateral approach involves approaching the lesion either through the temporal or parietal lobe. This approach is the shortest in distance, but potentially traverses critical language, motor and/or sensory cortex, and white matter tracts.

What was actually done

The patient underwent magnetic resonance imaging (MRI) for surgical navigation with diffusion tensor imaging, which demonstrated that the internal capsule was displaced anteriorly (Fig. 26.1). The patient was taken to surgery for an asleep left parietal craniotomy with tubular retractor for resection of the thalamic lesion through a transsulcal, superior parietal lobule approach with intraoperative monitoring. The patient was induced and intubated per routine. The head was fixed in pins, with two pins centered on the right external auditory meatus and one pin over the left external auditory meatus. The head was kept neutral and flexed. A linear incision was then planned in the coronal plane over the superior parietal lobule over an identified sulcus based on preoperative MRI surgical navigation. The patient was draped in the usual standard fashion and given dexamethasone, levetiracetam, and cefazolin. A linear incision was made, and the skin incision was retracted with cerebellar retractors. A left superior parietal craniotomy was done centered on the identified sulcus that was anterior to the parietal-occipital sulcus. Ultrasound and surgical navigation were used to confirm the trajectory toward the lesion. The dura was opened in a cruciate fashion and tacked up with sutures. Strip electrodes were placed in the subdural space, and a phase reversal was obtained anterior to the craniotomy confirming that the central sulcus was several gyri anterior to the planned approach. The exoscope was then brought in for the remainder of the case. The predetermined sulcus was opened sharply with microinstruments. Under navigation guidance, the 75-mm tubular retractor was placed through the opened sulcus and docked on the superficial aspect of the lesion. The tumor was debulked internally. After the majority of the tumor was removed, there was some decrease in the amplitude and latency of the somatosensory evoked potentials but no change in the motor evoked potentials, and the surgery was stopped. Preliminary diagnosis was infiltrating glioma. The dura, bone, and skin were closed in standard fashion.

The patient awoke near their neurologic baseline with intact speech but increased right upper extremity (3/5) weakness and was taken to the intensive care unit for recovery. Postoperative MRI done within 48 hours after surgery showed near total resection of the lesion with expected residual anterior and medial within the cavity (Fig. 26.2). The patient participated with physical and occupational therapy and was discharged to home on postoperative day 4 with improved 4/5 right upper extremity strength. The patient was prescribed 3 months of levetiracetam, and dexamethasone was tapered to off over 7 days after surgery. The patient was seen at 2 weeks postoperatively for staple removal and was full strength with intact speech. Pathology was a World Health Organization grade III anaplastic astrocytoma (IDH wild type, O6-methylguanine-DNA methyl-transferase methylated). The patient underwent adjuvant temozolomide chemotherapy with concurrent radiation therapy for 6 weeks followed by six adjuvant temozolomide cycles. The patient remains without recurrence and is neurologically intact 12 months after surgery.

Commonalities among the experts

The majority of surgeons opted for patients having diffusion tensor imaging to identify white matter tracts prior to surgery, and half requested functional MRI to identify

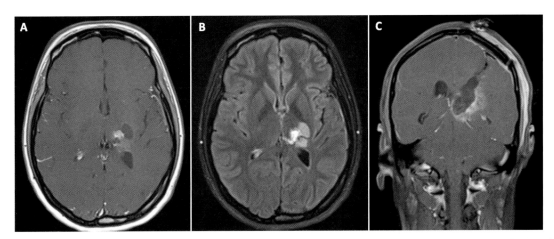

Fig. 26.2 Postoperative magnetic resonance imaging. (A) T1 axial image with gadolinium contrast; **(B)** T2 axial fluid attenuation inversion recovery image; **(C)** T1 coronal with gadolinium contrast magnetic resonance imaging scan demonstrating near total resection of the lesion involving the left thalamus through a transsulcal approach with a tubular retractor.

functional cortical areas. The majority of surgeons elected for performing this surgery through a left superior parietal approach, with the remaining surgeon choosing a supracerebellar infratentorial approach. Half of the surgeons chose to use intraoperative MRI to assess for need for additional resection, and one selected 5-aminolevulinic acid to help assist resection. The goal of surgery in all surgeons was extensive resection of the enhancing portion of the tumor. Most surgeons identified the importance of protecting the corticospinal tracts within the internal capsule, and the most feared complications were motor and language deficits. Surgery was generally pursued with surgical navigation, surgical microscope, brain retractor system (three fixed bladed and one tubular retractor), intraoperative monitoring, and ultrasonic aspirator with perioperative steroids and antiepileptics. The majority of surgeons relied on using a transsulcal approach to limit cortical and subcortical injury, as well as intraoperative monitoring to guide aggressiveness of resection. Following surgery, all patients were admitted to the intensive care unit, and imaging was obtained within 72 hours after surgery to assess extent of resection and/or potential complications. Two surgeons used intraoperative MRI. For a diagnosis of a high-grade glioma, regardless of O6-methylguanine-DNA methyl-transferase and IDH status, most surgeons favored the use of postoperative radiation and temozolomide.

SUMMARY OF QUALITY OF EVIDENCE TO GUIDE SPECIFIC INTERVENTIONS FOR THIS CASE

- Surgery as opposed to biopsy or observation for deep-seated high-grade gliomas—Class III.
- Increasing extent of resection associated with improved outcomes for high-grade gliomas—Class II-2.
- Intraoperative monitoring for intrinsic brain tumor surgery—Class II-3.
- Diffusion tensor imaging to avoid white matter injury—Class III.
- Use of tubular retractors for deep-seated brain tumors—Class III.

REFERENCES

1. McGirt MJ, Mukherjee D, Chaichana KL, Than KD, Weingart JD, Quinones-Hinojosa A. Association of surgically acquired motor and language deficits on overall survival after resection of glioblastoma multiforme. *Neurosurgery*. 2009;65:463–469; discussion 469–470.
2. Chaichana KL, Cabrera-Aldana EE, Jusue-Torres I, et al. When gross total resection of a glioblastoma is possible, how much resection should be achieved? *World Neurosurg*. 2014;82:e257–e265.
3. Chaichana KL, Garzon-Muvdi T, Parker S, et al. Supratentorial glioblastoma multiforme: the role of surgical resection versus biopsy among older patients. *Ann Surg Oncol*. 2011;18:239–245.
4. Iyer R, Chaichana KL. Minimally invasive resection of deep-seated high-grade gliomas using tubular retractors and exoscopic visualization. *J Neurol Surg A Cent Eur Neurosurg*. 2018;79:330–336.
5. Dziurzynski K, Blas-Boria D, Suki D, et al. Butterfly glioblastomas: a retrospective review and qualitative assessment of outcomes. *J Neurooncol*. 2012;109:555–563.
6. Balana C, Capellades J, Teixidor P, et al. Clinical course of high-grade glioma patients with a "biopsy-only" surgical approach: a need for individualised treatment. *Clin Transl Oncol*. 2007;9:797–803.
7. Rhoton AL Jr. The cerebrum. Anatomy. *Neurosurgery*. 2007;61:37–118; discussion 118–119.
8. Duffau H. The reliability of asleep-awake-asleep protocol for intraoperative functional mapping and cognitive monitoring in glioma surgery. *Acta Neurochir (Wien)*. 2013;155:1803–1804
9. Eseonu CI, Eguia F, Garcia O, Kaplan PW, Quinones-Hinojosa A. Comparative analysis of monotherapy versus duotherapy antiseizure drug management for postoperative seizure control in patients undergoing an awake craniotomy. *J Neurosurg*. 2018;128:1661–1667.
10. Eseonu CI, Eguia F, ReFaey K, et al. Comparative volumetric analysis of the extent of resection of molecularly and histologically distinct low grade gliomas and its role on survival. *J Neurooncol*. 2017;134:65–74.
11. Eseonu CI, Rincon-Torroella J, ReFaey K, et al. Awake craniotomy vs craniotomy under general anesthesia for perirolandic gliomas: evaluating perioperative complications and extent of resection. *Neurosurgery*. 2017;81:481–489.
12. Bertani G, Fava E, Casaceli G, et al. Intraoperative mapping and monitoring of brain functions for the resection of low-grade gliomas: technical considerations. *Neurosurg Focus*. 2009;27:E4.
13. Nossek E, Korn A, Shahar T, et al. Intraoperative mapping and monitoring of the corticospinal tracts with neurophysiological assessment and 3-dimensional ultrasonography-based navigation. Clinical article. *J Neurosurg*. 2011;114:738–746.

27

Recurrent high-grade glioma

Case reviewed by Orin Bloch, Javier Avendano Mendez-Padilla, Maryam Rahman, Walter Stummer

Introduction

Despite advances in medical and surgical therapy, the median survival for patients with high-grade gliomas remains approximately 1 year.[1–6] These tumors frequently invade and infiltrate the surrounding parenchyma, and therefore make curative resection unlikely.[6] Despite extensive resection, these tumors will also still recur.[7–10] For patients with recurrence, the management is controversial and includes repeat resection, radiation therapy, salvage chemotherapy, and/or clinical trials.[11,12] In this chapter, we present a case of a recurrent high-grade glioma.

Example case

Chief complaint: headaches with potential recurrent tumor
History of present illness
A 50-year-old, right-handed man with type 2 diabetes who underwent gross total resection of a left temporal IDH wild-type,

O6-methylguanine-DNA methyl-transferase nonmethylated glioblastoma 6 months prior, followed by 6 weeks of radiation and temozolomide, followed by three adjuvant cycles with worsening headaches and possible recurrence (Fig. 27.1). He was given steroids without improvement.
Medications: Metformin, dexamethasone.
Allergies: No known drug allergies.
Past medical and surgical history: Gross total resection of a left temporal glioblastoma resection 6 months prior.
Family history: No history of intracranial malignancies.
Social history: Professional speaker. No smoking and social alcohol.
Physical examination: Awake, alert, oriented to person, place, and time; *Language:* intact naming and repetition; Cranial nerves II to XII intact; No drift, moves all extremities with full strength.

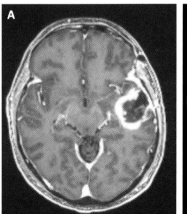 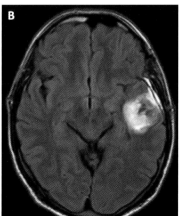 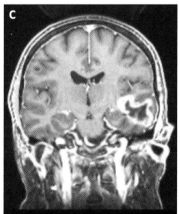

Fig. 27.1 Preoperative magnetic resonance imaging. (A) T1 axial image with gadolinium contrast; **(B)** T2 axial fluid attenuation inversion recovery image; **(C)** T1 coronal image with gadolinium contrast demonstrating increased enhancement and edema along the previous resection cavity consistent with tumor recurrence versus radiation necrosis.

	Orin Bloch, MD, University of California-Davis, Sacramento, CA, United States	Javier Avendano Mendez-Padilla, MD, National Institute of Neurology and Neurosurgery, Tlalpan, Mexico	Maryam Rahman, MD, University of Florida, Gainesville, FL, United States	Walter Stummer, MD, PhD, University of Munster, Munster, NRW, Germany
Preoperative				
Additional tests requested	MR perfusion fMRI DTI MRS	PET MRS fMRI DTI Neuropsychological assessment	fMRI DTI Neuropsychological assessment	FET PET to evaluate for pseudoprogression with biopsy fMRI DTI MRS Language evaluation
Surgical approach selected	Left fronto-temporal craniotomy with awake language, motor, and sensory mapping pending MRS	Left temporal awake craniotomy with language mapping	Left temporal craniotomy with awake mapping and 5-ALA resection and intraoperative MRI	Left temporal craniotomy with awake language mapping and 5-ALA
Anatomic corridor	Left fronto-temporal	Left temporal	Left temporal	Left temporal
Goal of surgery	Biopsy to determine recurrent tumor; then if positive, safe maximal resection of enhancing portion	GTR of enhancing portion and maximal FLAIR with brain mapping	Resection of contrast and FLAIR based on mapping	Resection of fluorescence
Perioperative				
Positioning	Left semi-lateral	Left supine with 90-degree right rotation	Left lateral	Left supine with right rotation
Surgical equipment	Stereotactic navigation IOM (EEG) Brain stimulator Ultrasonic aspirator	Stereotactic navigation Ultrasound Brain stimulator Fluorescein	Stereotactic navigation Surgical microscope Brain stimulator IOM (EEG) Intraoperative MRI	Stereotactic navigation Surgical microscope with 5-ALA Ultrasound Brain stimulator Ultrasonic aspirator
Medications	Steroids Antiepileptics Mannitol	Steroids Antiepileptics Fluorescein	Steroids Antiepileptics Mannitol Fluorescein	Steroids
Anatomic considerations	AF, temporal stem, MCA and lenticulostriates	AF, uncinate fasciculus, Sylvian fissure and vessels	Sylvian fissure, language cortical and subcortical regions	Wernicke, Ludders temporobasal language, IFOF, AF, internal capsule
Complications feared with approach chosen	Language deficit, stroke	Language deficit, venous injury, arterial injury, cerebral edema	Language deficit	Language deficit, dysphagia, visual field deficit
Intraoperative				
Anesthesia	Asleep-awake-asleep	Asleep-awake-asleep	Asleep-awake-asleep	Awake-awake-awake
Skin incision	Pterional (previous incision)	Pterional (previous incision)	Question mark	Pterional
Bone opening	Left fronto-temporal	Left fronto-temporal	Left temporal	Left fronto-temporal
Brain exposure	Left fronto-temporal	Left fronto-temporal	Left temporal	Left fronto-temporal

	Orin Bloch, MD, University of California-Davis, Sacramento, CA, United States	Javier Avendano Mendez-Padilla, MD, National Institute of Neurology and Neurosurgery, Tlalpan, Mexico	Maryam Rahman, MD, University of Florida, Gainesville, FL, United States	Walter Stummer, MD, PhD, University of Munster, Munster, NRW, Germany
Method of resection	Circumferential scalp block, craniotomy to include complete left temporal and inferior frontal region, expand prior craniotomy if necessary, open dura, biopsy through old corticectomy, awaken patient, motor and speech mapping and identify positive sites in temporal lobe, internal debulking while mapping if biopsy positive for recurrent tumor, maximal safe resection, insertion of subgaleal drain	Patient asleep with laryngeal mask, scalp block, craniotomy that extends 2–4 cm outside lesion boundary, dura opened largely to encompass mapping sites, patient awakened, simulation with brain stimulator at 2 mA up to 8 mA with language mapping by neuropsych, positive sites marked with tags, resection based on negative areas, subcortical mapping using semantics for AF, after resection patient is put under general anesthesia	Monitored anesthesia care, scalp block, myocutaneous flap, temporal craniotomy, awaken patient, ECoG and bipolar stimulation for brain mapping with language tasks (naming, repetition) by neuropsych, fluorescence-guided resection, intraoperative MRI to guide further resection	Monitored scalp block, position while patient responsive with no laryngeal mask, deepen sedation for craniotomy, left temporal craniotomy, reduce sedation, language mapping over exposed area with identification of the Broca, resect upper and medial and posterior margins of fluorescence while mapping, spare mesial temporal structures, remove temporobasal remnants
Complication avoidance	Awake language and motor mapping, internal debulking until margins met or positive mapping site encountered	Awake language mapping in cortical and subcortical space	Cortical and subcortical mapping, fluorescence, intraoperative MRI	Cortical and subcortical language mapping, fluorescence, spare mesial temporal structures
Postoperative				
Admission	ICU	ICU	ICU	ICU or intermediate care
Postoperative complications feared	Language deficit, seizure	Language deficit, motor deficit, seizures, cerebral edema	Language deficit	Language or visual field deficit
Follow-up testing	MRI within 48 hours after surgery	MRI within 72 hours after surgery	MRI within 48 hours after surgery	MRI within 48 hours after surgery
Follow-up visits	14 days after surgery with neurosurgery and neurooncology	2 weeks after surgery with neurosurgery and neurooncology	2 weeks after surgery with neurooncology 6 weeks after surgery with neurosurgery	3 months after surgery
Adjuvant therapies recommended				
IDH status	Mutant–clinical trial, CCNU or bevacizumab Wild type–clinical trial, CCNU or bevacizumab	Mutant–bevacizumab and/or irinotecan Wild type–bevacizumab and/or irinotecan	Mutant–radiation/ temozolomide Wild type–radiation/ temozolomide, TTF, consideration of clinical trials	Mutant–CCNU +/– TTF Wild type–CCNU +/– TTF, experimental therapy
MGMT status	Methylated–clinical trial, CCNU or bevacizumab Unmethylated–clinical trial, CCNU or bevacizumab	Methylated–bevacizumab and/or irinotecan Unmethylated–bevacizumab and/or irinotecan	Methylated–radiation/ temozolomide Unmethylated–radiation/ temozolomide, TTF, consideration of clinical trials	Methylated–CCNU +/– TTF Unmethylated–CCNU +/– TTF, experimental therapy

5-ALA, 5-aminolevulinic acid; AF, arcuate fasciculus; CCNU, lomustine; ECoG, electrocorticography; EEG, electroencephalogram; DTI, diffusion tensor imaging; FET, fluoro-O-(2) fluoroethyl-l-tyrosine; FLAIR, fluid attenuation inversion recovery; fMRI, functional magnetic resonance imaging; GTR, gross total resection; ICU, intensive care unit; IFOF, inferior frontal occipital fasciculus; IOM, intraoperative monitoring; MCA, middle cerebral artery; MGMT, O6-methylguanine-DNA methyl-transferase; MR, magnetic resonance; MRI, magnetic resonance imaging; MRS, magnetic resonance spectroscopy; PET, positron emission tomography; TTF, tumor treatment fields.

Differential diagnosis and actual diagnosis

- Recurrent high-grade glioma
- Radiation necrosis/treatment effect

Important anatomic and preoperative considerations

Patients who undergo resection of a high-grade glioma undergo postoperative radiation and temozolomide chemotherapy for 6 weeks followed by monthly adjuvant cycles.[13] The surgical cavity, regardless of extent of resection, is monitored with surveillance scans.[14,15] The differential diagnosis of progressive enhancement and edema include recurrent tumor or treatment effect.[14,15] These diagnoses have similar radiographic appearance on magnetic resonance imaging (MRI), and therefore may be difficult to differentiate.[14,15] Other modalities to help in differentiating between treatment effect and recurrent tumor include perfusion MRI, magnetic resonance spectroscopy, and positron emission tomography, among others.[14,15] In concerning circumstances and/or in inconclusive cases, brain biopsy or resection may be necessary.[14,15]

Approaches to this lesion

For evaluating for recurrence versus radiation necrosis, imaging may not be able to differentiate between the two, and therefore obtaining tissue may be necessary.[14,15] The treatment of recurrent tumor includes biopsy to guide adjuvant therapy or reresection for diagnosis and symptomatic improvement.[6,16,17] A biopsy can be done either via a needle biopsy or open biopsy, in which the advantages include being minimally invasive and can be applied to eloquent regions, whereas the disadvantages include potential sampling error and inability to improve symptomatic mass effect.[18,19] Surgical resection has the advantages of more tissue to minimize sampling error and improvement in mass effect, but the disadvantages include potential surgical risks and difficulty in

applying to eloquent regions.[6,16,17] Other options include laser interstitial therapy, hyperbaric oxygen, and bevacizumab chemotherapy for recurrent tumor and/or radiation necrosis.[20] When surgery is pursued, both asleep or awake surgery can be done (Chapter 1, Fig. 1.2).

What was actually done

The case was discussed in a multidisciplinary neurooncology conference, and the prevailing thought was to pursue repeat resection for diagnosis to guide adjuvant therapy and reduce symptomatic mass effect. The patient was taken to surgery for left temporal craniotomy for tumor resection with general anesthesia without intraoperative monitoring. The patient was induced and intubated per routine. The head was fixed in pins, with two pins centered on the inion and one pin on the right forehead in the midpupillary line. The head was turned 90 degrees to the right, and a bump was placed under the left shoulder to facilitate turning. The old linear incision was then identified. The patient was draped in the usual standard fashion and given dexamethasone, levetiracetam, and cefazolin. The linear incision was made, and a myocutaneous flap was formed and held in place with cerebellar retractors. The prior burr holes and craniotomy were removed, as these spanned the lesion based on preoperative MRI surgical navigation. The dura was opened in a semicircular fashion with the base along the sphenoid wing. Ultrasound and surgical navigation were used to confirm the lesion, and the lesion was removed piecemeal until white matter was seen on all the edges. The dura, bone, and skin were closed in standard fashion.

The patient awoke at his neurologic baseline with intact speech and full strength and was taken to the intensive care unit for recovery. Postoperative MRI done within 48 hours after surgery showed gross total resection of the contrast-enhancing portion of the lesion (Fig. 27.2). The patient participated with physical and occupational therapy and was discharged to home on postoperative day 2 with an intact neurologic examination. The patient was prescribed 1 week of levetiracetam, and dexamethasone was tapered to off over 7 days after surgery. The patient was seen at 2 weeks postoperatively for removal of stitches and remained

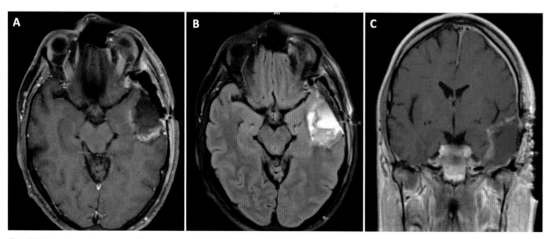

Fig. 27.2 **Postoperative magnetic resonance imaging.** **(A)** T1 axial with gadolinium contrast; **(B)** T2 axial fluid attenuation inversion recovery image; **(C)** T1 coronal image with gadolinium contrast demonstrating gross total resection of the enhancing portion of the tumor.

neurologically intact. Pathology was recurrent World Health Organization grade IV glioblastoma (IDH wild type, MGMT unmethylated). The patient underwent tumor treatment fields. The patient is without recurrence for 6 months following the repeat resection.

Commonalities among the experts

All surgeons opted for patients having diffusion tensor imaging to identify white matter tracts, and functional MRI to identify eloquent areas prior to surgery, whereas half requested magnetic resonance spectroscopy to help determine recurrence versus treatment effect. All surgeons elected for performing this surgery through a left temporal awake cortical and subcortical brain mapping approach with an asleep-awake-asleep anesthesia protocol, in which half used 5-aminolevulinic acid and one surgeon used intraoperative MRI to further guide resection. Half of the surgeons chose to use intraoperative MRI to assess for need for additional resection, and one surgeon selected 5-aminolevulinic acid to help assist resection. The goal of surgery in all surgeons was extensive resection of the enhancing portion of the tumor, and two surgeons also wanted to maximally resect the fluid attenuation inversion recovery component of the tumor. Most surgeons identified the importance of protecting the arcuate fasciculus and Sylvian fissure vessels, and the most feared complication was speech dysfunction. Surgery was generally pursued with surgical navigation, surgical microscope, brain stimulator, and ultrasonic aspirator with perioperative steroids and antiepileptics. All surgeons relied on cortical and subcortical mapping, whereas half relied on fluorescence to minimize the potential for iatrogenic injury. Following surgery, all patients were admitted to the intensive care unit, and imaging was obtained within 72 hours after surgery to assess extent of resection and/or potential complications. For a diagnosis of a recurrent glioblastoma, regardless of MGMT and IDH status, most surgeons favored the use of alternative therapies, including lomustine, bevacizumab, and/or tumor treatment fields.

SUMMARY OF QUALITY OF EVIDENCE TO GUIDE SPECIFIC INTERVENTIONS FOR THIS CASE

- Surgical resection of recurrent high-grade gliomas—Class II-2.
- Increasing extent of resection associated with improved outcomes for recurrent high-grade gliomas—Class III.
- Surgery for radiation necrosis—Class III.
- Tumor treatment fields for recurrent high-grade gliomas—Class I.

REFERENCES

1. DeAngelis LM. Brain tumors. *N Engl J Med*. 2001;344:114–123.
2. Gallia GL, Brem S, Brem H. Local treatment of malignant brain tumors using implantable chemotherapeutic polymers. *J Natl Compr Canc Netw*. 2005;3:721–728.
3. Chaichana K, Parker S, Olivi A, Quinones-Hinojosa A. A proposed classification system that projects outcomes based on preoperative variables for adult patients with glioblastoma multiforme. *J Neurosurg*. 2010;112:997–1004.
4. Chaichana KL, Cabrera-Aldana EE, Jusue-Torres I, et al. When gross total resection of a glioblastoma is possible, how much resection should be achieved. *World Neurosurg*. 2014;82:e257–e265.
5. Chaichana KL, Jusue-Torres I, Navarro-Ramirez R, et al. Establishing percent resection and residual volume thresholds affecting survival and recurrence for patients with newly diagnosed intracranial glioblastoma. *Neuro Oncol*. 2014;16:113–122.
6. Chaichana KL, Zadnik P, Weingart JD, et al. Multiple resections for patients with glioblastoma: prolonging survival. *J Neurosurg*. 2013;118:812–820.
7. Barker 2nd FG, S.M. Chang, Gutin PH, et al. Survival and functional status after resection of recurrent glioblastoma multiforme. *Neurosurgery*. 1998;42:709–720; discussion 720–730.
8. Hau P, Baumgart U, Pfeifer K, et al. Salvage therapy in patients with glioblastoma: is there any benefit. *Cancer*. 2003;98:2678–2686.
9. Helseth R, Helseth E, Johannesen TB, et al. Overall survival, prognostic factors, and repeated surgery in a consecutive series of 516 patients with glioblastoma multiforme. *Acta Neurol Scand*. 2010;122:159–167.
10. Stark AM, Nabavi A, Mehdorn HM, Blomer U. Glioblastoma multiforme-report of 267 cases treated at a single institution. *Surg Neurol*. 2005;63:162–169; discussion 169.
11. Sathornsumetee S, Rich JN. New treatment strategies for malignant gliomas. *Expert Rev Anticancer Ther*. 2006;6:1087–1104.
12. Nieder C, Grosu AL, Molls M. A comparison of treatment results for recurrent malignant gliomas. *Cancer Treat Rev*. 2000;26:397–409.
13. Stupp R, Mason WP, van den Bent MJ, et al. Radiotherapy plus concomitant and adjuvant temozolomide for glioblastoma. *N Engl J Med*. 2005;352:987–996.
14. Choi SH, Kim JW, Chang JS, et al. Impact of including peritumoral edema in radiotherapy target volume on patterns of failure in glioblastoma following temozolomide-based chemoradiotherapy. *Sci Rep*. 2017;7:42148.
15. Shah R, Vattoth S, Jacob R, et al. Radiation necrosis in the brain: imaging features and differentiation from tumor recurrence. *Radiographics*. 2012;32:1343–1359.
16. Bloch O, Han SJ, Cha S, et al. Impact of extent of resection for recurrent glioblastoma on overall survival: clinical article. *J Neurosurg*. 2012;117:1032–1038.
17. McGirt MJ, Chaichana KL, Attenello FJ, et al. Extent of surgical resection is independently associated with survival in patients with hemispheric infiltrating low-grade gliomas. *Neurosurgery*. 2008;63:700–707; author reply 707–708.
18. Iyer R, Chaichana KL. Minimally invasive resection of deep-seated high-grade gliomas using tubular retractors and exoscopic visualization. *J Neurol Surg A Cent Eur Neurosurg*. 2018;79:330–336.
19. Jackson C, Gallia GL, Chaichana KL. Minimally invasive biopsies of deep-seated brain lesions using tubular retractors under exoscopic visualization. *J Neurol Surg A Cent Eur Neurosurg*. 2017;78:588–594.
20. Silva D, Sharma M, Barnett GH. Laser ablation vs open resection for deep-seated tumors: evidence for laser ablation. *Neurosurgery*. 2016;63(Suppl 1):15–26.

28

Multifocal high-grade glioma

Case reviewed by Juan A. Barcia, Mohamed El-Fiki, Michael Lim, Michael E. Sughrue

Introduction

Patients with high-grade gliomas have poor prognoses, with median survival approximately 12 months.[1-4] A subset of patients with glioblastoma (GBM) have multifocal disease, whereby their lesions are separated by space.[5,6] These patients are considered to have poorer prognoses among patients with GBM.[5,6] These tumors are known to possess mutations in all three common GBM pathways, including RTK/PI3K, p53, and RB regulatory pathways with aberrations of epidermal growth factor receptor and CDKN2A/B.[7] The management of these lesions is therefore controversial and ranges from needle biopsies and resection of the most accessible lesion to resection of all lesions.[5,6,8] In this chapter, we present a case of a multifocal high-grade glioma.

Example case

Chief complaint: right arm and leg weakness
History of present illness
A 51-year-old, right-handed man with no significant past medical history presented with progressive right arm and leg weakness. Over the past 3 weeks, he has noted decreased dexterity in his right hand and now with an inability to walk (Fig. 28.1).
Medications: None.
Allergies: No known drug allergies.
Past medical and surgical history: None.
Family history: No history of intracranial malignancies.
Social history: Accountant. No smoking and no alcohol.
Physical examination: Awake, alert, oriented to person, place, and time; *Language*: intact naming and repetition; Cranial nerves II to XII intact; Right drift, right upper extremity 4/5, left upper extremity 5/5, right lower extremity 4/5, left lower extremity 5/5.
Imaging: Chest/abdomen/pelvis with no evidence of primary disease.

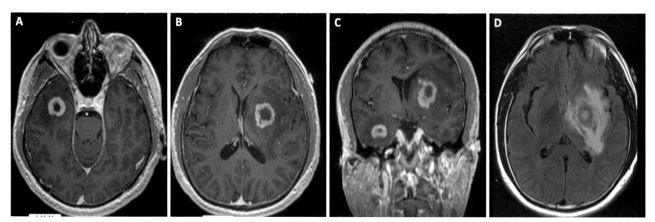

Fig. 28.1 Preoperative magnetic resonance imaging. (A) T1 axial image with gadolinium contrast through the temporal lobe; **(B)** T1 axial image with gadolinium contrast through the basal ganglia; **(C)** T1 coronal image with gadolinium contrast; **(D)** T2 axial fluid attenuation inversion recovery magnetic resonance imaging scan demonstrating multifocal, contrast-enhancing lesions involving the right temporal lobe and left basal ganglia.

	Juan A. Barcia, MD, PhD, Hospital Clínico San Carlos, Complutense University, Madrid, Spain	Mohamed El-Fiki, MBBCh, MS, MD, University of Alexandria, Alexandria, Egypt	Michael Lim, MD, Stanford University School of Medicine, Stanford, CA, United States	Michael E. Sughrue, MD, Prince of Wales Hospital, Sydney, Australia
Preoperative				
Additional tests requested	DTI Neuropsychological assessment for language dominance CT chest/abdomen/pelvis	DTI MRS Whole-body PET CT chest, abdominal ultrasound	DTI fMRI	DTI
Surgical approach selected	Right temporal stereotactic biopsy with local anesthetics followed by adjuvant therapy or left awake craniotomy if hemiparesis persists despite steroids pending patient's preference	Right temporal excisional biopsy with 5-ALA	Right temporal craniotomy	Right awake transcallosal contralateral transventricular approach for left basal lesion, LITT for remaining lesions
Anatomic corridor	Right temporal	Right temporal	Right temporal	Interhemispheric transventricular
Goal of surgery	Diagnosis if biopsy pursued, diagnosis and motor recovery if left basal ganglia lesion pursued	Diagnosis to guide adjuvant therapy	Gross total resection of right temporal lesion	Extensive resection of contrast-enhancing portion of left basal ganglia lesion to reduce mass effect
Perioperative				
Positioning	Right lateral	Right supine with left rotation	Right supine	Left lateral (surgical side down)
Surgical equipment	Surgical navigation Biopsy set	Surgical navigation Surgical microscope with 5-ALA Ultrasonic aspirator	Surgical navigation IOM (SSEP)	Surgical navigation Brain stimulator Surgical microscope
Medications	Antiepileptics	Steroids Mannitol/furosemide Antiepileptics	Steroids Mannitol Antiepileptics	Steroids Mannitol
Anatomic considerations	Right temporal lobe, Sylvian fissure, temporal horn of lateral ventricle	STA, zygomatic arch, MTG/ITG	Right anterior temporal lobe	ACA, cingulate gyrus, caudate nucleus, CST, basal ganglia, lenticulostriate artery
Complications feared with approach chosen	Hemorrhage, brain shifts	Increasing neurologic deficit	Motor and language deficit from left lesion	Avoiding laterally placed critical white matter tracts
Intraoperative				
Anesthesia	General	General	General	Asleep-awake-asleep
Skin incision	Linear	Reverse question mark	Reverse question mark	Linear bicoronal
Bone opening	Right temporal	Right temporal	Right temporal	Right frontal
Brain exposure	Right temporal	Right temporal	Right temporal	Right frontal

(continued on next page)

	Juan A. Barcia, MD, PhD, Hospital Clínico San Carlos, Complutense University, Madrid, Spain	Mohamed El-Fiki, MBBCh, MS, MD, University of Alexandria, Alexandria, Egypt	Michael Lim, MD, Stanford University School of Medicine, Stanford, CA, United States	Michael E. Sughrue, MD, Prince of Wales Hospital, Sydney, Australia
Method of resection	Linear incision, right temporal burr hole, open dura, stereotactic needle biopsy of right temporal lesion, obtain various samples at the periphery and core of the enhancing region, intraoperative pathology to confirm lesional tissue	Craniotomy guided by navigation, low temporal opening and removal of bone to reach temporal floor, suture holes for fixation, dural tack up sutures, U-shaped dural opening based on temporal floor, identify Sylvian fissure/STS/ITS, transsulcal approach, excisional biopsy with 5-ALA, dissect lesion from surrounding brain if possible and remove en bloc, avoid ventricular entry, watertight dural closure, insertion of subgaleal drain	Myocutaneous flap, craniotomy guided by navigation, large corticectomy in MTG over lesion, dissect capsule from surrounding brain, attempted en bloc resection	Patient sedated, scalp block, right frontal craniotomy under navigation guidance up to sagittal sinus, interhemispheric approach, left callosotomy, entry into the left lateral ventricle, enter tumor above caudate head, awake patient and perform language and motor mapping, resection of tumor preserving lenticulostriates at inferior aspect of the tumor, awareness that tumor can appear like basal ganglia, placement of EVD
Complication avoidance	Stereotactic needle biopsy, avoid left basal ganglia lesion, biopsy from different locations	Preserve STA, transsulcal, avoid left basal ganglia lesion, en bloc resection, avoid ventricular entry	Avoid left basal ganglia lesion, IOM	Awake cortical and subcortical language and motor mapping, contralateral approach, EVD
Postoperative				
Admission	ICU	ICU	ICU	ICU
Postoperative complications feared	Hemorrhage, seizures	Hematoma, seizures	Visual field deficit, memory loss	Hydrocephalus, injury to lenticulostriate arteries
Follow-up testing	CT immediately after surgery	Depends on pathology of lesion	MRI within 48 hours after surgery Visual field testing	MRI within 48 hours after surgery LITT therapy of remaining lesions if GBM in 1–2 weeks
Follow-up visits	When pathological diagnosis available	7 days, 1 month, and every three months after surgery	14 days after surgery	7–14 days after surgery
Adjuvant therapies recommended				
IDH status	Mutant–radiation/ temozolomide Wild type–radiation/ temozolomide	Mutant–radiation/ temozolomide Wild type–radiation/ temozolomide	Mutant–radiation/ temozolomide +/– TTF Wild type–radiation/ temozolomide +/– TTF	Mutant–radiation/ temozolomide Wild type–radiation/ temozolomide
MGMT status	Methylated– temozolomide, followed by radiation/ temozolomide Unmethylated– radiation/ temozolomide	Methylated–radiation/ temozolomide Unmethylated–radiation/ temozolomide	Methylated–radiation/ temozolomide +/– TTF Unmethylated–radiation/ temozolomide +/– TTF	Methylated–radiation/ temozolomide Unmethylated–radiation/ temozolomide

5-ALA, 5-aminolevulinic acid; *ACA*, anterior cerebral artery; *CST*, corticospinal tract; *CT*, computed tomography; *DTI*, diffusion tensor imaging; *EVD*, external ventricular drain; *fMRI*, functional magnetic resonance imaging; *GBM*, glioblastoma; *ICU*, intensive care unit; *IOM*, intraoperative monitoring; *ITG*, inferior temporal gyrus; *ITS*, inferior temporal sulcus; *LITT*, laser interstitial thermal therapy; *MGMT*, O6-methylguanine-DNA methyl-transferase; *MRI*, magnetic resonance imaging; *MRS*, magnetic resonance spectroscopy; *MTG*, middle temporal gyrus; *PET*, positron emission tomography; *SSEP*, somatosensory evoked potentials; *STA*, superficial temporal artery; *STS*, superior temporal sulcus; *TTF*, tumor treatment fields.

Differential diagnosis and actual diagnosis

- Metastatic brain cancer
- Multifocal high-grade glioma
- Cerebral abscess
- Lymphoma

Important anatomic and preoperative considerations

As discussed in Chapter 12, in cases in which tissue is needed for multifocal lesions, the goal of lesion selection is to obtain the highest yield tissue in the area with the least risk of neurologic deficit. Among these lesions in this case, the right temporal lesion possesses the highest yield tissue with the lowest risk. However, patients with multifocal lesions may be symptomatic from primarily one lesion, and therefore, if nonbiopsy surgical resection is pursued, resection generally should target the more symptomatic lesion. In this case, the more symptomatic lesion is the left basal ganglia lesion.

Approaches to this lesion

The approaches to multifocal lesions include needle biopsy, excisional biopsy, or surgical resection of one or more lesions.[5,6] Patients with multifocal disease include metastatic brain cancer[9] and multifocal high-grade glioma.[5,6] For patients with multifocal metastases, the surgical resection of all lesions have similar outcomes to single solitary lesions.[9] For multifocal high-grade gliomas, the management is more controversial.[5,6,8] This is because patients with multifocal high-grade gliomas typically have poor prognoses regardless of treatment algorithm.[5,6] A needle biopsy has the least risk and has a high yield of diagnosis, but the drawbacks include sampling error, inability to reduce mass effect, and lack of tissue for genomic analyses and tissue banking.[10] An excisional biopsy provides more tissue for pathology and less risk of sampling error but has higher surgical risks and does not improve mass effect.[10] Surgical resection has the highest inherent risk but yields more tissue for pathology and tissue banking and can provide symptomatic improvement.[10] In a study by Sawaya and colleagues, they found that patients who underwent resection of all multifocal high-grade gliomas in a single setting had similar outcomes to matched patients with solitary high-grade gliomas (median survival of 9.7 vs. 10.5 months, respectively, $P = 0.34$).[8]

What was actually done

The case was discussed in a multidisciplinary neurooncology conference, and the prevailing thought was that the patient had metastatic brain tumors despite negative systemic workup. The patient was taken to surgery for right temporal and left frontal craniotomies for tumor resection of the right temporal and left basal ganglia lesions with general anesthesia and intraoperative monitoring. The patient was induced and intubated per routine, and the patient underwent continuous electroencephalogram and somatosensory evoked potential monitoring. The head was placed in a headrest, and electromagnetic surgical navigation was used that obviated head pinning. The right temporal lesion was addressed first because it was the least eloquent. The head was turned 90 degrees to the left, and a bump was placed under the right shoulder to facilitate turning. A linear incision was then planned from the zygoma to the superior temporal line over the lesion based on surgical navigation. The patient was draped in the usual standard fashion and given dexamethasone, levetiracetam, and cefazolin. The linear incision was made, and a myocutaneous flap was formed and held in place with cerebellar retractors. A keyhole temporal craniotomy was made, and the dura was opened in a cruciate fashion. The lesion was accessed through the middle temporal gyrus and removed en bloc. Preliminary diagnosis was lesional but favored sarcoma. The dura, bone, and skin were closed in standard fashion. The patient was then placed supine on the headrest with the neck slightly flexed. A Kocher point incision was then planned with a linear incision in the sagittal plane over the midpupillary line. The patient was draped in the usual standard fashion. The linear incision was made, and the skin was retracted with Weitlaner retractors. A keyhole frontal craniotomy was made, and the dura was opened in a cruciate fashion. The sulcus was opened sharply under exoscopic visualization, and a 65-mm tubular retractor was placed through the sulcus and docked superficially on the lesion. The lesion was removed en bloc. The dura, bone, and skin were closed in standard fashion.

The patient awoke with intact speech but worsened right-sided weakness (2-3/5) and was taken to the intensive care unit for recovery. Postoperative magnetic resonance imaging done within 48 hours after surgery showed gross total resection of the right temporal and left basal ganglia lesions (Fig. 28.2). The patient participated with physical and occupational therapy and was discharged to rehabilitation on postoperative day 5 with improved right-sided strength (3/5). The patient was prescribed 3 months of levetiracetam, and dexamethasone was tapered to off over 10 days after surgery. The patient was seen at 2 weeks postoperatively for removal of staples and had improved right-sided strength (4-4+/5). Pathology for both lesions was a World Health Organization grade IV gliosarcoma (IDH wild type, O6-methylguanine-DNA methyl-transferase unmethylated). The patient underwent temozolomide and radiation therapy with four adjuvant cycles. The patient did well initially but developed lung lesions that were biopsied and consistent with gliosarcoma. The patient died 6 months after cranial surgery.

Commonalities among the experts

All surgeons opted for patients having diffusion tensor imaging to identify white matter tracts prior to surgery. Half of the surgeons elected for performing a biopsy through the temporal lobe of the lesion for diagnosis to guide adjuvant therapy, whereas the other half requested surgical resection (temporal approach in one and an awake contralateral transcallosal approach in the other) with the goal of extensive resection. Most surgeons identified the

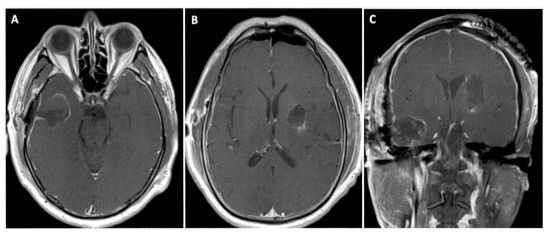

Fig. 28.2 **Postoperative magnetic resonance imaging. (A)** T1 axial image with gadolinium contrast through the temporal lobe; **(B)** T1 axial image with gadolinium contrast through the basal ganglia; **(C)** T1 coronal image with gadolinium contrast magnetic resonance imaging scan demonstrating gross total resection of multifocal, contrast-enhancing lesions involving the right temporal lobe and left basal ganglia.

importance of understanding temporal lobe anatomy, in which most feared causing progressive neurologic deficits in this patient. Surgery was pursued with surgical navigation in all, biopsy kits in half, and surgical microscopes in half, along with perioperative steroids and antiepileptics. Half of the surgeons utilized a biopsy approach to minimize risk of iatrogenic injury, whereas among those who pursued surgical resection, one avoided basal ganglia transgression and the other employed a contralateral approach with awake subcortical mapping. Following surgery, all patients were admitted to the intensive care unit, and most obtained imaging within 48 hours after surgery to assess extent of resection and/or potential complications. For a diagnosis of a high-grade glioma, regardless of O6-methylguanine-DNA methyl-transferase and IDH status, all surgeons favored the use of postoperative radiation and temozolomide, and one surgeon provided the additional option of tumor treatment fields.

SUMMARY OF QUALITY OF EVIDENCE TO GUIDE SPECIFIC INTERVENTIONS FOR THIS CASE

- Surgery resection of multifocal high-grade gliomas—Class III.
- Increasing extent of resection associated with improved outcomes for multifocal high-grade gliomas—Class III.
- Multidisciplinary care and brain tumor outcomes—Class III.

REFERENCES

1. DeAngelis LM. Brain tumors. *N Engl J Med*. 2001;344:114–123.
2. Hau P, Baumgart U, Pfeifer K, et al. Salvage therapy in patients with glioblastoma: is there any benefit? *Cancer*. 2003;98:2678–2686.
3. Chaichana KL, Jusue-Torres I, Navarro-Ramirez R, et al. Establishing percent resection and residual volume thresholds affecting survival and recurrence for patients with newly diagnosed intracranial glioblastoma. *Neuro Oncol*. 2014;16:113–122.
4. Chaichana KL, Zadnik P, Weingart JD, et al. Multiple resections for patients with glioblastoma: prolonging survival. *J Neurosurg*. 2013;118:812–820.
5. Ahmadipour Y, Jabbarli R, Gembruch O, et al. Impact of multifocality and molecular markers on survival of glioblastoma. *World Neurosurg*. 2019;122:e461–e466.
6. Paulsson AK, Holmes JA, Peiffer AM, et al. Comparison of clinical outcomes and genomic characteristics of single focus and multifocal glioblastoma. *J Neurooncol*. 2014;119:429–435.
7. Abou-El-Ardat K, Seifert M, Becker K, et al. Comprehensive molecular characterization of multifocal glioblastoma proves its monoclonal origin and reveals novel insights into clonal evolution and heterogeneity of glioblastomas. *Neuro Oncol*. 2017;19:546–557.
8. Hassaneen W, Levine NB, Suki D, et al. Multiple craniotomies in the management of multifocal and multicentric glioblastoma. Clinical article. *J Neurosurg*. 2011;114:576–584.
9. Kocher M, Soffietti R, Abacioglu U, et al. Adjuvant whole-brain radiotherapy versus observation after radiosurgery or surgical resection of one to three cerebral metastases: results of the EORTC 22952-26001 study. *J Clin Oncol*. 2011;29:134–141.
10. Jackson C, Gallia GL, Chaichana KL. Minimally invasive biopsies of deep-seated brain lesions using tubular retractors under exoscopic visualization. *J Neurol Surg A Cent Eur Neurosurg*. 2017;78:588–594.

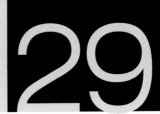

Butterfly high-grade glioma

Case reviewed by Chetan Bettegowda, Zvi Ram, Michael E. Sughrue, Shota Tanaka

Introduction

Patients with high-grade gliomas are known to have poor survival.[1–6] Among these patients, it is argued that butterfly lesions that cross the corpus callosum and involve both cerebral hemispheres have the worst prognoses.[7,8] Because of this presumed poor prognosis of butterfly lesions, patients with these lesions typically only undergo biopsy followed by adjuvant therapy.[7,8] However, more recent studies show that these patients may also benefit from extensive resection similar to their counterparts that only involve one hemisphere.[7,8] In this chapter, we present a case of a butterfly high-grade glioma.

Example case

Chief complaint: lethargy
History of present illness
A 29-year-old, right-handed woman with no significant past medical history who was transferred after a needle biopsy revealing glioblastoma for increasing lethargy. She initially presented with worsening headaches, and imaging revealed a large brain tumor. She underwent a right frontal needle biopsy consistent with glioblastoma 3 days prior. In the interim, she developed progressive lethargy and was transferred for further evaluation and management (Fig. 29.1).
Medications: Dexamethasone 4 mg every 6 hours, levetiracetam.
Allergies: No known drug allergies.
Past medical and surgical history: Right frontal needle biopsy 3 days prior.
Family history: No history of intracranial malignancies.
Social history: Graduate student. No smoking, social alcohol.
Physical examination: Sleepy, arouses to voice, oriented to person, place, and time; *Language:* intact naming and repetition; Cranial nerves II to XII intact; Unable to participate with drift, moves all extremities with good strength.

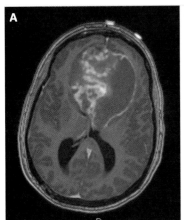 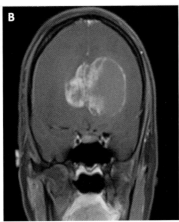 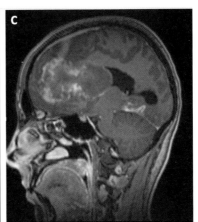

Fig. 29.1 Preoperative magnetic resonance imaging. (A) T1 axial image with gadolinium contrast; **(B)** T1 coronal image with gadolinium contrast; **(C)** T1 sagittal with gadolinium contrast magnetic resonance imaging scan demonstrating a bifrontal likely butterfly high-grade glioma.

	Chetan Bettegowda, MD, PhD, Johns Hopkins University, Baltimore, MD, United States	Zvi Ram, MD, Tel Aviv Medical Center, Tel Aviv, Israel	Michael E. Sughrue, MD, Prince of Wales Hospital, Sydney, Australia	Shota Tanaka, MD, PhD, The University of Tokyo, Tokyo, Japan
Preoperative				
Additional tests requested	None	DTI Neuropsychological assessment	DTI fMRI	PET methionine Ophthalmologic examination
Surgical approach selected	Bifrontal craniotomy	Left frontal craniotomy with 5-ALA	Left frontal craniotomy	Right frontal craniotomy with 5-ALA
Anatomic corridor	Bifrontal	Left MFG	Left MFG	Right frontal
Goal of surgery	Debulking	Gross total resection of enhancing component	Gross total resection	Debulking
Perioperative				
Positioning	Supine neutral	Supine neutral	Supine neutral	Supine neutral
Surgical equipment	Surgical navigation IOM (SSEP, EEG) Surgical microscope Ultrasound Ultrasonic aspirator	Surgical navigation Surgical microscope with 5-ALA Ultrasonic aspirator Brain stimulator IOM	Surgical navigation Surgical microscope	Surgical navigation IOM (MEP) Surgical microscope with 5-ALA Doppler
Medications	Mannitol Steroids Antiepileptics	Steroids	Mannitol Steroids	Mannitol Steroids Antiepileptics
Anatomic considerations	Frontal sinus, superior sagittal sinus, lateral ventricles, ACAs, internal capsule, basal ganglia, choroid vessels, fornices	ACA, lateral ventricles, CST	ACA, DMN/salience network, cingulum, caudate, contralateral cingulate gyrus	ACA
Complications feared with approach chosen	Vascular injury, injury to Sylvian vessels, forniceal injury	Motor deficits, intraventricular hemorrhage, ACA stroke	Preserving DMN/salience networks	Vascular injury to ACA
Intraoperative				
Anesthesia	General	General	General	General
Skin incision	Bifrontal	Bifrontal	Bifrontal	Curved
Bone opening	Bilateral frontal	Left frontal	Left frontal	Right frontal
Brain exposure	Bilateral frontal	Left SFG/MFG	Left SFG/MFG/IFG	Right frontal
Method of resection	Bifrontal incision with pericranial graft, right frontal and separate left frontal craniotomies, start on right side, open dura around biopsy sight and enter tumor along biopsy tract and tumor debulking, open left frontal dura, enter left side and debulk tumor, leave intraventricular component, EVD placement	Bifrontal incision, left frontal craniotomy to midline, U-shaped dural opening based on midline, expose SFG, access tumor through the SFG, debulk using ultrasonic aspirator, chase tumor to contralateral side with removal of genu, attempt to avoid ventricular entry and spare bilateral ACAs, stimulate posterior to avoid CST injury	Left frontal craniotomy, expose MFG, access tumor through superior/medial surface and expose tumor lateral to cingulate, resect posterior and deep areas avoiding caudate head, resect between callosal sulcus and ventricle, enter ventricle and section septum pellucidum, identify right caudate head and resect tumor medial to it, stay superior to rostrum to avoid septal nuclei, EVD placement	Right frontal craniotomy, dural opening, expose right SFG/MFG, entry into tumor under microscopic visualization, resection with careful attention to ACAs, further resection into genu and opening of left frontal cystic/necrotic component, reconstruction of ventricular wall if entered

	Chetan Bettegowda, MD, PhD, Johns Hopkins University, Baltimore, MD, United States	Zvi Ram, MD, Tel Aviv Medical Center, Tel Aviv, Israel	Michael E. Sughrue, MD, Prince of Wales Hospital, Sydney, Australia	Shota Tanaka, MD, PhD, The University of Tokyo, Tokyo, Japan
Complication avoidance	IOM, separate bifrontal craniotomies, follow previous surgical track, debulk tumor until reduction in mass effect, EVD	Expose SFG, stay within tumor, stimulate posterior aspect to avoid CST injury, avoid aggressive right-sided resection	Identify and avoid bilateral caudate heads, cingulate gyrus, callosal sulcus, EVD	Right frontal entry, IOM
Postoperative				
Admission	ICU	ICU	ICU	ICU
Postoperative complications feared	Hydrocephalus, intraventricular hemorrhage, ACA injury, seizures, weakness, language deficit	ACA injury, intraventricular hemorrhage, CST injury, SMA syndrome	Hydrocephalus, vasospasm	Vasospasm, infarction
Follow-up testing	HCT immediately after surgery MRI within 24 hours after surgery Physical/occupational/ speech therapy	CTA if motor deficit MRI within 48 hours after surgery	MRI within 24 hours after surgery	MRI within 48 hours after surgery
Follow-up visits	14 days after surgery	14 days after surgery	14 days after surgery 7 days after surgery for neurooncology	14–21 days after surgery
Adjuvant therapies recommended				
IDH status	Mutant–radiation/ temozolomide Wild type–radiation/ temozolomide	Mutant–radiation/ temozolomide + TTF Wild type– radiation + TTF	Mutant–radiation/ temozolomide Wild type–radiation/ temozolomide	Mutant–radiation/ temozolomide Wild type–radiation/ temozolomide
MGMT status	Methylated–radiation/ temozolomide Unmethylated–radiation/ temozolomide	Methylated–radiation/ temozolomide + TTF Unmethylated– radiation + TTF	Methylated–radiation/ temozolomide Unmethylated–radiation/ temozolomide	Methylated–radiation/ temozolomide Unmethylated–radiation/ temozolomide

5-ALA, 5-aminolevulinic acid; *ACA*, anterior cerebral artery; *DMN*, default mode network; *CST*, corticospinal tracts; *CTA*, computed tomography angiography; *DTI*, diffusion tensor imaging; *EEG*, electroencephalogram; *EVD*, external ventricular drain; *fMRI*, functional magnetic resonance imaging; *HCT*, head computed tomography; *ICU*, intensive care unit; *IFG*, inferior frontal gyrus; *IOM*, intraoperative monitoring; *MFP*, motor evoked potential; *MFG*, middle frontal gyrus; *MGMT*, O6-methylguanine-DNA methyl-transferase; *MRI,* magnetic resonance imaging; *PET*, positron emission tomography; *SFG*, superior frontal gyrus; *SMA*, supplementary motor area; *SSEP*, somatosensory evoked potential; *TTF*, tumor treatment fields.

Differential diagnosis and actual diagnosis

- High-grade glioma
- Cerebral abscess
- Lymphoma
- Metastatic brain cancer

Important anatomic and preoperative considerations

The corpus callosum consists of the rostrum, genu, body, and splenium.[9,10] It is separated from the overlying cingulate gyrus by the callosal sulcus.[9,10] The cingulate gyrus is separated from the medial frontal lobe by the cingulate sulcus.[9,10] The cingulum is a collection of white matter fibers that project from the cingulate gyrus to the entorhinal cortex as part of the limbic system, and also receives afferent fibers from the thalamus as part of the spinothalamic tract.[9,10] Butterfly gliomas typically cross the corpus callosum and are therefore in close juxtaposition to the cingulum and cingulate gyrus.[7,8] In addition, there are several white matter tracts that need to be considered, including the superior longitudinal fasciculus laterally, the frontal aslant tract on the dominant hemisphere posterolaterally, the cingulum medially, and the default mode network (DMN).[9–11] The DMN consists of connections between the medial and lateral parietal, anteromedial prefrontal, posterior cingulate cortex, and medial and lateral temporal cortices, and plays a role in several complex cognitive functions, including speech, theory of mind, and memory.[11] Injury to these areas can significantly affect quality of life and lead to symptoms including abulia.[11]

Approaches to this lesion

The management of butterfly gliomas is controversial and varied.[7,8] Butterfly gliomas are typically larger, more difficult to resect, and associated with more morbidity than gliomas located elsewhere.[7,8] As a result, the management of these lesions include biopsy, excisional biopsy, unilateral resection, and bilateral resections, among others.[7,8] The advantages of needle biopsy and excisional biopsies are that they are typically minimally invasive, short surgical duration, shortened hospital stay, and associated with minimal morbidity to facilitate initiation of adjuvant therapy; however, they do not improve mass effect or tumor burden and can be associated with sampling error.[12] Unilateral resections aim to debulk the tumor only on one side, whereby the chosen side typically has a greater tumor burden, involves the non-dominant hemisphere, and/or avoids critical neurovascular structures, including the DMN and/or anterior cerebral arteries. Bilateral resections aim to remove as much tumor as possible but has the inherent risk of bifrontal injury, injury to the DMN, and potentially more morbidity, longer hospital stays, and delay in adjuvant therapies. Recent studies have shown that anterior butterfly glioma resections can occur safely, and that more extensive resection can be associated with improved outcomes as compared with lesser resections for this subset of gliomas.[7,8]

What was actually done

The patient was too lethargic to participate in an awake brain mapping procedure, and because of the significant mass effect, it was determined to attempt extensive resection from the right, nondominant side first, but if significant lesion remained, then a contralateral approach would be done concurrently. The patient was therefore taken to surgery for bilateral frontal craniotomies for tumor resection with general anesthesia and intraoperative monitoring. The patient was induced and intubated per routine, and the patient underwent continuous electroencephalogram and somatosensory evoked potential monitoring. The head was fixed in pins, with two pins centered on the left external auditory meatus and one pin over the right external auditory meatus on the superior temporal line. The head was flexed and kept neutral. The old right linear incision was identified and extended, and a parallel left linear incision was planned in the sagittal plan over the midpupillary line at the Kocher point based on surgical navigation. The patient was draped in the usual standard fashion and given dexamethasone, levetiracetam, and cefazolin. The right frontal incision was opened and extended, and the skin was retracted with a Weitlaner retractor. The burr hole made during the previous biopsy was used to make a right frontal keyhole craniotomy, and the right frontal dura was opened in a cruciate fashion. The sulcus was opened under microscopic visualization, and a 65-mm tubular retractor was placed transsulcal into the center of the lesion based on surgical navigation. The tumor was debulked until white matter was seen on all the edges except the medial portion that could not be reached. At this point, the left frontal incision was made, skin retracted with a Weitlaner retractor, and a keyhole craniotomy was made. The dura was opened in a cruciate fashion, and the underlying sulcus was opened under microscopic visualization, and another 65-mm tubular retractor was placed into the center of the remaining left frontal lesion based on surgical navigation. The tumor was debulked until white matter was seen on all the edges. Once the tumor was thought to be completely resected and not exceeding the tumor boundaries, each retractor was withdrawn, and the cavities were inspected for hemostasis. The ventricles were never entered, and therefore an external ventricular drain was not placed. Preliminary diagnosis was high-grade glioma. The dura, bone, and skin were closed bilaterally in standard fashion.

The patient awoke at her neurologic baseline with intact speech and moved all extremities with good strength and was taken to the intensive care unit for recovery. Postoperative magnetic resonance imaging done within 48 hours after surgery showed near total resection with residual along the genu of the corpus callosum (Fig. 29.2). The patient participated with physical and occupational therapy and was discharged to home on postoperative day 3 with an intact examination and no signs of abulia. The patient was prescribed 3 months of levetiracetam, and dexamethasone was tapered to off over 10 days after surgery. The patient was seen at 2 weeks postoperatively for removal of staples and remained neurologically intact. Pathology was a

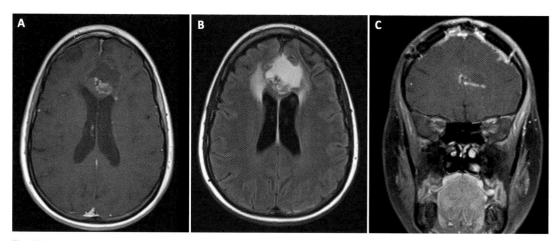

Fig. 29.2 Postoperative magnetic resonance imaging. (A) T1 axial image with gadolinium contrast; **(B)** T2 axial fluid attenuation inversion recovery image; **(C)** T1 coronal with gadolinium contrast magnetic resonance imaging scan demonstrating near total resection of the butterfly lesion with residual along the genu of the corpus callosum.

World Health Organization grade IV glioblastoma (IDH mutant, O6-methylguanine-DNA methyl-transferase methylated). The patient returned to school 4 weeks after surgery. The patient also underwent temozolomide and radiation therapy with six adjuvant cycles. The patient has been without recurrence 12 months after surgery.

Commonalities among the experts

Half of the surgeons opted for patients having diffusion tensor imaging to identify white matter tracts prior to surgery. All surgeons elected for resection of this lesion, in which two favored a left frontal craniotomy and left middle frontal gyrus approach, one a right frontal craniotomy, and another bifrontal craniotomy. Half of the surgeons chose to use 5-aminolevulinic acid to help guide resection. The goal of surgery in half of the surgeons was gross total resection of the lesion, whereas the other half aimed for debulking. All surgeons were concerned about the location of the anterior cerebral arteries, and half were concerned about injury to the basal ganglia. The most feared complication was injury to the anterior cerebral arteries. Surgery was generally pursued with surgical navigation, surgical microscope, ultrasonic aspirator, and intraoperative monitoring with perioperative steroids, antiepileptics, and mannitol. The majority of surgeons relied on internal debulking to minimize potential iatrogenic injury. Following surgery, all patients were admitted to the intensive care unit, and imaging was obtained within 48 hours after surgery to assess extent of resection and/or potential complications. For a diagnosis of a glioblastoma, regardless of O6-methylguanine-DNA methyl-transferase and IDH status, all surgeons chose to administer radiation and temozolomide chemotherapy, with one surgeon providing the option of tumor treatment fields.

SUMMARY OF QUALITY OF EVIDENCE TO GUIDE SPECIFIC INTERVENTIONS FOR THIS CASE

- Surgery resection of butterfly gliomas—Class II-3.
- Increasing extent of resection associated with improved outcomes for butterfly gliomas—Class II-3.

REFERENCES

1. Chaichana K, Parker S, Olivi A, Quinones-Hinojosa A. A proposed classification system that projects outcomes based on preoperative variables for adult patients with glioblastoma multiforme. *J Neurosurg.* 2010;112:997–1004.
2. Chaichana KL, Chaichana KK, Olivi A, et al. Surgical outcomes for older patients with glioblastoma multiforme: preoperative factors associated with decreased survival. Clinical article. *J Neurosurg.* 2011;114:587–594.
3. Chaichana KL, Halthore AN, Parker SL, et al. Factors involved in maintaining prolonged functional independence following supratentorial glioblastoma resection. Clinical article. *J Neurosurg.* 2011;114:604–612.
4. Lacroix M, Abi-Said D, Fourney DR, et al. A multivariate analysis of 416 patients with glioblastoma multiforme: prognosis, extent of resection, and survival. *J Neurosurg.* 2001;95:190–198.
5. Laws ER, Parney IF, Huang W. et al: Survival following surgery and prognostic factors for recently diagnosed malignant glioma: data from the Glioma Outcomes Project. *J Neurosurg.* 2003;99:467–473.
6. Sanai N, Polley MY, McDermott MW, Parsa AT, Berger MS. An extent of resection threshold for newly diagnosed glioblastomas. *J Neurosurg.* 2011;115:3–8.
7. Chaichana KL, Jusue-Torres I, Lemos AM, et al. The butterfly effect on glioblastoma: is volumetric extent of resection more effective than biopsy for these tumors? *J Neurooncol.* 2014;120:625–634.
8. Burks JD, Bonney PA, Conner AK, et al. A method for safely resecting anterior butterfly gliomas: the surgical anatomy of the default mode network and the relevance of its preservation. *J Neurosurg.* 2017;126:1795–1811.
9. Fernandez-Miranda JC, Rhoton Jr AL, Alvarez-Linera J, Kakizawa Y, Choi C, de Oliveira EP. Three-dimensional microsurgical and tractographic anatomy of the white matter of the human brain. *Neurosurgery.* 2008;62:989–1026; discussion 1026–1028.
10. Rhoton Jr AL. The cerebrum. Anatomy. *Neurosurgery.* 2007;61:37–118; discussion 118–119.
11. Raichle ME. The brain's default mode network. *Annu Rev Neurosci.* 2015;38:433–447.
12. Jackson CM, Lim M, Drake CG. Immunotherapy for brain cancer: recent progress and future promise. *Clin Cancer Res.* 2014;20:3651–3659.

30

Pontine high-grade glioma

Case reviewed by Bob S. Carter, Shlomi Constantini, Danil A. Kozyrev, Alessandro Olivi, Giuseppe Maria Della Pepa, Andrew E. Sloan

Introduction

Brainstem surgery can be associated with significant morbidity and mortality.[1,2] This high risk of neurologic injury is owing to the fact that the brainstem has a high density of eloquent gray and white matter structures, including cranial nerve nuclei, cranial nerve tracts, and craniospinal tracts, among others.[1,2] With improvements in neuroimaging, advances in surgical techniques, and improved mapping paradigms, surgery within the brainstem can occur with reduced morbidity.[1,2] In this chapter, we present a case of a likely high-grade lesion within the pons.

Example case

Chief complaint: double vision

History of present illness

A 46-year-old, right-handed man with no significant past medical history presented with double vision. Over the past 4 to 5 months, he has complained of progressive double vision to the point where he cannot drive. Imaging was done and revealed a brain lesion (Fig. 30.1).

Medications: None.

Allergies: No known drug allergies.

Past medical and surgical history: None.

Family history: No history of intracranial malignancies.

Social history: Farmer. No smoking or alcohol.

Physical examination: Awake, alert, oriented to person, place, and time; *Language*: intact naming and repetition; Cranial nerves II to XII intact except right eye abduction weakness and dysconjugate gaze; No drift, moves all extremities with full strength; Cerebellar: no finger-to-nose dysmetria.

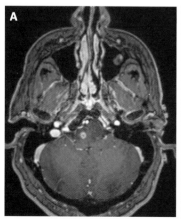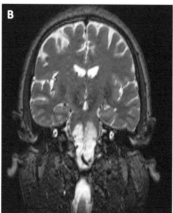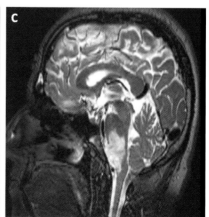

Fig. 30.1 Preoperative magnetic resonance imaging. (A) T1 axial image with gadolinium contrast; **(B)** T2 coronal image; **(C)** T2 sagittal magnetic resonance imaging scan demonstrating an enhancing lesion in the right pontine tegmentum.

	Bob S. Carter, MD, PhD, Massachusetts General Hospital, Boston, MA, United States	Shlomi Constantini, MD, Danil A. Kozyrev, MD, Tel Aviv Sourasky Medical Center, Tel Aviv, Israel	Alessandro Olivi, MD, Giuseppe Maria Della Pepa, MD, Fondazione Policlinico Universitario Agostino Gemelli IRCSS, Catholic University of Rome, Rome, Italy	Andrew E. Sloan, MD, University Hospital, Case Western Reserve Cleveland, OH, United States
Preoperative				
Additional tests requested	CSF analysis	MRI diffusion Spine MRI PET	DTI MRS	CT chest, abdomen, pelvis CSF analysis Hearing test Serum ACE levels DTI
Surgical approach selected	Right suboccipital stereotactic needle biopsy	No surgery, radiation therapy only	Right suboccipital retrosigmoid craniotomy for excisional biopsy with 5-ALA	Right suboccipital retrosigmoid craniotomy for excisional biopsy
Anatomic corridor	Right middle cerebellar peduncle		Lateral perimedullary cistern	Lateral perimedullary cistern
Goal of surgery	Diagnosis		Diagnosis	Diagnosis
Perioperative				
Positioning	Right supine		Right park bench	Right supine with 90 degree left rotation
Surgical equipment	Surgical navigation Biopsy kit		Surgical navigation IOM (MEP/SSEP), nerve stimulator Surgical microscope with 5-ALA Ultrasound	Surgical navigation IOM (MEP, EMG cranial nerves 7/8, BAERs) Surgical microscope
Medications	None		Steroids Possible mannitol	Steroids Mannitol Antiepileptics
Anatomic considerations	Pons, medulla		Vertebral artery, PICA, lower cranial nerves, transverse-sigmoid sinuses, jugular bulb	PICA, AICA, brainstem nuclei, cranial nerves 7/8
Complications feared with approach chosen	Corticospinal tract injury, cranial neuropathy	High risk of neurologic injury with surgical approaches	Vascular injury, CSF leak, cerebellar retraction injury	Brainstem manipulation
Intraoperative				
Anesthesia	General		General	General
Skin incision	Linear		Right paramedian linear	Right retrosigmoid
Bone opening	Right suboccipital burr hole		Suboccipital below transverse sinus and medial to sigmoid sinus	Suboccipital below transverse sinus and medial to sigmoid sinus
Brain exposure	Right cerebellar hemisphere		Lower suboccipital to expose lateral perimedullary cistern	Lower suboccipital to expose lateral perimedullary cistern

(continued on next page)

	Bob S. Carter, MD, PhD, Massachusetts General Hospital, Boston, MA, United States	Shlomi Constantini, MD, Danil A. Kozyrev, MD, Tel Aviv Sourasky Medical Center, Tel Aviv, Israel	Alessandro Olivi, MD, Giuseppe Maria Della Pepa, MD, Fondazione Policlinico Universitario Agostino Gemelli IRCSS, Catholic University of Rome, Rome, Italy	Andrew E. Sloan, MD, University Hospital, Case Western Reserve Cleveland, OH, United States
Method of resection	Linear incision 3–4 cm based on surgical navigation, burr hole based on navigation, open dura, single core biopsy targeting wispy enhancing area above main area of enhancement, review personally with pathology, avoid second pass if possible		Use cranial landmarks to identify transverse-sigmoid junction to plan incision, craniotomy based inferior to this centered over the enhancing region at the lower lateral perimedullary cistern, anterior-based dural flap to enter cerebellopontine cistern, confirm trajectory with navigation, stimulate lateral brainstem to find safe entry zone, sample both contrast-enhancing and nonenhancing areas aided with 5-ALA, watertight dural closure with pericranium if needed, inspection and waxing of mastoid air cells	Use navigation and cranial landmarks to identify transverse-sigmoid junction based on position of zygoma and asterion, craniotomy below the transverse-sigmoid junction, curvilinear dural opening, location of tumor confirmed with navigation, expose lateral perimedullary cistern, find transsulcal approach based on DTI to enter tumor and sample, stop resection once diagnosis confirmed
Complication avoidance	Needle biopsy, one core specimen		Brainstem mapping, 5-ALA, excisional biopsy	DTI, transsulcal entry, stop after diagnosis obtained
Postoperative				
Admission	ICU		ICU	ICU
Postoperative complications feared	Worsening double vision		Respiratory failure, dysphagia, tongue weakness, vocal cord dysfunction	Injury to cranial nerves 7 and 8, CSF leak, retraction injury
Follow-up testing	CT immediately after surgery		Swallow evaluation	MRI within 48 hours after surgery
Follow-up visits	7–10 days after surgery		10 days after surgery MRI 3 months after surgery	10–14 days after surgery
Adjuvant therapies recommended				
Diffuse astrocytoma (IDH mutant, retain 1p19q)	STR–radiation/ temozolomide GTR–radiation/ temozolomide	STR–radiation GTR–not possible	STR–temozolomide +/– radiation GTR–temozolomide +/– radiation	STR–radiation/ temozolomide or PCV GTR–radiation/ temozolomide or PCV
Oligodendroglioma (IDH mutant, 1p19q LOH)	STR–radiation/PCV GTR–radiation/PCV	STR–radiation GTR–not possible	STR–temozolomide GTR–temozolomide	STR–radiation/ temozolomide GTR–radiation/ temozolomide
Anaplastic astrocytoma (IDH wild type)	STR–radiation/ temozolomide GTR–radiation/ temozolomide	STR–radiation GTR–not possible	STR–radiation/temozolomide GTR–radiation/temozolomide	STR–radiation/ temozolomide GTR–radiation/ temozolomide

5-ALA, 5-aminolevulinic acid; *ACE*, angiotensin-converting enzymes; *AICA*, anterior inferior cerebellar artery; *BAERs*, brainstem auditory evoked responses; *CSF*, cerebrospinal fluid; *CT*, computed tomography; *DTI*, diffusion tensor imaging; *GTR*, gross total resection; *ICU*, intensive care unit; *IOM*, intraoperative monitoring; *LOH*, loss of heterozygosity; *MEP*, motor evoked potential; *MRI*, magnetic resonance imaging; *MRS*, magnetic resonance spectroscopy; *PCV*, procarbazine, lomustine, vincristine; *PET*, positron emission tomography; *PICA*, posterior inferior cerebellar artery; *SSEP*, somatosensory evoked potential; *STR*, subtotal resection.

Differential diagnosis and actual diagnosis

- Low-grade glioma (astrocytoma, oligodendroglioma)
- High-grade glioma
- Demyelinating disease (i.e., multiple sclerosis)

Important anatomic and preoperative considerations

For a full description of pontine and fourth ventricular anatomy, see Chapter 13. The pons has one anterior, two posterior-lateral, and one posterior faces.[3] The two posterolateral faces continue with the cerebellar peduncles, in which anteriorly is the middle cerebellar peduncle (MCP), superiorly is superior cerebellar peduncle, and inferiorly is the inferior cerebellar peduncle.[3] The posterior face corresponds to the floor of the fourth ventricle.[3] The nuclei of cranial nerves V, VI, VII, and VIII originate in the pons.[3] From ventral to dorsal at the level of the pons at the level of the sensory and motor nucleus of cranial nerve V resides the superficial pontine fibers, corticospinal tract, medial and deep transverse fibers, medial lemniscus (immediately dorsal to the crossed cerebellopontine fibers), central tegmental tract, nucleus ceruleus, and the mesencephalic nucleus of cranial nerve V.[3] Medial to the central tegmental tract is the tectospinal tract that is ventral to the middle longitudinal fasciculus.[3]

Approaches to this lesion

Lesions in the pons represent a challenging surgical entity. Surgical resection is typically offered for pontine lesions when the lesion extends to the dorsal surface and/or are exophytic.[1,2] Diffuse pontine lesions without dorsal extension are typically observed or biopsied to provide tissue to guide tailored adjuvant therapy.[4] When surgical resection is pursued, the most commonly used approaches are a direct posterior approach through the floor of the fourth ventricle via a telovelar approach, a posterolateral approach through the MCP via a retrosigmoid or transcerebellar approach, and a lateral approach through a transcavernous, anterior transpetrosal, or presigmoid approach.[1,2] When needle biopsies are pursued, the three most common approaches include a suboccipital transcerebellar, ipsilateral transfrontal transtentorial, and contralateral transfrontal transtentorial approaches.[4] The advantages of the suboccipital transcerebellar approach are it typically provides the shortest distance to the pons and minimizes exposure to ventricular spaces that would create brain shifts that alter targeting accuracy, but the primary disadvantages are that it requires a prone position, which makes navigation less accurate, and the biopsy path is via the MCP, which can cause significant deficits.[4] An alternative to a transcerebellar route is a transfrontal approach that can be done ipsilateral or contralaterally.[4] This approach allows a wider ability to target the lateral in addition to the medial pons, but the path trajectory is quite long and potentially can enter the ventricle, thus leading to targeting inaccuracies and can also involve the internal capsule, basal ganglia, and thalamus.[4]

What was actually done

The patient was taken to surgery for a right paramedian transcerebellar approach for a needle biopsy of the enhancing potion of the pontine lesion with general anesthesia without intraoperative monitoring. The patient was induced and intubated per routine. The head was fixed in neutral position, with two pins centered over the left external auditory meatus and one pin over the right external auditory meatus. The patient was then placed prone onto chest rolls with the neck flexed and reduced. The head was kept neutral to keep anatomic orientation. A right paramedian incision was planned based on surgical navigation in which the surgical path was through the cerebellar hemisphere into the enhancing portion of the right pontine lesion via the MCP. The patient was draped in the usual standard fashion and given dexamethasone and cefazolin. The right paramedian incision was made, dissection took place down to the periosteum, and the skin was retracted with a Weitlaner retractor. A burr hole was made, and the dura was opened. The core biopsy needle was passed under surgical navigation into the pons, and specimen was taken in all four quadrants. Preliminary pathology was infiltrating glioma. The needle was withdrawn, and no bleeding was seen. Gelfoam was placed in the epidural space, and a burr hole was used to cover the opening. The skin was closed in standard fashion.

The patient awoke at their neurologic baseline with right eye abduction weakness, intact speech, and full strength bilaterally and taken to the intensive care unit for recovery. A postoperative head computed tomography was done after surgery that showed good localization to the contrast-enhancing region of the pons and expected postoperative changes (Fig. 30.2). The patient participated with physical and occupational therapy and was discharged to home on postoperative day 1 with an intact neurologic examination. The patient was prescribed 24 hours of dexamethasone. The patient was seen at 2 weeks postoperatively for suture removal and remained neurologically intact except stable right eye abduction weakness. Pathology was a World Health Organization grade III anaplastic astrocytoma (IDH wild type, 1p/19q wild type). The patient underwent temozolomide and radiation therapy for 6 weeks followed by adjuvant cycles. The patient had progressive symptoms, including imbalance, dysphagia, and double vision approximately 4 months after the surgery, and serial MRI scans showed progression of the lesion. He was tried on bevacizumab without improvement. The patient died 6 months after surgery.

Commonalities among the experts

Half of the surgeons opted for patients having diffusion tensor imaging to identify white matter tracts and cerebrospinal fluid analysis to help aid diagnosis prior to surgery. The majority of surgeons elected for biopsy of this lesion, in which two favored an excisional biopsy (lateral perimedullary cistern), and the other a stereotactic needle biopsy (right MCP). The goal for these surgeons was diagnosis to guide potential adjuvant therapy. In those surgeons pursing surgery, all were concerned about the location of posterior circulation arteries (posterior inferior cerebellar artery, vertebral artery), as well as the lower cranial nerves. Most surgeons

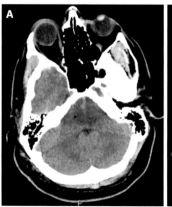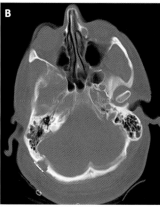

Fig. 30.2 Postoperative head computed tomography. (A) Axial brain windows; **(B)** axial bone windows demonstrating air in the region of the preoperative enhancement consistent with good localization of the biopsy.

For a diagnosis of oligodendroglioma, radiation and/or chemotherapy was requested by all surgeons. For a diagnosis of anaplastic astrocytoma, most surgeons requested radiation and temozolomide.

SUMMARY OF QUALITY OF EVIDENCE TO GUIDE SPECIFIC INTERVENTIONS FOR THIS CASE

- Biopsy versus surgical resection for pontine gliomas— Class III.
- Transcerebellar versus transfrontal approach for pontine biopsy—Class III.
- Temozolomide and radiation therapy for high-grade gliomas—Class I.

were concerned about brainstem injury. Surgery was generally pursued with surgical navigation, surgical microscope, intraoperative monitoring, and brainstem mapping with perioperative steroids and mannitol. The majority of surgeons relied on biopsy as opposed to resection, and half relied on brainstem mapping to minimize potential iatrogenic injury. Following surgery, all patients were admitted to the intensive care unit, and most pursing surgery requested imaging within 48 hours after surgery to assess for potential complications. For a diagnosis of diffuse astrocytoma, radiation and/or chemotherapy was requested by all surgeons.

REFERENCES

1. Cavalheiro S, Yagmurlu K, da Costa MD, et al. Surgical approaches for brainstem tumors in pediatric patients. *Childs Nerv Syst*. 2015; 31:1815–1840.
2. Jallo GI, Shiminski-Maher T, Velazquez L, Abbott R, Wisoff J, Epstein F. Recovery of lower cranial nerve function after surgery for medullary brainstem tumors. *Neurosurgery*. 2005;56:74–77; discussion 78.
3. Ribas EC. Yagmurlu K, de Oliveira E, Ribas GC, Rhoton A Jr. Microsurgical anatomy of the central core of the brain. *J Neurosurg*. 2018;129:752–769.
4. Amundson EW, McGirt MJ, Olivi A. A contralateral, transfrontal, extraventricular approach to stereotactic brainstem biopsy procedures. Technical note. *J Neurosurg*. 2005;102:565–570.

31

Medulloblastoma

Case reviewed by Steven Brem, George I. Jallo, James Rutka, Charles Teo

Introduction

The most common type of primary malignant brain tumor in children is medulloblastoma, in which it accounts for approximately 25% of childhood brain tumors.[1,2] Medulloblastomas can also occur in adults, but they comprise less than 1% of primary brain tumors, and their incidence decreases with patient age.[1,2] However, these behave similarly to pediatric medulloblastomas in which the 5-year overall survival rates range from 56% to 84%, median survivals range from 6 to 17.6 years, and the 5-year progression-free survival rates range from 40% to 61%.[1,2] As with children, the primary prognostic factors are extent of resection and presence of localized (nondisseminated) disease.[1,2] In this chapter, we present a case of a young adult with medulloblastoma.

Example case

Chief complaint: headaches

History of present illness

A 21-year-old, right-handed man with no significant past medical history presented with headaches. Over the past 4 to 5 months, he has complained of progressive headaches. More recently, he developed nausea and vomiting. He was seen in the emergency room where imaging revealed a brain lesion (Fig. 31.1).

Medications: None.

Allergies: No known drug allergies.

Past medical and surgical history: None.

Family history: No history of intracranial malignancies.

Social history: College student. No smoking or alcohol.

Physical examination: Awake, alert, oriented to person, place, and time; Cranial nerves (CN) II to XII intact; No drift, moves all extremities with full strength; Cerebellar: no finger-to-nose dysmetria, no truncal ataxia.

Magnetic resonance imaging spine: No lesions noted.

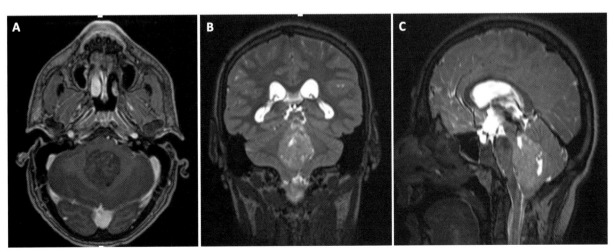

Fig. 31.1 Preoperative magnetic resonance imaging. (A) T1 axial image with gadolinium contrast; **(B)** T2 coronal image; **(C)** T2 sagittal magnetic resonance imaging scans demonstrating a heterogeneously enhancing lesion within the fourth ventricle.

	Steven Brem, MD, University of Pennsylvania, Philadelphia, PA, United States	George I. Jallo, MD, Johns Hopkins All Children's Hospital, St. Petersburg, FL, United States	James Rutka, MD, PhD, University of Toronto, Sick Kids Toronto, Canada	Charles Teo, MBBS, University of New South Wales, Sydney, Australia
Preoperative				
Additional tests requested	Complete spine MRI	Complete spine MRI	Complete spine MRI Neuroophthalmology evaluation	None
Surgical approach selected	Midline suboccipital craniotomy	Midline suboccipital craniotomy and endoscope-assisted	Midline suboccipital craniotomy	Midline suboccipital craniotomy and endoscope-assisted
Anatomic corridor	Telovelar	Telovelar, possible transvermian	Telovelar	Transvermian
Goal of surgery	Maximal safe resection	GTR	GTR	GTR
Perioperative				
Positioning	Prone-concorde	Prone	Prone	Prone
Surgical equipment	Surgical navigation IOM (SSEP, BAERs, cranial nerves 7–11) Ultrasonic aspirator	Surgical navigation IOM (MEP, SSEP, cranial nerve 5–12 EMG, BAERs) Surgical microscope Ultrasound Nerve stimulator Ultrasonic aspirator Endoscope	IOM Surgical microscope Ultrasonic aspirator	Central line Surgical microscope 30-degree endoscope
Medications	Steroids Mannitol	Steroids	None	Steroids
Anatomic considerations	Structures within floor of fourth ventricle, seventh nerve nuclei	Structures within floor of fourth ventricle	Structures within floor of fourth ventricle	Structures within floor of fourth ventricle, cerebral aqueduct
Complications feared with approach chosen	Hydrocephalus, brainstem injury, cranial neuropathy, pseudomeningocele	Ophthalmoplegia, facial palsy, hearing low, lower cranial nerve dysfunction, truncal/ appendicular ataxia, cerebellar mutism	Ophthalmoplegia, facial palsy, dysmetria/ ataxia	Brainstem injury
Intraoperative				
Anesthesia	General	General	General	General
Skin incision	Midline linear from inion to C2	Midline linear	Midline linear	Midline linear
Bone opening	Suboccipital craniotomy and C1 laminectomy	Suboccipital craniotomy and C1 laminectomy	Suboccipital craniotomy +/– C1 laminectomy	Suboccipital craniotomy and C1 laminectomy
Brain exposure	Cerebellar hemispheres, cerebellomedullary junction	Cerebellar hemispheres, cerebellomedullary junction	Cerebellar hemispheres, cerebellomedullary junction	Cerebellar hemispheres, cerebellomedullary junction

	Steven Brem, MD, University of Pennsylvania, Philadelphia, PA, United States	George I. Jallo, MD, Johns Hopkins All Children's Hospital, St. Petersburg, FL, United States	James Rutka, MD, PhD, University of Toronto, Sick Kids Toronto, Canada	Charles Teo, MBBS, University of New South Wales, Sydney, Australia
Method of resection	Place EVD, position prone, linear incision from inion to C2, bilateral suboccipital craniotomy from transverse sinus superiorly to posterior lip of foramen magnum inferiorly and make sufficiently wide, Y-shaped dural opening, telovelar approach to fourth ventricle with dynamic retraction under microscopic visualization, goal would be 100% resection, care taken at floor of fourth ventricle, watertight dural closure, reinforce with artificial dural graft, bone flap replacement or titanium mesh cranioplasty	Midline incision, bilateral suboccipital craniotomy and C1 laminectomy, Y-shaped dural opening, unilateral telovelar exposure, identify and ligate tela choroidea and inferior medullary velum, protect spinal canal with cottonoid, internal debulking, identify floor of fourth ventricle, stimulate if any residual remains to identify ability to sharply remove without transgressing floor, Frazier point burr hole and EVD if necessary, inspect for residual with endoscope, watertight dural closure with dural substitute	Midline incision, bilateral suboccipital craniotomy +/− C1 laminectomy, Y-shaped dural opening, tumor should present itself beneath tonsils, telovelar exposure if needed, debulk tumor early with ultrasonic aspirator, identify floor of the fourth ventricle, debulk tumor down to the ventricular floor, if tumor invades floor of ventricle do not transgress floor, remove tumor up to aqueduct, dural closure with dural substitute and Tisseel	Midline incision, limited occipital craniotomy/craniectomy and C1 laminectomy, Y-shaped dural opening monitoring and coagulation of midline and circular sinuses, identification of tumor below vermis and early protection of floor of ventricle, total resection and if necessary, midline split of vermis and endoscopic inspection including lateral recesses
Complication avoidance	EVD, telovelar approach, care at floor of fourth ventricle	Telovelar exposure, identify floor of fourth ventricle, stimulate to identify eloquence, sharply remove from floor, endoscope for inspection	Telovelar exposure, identify floor of fourth ventricle	Early protection of ventricular floor, vermian split if necessary, endoscope for inspection
Postoperative				
Admission	ICU	ICU	ICU	ICU
Postoperative complications feared	Hydrocephalus, cranial neuropathy (diplopia, facial diplegia, hearing loss, swallowing difficulty), apnea, pseudomeningocele, ataxia	CSF leak, lower cranial neuropathy (facial weakness, hearing loss, dysphagia), ataxia	CSF leak, hydrocephalus, brainstem injury, cranial nerve palsies	Hydrocephalus
Follow-up testing	MRI within 24 hours after surgery Spinal MRI 2 weeks after surgery	MRI within 48 hours after surgery	MRI within 24 hours after surgery	MRI within 24 hours after surgery
Follow-up visits	1 month after surgery 1 week after surgery with medical oncology 5 weeks after surgery with radiation oncology	14–21 days after surgery	4–6 weeks after surgery	6–8 weeks after surgery
Adjuvant therapies recommended	STR–reduced dose craniospinal radiation with chemotherapy GTR–craniospinal radiation, possible proton therapy	STR–possible repeat surgery NTR–radiation/chemotherapy GTR–radiation/chemotherapy	STR–possible repeat surgery NTR–radiation/chemotherapy GTR–radiation/chemotherapy	STR–possible repeat surgery NTR–per oncology GTR–per oncology

BAER, brainstem auditory evoked responses; CSF, cerebrospinal fluid; EMG, electromyography; EVD, external ventricular drain; GTR, gross total resection; ICU, intensive care unit; IOM, intraoperative monitoring; MEP, motor evoked potential; MRI, magnetic resonance imaging; NTR, near total resection; SSEP, somatosensory evoked potential; STR, subtotal resection.

Differential diagnosis and actual diagnosis

- Medulloblastoma
- Ependymoma
- Choroid plexus papilloma
- Hemangioblastoma

Important anatomic and preoperative considerations

There are many different classifications of medulloblastomas.[1,3] Histologically, the World Health Organization divided medulloblastomas into three major groups: classic (66%, composed of sheets of densely packed basophilic cells with high nuclear to cytoplasmic ratio, and moderate mitotic and apoptotic activity); desmoplastic/nodular (15%, most favorable prognosis, have reticulin-free areas with reticulin-rich stroma with immunopositivity for synaptophysin, and can occur laterally), and large cell/anaplastic (2%–4%, worst prognosis, monomorphous population of large cells with prominent nucleoli, high proliferative activity, abundant apoptosis).[1,3] More recently, medulloblastomas have been classified into four groups based on molecular profiling: Wnt (11%, best overall prognosis with overall survival of 90%, commonly possess mutations of the Wnt pathway CTNNB1 mutation that encodes β-catenin), Shh (28%, intermediate prognosis similar to group 4, commonly possess PTCH1 mutations in which Shh binds), group 3 (28%, worst prognosis and are frequently metastatic, associated with MYC amplification), and group 4 (34%, associated with isochromosome 17q, intermediate prognosis but frequently metastasize).[1,3] The historic classification, also called the Chang system, which is infrequently used grouped the tumors based on size and invasiveness of the tumors, as well as the presence of metastases, but this later evolved to classifying tumors based on risk in which standard risk were children aged 3 years or older at diagnosis, no evidence of metastatic spread, and have less than 1.5 cm^2 of residual disease after surgery, whereas high risk were children aged younger than 3 years, evidence of cerebrospinal fluid spread, and/or less complete resection ($\geq$1.5 cm^2).[1,3]

For a full discussion of fourth ventricular anatomy see Chapter 13. Medulloblastomas typically arise from the floor of the fourth ventricle, which is located over the dorsal surface of the brainstem.[4] The floor of the fourth ventricle is divided into a superior pontine triangle (line from the cerebral aqueduct to the line connecting the lateral recesses), intermediate triangle (between the superior and inferior boundaries of the lateral recesses), and inferior medullary triangle (inferolateral margin of the floor of the fourth ventricle or obex).[4] The floor also has well-formed sulci with a medial sulcus in the midline, and the sulcus limitans laterally on both sides of the medial sulcus.[4] The median eminence is in-between the medial sulcus and sulcus limitans, which is the location of the facial colliculus.[4] The superior limit of the facial colliculus is the superior intrapontine segment of the facial nerve, and the inferior limit is formed by the intrapontine portion of the facial nerves that curves beneath the nucleus of CN VI.[4] The sulcus limitans itself has two depressions or fovea, in which the superior fovea lies laterally to the facial colliculus, and the inferior fovea lies lateral to the hypoglossal triangle in the medullary portion of the ventricular floor.[4] Over the median eminence, caudal to the facial colliculus, lies the hypoglossal trigone medially, and the vagal trigone laterally.[4]

The cerebellum itself is divided into two hemispheres and the midline vermis.[4] The cerebellar cortex, like the cerebral cortex, consist of gray matter and overlies the white matter, which houses the deep cerebellar nuclei (dentate, emboliform, globose, and fastigii).[4] Grossly, the cerebellum can be divided into the flocculonodular, anterior, and posterior lobes, in which the anterior and posterior lobes are present in the vermis and hemispheres.[4] Functionally, the vermis plays a role in body posture and movement, especially of the trunk. Anatomically, it connects the cerebellar hemispheres, and consists of nine lobules (lingual, central, culmen, declive, folium, tuber, pyramid, uvula, and nodule).[4] The lingula is the upper portion of the vermis, and is separated from the central lobule by the precentral fissure.[4] The central lobule, which lies below the lingula, resides above the culmen.[4] The culmen itself is separated from the declive by the primary fissure.[4] The pyramid is separated from the tuber and uvula by the prepyramidal and secondary fissures, respectively.[4]

Approaches to this lesion

The approaches to fourth ventricular lesions can be divided into intra- and extraaxial approaches.[5] The primary intra-axial approach is a transvermian approach through the vermis. This approach is typically limited to the bottom half of the vermis, as an upper vermian approach is associated with a high risk of cerebellar mutism, which is associated with decreased or absent speech, abulia, hypotonia, and ataxia. The advantages of this approach are that it minimizes potential injury to the posterior inferior cerebellar artery (PICA) vessels and allows upper and fourth ventricular access; however, it is associated with cerebellar mutism and prolonged truncal ataxia. As opposed to an intraaxial approach, an extraaxial approach involves unilateral or bilateral telovelar approaches through a midline suboccipital craniotomy. The advantages of this approach are that it avoids parenchymal injury and minimizes risk of cerebellar mutism, but it exposes the PICA vessels to potential injury and can have limited visualization of the entire fourth ventricle without retraction.

What was actually done

The patient was taken to surgery for a midline suboccipital craniotomy for bilateral telovelar approach for fourth ventricular tumor with general anesthesia. The patient was induced and intubated per routine. Intraoperative monitoring was used to monitor somatosensory evoked potentials, as well as CNs V, VII, IX, X, XI, and XII. The head was fixed in neutral position, with two pins centered over the left external auditory meatus, and one pin over the right external auditory meatus. The patient was then placed prone onto chest rolls with the neck flexed and reduced. A midline incision was planned that spanned from just above the inion to the C2 spinous process. In addition, a Frazier burr hole site was planned in case it was needed for an external ventricular drain. The patient was draped in the usual standard fashion and given dexamethasone and cefazolin. A midline incision was made, and dissection took place in the avascular plane between the suboccipital muscles. The skin and muscles were retracted with a cerebellar retractor, and the C1 spinous process and occipital bone with foramen magnum were identified. A suboccipital craniotomy was made below the transverse sinus with incorporation of the foramen magnum. In addition, a C1 laminectomy was done to facilitate dural opening and closure. The dura was then opened in a Y-shape that extended down the midline to C1 and tacked up to the surrounding muscles. The microscope was brought in, and the arachnoid between the tonsils and the cerebellar hemispheres were opened with sharp dissection making sure to identify and protect the bilateral PICAs. The cerebellar tonsils were retracted laterally with dynamic retraction without fixed retractors to expose and open the tela choroidea and inferior medullary velum bilaterally. The spinal canal was protected with cottonoids to minimize potential tumor seeding. The tumor was debulked until the ventricular walls were seen on all edges. A small attachment to the floor of the fourth ventricle was identified and sharply removed after brainstem mapping to confirm no facial nerve involvement. No residual tumor was seen. A synthetic dural graft was used for watertight dural closure, and the bone and skin were closed in standard fashion.

The patient awoke at their neurologic baseline with intact speech, full strength bilaterally, and intact CNs, and was taken to the intensive care unit for recovery. Magnetic resonance imaging (MRI) was done within 48 hours after surgery and showed gross total resection (Fig. 31.2). The patient participated with physical and occupational therapy and was discharged to home on postoperative day 3 with an intact neurologic examination, except for some disequilibrium. The patient was prescribed dexamethasone that was tapered to off over 7 days after surgery. The patient was seen at 2 weeks postoperatively for suture removal

and remained neurologically intact with improved balance. Pathology was a World Health Organization grade IV medulloblastoma of the Shh subtype. The patient underwent craniospinal radiation (54 Gy to the tumor site and 30 Gy to the spine) and chemotherapy was deferred.[3] The lesion was observed with serial MRI examinations at 3 months, followed by 6-month intervals, and has been without recurrence for 12 months. The patient returned to work at 6 weeks postoperatively and remains without neurologic deficits with improved balance.

Commonalities among the experts

The majority of the surgeons opted for the patient having complete spine MRI to evaluate for drop or concurrent lesions prior to surgery. All the surgeons elected for a midline suboccipital approach, in which three surgeons chose telovelar (with one possible transvermian), and the other surgeons a transvermian approach to the fourth ventricle. The general goal for these surgeons was gross total resection. All surgeons were concerned about maintaining the integrity of the floor of the fourth ventricle, and most feared brainstem injury, namely facial palsy and ophthalmoplegia. Surgery was generally pursued with surgical navigation, surgical microscope, intraoperative monitoring, ultrasonic aspirator, and possible endoscopic assistance with perioperative steroids. The majority of surgeons relied on a telovelar approach to minimize cerebellar vermian injury, and being cognizant of the floor of the fourth ventricle to minimize potential iatrogenic injury. Following surgery, all patients were admitted to the intensive care unit, and all surgeons requested imaging within 48 hours after surgery to assess for extent of resection and/or potential complications. If subtotal resection of the medulloblastoma was achieved, the majority of surgeons advocated for second look surgery. If gross total resection of the medulloblastoma was achieved, radiation and/or chemotherapy was advocated by all surgeons.

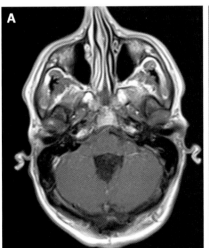 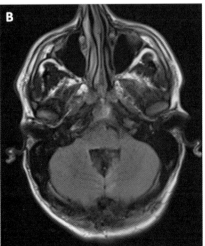 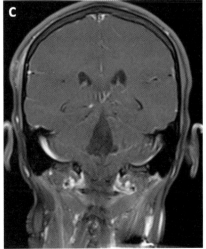

Fig. 31.2 **Postoperative magnetic resonance imaging. (A)** T1 axial image with gadolinium contrast; **(B)** T2 fluid attenuation inversion recovery axial image; **(C)** T1 coronal image with gadolinium contrast magnetic resonance imaging scans demonstrating gross total resection of the fourth ventricular tumor.

SUMMARY OF QUALITY OF EVIDENCE TO GUIDE SPECIFIC INTERVENTIONS FOR THIS CASE

- Extensive surgical resection of medulloblastoma—Class II-2.
- Craniospinal radiation for gross total resection of adult medulloblastoma—Class II-3.
- Chemotherapy for recurrence of medulloblastoma—Class II-3.
- Monitoring and brainstem mapping for brainstem surgery—Class III.

REFERENCES

1. Holgado BL, Guerreiro Stucklin A, Garzia L, Daniels C, Taylor MD. Tailoring medulloblastoma treatment through genomics: making a change, one subgroup at a time. *Annu Rev Genomics Hum Genet*. 2017;18:143–166.
2. Kieran MW. Targeted treatment for sonic hedgehog-dependent medulloblastoma. *Neuro Oncol*. 2014;16:1037–1047.
3. Prados MD, Warnick RE, Wara WM, Larson DA, Lamborn K, Wilson CB. Medulloblastoma in adults. *Int J Radiat Oncol Biol Phys*. 1995;32:1145–1152.
4. Ribas EC, Yagmurlu K, de Oliveira E, Ribas GC, Rhoton A Jr. Microsurgical anatomy of the central core of the brain. *J Neurosurg*. 2018;129:752–769.
5. Tomasello F, Conti A, Cardali S, La Torre D, Angileri FF. Telovelar approach to fourth ventricle tumors: highlights and limitations. *World Neurosurg*. 2015;83:1141–1147.

32

Language area metastatic brain cancer

Case reviewed by Orin Bloch, Francesco DiMeco, Massimiliano Del Bene, Fernando Hakim, Diego Gomez, Maciej S. Lesniak

Introduction

An estimated 25% to 45% of patients with cancer will develop brain metastases.[1,2] The management of patients who develop brain metastases includes some combination of surgery, radiation therapy, and/or chemotherapy.[1–5] Surgical resection of these lesions is typically offered for patients with good prognoses who have lesions that are large, accessible, and/or symptomatic.[6–8] In this chapter, we present a case of a patient with a language area metastatic brain tumor.

Example case

Chief complaint: speaking difficulties and right-sided weakness

History of present illness

A 46-year-old, right-handed woman with a history of melanoma presented with acute onset of speech difficulties and right-sided weakness. Her melanoma was resected from her back 5 years ago but had not undergone recent surveillance imaging. On returning home from work, she presented with progressive headaches, difficulty getting words out, and right-sided weakness. She was taken to the emergency room where imaging revealed a large brain tumor (Fig. 32.1).

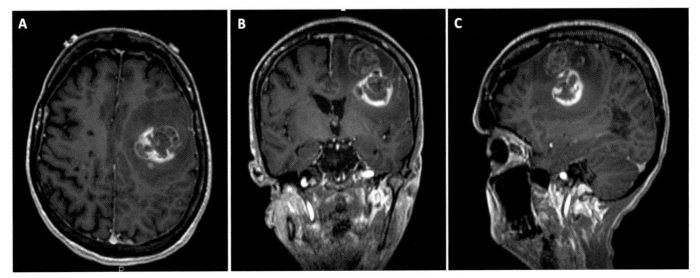

Fig. 32.1 Preoperative magnetic resonance imaging. (A) T1 axial image with gadolinium contrast; **(B)** T1 coronal image with gadolinium contrast; **(C)** T1 sagittal image with gadolinium contrast magnetic resonance imaging scan demonstrating a heterogeneously enhancing multicentric lesion within the left frontal lobe in close juxtaposition to the language areas.

Medications: None.

Allergies: No known drug allergies.

Past medical and surgical history: Melanoma back excision 5 years prior.

Family history: No history of intracranial malignancies.

Social history: Accountant. No smoking or alcohol.

Physical examination: Awake, alert, oriented to person, place, and time; Language: naming difficulties, impaired repetition; Cranial nerves I to XII intact, except slight right facial droop; Right upper extremity 4+/5, right lower extremity 5/5, left upper extremity 5/5, left lower extremity 5/5.

Computed tomography chest/abdomen/pelvis: Small punctate lesions with the lung and liver.

	Orin Bloch, MD, University of California–Davis, Sacramento, CA, United States	Francesco DiMeco, MD, Massimiliano Del Bene, MD, Carlo Besta Neurological Institute, Milan, Italy	Fernando Hakim, MD, Diego Gomez, MD, Hospital Universitario Fundacion Santafe de Bogota, Bogota, Colombia	Maciej S. Lesniak, MD, Northwestern University, Chicago, IL, United States
Preoperative				
Additional tests requested	DTI CT chest/abdomen/pelvis Oncology evaluation Radiation oncology evaluation	DTI if possible fMRI if possible	fMRI Oncology evaluation Radiation oncology evaluation	None
Surgical approach selected	Left frontal craniotomy with asleep motor mapping	Left fronto-parietal craniotomy with asleep cortical and subcortical motor mapping	Left frontal awake craniotomy with motor and language mapping	Left frontal craniotomy
Anatomic corridor	Superior frontal gyrus	Middle frontal gyrus	Left frontal	Left SFG
Goal of surgery	Safe debulking of tumor to relive mass effect as adjuvant therapies effective at tumor control	Complete resection with 5-mm margins, reduce mass effect, improve neurologic function	Gross total resection without neurologic deficit	Gross total resection
Perioperative				
Positioning	Left supine neutral	Left supine with right rotation	Left supine with 30-degree right rotation	Left supine
Surgical equipment	Surgical navigation IOM (MEP) Brain stimulator Surgical microscope Ultrasonic aspirator	Surgical navigation IOM (MEP/SSEP) Chisel Brain stimulator Surgical microscope Ultrasonic aspirator	Surgical navigation Brain stimulator Ultrasonic aspirator	Surgical navigation Ultrasonic aspirator
Medications	Mannitol Steroids Antiepileptics	Steroids Antiepileptics	Mannitol Steroids Antiepileptics	Mannitol Steroids
Anatomic considerations	Primary motor cortex, SMA, subcortical CST, AF	Central sulcus, precentral/postcentral gyri, CST, frontal operculum	Broca area, primary motor cortex, vein of Trolard	Broca area, primary motor cortex
Complications feared with approach chosen	Speech and motor deficit	Motor deficit from primary motor cortex or CST, language dysfunction	Speech and motor deficit	Speech and motor deficit
Intraoperative				
Anesthesia	General	General	Asleep-awake-asleep	General
Skin incision	Linear	Retrocoronal linear	Curvilinear	Linear
Bone opening	Left frontal	Left frontal-parietal	Left frontal	Left frontal
Brain exposure	Left SFG	Left frontal-parietal	Left frontal	Left SFG

	Orin Bloch, MD, University of California–Davis, Sacramento, CA, United States	Francesco DiMeco, MD, Massimiliano Del Bene, MD, Carlo Besta Neurological Institute, Milan, Italy	Fernando Hakim, MD, Diego Gomez, MD, Hospital Universitario Fundacion Santafe de Bogota, Bogota, Colombia	Maciej S. Lesniak, MD, Northwestern University, Chicago, IL, United States
Method of resection	Approximate 4-cm craniotomy based on navigation above SFG where tumor comes closest the surface, open dura, 2-cm transverse corticectomy anterior to SMA in SFG, subcortical dissection to tumor margin, central debulking of tumor with bipolar and ultrasonic aspirator, work through superior lesion into deeper lesion, identify boundary between tumor and normal parenchyma leaving small margin at posterior/deep/lateral aspects	Wide craniotomy without burr holes using drill and chisel, dural tack up sutures, ultrasound to identify lesion and tailor dural opening, C-shaped dural opening based on midline, cortical strip and phase reversal to identify central sulcus, corticectomy based on cortical mapping, en bloc resection trying to find interface between tumor and healthy parenchyma aided with cortical and subcortical mapping and ultrasound, resection of 5-mm margin if negative mapping with ultrasonic aspirator, final ultrasound scan, watertight dural closure	Craniotomy guided by navigation, U-shaped dural opening, awake and extubate patient, cortical stimulation mapping, corticectomy centered over lesion in areas of negative mapping sites, intralesional debulking with aid of ultrasonic aspirator and bipolar coagulation, continuous speech and motor evaluation, periodic navigation checks, find gliotic plane to achieve gross total resection with special attention to neurologic examination, watertight dural closure	Craniotomy based on navigation, identify shortest distance to the lesion, internal debulking with ultrasonic aspirator, capsular resection to achieve gross total resection
Complication avoidance	Limit opening to SFG, work anterior to SMA, asleep motor mapping to identify motor cortex and CST, leave small remnant at deep margin	Craniotomy without burr holes, ultrasound, continuous MEP with cortical strip, cortical and subcortical mapping, en bloc resection, 5-mm resection margin	Language and motor mapping, corticectomy over negative mapping site, intralesional debulking	Superior to the Broca, anterior to motor cortex, intralesional debulking
Postoperative				
Admission	ICU	Floor	ICU	ICU
Postoperative complications feared	Motor deficit, language deficit, seizure	Motor deficit, language deficit, SMA syndrome	Cerebral edema	Worsening speech deficit
Follow-up testing	MRI within 48 hours after surgery	CT within 24 hours after surgery MRI within 48 hours after surgery Radiation oncology evaluation	MRI within 72 hours after surgery	MRI within 24 hours after surgery
Follow-up visits	14 days after surgery	1 month after surgery prior to radiation therapy	7 days after surgery	14 days after surgery
Adjuvant therapies recommended	SRS Immunotherapy vs. BRAF inhibitor based on tumor genomics	SRS to cavity Oncology evaluation	SRS to cavity Chemotherapy per oncology	SRS to cavity

AF, arcuate fasciculus; *BRAF*, B-Raf protein mutation; *CST*, corticospinal tract; *CT*, computed tomography; *DTI*, diffusion tensor imaging; *fMRI*, functional magnetic resonance imaging; *ICU*, intensive care unit; *IOM*, intraoperative monitoring; *MEP*, motor evoked potential; *MRI*, magnetic resonance imaging; *SFG*, superior frontal gyrus; *SMA*, supplementary motor area; *SRS*, stereotactic radiosurgery; *SSEP*, somatosensory evoked potential.

Differential diagnosis and actual diagnosis

- Metastatic brain cancer
- High-grade glioma
- Lymphoma
- Cerebral abscess

Important anatomic and preoperative considerations

There are several classification schemes aimed at prognosticating outcomes for patients with metastatic brain tumors, and are therefore used as a guide for offering different forms of treatment.[9,10] The recursive partitioning analysis (RPA) classification system (Table 32.1) is a three-tiered system based on age, Karnofsky performance score (KPS), primary tumor control, and extracranial disease, in which RPA class 1 patients have a median survival of 7.1 months and are younger than age 65 years, good performance status (KPS ≥70), primary tumor control, and no extracranial disease; RPA class 2 patients have a median survival of 4.2 months and have good performance status (KPS ≥70), but are older than age 65 years, do not have primary tumor control, and/or presence of extracranial disease; and RPA class 3 patients have a median survival of 2.3 months and have poor performance status (KPS <70).[11] Surgery is typically offered to RPA class 1 and a select group of RPA class 2 patients, whereas other patients are typically offered palliative therapies, including stereotactic or whole-brain radiation therapy.[6] The patient in this case is RPA class 2, in which they are younger than age 65 years, has good KPS, and has primary tumor control, but has presence of extracranial disease.

For a full discussion of frontal lobe anatomy and language area cortical and subcortical white matter tracts in the left frontal lobe, see Chapters 2, 5, and 6. This lesion is within the left superior and middle frontal gyrus with involvement of the ventral premotor cortex and supplementary motor area, with additional involvement of the superior longitudinal fasciculus and arcuate fasciculus laterals and frontal aslant tract medially.

Table 32.1 RPA for patients with metastatic brain tumors		
RPA Class	**Characteristics**	**Median Survival (months)**
RPA class 1	Age <65 KPS ≥70 Primary tumor control No extracranial disease	7.1
RPA class 2	KPS ≥70 and one of the following: Age ≥65 Lack of primary tumor control Extracranial disease	4.2
RPA class 3	KPS <70	2.3
KPS, Karnofsky performance score; *RPA*, recursive partitioning analysis.		

Approaches to this lesion

As with any intraaxial lesion, surgery can either be done asleep or awake (Chapter 1, Fig. 1.2). With awake surgery, the cortical and subcortical regions are mapped to identify eloquence, and therefore requires a patient who is cooperative and possesses a high-quality neurologic examination to follow and monitor.[12] Metastatic lesions typically occur at the gray-white matter junction in the subcortical space, and therefore to access these lesions, the cortex and subcortical white matter must be transgressed.[13–16] For lesions below the level of the cortical sulci, the options for accessing the lesion is either transgyral or transsulcal.[13–16] A transgyral approach involves going through the pia, gray matter, and white matter to reach the lesion, thus avoiding the sulci and/or fissures, whereas a transsulcal approach involves opening the arachnoid over the sulci or fissures, entering the sulci, and eventually traversing the parenchyma.[13–16] The advantages of the transgyral approach is that it avoids the sulcal vessels, and therefore minimizes ischemic injuries and is the most commonly used method; however, its disadvantages include increasing distance of violated parenchyma, engages potential projection and association white matter tracts, and cannot be typically applied to eloquent regions.[13,17–18] The advantages of the transsulcal approach are that it minimizes the distance of parenchyma violated, engages less critical subcortical U-fibers, and can be applied in eloquent regions; however, its disadvantages include potential injury to sulcal arteries and veins, injury to two adjacent gyri from manipulation, and more technically challenging.[13,17–18]

What was actually done

The patient was taken for a left frontal craniotomy for resection of the multicentric metastatic brain tumor with general anesthesia without intraoperative monitoring. The patient did not have a good enough examination to undergo awake mapping surgery, and monitoring was not used because of the superficial location of the tumor obviating alternative approaches. The patient was induced and intubated per routine. The head was fixed in neutral position, with two pins centered over the right external auditory meatus and one pin posterior to the left external auditory meatus. The patient's head was flexed and kept neutral. A pterional incision was planned that spanned from the vertex to the ipsilateral superior temporal line based on surgical navigation. The patient was draped in the usual standard fashion and given dexamethasone, levetiracetam, and cefazolin. The incision was made, and the skin flap was reflected anteriorly with fishhooks attached to a retractor arm. The margins of the tumor were identified with surgical navigation, and a left frontal craniotomy was made. The dura was opened in a cruciate fashion and tacked up. Ultrasound and surgical navigation were used to identify the borders of the superior lesion. A corticectomy was made overlying the lesion in the gyrus, and the superficial tumor was identified; it was dissected from the surrounding parenchyma and removed en bloc. The inferior lesion was then identified and connected with the superficial lesion. The microscope was brought in for the deeper lesion to provide illumination and visualization. The tumor was removed en bloc. The cavity was

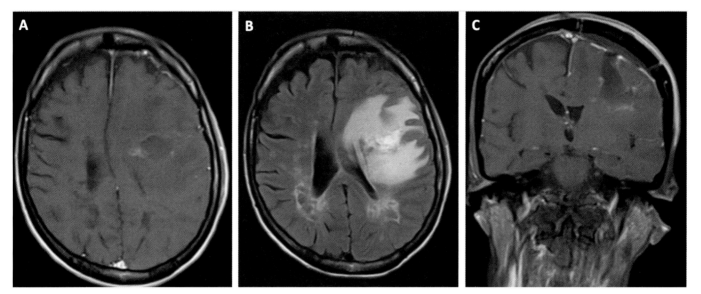

Fig. 32.2 Postoperative magnetic resonance imaging. (A) T1 axial image with gadolinium contrast; **(B)** T2 fluid attenuation inversion recovery axial image; **(C)** T1 coronal image with gadolinium contrast magnetic resonance imaging scan demonstrating gross total resection of the multicentric lesion within the left frontal lobe in close juxtaposition to the language areas.

inspected with direct visualization and ultrasound showed no residual tumor. The dura, bone, and skin were closed in standard fashion.

The patient awoke at their neurologic baseline with improved speech and strength and was taken to the intensive care unit for recovery. Magnetic resonance imaging (MRI) was done within 48 hours after surgery and showed gross total resection (Fig. 32.2). The patient participated with physical and occupational therapy and was discharged to home on postoperative day 2 with an intact neurologic examination. The patient was prescribed dexamethasone that was tapered to off over 10 days after surgery. The patient was seen at 2 weeks postoperatively for staple removal and remained neurologically intact. Pathology was metastatic melanoma that was positive for BRAF+ mutation, and the patient underwent postoperative stereotactic radiosurgery to the cavity followed by pembrolizumab immunotherapy. The lesion was observed with serial MRI examinations at 3 to 6 months intervals and has been without local or distal recurrence for 18 months. The patient returned to work at 5 weeks postoperatively and remains without neurologic deficits.

Commonalities among the experts

Half of the surgeons opted for the patient having diffusion tensor imaging to evaluate for white matter tracts, functional MRI to evaluate for eloquent cortical areas, and oncology and radiation oncology evaluation prior to pursuing surgery. All the surgeons elected for a left frontal approach (half via the superior frontal gyrus), with the majority of surgeons employing cortical and subcortical mapping (two asleep motor, one awake language and motor). The general goal for these surgeons was gross total resection. All surgeons were concerned about the primary motor cortex, and half were concerned about the Broca area. The most feared complications were motor and speech deficits. Surgery was generally pursued with surgical navigation, surgical microscope, intraoperative monitoring, and ultrasonic aspirator

with perioperative steroids, antiepileptics, and mannitol. All surgeons relied on a mapping or anatomy to stay anterior to the primary motor cortex, and the majority advocated for intralesional debulking to minimize potential iatrogenic injury. Following surgery, the majority of surgeons admitted their patients to the intensive care unit (one to the floor), and all requested imaging within 72 hours after surgery to assess for extent of resection and/or potential complications. All surgeons advocated for stereotactic radiosurgery to the lesion and cavity after the surgery.

SUMMARY OF QUALITY OF EVIDENCE TO GUIDE SPECIFIC INTERVENTIONS FOR THIS CASE

- Surgical resection plus radiation therapy versus radiation therapy alone for metastatic brain tumors—Class I.
- En bloc versus piecemeal resection of metastatic brain tumors—Class II-3.
- Resection of multiple metastatic brain tumors—Class II-2.
- Postoperative stereotactic radiosurgery following surgical resection of a metastatic brain tumor—Class I
- Immunotherapy for metastatic melanoma—Class I.

REFERENCES

1. Eichler AF, Loeffler JS. Multidisciplinary management of brain metastases. *Oncologist.* 2007;12:884–898.
2. Ewend MG, Morris DE, Carey LA, Ladha AM, Brem S. Guidelines for the initial management of metastatic brain tumors: role of surgery, radiosurgery, and radiation therapy. *J Natl Compr Canc Netw.* 2008;6:505–513; quiz 514.
3. Barnholtz-Sloan JS, Yu C, Sloan AE, et al. A nomogram for individualized estimation of survival among patients with brain metastasis. *Neuro Oncol.* 2012;14:910–918.
4. Ewend MG, Brem S, Gilbert M, et al. Treatment of single brain metastasis with resection, intracavity carmustine polymer wafers, and radiation therapy is safe and provides excellent local control. *ClinCancer Res.* 2007;13:3637–3641.

5. Ewend MG, Williams JA, Tabassi K, et al. Local delivery of chemotherapy and concurrent external beam radiotherapy prolongs survival in metastatic brain tumor models. *Cancer Res.* 1996;56:5217–5223.
6. Chaichana KL, Acharya S, Flores M, et al. Identifying better surgical candidates among recursive partitioning analysis class 2 patients who underwent surgery for intracranial metastases. *World Neurosurg.* 2014;82:e267–e275.
7. Chaichana KL, Gadkaree S, Rao K, et al. Patients undergoing surgery of intracranial metastases have different outcomes based on their primary pathology. *Neurol Res.* 2013;35:1059–1069.
8. Chaichana KL, Rao K, Gadkaree S, et al. Factors associated with survival and recurrence for patients undergoing surgery of cerebellar metastases. *Neurol Res.* 2014;36:13–25.
9. Patchell RA, Tibbs PA, Regine WF, et al. Postoperative radiotherapy in the treatment of single metastases to the brain: a randomized trial. *JAMA.* 1998;280:1485–1489.
10. Patchell RA, Tibbs PA, Walsh JW, et al. A randomized trial of surgery in the treatment of single metastases to the brain. *N Engl J Med.* 1990;322:494–500.
11. Gaspar L, Scott C, Rotman M, et al. Recursive partitioning analysis (RPA) of prognostic factors in three Radiation Therapy Oncology Group (RTOG) brain metastases trials. *Int J Radiat Oncol Biol Phys.* 1997;37:745–751.
12. Duffau H, Mandonnet E. The "onco-functional balance" in surgery for diffuse low-grade glioma: integrating the extent of resection with quality of life. *Acta Neurochir (Wien).* 2013;155:951–957.
13. Jackson C, Gallia GL, Chaichana KL. Minimally invasive biopsies of deep-seated brain lesions using tubular retractors under exoscopic visualization. *J Neurol Surg A Cent Eur Neurosurg.* 2017;78:588–594.
14. Day JD. Transsulcal parafascicular surgery using Brain Path(R) for subcortical lesions. *Neurosurgery.* 2017;64:151–156.
15. Harkey HL, Al-Mefty O, Haines DE, Smith RR. The surgical anatomy of the cerebral sulci. *Neurosurgery.* 1989;24:651–654.
16. Ribas GC, Yasuda A, Ribas EC, Nishikuni K, Rodrigues AJ Jr. Surgical anatomy of microneurosurgical sulcal key points. *Neurosurgery.* 2006;59:ONS177–ONS210; discussion ONS210–ONS171.
17. Gassie K, Wijesekera O, Chaichana KL. Minimally invasive tubular retractor-assisted biopsy and resection of subcortical intra-axial gliomas and other neoplasms. *J Neurosurg Sci.* 2018;62:682–689.
18. Iyer R, Chaichana KL. Minimally invasive resection of deep-seated high-grade gliomas using tubular retractors and exoscopic visualization. *J Neurol Surg A Cent Eur Neurosurg.* 2018;79:330–336.

33

Left perirolandic metastatic brain cancer

Case reviewed by Sunit Das, Peter E. Fecci, Alessandro Olivi, Giuseppe Maria Della Pepa, Ganesh Rao

Introduction

The most common type of brain tumor in adults is metastatic brain tumors, with an incidence 3 to 14 per 100,000 people per year.[1,2] Approximately 10% to 20% of these metastatic brain tumors occur in eloquent locations, which include primary motor, somatosensory, speech, and/or visual cortices.[3] The general management of large, symptomatic metastatic brain tumors is surgery followed by radiation therapy.[1,2,4–6] However, lesions in eloquent regions are surgically more challenging, and therefore typically undergo radiation therapy to minimize the risk of surgically induced morbidity.[3] Radiation without surgical therapy, however, does little to improve symptomatic mass effect in the immediate period.[1,2,4–6] In this chapter, we present a case of a patient with a dominant hemisphere perirolandic metastatic brain tumor.

Example case

Chief complaint: headaches and right-hand weakness
History of present illness
An 80-year-old, right-handed man with a history of hypertension, coronary artery disease, and bladder cancer status postresection and radiation therapy presented with headaches over the past couple of weeks unresponsive to pain medications, and difficulties with writing and buttoning his shirts over the same time frame. He saw his oncologist who ordered systemic imaging, and a brain lesion was seen (Fig. 33.1).
Medications: Aspirin, irbesartan, hydrochlorothiazide.
Allergies: No known drug allergies.
Past medical and surgical history: Hypertension, coronary artery disease, bladder cancer status postresection 5 years prior.
Family history: No history of intracranial malignancies.

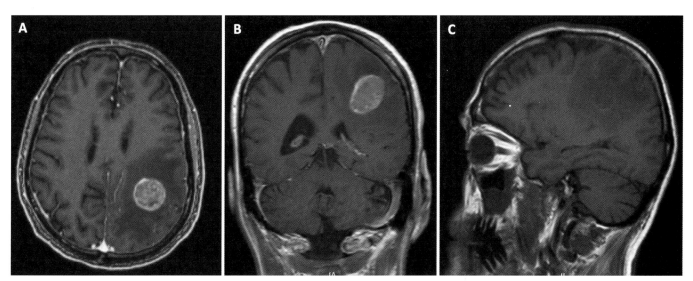

Fig. 33.1 Preoperative magnetic resonance imaging. (A) T1 axial image with gadolinium contrast; **(B)** T1 coronal image with gadolinium contrast; **(C)** T1 sagittal image without gadolinium contrast magnetic resonance imaging scans demonstrating a heterogeneously enhancing lesion in close proximity to the precentral cortex and rolandic fissure.

Social history: Retired, independent with activities of daily living, remote smoking history, and no alcohol.

Physical examination: Awake, alert, oriented to person, place, and time; Language: naming difficulties, impaired repetition; Cranial nerves II to XII intact, except slight right facial droop;

Right upper extremity 4+/5, Right lower extremity 5/5, Left upper extremity 5/5, Left lower extremity 5/5.

Computed tomography chest/abdomen/pelvis: Several liver lesions concerning for metastatic disease.

	Sunit Das, MD, PhD, St. Michael's Hospital, University of Toronto, Toronto, Canada	Peter E. Fecci, MD, PhD, Duke University, Durham, NC, United States	Alessandro Olivi, MD, Giuseppe Maria Della Pepa, MD, A. Gemelli University Hospital, Rome, Italy	Ganesh Rao, MD, Baylor College of Medicine, Houston, TX, United States
Preoperative				
Additional tests requested	DTI fMRI	DTI Oncology evaluation for prognosis	DTI fMRI	DTI
Surgical approach selected	Left parietal craniotomy or SRS	Left fronto-parietal craniotomy with awake speech and motor mapping	Left fronto-parietal craniotomy with asleep motor mapping	Left parieto-occipital craniotomy with asleep motor mapping
Anatomic corridor	Left parietal, transsulcal, MIPS	Left parietal	Left fronto-parietal	Left parieto-occipital
Goal of surgery	Gross total resection and neurologic preservation	Gross total resection, local disease control, palliative symptom control	Gross total resection and neurologic preservation	Gross total resection
Perioperative				
Positioning	Left supine semilateral	Left lateral	Left supine with right rotation	Left three-quarter prone
Surgical equipment	Surgical navigation Surgical microscope Ultrasonic aspirator Ultrasound	Surgical navigation Surgical microscope Brain stimulator	Surgical navigation IOM (SSEP/MEP) Brain stimulator	Surgical navigation Ultrasound Brain stimulator IOM (SSEP, EMG)
Medications	Steroids	Steroids Antiepileptics Mannitol	Steroids Antiepileptics	Steroids
Anatomic considerations	Motor and somatosensory cortex, CST	Receptive speech area, motor cortex, CST, AF, optic radiations	Central sulcus, motor and sensory cortices, CST, IFOF	Motor and somatosensory cortex, CST
Complications feared with approach chosen	Motor and sensory deficits	Language dysfunction, motor deficit	CST injury	Injury to motor cortex and CST, Gerstmann syndrome
Intraoperative				
Anesthesia	General	Asleep-awake-asleep	General	General
Skin incision	Linear	Linear	Linear	Linear/curvilinear
Bone opening	Left parietal	Left parietal	Left parietal	Left parietal
Brain exposure	Left fronto-parietal	Left fronto-parietal	Left parietal and possible central lobe	Left parieto-occipital

	Sunit Das, MD, PhD, St. Michael's Hospital, University of Toronto, Toronto, Canada	Peter E. Fecci, MD, PhD, Duke University, Durham, NC, United States	Alessandro Olivi, MD, Giuseppe Maria Della Pepa, MD, A. Gemelli University Hospital, Rome, Italy	Ganesh Rao, MD, Baylor College of Medicine, Houston, TX, United States
Method of resection	Craniotomy based on navigation, ultrasound to identify lesion, dural opening, determine suitability of sulcal opening, sulcal dissection under microscopic visualization, pial opening to access tumor, sequential mobilization with internal debulking, goal of gross total resection, ultrasound assessment, dural tack up sutures	Craniotomy based on navigation while patient asleep, patient awakened and following commands, dura opened, cortical stimulation of speech and motor areas starting at 1 mA, corticectomy planned based on negative mapping sites, en bloc vs. piecemeal resection depending on tumor consistency, patient sedated for closure	Craniotomy based on navigation with preoperative identification of planned trajectory posterior to somatosensory cortex, C-shaped dural opening, place strip electrode for MEP or phase reversal to identify central sulcus, stimulate electrode to find negative mapping area to enter tumor, corticectomy but ideally transsulcal, internal debulking of tumor, tumor margins dissected from parenchyma, ultrasound to check for residual, dural closure with pericranium if necessary	Craniotomy based on navigation, dura opened, cortical mapping to identify motor and sensory cortices, transcortical approach based on negative mapping sites, subcortical stimulation along trajectory, intralesional resection because of the size of the lesion, ultrasound to verify extent of resection
Complication avoidance	Transsulcal, ultrasound assessment, internal debulking	Cortical and subcortical mapping, method of resection depending on tumor consistency	Trajectory posterior to sensory cortex, internal debulking to minimize manipulation, ultrasound	Cortical and subcortical mapping, intralesional resection, ultrasound
Postoperative				
Admission	Floor	ICU	ICU	ICU
Postoperative complications feared	Motor and sensory deficit	Language dysfunction, motor deficit	Seizures, ischemia	Motor deficit
Follow-up testing	MRI within 48 hours after surgery	MRI within 24 hours after surgery	MRI within 24 hours after surgery	MRI within 24 hours after surgery
Follow-up visits	1 month after surgery	14 days after surgery and 4 weeks after surgery	10 days and 1 month after surgery	7–10 days after surgery and 1 month after surgery for MRI
Adjuvant therapies recommended	SRS or hypofractionated radiation to cavity	SRS	Radiation therapy	SRS or hypofractionated radiotherapy

AF, arcuate fasciculus; *CST*, corticospinal tracts; *DTI*, diffusion tensor imaging; *EMG*, electromyography; *fMRI*, functional magnetic resonance imaging; *ICU*, intensive care unit; *IFOF*, inferior frontal occipital fasciculus; *IOM*, intraoperative monitoring; *MEP*, motor evoked potential; *MIPS*, minimally invasive parafascicular surgery; *MRI*, magnetic resonance imaging; *SRS*, stereotactic radiosurgery; *SSEP*, somatosensory evoked potential,

Differential diagnosis and actual diagnosis

- Metastatic brain cancer
- High-grade glioma
- Lymphoma
- Cerebral abscess

Important anatomic and preoperative considerations

The recursive partitioning analysis (RPA) classification system is the most commonly used classification system to prognosticate outcomes for patients with metastatic brain tumors.[7] For a full description of the RPA classification, see Chapter 32, Fig. 32.2. The patient in this case is an RPA class 2 because of age older than 65 years and presence of extracranial disease, but has good functioning status (Karnofsky performance score ≥70). For a full discussion of the central sulcus and perirolandic anatomy, see Chapters 3 and 4. This lesion involves the pre- and postcentral gyrus and underlies the central sulcus or rolandic fissure.

Approaches to this lesion

For metastatic brain tumors, the treatment options include surgery and/or radiation therapy, in which the conventional radiation therapy is stereotactic radiosurgery (SRS) (Table 33.1).[1,2,4–6,8] For solitary lesions that are large (>2.0 cm) and symptomatic, the conventional approach is surgical

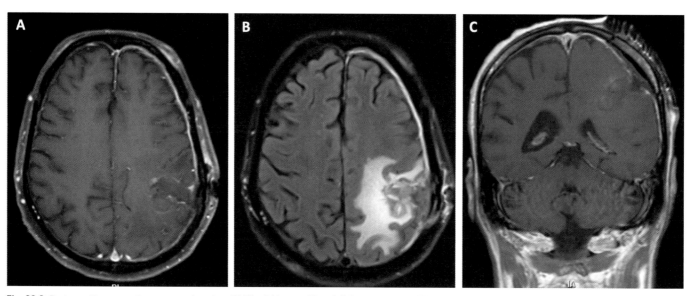

Fig. 33.2 Postoperative magnetic resonance imaging. (A) T1 axial image with gadolinium contrast; **(B)** T2 fluid attenuation inversion recovery axial image; **(C)** T1 coronal image with gadolinium contrast magnetic resonance imaging scans demonstrating gross total resection of the left perirolandic lesion.

Table 33.1 Advantages of stereotactic radiosurgery versus surgical resection

Characteristics	Stereotactic Radiosurgery	Surgical Resection
Tumor size <3cm	++	–
Tumor size >3 cm	+	++
Mass effect/edema	–	+
Immediate relief of symptoms	–	++
Eloquent location	++	+
Deep-seated location	++	+
Multiple lesions	++	–
++ Advantageous, + mildly advantageous, – not advantageous.		

resection followed by SRS after wound healing.[1,2,4–6] Postoperative SRS has been shown to decrease local recurrence even in cases with gross total resection.[1,2,4–6,8] An alternative to postoperative SRS is preoperative SRS.[9–11] The theoretical advantage of preoperative SRS is that it avoids delay in radiation for nonoperated lesions in cases with multiple brain metastases, sterilizes cells to minimize chance of leptomeningeal disease, and provides better delineated tumor margins for radiation therapy to minimize risk of radiation necrosis, whereas the potential drawbacks include wound healing and increased edema.[9–11] In terms of surgical approach, surgery can be done asleep with general anesthesia or awake with brain mapping (Chapter 1, Fig. 1.2). In addition, eloquent cortex and white matter tracts, including the primary motor and sensory cortices and corticospinal tracts, can be identified and monitored with indirect and direct methods inside and outside of the operating room (Chapter 3, Fig. 3.2). Furthermore, when surgery is pursued, accessing lesions in the subcortical space can be done transgyral or transsulcal (Chapter 32). This lesion is in the subcortical space below the central sulcus based on anatomic definitions, and in close proximity to not only the corticospinal tracts but also the superior longitudinal fasciculus and arcuate fasciculus.

What was actually done

The patient was admitted and underwent preoperative SRS to the lesion. In the afternoon of the same day as SRS, the patient was taken to surgery for a left frontal-parietal craniotomy with awake motor and language mapping for resection of the lesion. The patient was intubated with a laryngeal mask airway. The scalp was blocked bilaterally with local anesthetic, and the head was fixed in pins, with two pins centered on the inion and one pin on the right forehead in the midpupillary line. The head was turned 60 degrees to the right, and a bump was placed under the left shoulder and hip to facilitate turning and patient comfort. A linear incision was planned over the center of the lesion in the coronal plane based on preoperative magnetic resonance imaging (MRI) navigation. The patient was draped in the usual standard fashion and given mannitol (1 g/kg), dexamethasone, levetiracetam, and cefazolin. The flap was made and held in place with self-retaining cerebellar retractors. A left frontal-parietal craniotomy was done to encompass the lesion. Ultrasound and surgical navigation were used to confirm lesion boundaries, and the boundaries were designated with letter tags once the dura was opened. The dura was anesthetized with local anesthetics between the leaflets adjacent to the middle meningeal vessels. The patient was awakened, and the dura was opened once the patient followed commands consistently. Strip electrodes were placed in the subdural space for after-discharge monitoring. The cortex was initially stimulated at 2 mA, and hand dysfunction was achieved at 3 mA with an Ojemann stimulator (Integra, Princeton, NJ) over the precentral gyrus. The rest of the cortical and subcortical mapping took place at 3 mA. The patient participated in continuous motor movement of the right face, arm, and leg with picture naming. The primary motor and sensory cortices were identified based on cortical stimulation with hand weakness and paresthesias, respectively. The lesion was confirmed to be below the central sulcus. The microscope was brought in, and the sulcus was opened sharply with microdissection. Once the sulcus was opened, a tubular retractor was placed under navigation guidance into the lesion to provide retraction of the surrounding parenchyma. The lesion was removed piecemeal until white matter was seen on all the edges. The patient had no change in motor or language function during the resection. Preliminary diagnosis was consistent with metastatic carcinoma. The retractor was withdrawn, and the patient was put under sedation. The dura, bone, and skin were closed in standard fashion.

The patient awoke at their neurologic baseline with full strength bilaterally and was taken to the intensive care unit for recovery. Postoperative MRI done within 48 hours after surgery showed gross total resection (Fig. 33.2). The patient participated with physical and occupational therapy and was discharged to home on postoperative day 2 with an intact neurological examination. The patient was prescribed 3 months of levetiracetam, and dexamethasone was tapered to off over 14 days after surgery. The patient was seen at 2 weeks postoperatively for staple removal and was full strength. Pathology was consistent with transition cell bladder carcinoma. The lesion was observed with serial MRI examinations at 3-month intervals, and the patient has been without recurrence or systemic disease for 12 months and has been neurologically intact.

Commonalities among the experts

All of the surgeons opted for the patient having diffusion tensor imaging to evaluate for white matter tracts, and half opted for functional MRI to evaluate for eloquent cortical areas prior to pursuing surgery. All the surgeons elected for a left parietal-based approach, in which three employed cortical and subcortical mapping (two asleep motor, one awake language and motor). The goal for all surgeons was gross total resection. All surgeons were concerned about the primary motor and sensory cortices, as well as the corticospinal tract. The most feared complication was a motor deficit. Surgery was generally pursued with surgical navigation, surgical microscope, ultrasound, and brain stimulator with perioperative steroids and antiepileptics. Most surgeons advocated for cortical and subcortical mapping, as well as intralesional debulking to minimize potential iatrogenic injury. Following surgery, the majority of surgeons admitted their patients to the intensive care unit (one to the floor), and all requested imaging within 48 hours after surgery to assess for extent of resection and/or potential complications. All surgeons advocated for SRS to the lesion and cavity after the surgery.

SUMMARY OF QUALITY OF EVIDENCE TO GUIDE SPECIFIC INTERVENTIONS FOR THIS CASE

- Surgical resection plus radiation therapy versus radiation therapy alone for metastatic brain tumors—Class I.
- Preoperative versus postoperative stereotactic radiation therapy—Class II-2.
- En bloc versus piecemeal resection of metastatic brain tumors—Class II-3.
- Transsulcal versus transgyral approach for subcortical metastatic tumors—Class III.
- Tubular retractors for subcortical metastatic tumors—Class III.

REFERENCES

1. Eichler AF, Loeffler JS. Multidisciplinary management of brain metastases. *Oncologist.* 2007;12:884–898.
2. Ewend MG, Morris DE, Carey LA, Ladha AM, Brem S. Guidelines for the initial management of metastatic brain tumors: role of surgery, radiosurgery, and radiation therapy. *J Natl Compr Canc Netw.* 2008;6:505–513; quiz 514.
3. Dea N, Borduas M, Kenny B, Fortin D, Mathieu D. Safety and efficacy of Gamma Knife surgery for brain metastases in eloquent locations. *J Neurosurg.* 2010;113(Suppl):79–83.
4. Barnholtz-Sloan JS, Yu C, Sloan AE, et al. A nomogram for individualized estimation of survival among patients with brain metastasis. *Neuro Oncol.* 2012;14:910–918.
5. Ewend MG, Brem S, Gilbert M, et al. Treatment of single brain metastasis with resection, intracavity carmustine polymer wafers, and radiation therapy is safe and provides excellent local control. *Clin Cancer Res.* 2007;13:3637–3641.
6. Ewend MG, Williams JA, Tabassi K, et al. Local delivery of chemotherapy and concurrent external beam radiotherapy prolongs survival in metastatic brain tumor models. *Cancer Res.* 1996;56:5217–5223.
7. Gaspar L, Scott C, Rotman M, et al. Recursive partitioning analysis (RPA) of prognostic factors in three Radiation Therapy Oncology Group (RTOG) brain metastases trials. *Int J Radiat Oncol Biol Phys.* 1997;37:745–751.
8. Marchan EM, Peterson J, Sio TT, et al. Postoperative cavity stereotactic radiosurgery for brain metastases. *Front Oncol.* 2018;8:342.
9. Patel KR, Burri SH, Asher AL, et al. Comparing preoperative with postoperative stereotactic radiosurgery for resectable brain metastases: a multi-institutional analysis. *Neurosurgery.* 2016;79:279–285.
10. Prabhu RS, Miller KR, Asher AL, et al. Preoperative stereotactic radiosurgery before planned resection of brain metastases: updated analysis of efficacy and toxicity of a novel treatment paradigm. *J Neurosurg.* 2018:1–8.
11. Routman DM, Yan E, Vora S, et al. Preoperative stereotactic radiosurgery for brain metastases. *Front Neurol.* 2018;9:959.

34

Multiple accessible metastatic brain tumors

Case reviewed by Lucas Alverne Freitas de Albuquerque, Francesco DiMeco, Massimiliano Del Bene, Fredric B. Meyer, Robert E. Wharen

Introduction

The most common type of brain tumor in adults is metastatic brain tumors, with an incidence of 3 to 14 per 100,000 people per year.[1,2] Surgical resection is generally offered to patients with solitary, large, symptomatic lesions who have good prognoses, which is dependent on age, functional status, primary tumor control, and presence of extracranial disease.[1-5] However, a significant number of patients present with multiple metastatic brain tumors.[6-8] These lesions can sometimes all be accessible for surgical resection, whereas other times only a select few. In this chapter, we present a case of a patient with multiple metastatic brain lesions that are all relatively accessible.

Example case

Chief complaint: imbalance

History of present illness

A 47-year-old, right-handed man with a history of hypertension and lung adenocarcinoma status post resection and radiation therapy 2 years prior presented with imbalance over several weeks. He underwent resection of a lung adenocarcinoma followed by radiation for localized disease. He had been well but had increasing difficulty with balance in which he felt as though he was intoxicated over the past 3 to 4 weeks. He denies headaches, nausea, vomiting, or weakness (Fig. 34.1).

Medications: Lisinopril.

Allergies: No known drug allergies.

Past medical and surgical history: Hypertension, lung adenocarcinoma status postresection 2 years prior.

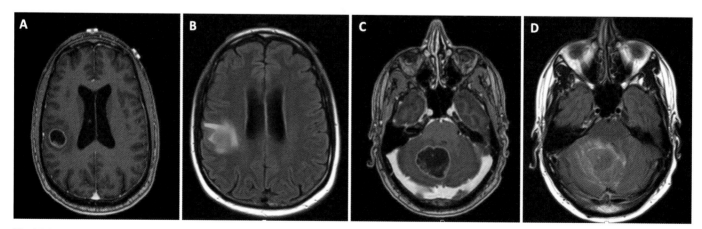

Fig. 34.1 Preoperative magnetic resonance imaging. (A) T1 axial image with gadolinium contrast above the Sylvian fissure; **(B)** T2 axial fluid attenuation inversion recovery image above the Sylvian fissure; **(C)** T1 axial image with gadolinium contrast at the level of middle cerebellar peduncle; **(D)** T2 axial fluid attenuation inversion recovery image at the level of middle cerebellar peduncle magnetic resonance imaging scans demonstrating a right perirolandic and an additional posterior fossa metastatic brain tumor.

Family history: No history of intracranial malignancies.
Social history: Mail delivery worker, remote smoking history, no alcohol.
Physical examination: Awake, alert, oriented to person, place, and time; Language: intact naming and repetition; Cranial nerve II to XII intact; No drift, moves all extremities with full strength; Cerebellar: truncal ataxia and bilateral finger-to-nose dysmetria.
Computed tomography chest/abdomen/pelvis: No evidence of systemic disease.

	Lucas Alverne Freitas de Albuquerque, MD, Hospital Geral de Fortaleza, Ceara, Brazil	Francesco DiMeco, MD, Massimiliano Del Bene, MD, Carlo Besta Neurological Institute, Milan, Italy	Fredric B. Meyer, MD, Mayo Clinic, Rochester, MN, United States	Robert E. Wharen, MD, Mayo Clinic, Jacksonville, FL, United States
Preoperative				
Additional tests requested	Anesthesiology evaluation Palliative care evaluation Psychological evaluation	Transcranial doppler ultrasound with micro bubbles to assess for right-to-left cardiac shunt	Oncology evaluation	Radiation oncology evaluation Oncology evaluation
Surgical approach selected	Midline suboccipital craniotomy	Median/right paramedial suboccipital craniotomy in sitting position	Midline suboccipital craniotomy	Preoperative SRS to right perirolandic lesion and right suboccipital craniectomy for cerebellar lesion
Anatomic corridor	Cerebellar vermis	Cerebellar hemisphere	Cerebellar vermis	Cerebellar hemisphere
Goal of surgery	Improve overall survival, avoid hydrocephalus	Complete resection with 5-mm margins, preserve CSF pathways	Complete resection of cerebellar tumor, decompression of fourth ventricle	Relief of posterior fossa mass effect
Perioperative				
Positioning	Prone Concorde, no pins	Semisitting, neutral	Prone neutral	Right supine
Surgical equipment	Surgical microscope	Precordial Doppler Central catheter Surgical navigation Surgical microscope Chisel Ultrasound Ultrasonic aspirator	Surgical microscope +/− Ultrasound +/− Ultrasonic aspirator	Surgical navigation Surgical microscope
Medications	Steroids Hypertonic saline	Steroids, high fluids	Steroids	Steroids +/− Mannitol
Anatomic considerations	Cerebellar vermis, dentate nucleus	Suboccipital muscles, occipital/transverse/torcular sinuses, cerebellar hemispheres, vermis, tentorium, cisterna magna, cerebellar draining veins	Transverse sinus, torcula, fourth ventricular floor, middle cerebellar peduncle	Cerebellar hemisphere Shortest working distance
Complications feared with approach chosen	Akinetic mutism, hydrocephalus	Venous air embolism, hydrocephalus, venous engorgement, CSF leak, posterior fossa syndrome	Cerebellar edema, wound healing issues, cerebellar mutism	Injury to cerebellum, hydrocephalus
Intraoperative				
Anesthesia	General	General	General	General
Skin incision	Midline linear	Midline linear	Midline linear from inion to C2	Linear paramedian

(continued on next page)

	Lucas Alverne Freitas de Albuquerque, MD, Hospital Geral de Fortaleza, Ceara, Brazil	Francesco DiMeco, MD, Massimiliano Del Bene, MD, Carlo Besta Neurological Institute, Milan, Italy	Fredric B. Meyer, MD, Mayo Clinic, Rochester, MN, United States	Robert E. Wharen, MD, Mayo Clinic, Jacksonville, FL, United States
Bone opening	Midline suboccipital	Median/right paramedial suboccipital	Midline suboccipital	Right suboccipital over tumor
Brain exposure	Bilateral cerebellar hemisphere and vermis	Bilateral cerebellar hemisphere eccentric to the right	Bilateral cerebellar hemisphere and vermis	Right cerebellar hemisphere
Method of resection	Midline incision, dissect in avascular plane, midline suboccipital craniotomy, Y-shaped dural opening, identify vermis, transvermian resection over shortest distance to lesion, watertight dural closure, subcutaneous drain	Muscle incision and detachment in one layer, bilateral occipital craniotomy eccentric to right without C1 laminectomy up to inferior edge of transverse sinus, craniotomy without burr hole, V-shaped dural opening, occipital sinus section at bottom, ultrasound-guided resection of lesion through parenchyma, en bloc resection, removal of 5-mm margin with ultrasonic aspirator, watertight dural closure	Craniotomy or craniectomy, bone opening close to torcula and transverse sinus, T-shaped dural opening, drainage of CSF for cisterna magna, work along top of vermis to identify entry point, 1.0-cm vertical incision in the vermis to locate tumor, infernally debulk tumor, infold and remove capsule, inspect cavity to confirm gross total resection, watertight dural closure	Craniotomy encompassing lesion, cruciate dural opening, transcerebellar approach through shortest distance, identification of capsule, internal decompression, mobilization of capsule from surrounding parenchyma, gross total resection, dural closure with synthetic graft
Complication avoidance	Shortest working distance, strict hemostasis	Ultrasound-guided resection, en bloc resection, removal of margin	Bony opening up to transverse sinus/torcula, small corticectomy in vermis, internally debulk tumor prior to mobilizing capsule	Shortest working distance, internal debulking, dural graft
Postoperative				
Admission	ICU	ICU	ICU	ICU
Postoperative complications feared	Hydrocephalus, CSF leak, akinetic mutism	Hydrocephalus, venous engorgement, CSF leak, posterior fossa syndrome	Cerebellar edema, wound healing issues, cerebellar mutism	Cerebellar edema, hydrocephalus
Follow-up testing	MRI within 48 hours after surgery Molecular testing of tumor	CT within 24 hours after surgery MRI within 48 hours after surgery Radiation oncology evaluation	Possible second stage surgery for perirolandic lesion MRI within 48 hours after surgery	MRI within 48 hours after surgery
Follow-up visits	14 days after surgery, 1 and 3 months after surgery and every 3 months after	4 weeks after surgery prior to radiation therapy	6 weeks after surgery with neurosurgery 2 weeks after surgery with radiation and neurooncology	2 weeks after surgery with radiation and neurooncology
Adjuvant therapies recommended	Postop SRS to cerebellar lesion cavity and other lesion, chemotherapy based on tumor markers	Postop SRS to cerebellar lesion cavity and other lesion	Radiation oncology evaluation for SRS vs. WBRT	Systemic therapy per oncology

CSF, cerebrospinal fluid; *CT*, computed tomography; *ICU*, intensive care unit, *MRI*, magnetic resonance imaging; *SRS*, stereotactic radiosurgery; *WBRT*, whole-brain radiation therapy.

Differential diagnosis and actual diagnosis

- Metastatic brain cancer
- High-grade glioma
- Lymphoma
- Cerebral abscess

Important anatomic and preoperative considerations

The recursive partitioning analysis classification system is the most commonly used classification system to prognosticate outcomes for patients with metastatic brain tumors (Chapter 32, Fig. 32.2).[9] The patient in this case is a recursive partitioning analysis class 1 because of age younger than 65 years, good functioning status (Karnofsky performance score ≥70), primary tumor control, and no extracranial systemic disease. The full description of the pre- and postcentral gyrus is in Chapters 3 and 4, and the full description of cerebellar anatomy is in Chapter 31. The supratentorial lesion is in close proximity to the precentral gyrus on the right, and the infratentorial lesion involves both the right cerebellar hemisphere and the vermis.

Approaches to this lesion

The majority of patients who develop metastatic brain tumors have multiple lesions.[6–8] The surgical management of solitary lesions and symptomatic lesions is well defined for metastatic brain tumors.[10–14] However, the management of patients with multiple lesions, in which not all lesions are symptomatic, is more controversial, especially in the modern radiosurgery era.[6–8] Bindal et al.[8] in 1993 performed a retrospective analysis of 56 patients who underwent surgery for multiple metastatic brain tumors, in which patients who had one or more lesions left unresected were compared with patients who underwent resection of all lesions, and matched to patients who had a solitary brain metastasis. They found that the outcomes for patients who had all of their metastatic brain tumors resected had increased survival times and prognoses comparable to patients who underwent resection of a solitary brain metastasis.[8] However, with the widespread availability and known efficacy of stereotactic radiosurgery, many advocate for the resection of only symptomatic lesions in patients with multiple brain metastases to minimize risk of surgically induced morbidity.[15]

What was actually done

The patient was taken to surgery for a midline suboccipital craniotomy followed by a right fronto-parietal craniotomy for metastatic brain tumors with general anesthesia and intraoperative monitoring for the supratentorial lesion. The posterior fossa lesion was chosen first, as the patient was most symptomatic from this lesion. The patient was induced and intubated per routine. The head was fixed in neutral position, with two pins centered over the left external auditory meatus and one pin over the right external auditory meatus. The patient was then placed prone onto chest rolls with the neck flexed and reduced. A midline incision was planned that spanned from just above the inion to the C2 spinous process. In addition, a left Frazier burr hole site was planned in case it was needed for an external ventricular drain. The patient was draped in the usual standard fashion and given dexamethasone and cefazolin. A midline incision was made, and dissection took place in the avascular plane between the suboccipital muscles. The skin and muscles were retracted with a cerebellar retractor, and the C1 spinous process and occipital bone with foramen magnum were identified. A midline suboccipital craniotomy that was eccentric to the right was made below the transverse sinus but above the lip of the foramen magnum. The ultrasound was used to confirm lesion boundaries before the dura was opened to evaluate if more bone needed to be removed. Once the opening was confirmed to be large enough, the dura was opened in a cruciate fashion. The cisterna manga and craniotomy were lined with cottonoids to minimize tumor spillage. A corticectomy was done over the medial aspect of the right cerebellar hemisphere. An attempt was made at removing the lesion en bloc, however, the tumor was soft in texture and cystic making it difficult to achieve a complete en bloc resection, and therefore it was removed in piecemeal. Preliminary pathology was adenocarcinoma. Once white matter was seen on all the edges, the cavity was inspected for residual, and hemostasis was obtained. The dura, bone, and skin were closed in standard fashion. After this was done, the patient was then positioned for a right frontal-parietal craniotomy with general anesthesia and intraoperative monitoring with somatosensory evoked potentials and electroencephalography. The patient was placed on a horseshoe with the head turned 90 degrees to the left, and a bump was placed underneath the right shoulder to facilitate turning. The electromagnetic stereotactic navigation was used to obviate the need for pinning. A linear incision was then planned in the coronal plane over the center of the lesion based on surgical navigation. The patient was draped in the usual standard fashion and given levetiracetam and cefazolin. An incision was made, and the scalp was retracted with Weitlaner retractors. A keyhole craniotomy was made over the targeted sulcus. The dura was opened in a cruciate fashion and tacked up after confirming lesion localization with ultrasound and surgical navigation. A strip electrode was placed in the subdural space, and a phase reversal confirmed that the central sulcus was anterior to the lesion. In addition, the cortex was stimulated around the identified sulcus to confirm no electrical activity in the contralateral face and hand muscles. The surgical microscope was brought in, and the sulcus was opened sharply with microdissection. Once the bottom of the sulcus was identified, the subcortical U-fibers were opened with bipolar cautery, and the lesion was identified. The lesion was then removed en bloc. The cavity was inspected with direct visualization and ultrasound to confirm no residual tumor. The dura, bone, and skin were closed in standard fashion.

The patient awoke at their neurologic baseline with full strength bilaterally and was taken to the intensive care unit for recovery. Magnetic resonance imaging was done within 48 hours after surgery and showed gross total resection of both lesions (Fig. 34.2). The patient participated with physical and occupational therapy and was discharged to home on postoperative day 3 with an intact neurologic

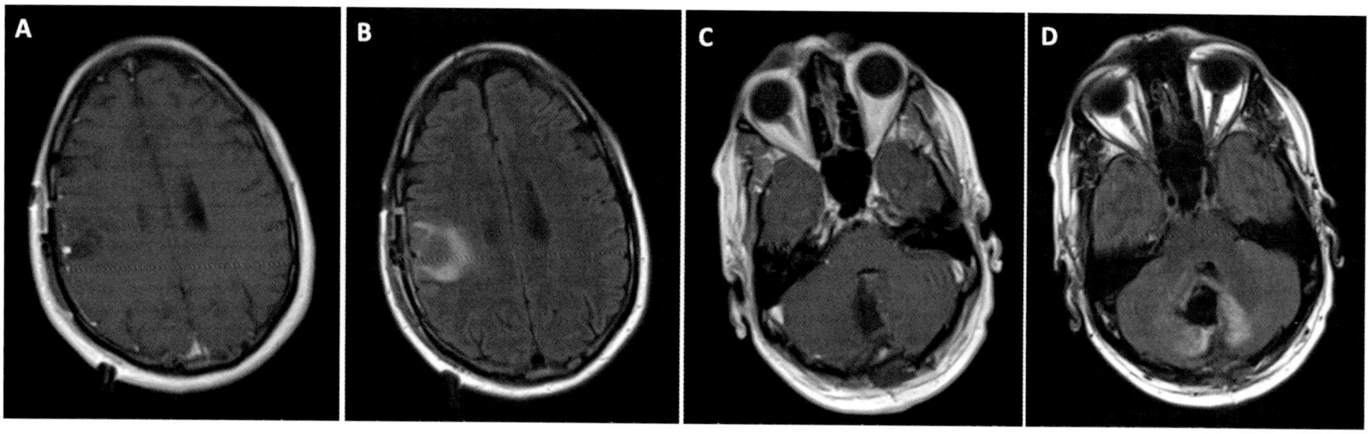

Fig. 34.2 Postoperative magnetic resonance imaging. (A) T1 axial image with gadolinium contrast above the Sylvian fissure; **(B)** T2 axial fluid attenuation inversion recovery image above the Sylvian fissure; **(C)** T1 axial image with gadolinium contrast at the level of middle cerebellar peduncle; **(D)** T2 axial fluid attenuation inversion recovery image at the level of middle cerebellar peduncle magnetic resonance imaging scans demonstrating gross total resection of the right perirolandic and posterior fossa metastatic brain tumors.

examination, except for some disequilibrium. The patient was prescribed dexamethasone that was tapered to off over 10 days after surgery. The patient was seen at 2 weeks postoperatively for suture removal and remained neurologically intact with improved balance. Final pathology was consistent with lung adenocarcinoma. The patient then underwent postoperative stereotactic radiosurgery to both surgical cavities. The lesion was observed with serial magnetic resonance imaging examinations at 3 month intervals, and has been without local or distal recurrence for 12 months. The patient returned to work at 6 weeks postoperatively and remains without neurologic deficits with improved balance.

Commonalities among the experts

Half of the surgeons opted for the patient having oncology and/or radiation oncology evaluations prior to pursuing surgery. All the surgeons elected for resection of only the cerebellar lesion, in which half preferred a cerebellar vermian approach and the other half a cerebellar hemispheric approach. The majority of surgeons utilized a midline suboccipital craniotomy. The goal for all surgeons was gross total resection of the cerebellar lesion. All surgeons were concerned about the cerebellar hemisphere and vermis. The most feared complication was cerebellar injury. Surgery was generally pursued with surgical navigation and surgical microscope with perioperative steroids. Most surgeons advocated for using the shortest working distance to access the tumor, and intralesional debulking to minimize potential iatrogenic injury. Following surgery, all patients were admitted to the intensive care unit, and all surgeons requested imaging within 72 hours after surgery to assess for extent of resection and/or potential complications. All surgeons advocated for stereotactic radiosurgery to the lesion and cavity after the surgery, as well as the remaining supratentorial lesion.

SUMMARY OF QUALITY OF EVIDENCE TO GUIDE SPECIFIC INTERVENTIONS FOR THIS CASE

- Surgical resection plus radiation therapy versus radiation therapy alone for metastatic brain tumors—Class I.
- Surgical resection of all brain metastases in one setting—Class II-2.
- En bloc versus piecemeal resection of metastatic brain tumors—Class II-3.
- Transsulcal versus transgyral approach for subcortical metastatic tumors—Class III.
- Asleep motor mapping for perirolandic tumors—Class III.

REFERENCES

1. Eichler AF, Loeffler JS. Multidisciplinary management of brain metastases. *Oncologist.* 2007;12:884–898.
2. Ewend MG, Morris DE, Carey LA, Ladha AM, Brem S. Guidelines for the initial management of metastatic brain tumors: role of surgery, radiosurgery, and radiation therapy. *J Natl Compr Canc Netw.* 2008;6:505–513; quiz 514.
3. Barnholtz-Sloan JS, Yu C, Sloan AE, et al. A nomogram for individualized estimation of survival among patients with brain metastasis. *Neuro Oncol.* 2012;14:910–918.
4. Ewend MG, Brem S, Gilbert M, et al. Treatment of single brain metastasis with resection, intracavity carmustine polymer wafers, and radiation therapy is safe and provides excellent local control. *Clin Cancer Res.* 2007;13:3637–3641.
5. Ewend MG, Williams JA, Tabassi K, et al. Local delivery of chemotherapy and concurrent external beam radiotherapy prolongs survival in metastatic brain tumor models. *Cancer Res.* 1996;56:5217–5223.
6. Auslands K, Apskalne D, Bicans K, Ozols R, Ozolins H. Postoperative survival in patients with multiple brain metastases. *Medicina (Kaunas).* 2012;48:281–285.
7. Baker CM, Glenn CA, Briggs RG, et al. Simultaneous resection of multiple metastatic brain tumors with multiple keyhole craniotomies. *World Neurosurg.* 2017;106:359–367.
8. Bindal RK, Sawaya R, Leavens ME, Lee JJ. Surgical treatment of multiple brain metastases. *J Neurosurg.* 1993;79:210–216.

9. Gaspar L, Scott C, Rotman M, et al. Recursive partitioning analysis (RPA) of prognostic factors in three Radiation Therapy Oncology Group (RTOG) brain metastases trials. *Int J Radiat Oncol Biol Phys*. 1997;37:745–751.

10. Chaichana KL, Acharya S, Flores M, et al. Identifying better surgical candidates among recursive partitioning analysis class 2 patients who underwent surgery for intracranial metastases. *World Neurosurg*. 2014;82:e267–e275.

11. Chaichana KL, Gadkaree S, Rao K, et al. Patients undergoing surgery of intracranial metastases have different outcomes based on their primary pathology. *Neurol Res*. 2013;35:1059–1069.

12. Chaichana KL, Rao K, Gadkaree S, et al. Factors associated with survival and recurrence for patients undergoing surgery of cerebellar metastases. *Neurol Res*. 2014;36:13–25.

13. Patchell RA, Tibbs PA, Regine WF, et al. Postoperative radiotherapy in the treatment of single metastases to the brain: a randomized trial. *JAMA*. 1998;280:1485–1489.

14. Patchell RA, Tibbs PA, Walsh JW, et al. A randomized trial of surgery in the treatment of single metastases to the brain. *N Engl J Med*. 1990;322:494–500.

15. Blomain ES, Kim H, Garg S, et al. Stereotactic radiosurgery practice patterns for brain metastases in the United States: a national survey. *J Radiat Oncol*. 2018;7:241–246.

35

Multiple metastases but not all accessible

Case reviewed by Miguel A. Arraez, Mark Bernstein, Michael Lim, Gabriel Zada

Introduction

Metastatic brain tumors are the most common type of brain tumors in adults, in which approximately 30% of cancer patients will develop metastatic brain tumors.[1,2] This number is expected to rise as systemic disease control continues to improve.[1,2] However, despite improvement in cancer diagnosis and treatment, the median survival remains 4 months, with 2-year survival rates less than 6%.[3] The current treatment paradigm for patients with metastatic brain tumors is heavily dependent on individual patient characteristics, including age, functional status, disease control, and tumor molecular characteristics, among others.[1,2,4–6] Surgery has been shown to play an important role in certain circumstances, namely for lesions causing significant neurologic symptoms, as tumor resection remains the only effective method in providing immediate relief of mass effect.[7–9] This usually applies to large tumors (>3 cm), as well as tumors causing mass effect, neurologic deficits, and seizures.[7–9] A relative contraindication to surgery is the presence of multiple lesions, as surgery may not improve the natural history of the individual's disease, and there may be significant morbidity associated with accessing and resecting some of the lesions with little added benefit.[10] In cases with multiple brain tumors in which there is a large dominant lesion, surgical resection of the more symptomatic lesion may be warranted.[10] In this chapter, we present a case of multiple brain lesions in which some may not be surgically accessible without inherent risks.

Example case

Chief complaint: headache, imbalance, and speaking difficulties

History of present illness

A 35-year-old, right-handed woman with a history of metastatic breast cancer status post bilateral mastectomy and local radiation therapy and chemotherapy who presented with progressive headaches, imbalance, and speaking difficulties. These headaches are diffuse, bifrontal, and exacerbated with straining. She also complained of imbalance and decreased coordination with both hands but denies any focal weakness. She also complained of difficulty getting her words out. These symptoms have been going on for the past week. She saw her oncologist, and imaging was done (Fig. 35.1).

Medications: Lisinopril.

Allergies: No known drug allergies.

Past medical and surgical history: Metastatic breast adenocarcinoma status bilateral mastectomy.

Family history: Strong family of history of breast cancer.

Social history: Teacher, no smoking or alcohol history.

Physical examination: Awake, alert, oriented to person, place, and time; Language: dysarthric and slowness with speech; Cranial nerves II to XII intact; No drift, moves all extremities with full strength; Cerebellar: right > left finger-to-nose dysmetria.

Computed tomography chest/abdomen/pelvis: Two small lung nodules and one liver lesion suspicious for metastatic disease.

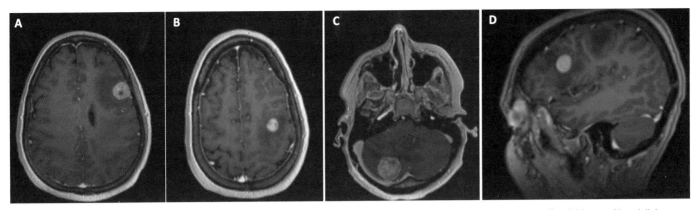

Fig. 35.1 Preoperative magnetic resonance imaging. (A) T1 axial image with gadolinium contrast through the middle frontal gyrus; **(B)** T1 axial image with gadolinium contrast through the superior frontal gyrus; **(C)** T1 axial image with gadolinium contrast through the traverse sinus; **(D)** T1 sagittal image with gadolinium contrast demonstrating three metastatic lesions involving the left middle frontal gyrus, the left precentral gyrus at the level of the hand, and the right superior cerebellar hemisphere.

	Miguel A. Arraez, MD, PhD, Carlos Haya University, Hospital Malaga, Spain	Mark Bernstein, MD, University of Toronto, Toronto, Canada	Michael Lim, MD, Stanford University School of Medicine, Stanford, CA, United States	Gabriel Zada, MD, University of Southern California, Los Angeles, CA, United States
Preoperative				
Additional tests requested	Oncology evaluation	Neuropsychological assessment fMRI		Full-body PET Physical therapy Radiation Oncology/oncology evaluation
Surgical approach selected	Right suboccipital +/– left frontal craniotomy	Right posterior fossa and left frontal craniotomies if symptoms do not respond with steroids, SRS for left paracentral lesion	Right suboccipital craniotomy and left frontal craniotomy for tumor with IOM	SRS for all three lesions
Anatomic corridor	Right cerebellar hemisphere	Right cerebellar hemisphere and left frontal	Right cerebellar hemisphere and left frontal	SRS
Goal of surgery	Gross total resection of posterior fossa lesion	Gross total resection of both lesions	Maintaining quality of life	Tumor control
Perioperative				
Positioning	Right park bench	Right park bench followed by left supine	Prone followed by left supine	Leksell frame
Surgical equipment	Surgical navigation Surgical microscope with 5-ALA Ultrasonic aspirator	Surgical navigation Surgical microscope IOM (BAERs)	IOM (SSEP)	Gamma knife
Medications	Steroids	Steroids	Steroids Mannitol Hyperventilation	Steroids
Anatomic considerations	Transverse sinus, tentorium, cerebellar surface	Cerebellar lesion: transverse sinus Frontal lesion: speech cortex	Cerebellar lesion: swelling Frontal lesion: speech cortex	Cerebellar lesion: swelling Frontal lesion: speech and motor cortex
Complications feared with approach chosen	Injury to transverse sinus and cerebellum	Neurologic worsening, language dysfunction	Language dysfunction	Language dysfunction, motor deficit

(continued on next page)

	Miguel A. Arraez, MD, PhD, Carlos Haya University, Hospital Malaga, Spain	Mark Bernstein, MD, University of Toronto, Toronto, Canada	Michael Lim, MD, Stanford University School of Medicine, Stanford, CA, United States	Gabriel Zada, MD, University of Southern California, Los Angeles, CA, United States
Intraoperative				
Anesthesia	General	General	General	Conscious sedation
Skin incision	Right paramedian	Cerebellar lesion: curvilinear Frontal lesion: linear	Cerebellar lesion: linear paramedian Frontal lesion: linear	None
Bone opening	Right suboccipital	Cerebellar lesion: right posterior fossa up to transverse sinus above foramen magnum Frontal lesion: left frontal	Cerebellar lesion: overlying lesion Frontal lesion: left MFG	None
Brain exposure	Cerebellum overlying lesion	Cerebellar lesion: right cerebellar hemisphere up to transverse sinus Frontal lesion: left MFG	Cerebellar lesion: overlying lesion Frontal lesion: left MFG	None
Method of resection	Right suboccipital craniotomy based on navigation, dural opening and reflected toward transverse sinus, microsurgical intralesional removal with ultrasonic aspirator, watertight dural closure	Cerebellar lesion first, suboccipital craniectomy with bur holes and rongeurs up to transverse sinus but maintaining foramen magnum based on navigation, dural opening based on transverse sinus, resection with microscopic visualization, dural closure with dural substitute if necessary, cranioplasty with mesh. Head refixed for left frontal lesion, craniotomy based on navigation, dural opening, microsurgical removal of tumor	Cerebellar lesion first, suboccipital craniotomy guided by navigation, cruciate dural opening, corticectomy over most superficial aspect of tumor, internal debulking of tumor, mobilize capsule, gross total resection. Head refixed, left MFG craniotomy based on navigation, cruciate dural opening, en bloc resection	None
Complication avoidance	Awareness of transverse sinus, intralesional resection	Cerebellar lesion: large opening Frontal lesion: access lesion where lesion comes to surface	Cerebellar lesion: opening confined to tumor Frontal lesion: en bloc resection	Avoidance of surgery
Postoperative				
Admission	ICU	Floor	ICU	Home
Postoperative complications feared	Cerebellar edema	Cerebellar edema, language dysfunction	CSF leak, language dysfunction	Peritumoral edema, radiation effect, language dysfunction, right-sided weakness, hydrocephalus
Follow-up testing	CT within 24 hours after surgery MRI within 72 hours after surgery	CT within 24 hours after surgery MRI prior to radiation	MRI within 48 hours after surgery	MRI 2 months after SRS
Follow-up visits	7 days after surgery	14 days after surgery	14 days after surgery	14 days after surgery
Adjuvant therapies recommended	SRS for left frontal and perirolandic lesions	SRS for all resected and nonresected lesions	SRS boost for all resected and nonresected lesions or WBRT	Chemotherapy per oncology

5-ALA, 5-aminolevulinic acid; *BAERs*, brainstem auditory evoked recordings; *CSF*, cerebrospinal fluid; *CT*, computed tomography; *fMRI*, functional magnetic resonance imaging; *ICU*, intensive care unit; *IOM*, intraoperative monitoring; *MFG*, middle frontal gyrus; *MRI*, magnetic resonance imaging; *PET*, positron emission tomography; *SRS*, stereotactic radiosurgery; *SSEP*, somatosensory evoked potential; *WBRT*, whole-brain radiation therapy.

Differential diagnosis and actual diagnosis

- Metastatic brain cancer
- Lymphoma
- Cerebral abscess
- High-grade glioma

Important anatomic and preoperative considerations

The recursive partitioning analysis classification system is the most commonly used classification system to prognosticate outcomes for patients with metastatic brain tumors (Chapter 32, Fig. 32.2).[11] The patient in this case is a recursive partitioning analysis class 2 because of the presence of extracranial systemic disease, but is young (age <65), good functioning status (Karnofsky performance score ≥70), and has primary tumor control. The patient has three metastatic brain tumors, with one right superior cerebellar hemisphere, one left middle frontal gyrus, and one precentral gyrus lesion. The patient is likely symptomatic from the right cerebellar hemisphere lesion with imbalance, and the left middle frontal gyrus lesion with speech difficulties. The patient does not appear to be symptomatic from the left precentral lesion, as the patient has full strength and no sensory abnormalities. For a full description of the cerebellar hemisphere, see Chapter 31, left frontal lobe see Chapters 5 and 6, and the perirolandic region see Chapters 3 and 4.

Approaches to this lesion

The majority of patients who develop metastatic brain tumors have multiple lesions.[12–14] For patients with a limited number of brain lesions, the options include surgical resection and/or radiation therapy in the form of stereotactic radiation or whole-brain radiation therapy (Chapter 33, Fig. 33.2).[12–15] From retrospective case–control studies, surgical resection of all lesions have similar outcomes to patients with solitary lesions.[14] However, these studies likely have a surgical bias in which patients have good functional status and prognosis, and lesions are accessible with minimal morbidity.[14] Radiation therapy can also be pursued, and most prefer stereotactic radiosurgery (SRS) because of its good local control profile with less cognitive side effects as compared with whole-brain radiation therapy.[15,16] SRS has been traditionally reserved for the treatment of smaller lesions (≤3 cm), because larger tumors have higher local recurrence rates following radiation therapy, but does not affect overall survival.[15,16] Additionally, even for patients who are considered good candidates for surgery, the local control rates following SRS is high, and the survival rates are similar between SRS and surgery patients in a study on metastatic non–small cell lung cancer.[17] SRS, however, does not provide immediate relief of mass effect or symptoms.[12–15] In this case, there are three lesions. The posterior fossa lesion has the lowest surgical morbidity profile, followed by the middle frontal gyrus, which can have aphasic complications, and then the perirolandic lesion, which can result in hemiparesis. The treatment options include SRS only, preoperative SRS followed by surgical resection, or surgical resection followed by postoperative SRS. Surgical resection can involve none, one, two, or three of the lesions. The advantages of SRS only are that it avoids potential surgical morbidity and avoids potential delay in adjuvant therapies, whereas its primary disadvantage is an immediate lack of symptomatic improvement. Preoperative SRS followed by surgical resection has the advantages of providing potential tumor control for nonresected lesions, minimizes potential delay in adjuvant therapy, potentially reduces risk of leptomeningeal disease with surgical resection, and radiation planning is better defined to minimize radiation necrosis, whereas its primary disadvantages include wound healing and increased edema until surgical resection occurs.[9,18,19] The utility of preoperative SRS, however, is not as well established as postoperative SRS.[9,15,18,19] Surgical resection followed by SRS is well established in providing local control, but requires wound healing before radiation can occur, which predisposes nonoperated lesions to increase in size and/or mass effect.[12–14]

What was actually done

The patient was admitted and underwent preoperative SRS of all three lesions. On the following day, the patient was taken to surgery for a midline suboccipital craniotomy, followed by a left frontal craniotomy for metastatic brain tumors with general anesthesia without intraoperative monitoring. The posterior fossa lesion was chosen first, as the patient was most symptomatic from this lesion. The patient was induced and intubated per routine. The head was fixed in neutral position, with two pins centered over the left external auditory meatus and one pin over the right external auditory meatus. The patient was then placed prone onto chest rolls with the neck flexed and reduced. A right paramedian incision over the center of the lesion was planned based on surgical navigation. In addition, a left Frazier burr hole site was planned in case it was needed for an external ventricular drain. The patient was draped in the usual standard fashion and given dexamethasone and cefazolin. The paramedian incision was made down to the periosteum, and the skin and muscles were retracted with a cerebellar retractor. A right suboccipital keyhole craniotomy that encompassed the lesion based on surgical navigation was made below the transverse sinus. Ultrasound was used to confirm lesion boundaries before the dura was opened to evaluate if more bone was needed to be removed. Once the opening was confirmed to be large enough, the dura was opened in a cruciate fashion. The cerebellum was lined with cottonoids to minimize tumor spillage. A corticectomy was done over the medial aspect of the right superior cerebellar hemisphere. The tumor was then removed en bloc. Preliminary pathology was adenocarcinoma. The cavity was inspected for residual and hemostasis was obtained. The dura, bone, and skin were closed in standard fashion. After this was done, the patient was then positioned for a left frontal craniotomy. The patient was placed on a horseshoe with the head turned 90 degrees to the right, and a bump was placed underneath the left shoulder to facilitate turning. The electromagnetic stereotactic navigation was used to obviate the need for pinning. A linear incision was then planned in the coronal plane over the center of the lesion based on surgical navigation. The patient was draped in the usual standard fashion and given levetiracetam and cefazolin. An incision was made, and the scalp was retracted

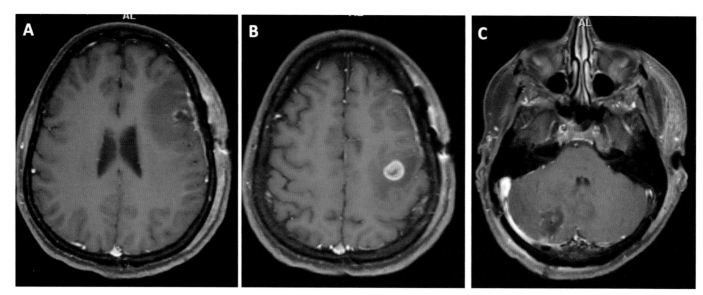

Fig. 35.2 Postoperative magnetic resonance imaging. (A) T1 axial image with gadolinium contrast through the middle frontal gyrus; **(B)** T1 axial image with gadolinium contrast through the superior frontal gyrus; **(C)** T1 axial image with gadolinium contrast through the traverse sinus, magnetic resonance imaging scans demonstrating gross total resection of the left middle frontal gyrus and right superior cerebellar hemisphere lesions, with unchanged appearance of the left precentral gyrus lesion.

with Weitlaner retractors. A keyhole craniotomy was made over the lesion. The dura was opened in a cruciate fashion and tacked up after confirming lesion localization with ultrasound and surgical navigation. Ultrasound was used to confirm the lesion, as the lesion could be seen adjacent to the pia. A small corticectomy was done, and the lesion was removed en bloc. The cavity was inspected with direct visualization, and hemostasis was obtained. The dura, bone, and skin were closed in standard fashion.

The patient awoke at their neurologic baseline with full strength bilaterally and intact speech and was taken to the intensive care unit for recovery. Magnetic resonance imaging was done within 48 hours after surgery and showed gross total resection of the right cerebellar and the left middle frontal gyrus lesions and stability of the left precentral gyrus lesion (Fig. 35.2). The patient participated with physical and occupational therapy and was discharged to home on postoperative day 2 with an intact neurologic examination. The patient was prescribed dexamethasone that was tapered to off over 10 days after surgery and levetiracetam for 3 months. The patient was seen at 2 weeks postoperatively for staple removal and remained neurologically intact with improved balance. Final pathology was consistent with breast adenocarcinoma (ER−, PR−, HER2+). The lesion was observed with serial magnetic resonance imaging examinations at 3-month intervals and has been without local or distal recurrence for 6 months. The precentral gyrus lesion decreased in size by approximately 60% at 6 months. The patient returned to work at 4 weeks postoperatively and remains without neurologic deficits with improved balance.

Commonalities among the experts

Half of the surgeons opted for the patient having oncology and/or radiation oncology evaluations prior to pursuing surgery. The majority of surgeons elected for resection of the right cerebellar lesion and likely concurrent resection of

the left frontal lesion. The goal for those surgeons pursuing surgery was gross total resection of the addressed lesions. All surgeons were concerned about the posterior fossa swelling of the cerebellar lesion, and the Broca area for the left frontal lesion. The surgeons most feared complication was language dysfunction. Surgery was generally pursued with surgical navigation and surgical microscope with perioperative steroids. Following surgery, the majority of patients were admitted to the intensive care unit (one to the floor), and most surgeons requested imaging within 72 hours after surgery to assess for extent of resection and/or potential complications. All surgeons advocated for SRS to the lesion and cavity after the surgery, as well as the remaining lesions.

SUMMARY OF QUALITY OF EVIDENCE TO GUIDE SPECIFIC INTERVENTIONS FOR THIS CASE

- Surgical resection plus radiation therapy versus radiation therapy alone for metastatic brain tumors—Class I.
- Preoperative versus postoperative stereotactic radiation therapy—Class II-2.
- Surgical resection of only symptomatic brain metastases in patients with multiple brain metastases—Class II-2.
- En bloc versus piecemeal resection of metastatic brain tumors—Class II-3.

REFERENCES

1. Eichler AF, Loeffler JS. Multidisciplinary management of brain metastases. *Oncologist.* 2007;12:884–898.
2. Ewend MG, Morris DE, Carey LA, Ladha AM, Brem S. Guidelines for the initial management of metastatic brain tumors: role of surgery, radiosurgery, and radiation therapy. *J Natl Compr Canc Netw.* 2008;6:505–513; quiz 514.
3. Lutterbach J, Bartelt S, Ostertag C. Long-term survival in patients with brain metastases. *J Cancer Res Clin Oncol.* 2002;128:417–425.

4. Barnholtz-Sloan JS, Yu C, Sloan AE, et al. A nomogram for individualized estimation of survival among patients with brain metastasis. *Neuro Oncol.* 2012;14:910–918.

5. Ewend MG, Brem S, Gilbert M, et al. Treatment of single brain metastasis with resection, intracavity carmustine polymer wafers, and radiation therapy is safe and provides excellent local control. *Clin Cancer Res.* 2007;13:3637–3641.

6. Ewend MG, Williams JA, Tabassi K, et al. Local delivery of chemotherapy and concurrent external beam radiotherapy prolongs survival in metastatic brain tumor models. *Cancer Res.* 1996;56:5217–5223.

7. Patchell RA, Tibbs PA, Regine WF, et al. Postoperative radiotherapy in the treatment of single metastases to the brain: a randomized trial. *JAMA.* 1998;280:1485–1489.

8. Patchell RA, Tibbs PA, Walsh JW, et al. A randomized trial of surgery in the treatment of single metastases to the brain. *N Engl J Med.* 1990;322:494–500.

9. Prabhu RS, Miller KR, Asher AL, et al. Preoperative stereotactic radiosurgery before planned resection of brain metastases: updated analysis of efficacy and toxicity of a novel treatment paradigm. *J Neurosurg.* 2019;131:1387–1394.

10. Chaichana KL, Acharya S, Flores M, et al. Identifying better surgical candidates among recursive partitioning analysis class 2 patients who underwent surgery for intracranial metastases. *World Neurosurg.* 2014;82:e267–e275.

11. Gaspar L, Scott C, Rotman M, et al. Recursive partitioning analysis (RPA) of prognostic factors in three Radiation Therapy Oncology Group (RTOG) brain metastases trials. *Int J Radiat Oncol Biol Phys.* 1997;37:745–751.

12. Auslands K, Apskalne D, Bicans K, Ozols R, Ozolins H. Postoperative survival in patients with multiple brain metastases. *Medicina (Kaunas).* 2012;48:281–285.

13. Baker CM, Glenn CA, Briggs RG, et al. Simultaneous resection of multiple metastatic brain tumors with multiple keyhole craniotomies. *World Neurosurg.* 2017;106:359–367.

14. Bindal RK, Sawaya R, Leavens ME, Lee JJ. Surgical treatment of multiple brain metastases. *J Neurosurg.* 1993;79:210–216.

15. Marchan EM, Peterson J, Sio TT, et al. Postoperative cavity stereotactic radiosurgery for brain metastases. *Front Oncol.* 2018;8:342.

16. Hartford AC, Paravati AJ, Spire WJ, et al. Postoperative stereotactic radiosurgery without whole-brain radiation therapy for brain metastases: potential role of preoperative tumor size. *Int J Radiat Oncol Biol Phys.* 2013;85:650–655.

17. Xu Z, Elsharkawy M, Schlesinger D, Sheehan J. Gamma knife radiosurgery for resectable brain metastasis. *World Neurosurg.* 2013;80:351–358.

18. Patel KR, Burri SH, Asher AL, et al. Comparing preoperative with postoperative stereotactic radiosurgery for resectable brain metastases: a multi-institutional analysis. *Neurosurgery.* 2016;79:279–285.

19. Routman DM, Yan E, Vora S, et al. Preoperative stereotactic radiosurgery for brain metastases. *Front Neurol.* 2018;9:959.

36

Deep-seated metastatic brain tumors

Case reviewed by Omar Arnaout, Mohamed El-Fiki, John S. Kuo, Charles Teo

Introduction

Metastatic brain cancer is the most common type of brain tumor in adults, with an estimated 200,000 new cases each year in the United States alone.[1,2] The treatment options for patients with metastatic brain cancer include some combination of surgical resection, radiation therapy, and/or chemotherapy, in which the goal is to prevent local tumor progression.[3–6] The majority of brain metastases occur at the gray-white junction, and as a result, most of these lesions are in close juxtaposition to the cortical surface.[7,8] When surgery is pursued for these typical lesions, the distance of traversed brain parenchyma is relatively short, and thus minimizes potential surgical morbidity.[3–6] However, some metastases occur in deep-seated regions, such as the thalamus, basal ganglia, and deep cerebellar nuclei.[7–10] Surgical resection of

these deep-seated lesions is more challenging because of the morbidity associated with accessing and resecting these lesions.[9,11–13] In this chapter, we present a case of a deep-seated, basal ganglia metastatic brain tumor.

Example case

Chief complaint: headache
History of present illness
A 60-year-old, right-handed man with a history of hypertension, hypercholesterolemia, lung adenocarcinoma status post right upper lung lobectomy and radiation therapy 12 months prior who presented with worsening headaches. For the prior 3 weeks, he complained of worsening headaches, especially in the morning and with activity. He denied any weakness or any speaking problems (Fig. 36.1).
Medications: Aspirin, lisinopril, atorvastatin.

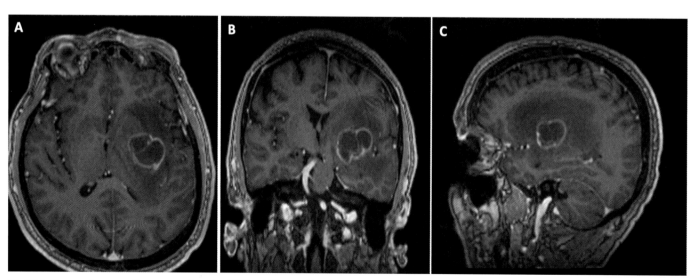

Fig. 36.1 Preoperative magnetic resonance imaging. (A) T1 axial image with gadolinium contrast; **(B)** T1 coronal image with gadolinium contrast; **(C)** T1 sagittal image with gadolinium contrast magnetic resonance imaging demonstrating a lesion involving the left basal ganglia that more specifically involves the putamen, globus pallidus, posterior limb of the internal capsule, and anterior thalamus.

Allergies: No known drug allergies.

Past medical and surgical history: Hypertension, hypercholesterolemia, lung adenocarcinoma status post right upper lung lobectomy 12 months prior.

Family history: No family of intracranial malignancies.

Social history: Military, remote smoking and no alcohol.

Physical examination: Awake, alert, oriented to person, place, and time; Language: slight dysarthria but intact naming and repetition; Cranial nerves II to XII intact; Right drift, moves all extremities with full strength.

Computed tomography chest/abdomen/pelvis: No evidence of systemic disease.

	Omar Arnaout, MD, Brigham and Women's Hospital, Boston, MA, United States	Mohamed El-Fiki, MBBCh, MS, MD, University of Alexandria, Alexandria, Egypt	John S. Kuo, MD, PhD, University of Texas at Austin, Austin, TX, United States	Charles Teo, MBBS, University of New South Wales, Sydney, Australia
Preoperative				
Additional tests requested	fMRI DTI CT chest, abdomen, pelvis	Oncology and radiation oncology evaluation MRS fMRI DTI PET	fMRI Wada (sodium amytal) test Neuropsychological assessment Radiation oncology evaluation	DTI
Surgical approach selected	Left fronto-temporal craniotomy	Left temporal awake craniotomy	Left fronto-temporal craniotomy	Left fronto-temporal craniotomy
Anatomic corridor	Left trans-Sylvian	Left trans-Sylvian	Left trans-Sylvian	Left trans-Sylvian, preservation of IFOF and CST
Goal of surgery	Diagnosis, relief of mass effect	Diagnosis, relief of mass effect	Diagnosis, relief of mass effect	GTR
Perioperative				
Positioning	Left supine with 45-degree right head rotation	Left supine with right head rotation	Left supine with right head rotation	Left supine with right head rotation
Surgical equipment	Surgical navigation IOM Ultrasound	Surgical navigation Surgical microscope Ultrasonic aspirator	Surgical navigation Surgical microscope Ultrasound	Central line Surgical navigation Surgical microscope
Medications	Steroids Antiepileptics	Steroids Mannitol, furosemide Antiepileptics	Steroids Mannitol, furosemide Antiepileptics	Steroids Antiepileptic
Anatomic considerations	Frontal opercular speech centers, SLF/AF, insula, MCA branches and lenticulostriate	Speech centers, insular branches of MCA, left putamen, PCA, striatum, anterior capsule, amygdaloid body and tail, thalamus, commissural fibers of temporal lobe, uncus, superior peduncle	Sylvian fissure, MCA branches	Sylvian fissure, MCA and branches, temporal stem, IFOF, CST
Complications feared with approach chosen	Language dysfunction, injury to MCA branches and lenticulostriate	Expressive and mixed aphasia, right hemiparesis	Language deficits	Language dysfunction, visual field deficit, memory deficits, IFOF injury
Intraoperative				
Anesthesia	General	Awake	General	General
Skin incision	Curvilinear	Linear	Curvilinear	Curvilinear behind hairline
Bone opening	Left fronto-temporal	Left fronto-temporal	Left fronto-temporal	Left fronto-temporal
Brain exposure	Left fronto-temporal	Left fronto-temporal	Left fronto-temporal	Left fronto-temporal

(continued on next page)

	Omar Arnaout, MD, Brigham and Women's Hospital, Boston, MA, United States	Mohamed El-Fiki, MBBCh, MS, MD, University of Alexandria, Alexandria, Egypt	John S. Kuo, MD, PhD, University of Texas at Austin, Austin, TX, United States	Charles Teo, MBBS, University of New South Wales, Sydney, Australia
Method of resection	Pterional craniotomy exposing Sylvian fissure, drill sphenoid ridge flat, C-shaped dural opening, wide Sylvian fissure opening under microscopic visualization, entry point determined based on ultrasound and navigation avoiding and minimizing injury to white matter tracts and normal cortex, debulk tumor internally, dissect along brain-tumor interface, avoid hemostatic absorbable material to facilitate image interpretation	Left posterior temporal craniotomy based on navigation, open dura, microscopic trans-Sylvian dissection, transinsular transcortical to access lesion with monitoring according to tractography, open pia at depth of sulcus and avoid insular vessels, ultrasonic aspirator, piecemeal resection without fixed retractors, repetitive cortical and subcortical stimulation, dural closure, subgaleal drain	Left fronto-temporal craniotomy centered on Sylvian fissure and based on navigation, ultrasound to confirm lesion, dural opening with concurrent irrigation of antibiotic-impregnated irrigation, navigation to confirm trajectory through Sylvian fissure, open Sylvian fissure under microscopic visualization, biopsy specimen, decompress cyst with needle or syringe, ultrasound to confirm resection, watertight dural closure	Meticulous positioning with surgical trajectory perpendicular to floor to minimize need for retraction at the deepest portion of the tumor, keyhole craniotomy (<2 cm) over Sylvian fissure based on navigation, GTR with awareness of IFOF and CST, watertight dural closure
Complication avoidance	Trans-Sylvian approach, insular entry based on navigation and ultrasound, debulk tumor internally	Awake brain mapping, trans-Sylvian, avoid vessels, piecemeal resection with monitoring, avoiding retractors	Ultrasound to guide trajectory and resection, decompress cyst early	Keyhole craniotomy, Sylvian fissure openings, awareness of white matter tracts medially to the lesion
Postoperative				
Admission	ICU	ICU	ICU	ICU
Postoperative complications feared	Language dysfunction, arterial or venous infarction, residual tumor	Aphasia, increased motor weakness, cognitive dysfunction	Seizure, language dysfunction, failure to extubate	Progressive motor weakness, language dysfunction, seizures
Follow-up testing	MRI within 48 hours after surgery	CT within 24 hours after surgery MRI immediately after and 3 months after surgery	MRI within 24 hours after surgery	MRI within 24 hours after surgery
Follow-up visits	7–10 days after surgery	7 days after surgery and 2 weeks after starting radiation 1 month and every 3 months after surgery	2 weeks after surgery	6–8 weeks after surgery
Adjuvant therapies recommended	Consultation with medical and radiation oncology	Chemotherapy and radiation therapy	SRS to tumor bed, evaluation by oncology for chemotherapy	No radiation for GTR, SRS for STR

AF, arcuate fasciculus; *CST*, corticospinal tract; *CT*, computed tomography; *DTI*, diffusion tensor imaging; *fMRI*, functional magnetic resonance imaging; *GTR*, gross total resection; *ICU*, intensive care unit; *IFOF*, inferior frontal occipital fasciculus; *IOM*, intraoperative monitoring; *MCA*, middle cerebral artery; *MRI*, magnetic resonance imaging; *MRS*, magnetic resonance spectroscopy; *PCA*, posterior cerebral artery; *PET*, positron emission tomography; *SLF*, superior longitudinal fasciculus; *SRS*, stereotactic radiosurgery; *STR*, subtotal resection.

Differential diagnosis and actual diagnosis

- Metastatic brain cancer
- High-grade glioma
- Lymphoma
- Cerebral abscess

Important anatomic and preoperative considerations

The recursive partitioning analysis classification system is the most commonly used classification system to prognosticate outcomes for patients with metastatic brain tumors (Chapter 32, Fig. 32.2).[14] The patient in this case is a recursive partitioning analysis class 1 because of the younger age (<65 years), good functioning status (Karnofsky performance score ≥70), primary tumor control, and absence of extracranial disease. The patient has a left basal ganglia tumor that more specifically involves the putamen, globus pallidus, posterior limb of the internal capsule, and anterior thalamus. The basal ganglia is a group of subcortical nuclei and white matter structures above the midbrain.[15] The brain structures that are typically included in the basal ganglia delineation include the striatum, pallidum, subthalamic nucleus, and substantia nigra.[15] The striatum includes the caudate nucleus, putamen, and nucleus accumbens, whereas the pallidum includes the internal, external, and ventral segments.[15] The basal ganglia is a major component of the extrapyramidal motor system that plays a role in emotion, motivation, associative, and cognitive functions, as well as motor planning in which they form major critical circuits with the thalamus, motor cortex, frontal cortex, and cingulate gyrus, among others.[15] Injury to the basal ganglia can cause various debilitating symptoms and include abulia, dystonia, and hemiparesis, among others.[15]

Approaches to this lesion

The treatment options for this lesion include radiation therapy and/or surgical resection (Chapter 33, Fig. 33.2).[16–18] The most commonly pursued radiation therapy is stereotactic radiosurgery (SRS) because of its good local control profile with less cognitive side effects as compared with whole-brain radiation therapy.[19] SRS has been traditionally reserved for the treatment of lesions in difficult-to-access locations, as well as smaller lesions (≤3 cm), because larger tumors have higher local recurrence rates following radiation therapy.[19] The disadvantage of SRS is that it does not provide immediate relief of mass effect or symptoms.[16–18] Surgical resection is typically offered for larger lesions (>3 cm), symptomatic lesions, and lesions with significant mass effect, as surgery is the only modality to provide immediate relief of symptoms, but can be associated with morbidity.[16–18] For nonbiopsy surgical resection of deep-seated lesions, the convention approach is a large craniotomy with large dural openings to accommodate bladed retractor systems.[11–13] The bladed retractor systems are needed to part the cortex and subcortical white matter superficial to the lesion, which puts the surrounding brain parenchyma at risk.[11–13] These retractor systems can cause damage by providing constant pressure and ischemia on the parenchyma, inducing sheer forces to white matter tracts during retraction and inequivalent pressures, and leaving the parenchyma unprotected between the blades.[11–13] An alternative method is the use of tubular retractors.[9–12] These retractors provide a protected corridor for accessing and resecting lesions in which they provide equivalent circumferential retraction forces.[9–12] The disadvantages of these retractors is that the corridor is small (<15 mm), which limits visualization, maneuverability, and available useable instruments.[9–12] Regardless of retractor system, these lesions can be approached via transgyral versus transsuclal.[11–13] For a full description of the transgyral versus transsulcal approach, see Chapter 32.

In terms of directionality, the lesion can be approached from an anterior, posterior, or lateral direction. An anterior approach through the Kocher point has the advantage of keeping the superior longitudinal fasciculus (SLF) and language cortices lateral and the cingulum medial, but its disadvantage is a long working corridor. The posterior approach through the superior parietal lobule has the same advantages of the anterior approach of keeping SLF and language cortices laterally and cingulum medially, but its disadvantage would be that it would involve the posterior limb of the internal capsule in addition to the long working distance. The lateral approach has the advantage of the shortest working distance; however, it incorporates several critical cortical and subcortical structures, including the SLF, arcuate fasciculus, language cortices, and insula.

What was actually done

The patient was taken for a left frontal craniotomy for resection of the left basal ganglia lesion with general anesthesia and intraoperative monitoring (motor evoked potential, somatosensory evoked potentials, and electroencephalography). The patient was induced and intubated per routine. The head was fixed in neutral position, with two pins centered over the right external auditory meatus and one pin over the left external auditory meatus. The patient's head was flexed and kept neutral. A linear incision was planned in the sagittal plane over the Kocher point based on surgical navigation. The patient was draped in the usual standard fashion and given dexamethasone, levetiracetam, and cefazolin. The incision was made, and the skin was retracted with a Weitlaner retractor. A keyhole craniotomy was made over the Kocher point in the midpupillary line. The dura was opened in a cruciate fashion and tacked up. The sulcus overlying accessing the lesion was identified and opened under exoscopic visualization. The 65-mm tubular retractor was passed under navigation and ultrasound guidance into the lesion. The lesion was then removed piecemeal until white matter was seen on all the edges. Preliminary pathology was adenocarcinoma. The retractor was then withdrawn, and hemostasis was obtained. The dura, bone, and skin were closed in standard fashion.

The patient awoke at near their neurologic baseline with slightly worsened right upper extremity strength (4/5) and was taken to the intensive care unit for recovery. Magnetic resonance imaging (MRI) was done within 48 hours after surgery and showed gross total resection (Fig. 36.2). The patient participated with physical and occupational therapy and was discharged to home on postoperative day 3 with an improved right upper extremity strength (4+/5). The patient was prescribed levetiracetam for 1 month, and dexamethasone that was tapered to off over 10 days. The patient was seen at 2 weeks postoperatively for staple removal and was neurologically intact. Pathology was lung adenocarcinoma consistent with their primary cancer. The patient underwent postoperative SRS to the cavity 2 weeks after surgery. The lesion was observed with serial MRI examinations at 3 to 6 month intervals and has been without local or distal recurrence for 15 months. The patient returned to work at 6 weeks postoperatively and remains without neurologic deficits.

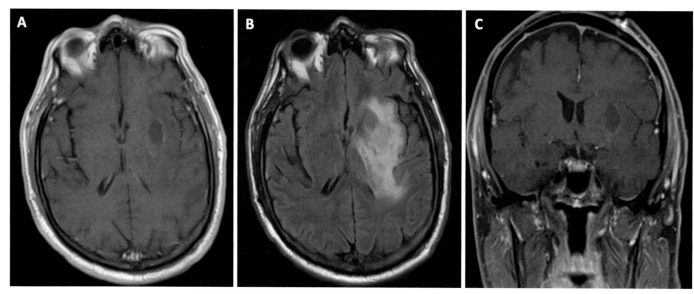

Fig. 36.2 Postoperative magnetic resonance imaging. (A) T1 axial image with gadolinium contrast; **(B)** T2 axial image fluid attenuation inversion recovery image; **(C)** T1 coronal image with gadolinium contrast demonstrating gross total resection of the left basal ganglia lesion.

Commonalities among the experts

The majority of the surgeons opted for the patient undergoing functional MRI to identify eloquent cortical regions, and diffusion tensor imaging to identify white matter tracts prior to pursuing surgery. All the surgeons elected for resection of the lesion, in which the majority performed the surgery under general anesthesia using a left fronto-temporal craniotomy through a trans-Sylvian approach. The goals for the majority of the surgeons were diagnosis and relief of mass effect. All surgeons were concerned about the language centers and the middle cerebral artery vessels and perforators. The most feared complications were language dysfunction followed by motor deficits. Surgery was generally pursued with surgical navigation, surgical microscope, and ultrasound with perioperative steroids, antiepileptics, and diuretics. Most surgeons advocated for using the trans-Sylvian approach and intralesional debulking to minimize potential iatrogenic injury. Following surgery, all patients were admitted to the intensive care unit, and all surgeons requested imaging within 48 hours after surgery to assess for extent of resection and/or potential complications. Most surgeons advocated for SRS to the lesion and cavity after the surgery regardless of extent of resection.

SUMMARY OF QUALITY OF EVIDENCE TO GUIDE SPECIFIC INTERVENTIONS FOR THIS CASE

- Surgical resection plus radiation therapy versus radiation therapy alone for metastatic brain tumors—Class I.
- En bloc versus piecemeal resection of metastatic brain tumors—Class II-3.
- Use of tubular retractors for deep-seated metastatic brain tumors—Class III.
- Postoperative stereotactic radiation therapy after metastatic tumor resection—Class I.

REFERENCES

1. Eichler AF, Loeffler JS. Multidisciplinary management of brain metastases. *Oncologist*. 2007;12:884–898.
2. Ewend MG, Morris DE, Carey LA, Ladha AM, Brem S. Guidelines for the initial management of metastatic brain tumors: role of surgery, radiosurgery, and radiation therapy. *J Natl Compr Canc Netw*. 2008;6:505–513; quiz 514.
3. Chaichana KL, Acharya S, Flores M, et al. Identifying better surgical candidates among recursive partitioning analysis class 2 patients who underwent surgery for intracranial metastases. *World Neurosurg*. 2014;82:e267–e275.
4. Chaichana KL, Gadkaree S, Rao K, et al. Patients undergoing surgery of intracranial metastases have different outcomes based on their primary pathology. *Neurol Res*. 2013;35:1059–1069.
5. Chaichana KL, Pradilla G, Huang J, Tamargo RJ. Role of inflammation (leukocyte-endothelial cell interactions) in vasospasm after subarachnoid hemorrhage. *World Neurosurg*. 2010;73:22–41.
6. Chaichana KL, Rao K, Gadkaree S, et al. Factors associated with survival and recurrence for patients undergoing surgery of cerebellar metastases. *Neurol Res*. 2014;36:13–25.
7. Carbonell WS, Ansorge O, Sibson N, Muschel R. The vascular basement membrane as "soil" in brain metastasis. *PLoS One*. 2009;4:e5857.
8. Pompili A, Carapella CM, Cattani F, et al. Metastases to the cerebellum. Results and prognostic factors in a consecutive series of 44 operated patients. *J Neurooncol*. 2008;88:331–337.
9. Bakhsheshian J, Strickland BA, Jackson C, et al. Multicenter investigation of channel-based subcortical trans-sulcal exoscopic resection of metastatic brain tumors: a retrospective case series. *Oper Neurosurg (Hagerstown)*. 2019;16:159–166.
10. Marenco-Hillembrand L, Alvarado-Estrada K, Chaichana KL. Contemporary surgical management of deep-seated metastatic brain tumors using minimally invasive approaches. *Front Oncol*. 2018;8:558.
11. Gassie K, Wijesekera O, Chaichana KL. Minimally invasive tubular retractor-assisted biopsy and resection of subcortical intra-axial gliomas and other neoplasms. *J Neurosurg Sci*. 2018;62:682–689.
12. Iyer R, Chaichana KL. Minimally invasive resection of deep-seated high-grade gliomas using tubular retractors and exoscopic visualization. *J Neurol Surg A Cent Eur Neurosurg*. 2018;79:330–336.
13. Jackson C, Gallia GL, Chaichana KL. Minimally invasive biopsies of deep-seated brain lesions using tubular retractors under exoscopic visualization. *J Neurol Surg A Cent Eur Neurosurg*. 2017;78:588–594.

14. Gaspar L, Scott C, Rotman M, et al. Recursive partitioning analysis (RPA) of prognostic factors in three Radiation Therapy Oncology Group (RTOG) brain metastases trials. *Int J Radiat Oncol Biol Phys.* 1997;37:745–751.

15. Schmitt O, Eipert P, Kettlitz R, Lessmann F, Wree A. The connectome of the basal ganglia. *Brain Struct Funct.* 2016;221:753–814.

16. Auslands K, Apskalne D, Bicans K, Ozols R, Ozolins H. Postoperative survival in patients with multiple brain metastases. *Medicina (Kaunas).* 2012;48:281–285.

17. Baker CM, Glenn CA, Briggs RG, et al. Simultaneous resection of multiple metastatic brain tumors with multiple keyhole craniotomies. *World Neurosurg.* 2017;106:359–367.

18. Bindal RK, Sawaya R, Leavens ME, Lee JJ. Surgical treatment of multiple brain metastases. *J Neurosurg.* 1993;79:210–216.

19. Hartford AC, Paravati AJ, Spire WJ, et al. Postoperative stereotactic radiosurgery without whole-brain radiation therapy for brain metastases: potential role of preoperative tumor size. *Int J Radiat Oncol Biol Phys.* 2013;85:650–655.

37

Intraventricular metastatic brain cancer

Case reviewed by Bernard R. Bendok, Devi Prasad Patra, Shlomi Constantini, Danil A. Kozyrev, Maryam Rahman, Charles Teo

Introduction

Metastatic brain cancer is the most common type of brain tumor in adults, in which 30% of cancer patients will develop brain tumors, with an estimated incidence of 200,000 new cases each year in the United States alone.[1,2] The majority of brain metastases occur at the gray-white junction, and as a result, most of these lesions are in close juxtaposition to the cortical surface.[3,4] An uncommon location is within the ventricular system, which accounts for 1% to 2% in most series.[5–7] In this chapter, we present a case of a metastatic brain tumor within the lateral ventricles.

Example case

Chief complaint: confusion
History of present illness
A 59-year-old, right-handed man with a history of renal cell cancer (RCC) status post nephrectomy and hypertension who presented with confusion. He underwent right nephrectomy followed by radiation and chemotherapy 2 years prior for RCC. His last positron emission tomography scan was 4 months prior and was negative for systemic disease. More recently, he presented with increasing confusion in which he forgot how to get home from work while driving. He saw his oncologist who ordered a magnetic resonance imaging (MRI) scan (Fig. 37.1).
Medications: Metoprolol.

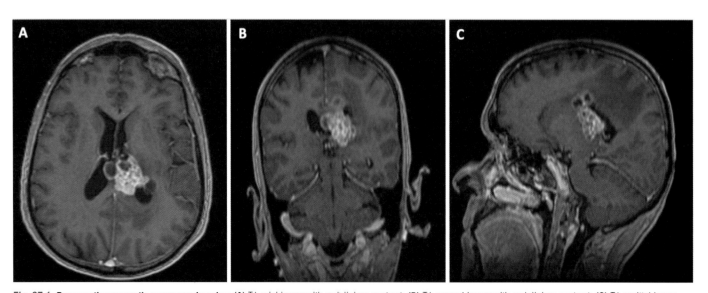

Fig. 37.1 Preoperative magnetic resonance imaging. (A) T1 axial image with gadolinium contrast; **(B)** T1 coronal image with gadolinium contrast; **(C)** T1 sagittal image with gadolinium contrast magnetic resonance imaging scan demonstrating a lesion involving the body and atrium of the left lateral ventricle.

Allergies: No known drug allergies.
Past medical and surgical history: RCC status post nephrectomy, radiation, and chemotherapy; hypertension.
Family history: No family of intracranial malignancies.
Social history: Sales executive, remote smoking and no alcohol.

Physical examination: Awake, alert, oriented to person, place, and time; Language: intact naming and repetition; Cranial nerves II to XII intact; Right drift, moves all extremities with full strength.
Computed tomography chest/abdomen/pelvis: Small lung lesions concerning for metastatic disease.

	Bernard R. Bendok, MD, Devi Prasad Patra, MD, Mayo Clinic, Scottsdale, AZ, United States	Shlomi Constantini, MD, Danil A. Kozyrev, MD, Tel Aviv Sourasky Medical Center, Tel Aviv, Israel	Maryam Rahman, MD, University of Florida, Gainesville, FL, United States	Charles Teo, MBBS, University of New South Wales, Sydney, Australia
Preoperative				
Additional tests requested	DTI fMRI Neurooncology evaluation Oncology evaluation Radiation oncology evaluation	Diffusion MRI DTI Spine MRI	None	None
Surgical approach selected	Left fronto-parietal craniotomy for tumor with EVD	Left parietal craniotomy interhemispheric approach	Left occipital-parietal craniotomy	Right frontal craniotomy
Anatomic corridor	Middle one-third interhemispheric transcallosal	Left parietal interhemispheric	Left occipital-parietal transventricular	Right interhemispheric, transcallosal
Goal of surgery	Maximal safe volume reduction	GTR	Near total resection, relief of hydrocephalus	Complete resection with preservation of fornices
Perioperative				
Positioning	Right lateral	Left supine with 45-degree rotation	Left three-quarter prone	Left lateral
Surgical equipment	Surgical navigation IOM Surgical microscope Ultrasonic aspirator	Ultrasound IOM Surgical microscope Electrified ultrasonic aspirator	Surgical navigation Surgical microscope Brain retractors	Central line Surgical navigation 30-degree rigid endoscope
Medications	Mannitol Steroids Antiepileptics	Mannitol Steroids	Mannitol Steroids Antiepileptics	Steroids Antiepileptics
Anatomic considerations	Bridging veins, pericallosal and callosomarginal ACA branches, corpus callosum, fornix, thalamus, thalamostriate veins, internal cerebral veins, choroid plexus, motor cortex	Interhemispheric fissure, cingulate gyrus, corpus callosum, pericallosal arteries	Thalamus	Superior sagittal sinus and draining veins, ACA and branches, corpus callosum, both fornices, thalamus, choroid plexus, and arteries
Complications feared with approach chosen	Cortical injury, thalamic injury , ACA injury, injury to superior sagittal sinus and/or bridging veins, intraventricular hemorrhage	Cerebral edema, venous infarct, hydrocephalus	Avoid interhemispheric veins around motor cortex	Ipsilateral approach would lead to SMA syndrome and injury to primary motor cortex, brain retraction
Intraoperative				
Anesthesia	General	General	General	General
Skin incision	Horseshoe	Linear bicoronal posterior to coronal suture	Linear	Right linear paramedian

(continued on next page)

	Bernard R. Bendok, MD, Devi Prasad Patra, MD, Mayo Clinic, Scottsdale, AZ, United States	Shlomi Constantini, MD, Danil A. Kozyrev, MD, Tel Aviv Sourasky Medical Center, Tel Aviv, Israel	Maryam Rahman, MD, University of Florida, Gainesville, FL, United States	Charles Teo, MBBS, University of New South Wales, Sydney, Australia
Bone opening	Left fronto-parietal	Left parietal	Left occipital-parietal	Right frontal
Brain exposure	Left fronto-parietal	Left parietal	Left occipital-parietal	Right frontal up to SSS
Method of resection	Lumbar drain placement, horseshoe skin flap raised with preservation of pericranium, two pairs of burr holes on both sides of sagittal sinus anteriorly and posteriorly, sinus separated and craniotomy on left side, exposed sinus covered with gelfoam, U-shaped dural opening based on sagittal sinus with preservation of bridging veins, identify falx and interhemispheric fissure, drain from EVD to facilitate openings, retract with cotton balls, identify ACA branches, divide arachnoid between pericallosal arteries and identify corpus callosum, 1- to 2-cm corpus callosotomy based on navigation, coagulate and shrink tumor because of anticipated vascularity, debulk tumor and avoid tumor spillage, dissect along cleavage plane between tumor and brain parenchyma, if good plane not evident then maximal safe debulking with avoidance of injury deep drainage veins/thalamus/fornix, copious irrigation, placement of EVD, dural closure with pericranium	Burr holes on sagittal sinus, left parietal craniotomy, administer mannitol and hyperventilation, C-shaped dural opening based on sinus, interhemispheric approach, CSF drained from cistern and drainage of tumor cyst, tumor should be identified at area of corpus callosum, mapping of tumor with electrified ultrasonic aspirator to guide resection, leave EVD for 2–3 days for CSF drainage and ICP measurement	Craniotomy over occipital-parietal area guided by navigation, dural opening, stereotactic-guided corticectomy, placement of EVD under navigation into atrium, place fixed brain retractors around EVD, resect tumor, leave EVD	Perpendicular positioning guided by stereotaxis, burr holes on SSS, right fontal craniotomy exposing SSS, identify bilateral pericallosal arteries, blunt dissection through corpus callosum left of midline using navigation, visualize tumor as it bulges into the cingulate gyrus, minimize corticectomy if possible, remove tumor totally if edges are well defined, identify choroidal artery blood supply if possible, inspection of cavity with 30-degree endoscope for residual with possible need for angled sucker-bipolar instrument, especially superolateral portion, watertight dural closure
Complication avoidance	Lumbar drain placement, interhemispheric approach, drain CSF, extent of resection based on cleavage planes, placement of EVD	Interhemispheric approach, drain CSF, electrified ultrasonic aspirator for mapping, care taken at inferolateral wall of tumor, EVD for ICP measurement and CSF drainage	EVD to guide trajectory, avoid thalamus	Anterior contralateral approach, ideal positioning, operative side down, identification of choroidal arteries, inspection with endoscope

	Bernard R. Bendok, MD, Devi Prasad Patra, MD, Mayo Clinic, Scottsdale, AZ, United States	Shlomi Constantini, MD, Danil A. Kozyrev, MD, Tel Aviv Sourasky Medical Center, Tel Aviv, Israel	Maryam Rahman, MD, University of Florida, Gainesville, FL, United States	Charles Teo, MBBS, University of New South Wales, Sydney, Australia
Postoperative				
Admission	ICU	ICU	ICU	ICU
Postoperative complications feared	Cognitive dysfunction, disconnection syndrome, thalamic edema, intraventricular hemorrhage, seizures, venous infarct	Disconnection syndrome, cognitive deficit, hydrocephalus	Visual deficit, thalamic injury, hydrocephalus	Venous hypertension, short-term memory loss, delayed intraventricular hemorrhage, seizures
Follow-up testing	CT within 24 hours after surgery MRI within 72 hours after surgery	MRI within 48 hours after surgery MRI 1 month after surgery	MRI 4 weeks after surgery prior to radiation	MRI within 24 hours after surgery
Follow-up visits	14 days after surgery	14 days after surgery	4 weeks after surgery	6–8 weeks after surgery
Adjuvant therapies recommended	Radiation therapy 3–6 weeks after surgery	Oncology board discussion	SRS to brain lesion	Observation with GTR, SRS with residual

ACA, anterior cerebral artery; *CSF*, cerebrospinal fluid; *CT*, computed tomography; *DTI*, diffusion tensor imaging; *EVD*, external ventricular drain; *fMRI*, functional magnetic resonance imaging; *GTR*, gross total resection; *ICP*, intracranial pressure; *ICU*, intensive care unit; *IOM*, intraoperative monitoring; *MRI*, magnetic resonance imaging; *SMA*, supplementary motor area; *SRS*, stereotactic radiosurgery; *SSS*, superior sagittal sinus.

Differential diagnosis and actual diagnosis

- Metastatic brain cancer
- High-grade glioma
- Meningioma
- Choroid plexus papilloma
- Ependymoma

Important anatomic and preoperative considerations

The recursive partitioning analysis classification system is the most commonly used classification system to prognosticate outcomes for patients with metastatic brain tumors (Chapter 32, Fig. 32.2).[8] The patient in this case is a recursive partitioning analysis class 2 because of the presence of likely systemic disease even though he is younger age (<65 years), has good functioning status (Karnofsky performance score ≥70), and primary tumor control. The patient has a lesion involving the left lateral ventricle within the body and atrium. Each lateral ventricle has a C-shape structure that wraps around the thalamus and has five components: frontal horn, body, atrium, occipital horn, and temporal horn.[9,10] The frontal horn lies deep to the pars triangularis and opercularis of the inferior frontal gyrus; the body lies below the inferior portion of the pre- and postcentral gyri; the atrium and occipital horn lies deep to the supramarginal and angular gyri of the parietal lobe, the posterior portion of the superior and middle temporal gyri, and the anterior part of the middle occipital gyrus; and the temporal horn is underneath the middle temporal gyrus.[9,10] Although the ventricle provides a protected corridor for surgery, the cortical and subcortical structures superficial to the ventricles have important critical functions that dictate surgical approach.[9,10] The superior longitudinal fasciculus (SLF) plays a role in the dorsal stream of language processing and, more specifically, phonetics.[9,10] SLF II connects the angular with the middle and inferior fontal gyri and is located superolateral to the frontal horn, body, and atrium; SLF III courses inferior and lateral to SLF II and connects the supramarginal and the inferior frontal gyri and is located lateral to the superior portion of the frontal horn and body.[9,10] On the medial aspect of the SLF is the arcuate fasciculus (AF), in which the superior portion is lateral to the superior portion of the frontal horn and body; central portion is lateral to the anterior part of the atrium; and the inferior portion runs lateral to the temporal horn.[9,10] The vertical occipital fasciculus plays a role in reading and facial recognition and has a close relationship with the posterior part of the AF in which it ascends obliquely to connect the inferior occipital lobe to the lateral superior occipital lobe and angular gyrus.[9,10] The inferior longitudinal fasciculus plays a role in facial recognition in which it connects the temporal pole with the dorsolateral occipital cortex and runs inferolateral to the temporal horn and atrium.[9,10] The inferior frontal occipital fasciculus plays a role in the ventral language stream with semantics in which it connects the middle and inferior frontal gyri with the temporal and occipital lobes and runs lateral to the inferior portion of the frontal horn, as well as lateral to the temporal horn and inferior portion of the atrium.[9,10]

Approaches to this lesion

The treatment options for this lesion include radiation therapy and/or surgical resection.[11–13] For a full detail of the advantages and disadvantages of each, see Chapter 33 (Fig. 33.2). The favorable characteristic for this lesion for stereotactic radiosurgery is a deep-seated location, whereas the advantages of surgical resection are tissue for diagnosis, as it is unclear if this is a brain metastasis, large tumor size (>3 cm), and immediate relief of mass effect.

In terms of directionality, the lesion can be approached from an anterior, posterior, or lateral direction. An anterior approach through the Kocher point has the advantage of keeping the SLF and language cortices lateral and the cingulum medial, but its disadvantage is a long working corridor, as the lesion is primarily in the body and atrium of the lateral ventricle. The posterior approach through the superior parietal lobule has the same advantages of the anterior approach of keeping SLF and language cortices laterally and cingulum medially, but its disadvantage would be that it can potentially damage the superior parietal lobule (coordination, reading, and Gerstmann syndrome). The lateral approach has the advantage of the shortest working distance; however, it incorporates several critical cortical and subcortical structures, including the SLF, AF, and language cortices.

Because this lesion is deep-seated, retractors would be needed to provide a corridor for visualization and resection. The options include the conventional bladed retractor systems or a tubular retractor.[14–17] The bladed retractor system consists of applying 1 to 4 retractor blades on the cortical and subcortical brain parenchyma, which can create a large corridor, with the drawbacks of potential damage to the involved parenchyma because of venous pressure from retractor pressure, shear injury to tissue from retractor forces, and potential for inadvertent injury due to tissue creep in-between the retractor blades.[16–18] An alternative method is the use of tubular retractors or channel-based resections, whereby cylindrical tubes are placed into the parenchyma, which creates a protected corridor with symmetric retraction forces, with the drawbacks of a small corridor that limits visualization, maneuverability, and available useable instruments.[14–17]

What was actually done

The patient was taken for a left parietal keyhole craniotomy for resection of the left lateral ventricular brain tumor with general anesthesia and intraoperative monitoring (motor evoked potential, somatosensory evoked potentials, and electroencephalography). The patient was induced and intubated per routine. The head was fixed in neutral position, with two pins centered over the right external auditory meatus, and one pin over the left external auditory meatus. The patient's head was flexed and kept neutral. A linear incision was planned in the coronal plane over the superior parietal lobule in the midpupillary line based on surgical navigation. The patient was draped in the usual standard fashion and given dexamethasone, levetiracetam, and cefazolin. The incision was made, and the skin was retracted with a Weitlaner retractor. A keyhole craniotomy was made over the superior parietal lobe. The dura was opened in a cruciate fashion and tacked up. The sulcus overlying accessing the atrium and posterior body of the lateral ventricle was identified and opened under exoscopic visualization. The 65-mm tubular retractor was passed under navigation into the superficial aspect of the ventricle. The lesion was then identified. It was coagulated and removed in piecemeal with a suction/cutting device (Myriad, NICO Corporation, Indianapolis, IN). The lesion was quite vascular, and therefore several rounds of coagulation with resection were done. Near the end of the resection, there was a 50% decrease in motor evoked potential and the resection was stopped. An external ventricular drain was placed through the retractor, and the retractor was withdrawn. Preliminary pathology was renal cell carcinoma. The dura, bone, and skin were closed in standard fashion.

The patient awoke with increased right-sided weakness (3/5) and dysarthria and was taken to the intensive care unit for recovery. An MRI was done within 48 hours after surgery and showed subtotal resection with residual in the vicinity of the thalamus (Fig. 37.2). The patient participated with

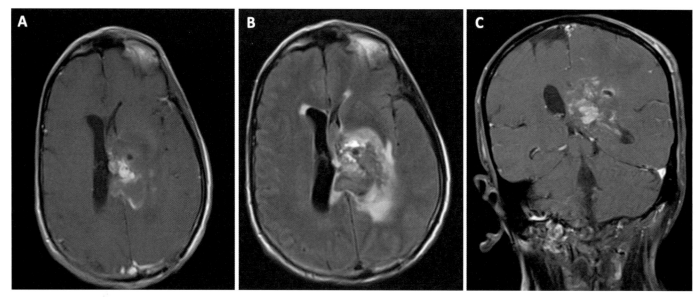

Fig. 37.2 Postoperative magnetic resonance imaging. (A) T1 axial image with gadolinium contrast; **(B)** T2 axial fluid attenuation inversion recovery image; **(C)** T1 coronal image with gadolinium contrast demonstrating subtotal resection of the lesion in the lateral ventricle, with some residual in close proximity to the thalamus with increased vasogenic edema.

physical, occupational, and speech therapy. The external ventricular drain was allowed to drain for 24 hours and then clamped and removed on postoperative day 3. The patient was discharged to inpatient rehabilitation on postoperative day 5 with improved right upper extremity strength (4/5) but persistent dysarthria. The patient was prescribed levetiracetam for 3 month and dexamethasone that was tapered to off over 14 days. The patient was seen at 2 weeks postoperatively for staple removal and remained weak in the right upper extremity (4/5) with dysarthria. Pathology was renal cell carcinoma consistent with their primary cancer. The patient underwent postoperative stereotactic radiosurgery to the cavity 3 weeks after surgery. The lesion was observed with serial MRI examinations at 3- to 6-month intervals and had been stable for 6 months. The patient, however, developed progressive systemic metastases despite chemotherapy and died 9 months after surgery.

Commonalities among the experts

Half of the surgeons opted for the patient to undergo diffusion tensor imaging to identify white matter tracts prior to pursuing surgery. All the surgeons elected for resection of the lesion, in which the majority chose an interhemispheric approach (two ipsilateral and one contralateral, two frontal and one parietal). The goals for half of the surgeons was gross total resection, and the other half was maximal safe resection. The majority of surgeons were concerned about the sagittal sinus and bridging veins, as well as the thalamus and fornices. The most feared complications varied from venous injury to thalamic injury to motor deficit. Surgery was generally pursued with surgical navigation, surgical microscope, and ultrasonic aspirator with perioperative steroids and mannitol. Most surgeons advocated for using the interhemispheric approach to minimize parenchyma transgression, as well as placement of an external ventricular drain for hydrocephalus. Following surgery, all patients were admitted to the intensive care unit, and most surgeons requested imaging within 72 hours after surgery to assess for extent of resection and/or potential complications. Most surgeons advocated for stereotactic radiosurgery to the lesion and cavity after the surgery regardless of extent of resection.

SUMMARY OF QUALITY OF EVIDENCE TO GUIDE SPECIFIC INTERVENTIONS FOR THIS CASE

- Surgical resection plus radiation therapy versus radiation therapy alone for metastatic brain tumors—Class I.
- En bloc versus piecemeal resection of metastatic brain tumors—Class II-3.
- Use of tubular retractors for deep-seated metastatic brain tumors—Class III.

- Postoperative stereotactic radiation therapy after metastatic tumor resection—Class I.

REFERENCES

1. Eichler AF, Loeffler JS. Multidisciplinary management of brain metastases. *Oncologist.* 2007;12:884–898.
2. Ewend MG, Morris DE, Carey LA, Ladha AM, Brem S. Guidelines for the initial management of metastatic brain tumors: role of surgery, radiosurgery, and radiation therapy. *J Natl Compr Canc Netw.* 2008;6:505–513; quiz 514.
3. Carbonell WS, Ansorge O, Sibson N, Muschel R. The vascular basement membrane as "soil" in brain metastasis. *PLoS One.* 2009;4:e5857.
4. Pompili A, Carapella CM, Cattani F, et al. Metastases to the cerebellum. Results and prognostic factors in a consecutive series of 44 operated patients. *J Neurooncol.* 2008;88:331–337.
5. Chaichana KL, Acharya S, Flores M, et al. Identifying better surgical candidates among recursive partitioning analysis class 2 patients who underwent surgery for intracranial metastases. *World Neurosurg.* 2014;82:e267–e275.
6. Chaichana KL, Gadkaree S, Rao K, et al. Patients undergoing surgery of intracranial metastases have different outcomes based on their primary pathology. *Neurol Res.* 2013;35:1059–1069.
7. Chaichana KL, Rao K, Gadkaree S, et al. Factors associated with survival and recurrence for patients undergoing surgery of cerebellar metastases. *Neurol Res.* 2014;36:13–25.
8. Gaspar L, Scott C, Rotman M, et al. Recursive partitioning analysis (RPA) of prognostic factors in three Radiation Therapy Oncology Group (RTOG) brain metastases trials. *Int J Radiat Oncol Biol Phys.* 1997;37:745–751.
9. Gungor A, Baydin S, Middlebrooks EH, Tanriover N, Isler C, Rhoton AL, Jr. The white matter tracts of the cerebrum in ventricular surgery and hydrocephalus. *J Neurosurg.* 2017;126:945–971.
10. Rhoton AL, Jr. The lateral and third ventricles. *Neurosurgery.* 2002;51:S207–S271.
11. Auslands K, Apskalne D, Bicans K, Ozols R, Ozolins H. Postoperative survival in patients with multiple brain metastases. *Medicina (Kaunas).* 2012;48:281–285.
12. Baker CM, Glenn CA, Briggs RG, et al. Simultaneous resection of multiple metastatic brain tumors with multiple keyhole craniotomies. *World Neurosurg.* 2017;106:359–367.
13. Bindal RK, Sawaya R, Leavens ME, Lee JJ. Surgical treatment of multiple brain metastases. *J Neurosurg.* 1993;79:210–216.
14. Bakhsheshian J, Strickland BA, Jackson C, et al. Multicenter investigation of channel-based subcortical trans-sulcal exoscopic resection of metastatic brain tumors: a retrospective case series. *Oper Neurosurg (Hagerstown).* 2019;16:159–166.
15. Marenco-Hillembrand L, Alvarado-Estrada K, Chaichana KL. Contemporary surgical management of deep-seated metastatic brain tumors using minimally invasive approaches. *Front Oncol.* 2018;8:558.
16. Gassie K, Wijesekera O, Chaichana KL. Minimally invasive tubular retractor-assisted biopsy and resection of subcortical intra-axial gliomas and other neoplasms. *J Neurosurg Sci.* 2018;62:682–689.
17. Iyer R, Chaichana KL. Minimally invasive resection of deep-seated high-grade gliomas using tubular retractors and exoscopic visualization. *J Neurol Surg A Cent Eur Neurosurg.* 2018;79:330–336.
18. Jackson C, Gallia GL, Chaichana KL. Minimally invasive biopsies of deep-seated brain lesions using tubular retractors under exoscopic visualization. *J Neurol Surg A Cent Eur Neurosurg.* 2017;78:588–594.

38

Skull base metastatic brain cancer

Case reviewed by Peter E. Fecci, Kenji Ohata, Jamie J. Van Gompel, Graeme F. Woodworth

Introduction

The most common type of brain malignancy in adults is metastatic brain tumor, in which approximately 30% of patients with primary cancers will develop brain disease.[1,2] Because of improvements in systemic therapies, there are more patients surviving with primary cancers, and thus a higher incidence of metastatic brain tumors.[1,2] This has resulted in more patients presenting with metastases in atypical cranial locations.[3–5] An uncommon location for metastases is the skull base.[5–7] These skull base metastases are challenging to manage because they are in close proximity to several critical neural and vascular structures.[5] In this chapter, we present a case of a metastatic brain tumor involving the skull base.

Example case

Chief complaint: double vision and headaches
History of present illness
A 39-year-old, right-handed woman with a history of synovial sarcoma status post right renal and adrenal resection with negative margins for synovial sarcoma 2 years prior presented with headaches and double vision. Over 2 weeks, she complained of bifrontal headaches and double vision in which her left eye was unable to move outward. She denies any visual field deficits (Fig. 38.1).
Medications: None.
Allergies: No known drug allergies.
Past medical and surgical history: Synovial sarcoma status post right nephrectomy/adrenalectomy with negative margins.

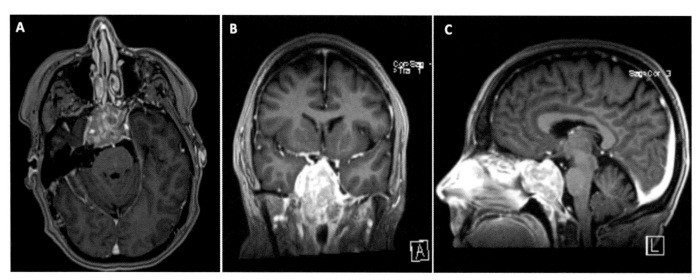

Fig. 38.1 Preoperative magnetic resonance imaging. (A) T1 axial image with gadolinium contrast; **(B)** T1 coronal image with gadolinium contrast; **(C)** T1 sagittal image with gadolinium contrast magnetic resonance imaging scan demonstrating a lesion involving sphenoid sinus, sella, and right cavernous sinus with circumferential internal carotid artery involvement.

Family history: No history of intracranial malignancies.
Social history: Homemaker, no smoking and no alcohol.
Physical examination: Awake, alert, oriented to person, place, and time; Language: intact naming and repetition; Cranial nerves

II to XII intact except cranial nerve VI palsy; No drift, moves all extremities with full strength.
Computed tomography chest/abdomen/pelvis: No evidence of systemic disease.

	Peter E. Fecci, MD, PhD, Duke University, Durham, NC, United States	Kenji Ohata, MD, PhD, Osaka City University, Osaka, Japan	Jamie J. Van Gompel, MD, Mayo Clinic, Rochester, MN, United States	Graeme F. Woodworth, MD, University of Maryland, Baltimore, MD, United States
Preoperative				
Additional tests requested	CT/CT angiography Neuroophthalmology (visual fields) Endocrinology evaluation	CT angiography CT venography Angiogram (right ICA BTO) Thin slice CT	Angiogram (right ICA BTO) PET full body	Thin slice CT Angiogram Otolaryngology evaluation for biopsy
Surgical approach selected	Endoscopic endonasal	Endoscopic endonasal	Endoscopic endonasal	Endoscopic endonasal
Anatomic corridor	Endoscopic endonasal	Endoscopic endonasal transpterygoid	Endoscopic endonasal with right transpterygoid	Endoscopic endonasal trans-sphenoidal, trans-tuberculum
Goal of surgery	Diagnosis, relief of mass effect	Maximal resection, followed by possible adjuvant therapy	Maximal resection with inability to obtain negative margins	Maximal resection with cranial nerve decompression
Perioperative				
Positioning	Supine, no pins	Supine, right 15-degree rotation	Supine	Supine
Surgical equipment	Surgical navigation Endoscope Coblator Micro Doppler	Surgical navigation Endoscope Doppler IOM (VEP)	Surgical navigation Endoscope Endoscopic clips Retractable knife Endonasal drill Specialty suctions	Lumbar drain Surgical navigation Endoscope Surgical microscope available
Medications	Steroids	None	Tranexamic acid	Steroids
Anatomic considerations	ICA and branches, optic nerves, vidian nerves, pituitary gland, diaphragma sella, cavernous sinus walls, and cranial nerves	Maxillary sinus, vidian canal, pterygoid plate, sellar floor, optic canal, paraclival ICA, cavernous sinus, pituitary gland	ICA	Sinonasal anatomy, including sphenoid sinus, planum sphenoidale, tuberculum sella, cavernous/paraclival ICA, optic nerves, other cranial nerves
Complications feared with approach chosen	ICA injury, CSF leak	ICA injury, CSF leak	ICA and basilar artery injuries	ICA injury, optic apparatus injury, pituitary injury, CSF leak
Intraoperative				
Anesthesia	General	General	General	General
Skin incision	None	None	None	None
Bone opening	Transsphenoidal	Transpterygoid, transsphenoidal	Transpterygoid, transsphenoidal	Transsphenoidal, transtubercular, transplanum

(continued on next page)

	Peter E. Fecci, MD, PhD, Duke University, Durham, NC, United States	Kenji Ohata, MD, PhD, Osaka City University, Osaka, Japan	Jamie J. Van Gompel, MD, Mayo Clinic, Rochester, MN, United States	Graeme F. Woodworth, MD, University of Maryland, Baltimore, MD, United States
Brain exposure	Pituitary gland	Pituitary gland	Pituitary gland	Pituitary gland, parasellar, anterior cranial fossa
Method of resection	Sphenoidotomy, preservation of bilateral nasoseptal flaps, micro Doppler probe and navigation to identify ICA and cavernous sinus, debulk with curettes and dissectors, maximal safe debulking; if CSF leak, abdominal fat, layered dural closure, nasoseptal flap, lumbar drain	Lateralize turbinates, harvest nasoseptal flap, complete sphenoidotomy, removal of right posteromedial wall of maxillary sinus and anteromedial portion of right pterygoid plate, ligation of SPA, follow right vidian canal, removal of tumor, removal of tuberculum sellae and medial part of optic canal, exposure and mobilization of right paraclival ICA, resect in sella, cavernous sinus, multilayer reconstruction with collagen matrix, abdominal fat, nasoseptal flap	Harvest large nasoseptal flap, right middle turbinate resection, posterior ethmoidectomies, large sphenoid antrostomy, removal of tumor, drill out involved bone, fat in clival recess, nasoseptal flap, lumbar drain if CSF leak	Lumbar drain insertion, hinarial access, bimanual dissection, posterior septectomy, expanded parasellar exposure, bimanual resection of tumor, nasal septal flap
Complication avoidance	Micro Doppler, limit to safe resection, nasoseptal flap for CSF leak	Wide exposure, mobilization of right paraclival ICA, large nasoseptal flap	Wide exposure, large nasoseptal flap	Lumbar drain insertion, wide exposure, nasoseptal flap
Postoperative				
Admission	ICU	ICU	ICU or floor depending on dural entry	ICU
Postoperative complications feared	CSF leak, ICA injury, endocrinopathy, diplopia, visual decline	Extraocular movement disorders, pituitary dysfunction	CSF leak, carotid artery injury	CSF leak, carotid artery injury, cranial neuropathy
Follow-up testing	MRI within 48 hours after surgery 1 day after surgery morning cortisol, electrolytes	CT immediately after surgery MRI within 1 week after surgery Pituitary function 1 week after surgery	MRI within 24 hours after surgery and 3 months after surgery	CT immediately after surgery
Follow-up visits	6 weeks after surgery 1 week with endocrine and ENT	1 week after surgery	2 weeks after surgery	2 and 6 weeks after surgery
Adjuvant therapies recommended	Fractionated radiotherapy	Radiation/chemotherapy	Proton beam therapy	Radiation therapy

BTO, balloon test occlusion; *CSF*, cerebrospinal fluid; *CT*, computed tomography; *ENT*, ear, nose, and throat; *ICA*, internal carotid artery; *ICU*, intensive care unit; *IOM*, intraoperative monitoring; *MRI*, magnetic resonance imaging; *PET*, positron emission tomography; *SPA*, sphenopalatine artery; *VEP*, visual evoked potential.

Differential diagnosis and actual diagnosis

- Metastatic brain cancer
- Chordoma
- Chondrosarcoma
- Pituitary adenoma
- Sinonasal malignancy

Important anatomic and preoperative considerations

The recursive partitioning analysis classification system is the most commonly used classification system to prognosticate outcomes for patients with metastatic brain tumors (Chapter 32, Fig. 32.2).[8] The patient in this case is a recursive partitioning analysis class 1 because of the presence of young age (<65 years), good functioning status (Karnofsky performance score ≥70), primary tumor control, and absence of systemic disease. The patient has a lesion involving the skull base, and more specifically the sphenoid sinus, with invasion into the sella and right cavernous sinus with circumferential involvement of the internal carotid artery. For a full discussion of sphenoid anatomy, see Chapter 56.

Approaches to this lesion

The treatment options for this lesion include radiation therapy and/or surgical resection.[9–11] For full details of the advantages and disadvantages of radiation therapy and surgical resection, see Chapter 33, Fig. 33.2. The favorable characteristics for stereotactic radiosurgery for this lesion are that the lesion is below the optic apparatus and extends into the cavernous sinus possibly precluding gross total resection, whereas the advantages of surgical resection include obtaining tissue for diagnosis, lesion has mass effect on the cavernous sinus causing a sixth nerve palsy, and symptomatic headaches. This lesion involves the sphenoid sinus with invasions in the right cavernous sinus and sella. The best access to this lesion is therefore through a transsphenoidal approach. This can be done through an endonasal or a sublabial approach, as the more conventional approach is through an endonasal route because it requires less mucosal incisions and less pain, with possibly shorter operating room times and hospital stays.[12]

What was actually done

The patient was taken for an endoscopic endonasal transsphenoidal resection of skull base tumor with the aim of debulking the lesion rather than gross total resection without intraoperative monitoring. The patient was induced and intubated per routine. The head was placed in a neutral position in a horseshoe headrest. An electromagnetic navigation system was used to avoid the need for head pinning. The left lower abdominal quadrant was prepped in case a fat graft was needed. The patient was draped in the usual standard fashion and given cefazolin. With the assistance of a rhinologist, the right middle and inferior turbinates were displaced laterally. A right nasal septal flap was raised and placed into the nasopharynx. A posterior septectomy was done to allow bilateral nasal access. The tumor was encountered in the sphenoid sinus, and the face of the sphenoid sinus was expanded with drilling. The tumor was removed until the sphenoid sinus was clear of obvious tumor using a combination of suction, ring curette, and a side-cutting tissue biting device (NICO Myriad, NICO Corporation, Indianapolis, IN). The tumor continued to be followed into the sella and right cavernous sinus. After debulking the tumor from the cavernous sinus with some venous bleeding, a Doppler was placed to confirm location of the carotid artery. The area was packed with gelfoam and irrigated. No cerebrospinal fluid leak occurred. Preliminary pathology was metastatic sarcoma. The nasoseptal flap was replaced and sewed back to the nasal septum. Doyle splints were placed bilaterally.

The patient awoke at their neurologic baseline with right sixth nerve palsy and was taken to the postoperative

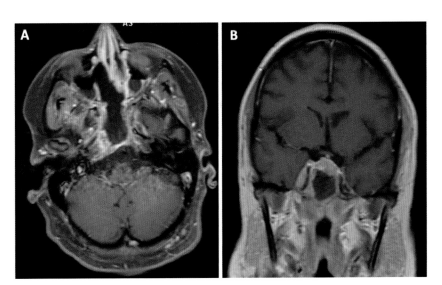

Fig. 38.2 Postoperative magnetic resonance imaging. (A) T1 axial image with gadolinium contrast; **(B)** T1 coronal image with gadolinium contrast demonstrating subtotal resection of the lesion with residual in the right cavernous sinus with circumferential involvement of the internal carotid artery.

recovery area and then a regular room. Magnetic resonance imaging was done within 24 hours after surgery and showed subtotal resection with residual in the right cavernous sinus (Fig. 38.2). The patient participated with physical therapy and was discharged to home on postoperative day 1 with 7 days of cefdinir. The patient was seen in the ear, nose, and throat clinic for Doyle splint removal on postoperative day 5. The patient was seen at 2 weeks postoperatively and had improved right cranial nerve VI function (90% abduction). Pathology was metastatic synovial sarcoma. The patient underwent postoperative stereotactic radiosurgery to the cavity 3 weeks after surgery. The lesion was observed with serial magnetic resonance imaging examinations at 3-month intervals and had been stable for 9 months.

Commonalities among the experts

The majority of the surgeons opted for the patient undergoing vascular imaging to help identify the course of the parasellar and paraclival carotid arteries prior to pursuing surgery. All the surgeons elected for resection of the lesion through an endonasal route, in which two advocated for additional transpterygoid supplementation. The goals in all surgeons was to achieve maximal resection with debulking with no intentions of negative margins. The majority of surgeons were concerned about the course of the carotid arteries, the optic apparatus, and the vidian canal. The most feared complications were carotid artery injury and cerebrospinal fluid leak. Surgery was generally pursued with surgical navigation, endoscope, and Doppler. Most surgeons advocated for using a wide skull base exposure and harvesting of a nasal septal flap to minimize potential iatrogenic injury. Following surgery, all patients were admitted to the intensive care unit, and most surgeons requested imaging within 48 hours after surgery to assess for extent of resection and/or potential complications. Most surgeons advocated for radiation therapy that varied from fractionated radiation to proton beam radiation therapy.

SUMMARY OF QUALITY OF EVIDENCE TO GUIDE SPECIFIC INTERVENTIONS FOR THIS CASE

- Surgical resection plus radiation therapy versus radiation therapy alone for metastatic brain tumors—Class I.
- Postoperative stereotactic radiation therapy after metastatic tumor resection—Class I.
- Endoscopic resection of skull base metastases—Class III.

REFERENCES

1. Eichler AF, Loeffler JS. Multidisciplinary management of brain metastases. *Oncologist*. 2007;12:884–898.
2. Ewend MG, Morris DE, Carey LA, Ladha AM, Brem S. Guidelines for the initial management of metastatic brain tumors: role of surgery, radiosurgery, and radiation therapy. *J Natl Compr Canc Netw*. 2008;6:505–513; quiz 514.
3. Claus EB. Neurosurgical management of metastases in the central nervous system. *Nat Rev Clin Oncol*. 2012;9:79–86.
4. Grossman R, Mukherjee D, Chang DC, et al. Predictors of inpatient death and complications among postoperative elderly patients with metastatic brain tumors. *Ann Surg Oncol*. 2011;18:521–528.
5. Chaichana KL, Flores M, Acharya S, et al. Survival and recurrence for patients undergoing surgery of skull base intracranial metastases. *J Neurol Surg B Skull Base*. 2013;74:228–235.
6. Barajas Jr RF, Cha S. Imaging diagnosis of brain metastasis. *Prog Neurol Surg*. 2012;25:55–73.
7. Delattre JY, Krol G, Thaler HT, Posner JB. Distribution of brain metastases. *Arch Neurol*. 1988;45:741–744.
8. Gaspar L, Scott C, Rotman M, et al. Recursive partitioning analysis (RPA) of prognostic factors in three Radiation Therapy Oncology Group (RTOG) brain metastases trials. *Int J Radiat Oncol Biol Phys*. 1997;37:745–751.
9. Auslands K, Apskalne D, Bicans K, Ozols R, Ozolins H. Postoperative survival in patients with multiple brain metastases. *Medicina (Kaunas)*. 2012;48:281–285.
10. Baker CM, Glenn CA, Briggs RG, et al. Simultaneous resection of multiple metastatic brain tumors with multiple keyhole craniotomies. *World Neurosurg*. 2017;106:359–367.
11. Bindal RK, Sawaya R, Leavens ME, Lee JJ. Surgical treatment of multiple brain metastases. *J Neurosurg*. 1993;79:210–216.
12. Cho DY, Liau WR. Comparison of endonasal endoscopic surgery and sublabial microsurgery for prolactinomas. *Surg Neurol*. 2002;58:371–375; discussion 375–376.

39

Radiation necrosis metastatic brain cancer

Case reviewed by Peter E. Fecci, Fernando Hakim, Diego Gomez, Michael Lim, Claudio Gustavo Yampolsky

Introduction

Metastatic brain cancer is the most common type of brain tumor in adults, in which 30% of cancer patients will develop brain tumors.[1,2] This rate is expected to increase as the management of metastatic brain tumors and systemic disease improves with the use of radiation therapy, surgical resection, targeted therapy, and/or immunotherapy, among others.[3–6] Because of an increase in long-term survivors, there will be an increase in the number of late toxicities, including radiation necrosis.[7–9] The risk of radiation necrosis varies between 5% and 25% in most series.[7–9] In this chapter, we present a case of a metastatic brain tumor that was treated with stereotactic radiosurgery (SRS) and had symptomatic growth with increased vasogenic edema concerning for local tumor recurrence versus radiation necrosis.

Example case

Chief complaint: double vision and headaches

History of present illness

A 69-year-old, right-handed woman with a history of non–small cell lung cancer status post right upper lobectomy and chemoradiation 3 years prior, and two metastatic brain tumors treated with SRS 8 months prior, who presented with worsening headaches over 3 weeks. These headaches were constant, associated with nausea, vomiting, and double vision. She was given high-dose steroids with minimal improvement. Imaging showed progression of both lesions, more so on the right than the left (Fig. 39.1).

Medications: None.

Allergies: No known drug allergies.

Past medical and surgical history: non–small cell lung cancer status post right upper lobectomy and chemoradiation

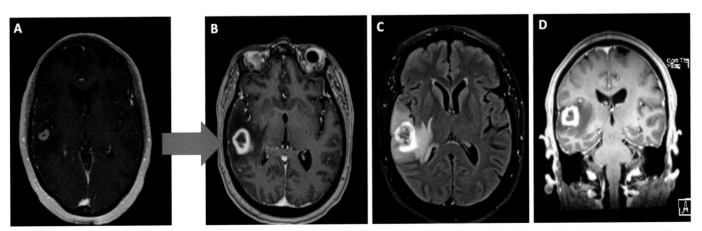

Fig. 39.1 Preoperative magnetic resonance imaging. (A) T1 axial image with gadolinium contrast (3 months prior); **(B)** T1 axial image with gadolinium contrast; **(C)** T2 axial fluid attenuation inversion recovery image; (D) T1 coronal image with gadolinium contrast magnetic resonance imaging scan demonstrating a growing lesion within the right superior temporal gyrus and left middle temporal gyrus, with increased edema following stereotactic radiosurgery.

3 years prior, two brain metastases status post SRS 8 months prior.

Family history: No history of intracranial malignancies.

Social history: Homemaker, no smoking and no alcohol.

Physical examination: Awake, alert, oriented to person, place, and time; Language: intact naming and repetition; Cranial nerves II to XII intact; No drift, moves all extremities with full strength.

Computed tomography chest/abdomen/pelvis: No evidence of systemic disease. Magnetic resonance (MR) perfusion unable to distinguish between radiation necrosis versus recurrent tumor.

	Peter E. Fecci, MD, PhD, Duke University, Durham, NC, United States	Fernando Hakim, MD, Diego Gomez, MD, Hospital Universitario Fundacion Santafe de Bogota, Bogota, Colombia	Michael Lim, MD, Stanford University School of Medicine, Stanford, CA, United States	Claudio Gustavo Yampolsky, MD, Hospital Italiano de Buenos Aires, Buenos Aires, Argentina
Preoperative				
Additional tests requested	None	MRS PET	None	MRS Neurooncology evaluation
Surgical approach selected	LITT for steroid responder, craniotomy for nonresponders	Right and left temporal craniotomies	Right craniotomy	Right fronto-temporal and left temporal craniotomies
Anatomic corridor	Right temporal	Right and left temporal	Right temporal	Right and left temporal
Goal of surgery	Diagnosis, local and symptom control	Gross total resection of both lesions	Diagnosis and decompression	Maximal safe resection without affecting function
Perioperative				
Positioning	Right supine	Right lesion: right supine with 30-degree left rotation Left lesion: left supine with 30-degree left rotation	Right supine	Right lesion: right semilateral Left lesion: right lateral
Surgical equipment	Surgical navigation Intraoperative MRI Biopsy frame LITT	Surgical navigation Ultrasonic aspirator	Surgical navigation IOM (SSEP)	Right lesion: none Left lesion: surgical navigation, surgical microscope
Medications	Steroids Antiepileptics Mannitol	Steroids Mannitol	Steroids Antiepileptics	Steroids Antiepileptics
Anatomic considerations	Vein of Labbe, temporal horn, optic radiation	Right lesion: vein of Labbe, M3 branches Left lesion: vein of Labbe	Optic radiations	Right lesion: Sylvian fissure, MCA, temporal lobe Left lesion: temporal lobe
Complications feared with approach chosen	Venous infarct, visual field cut, cerebral edema, pseudomeningocele	Right lesion: hemorrhage Left lesion: language deficit	Visual field cuts	Speech deficit, motor complications
Intraoperative				
Anesthesia	General	General	General	General
Skin incision	Linear	Right lesion: reverse question mark Left lesion: preauricular curvilinear	Linear	Right lesion: curvilinear Left lesion: linear
Bone opening	Right temporal burr hole	Right lesion: right temporal Left lesion: left temporal	Right temporal	Right lesion: right fronto-temporal Left lesion: left temporal
Brain exposure	STG	Right lesion: right temporal Left lesion: left temporal	Right temporal	Right lesion: right temporal Left lesion: left temporal

	Peter E. Fecci, MD, PhD, Duke University, Durham, NC, United States	Fernando Hakim, MD, Diego Gomez, MD, Hospital Universitario Fundacion Santafe de Bogota, Bogota, Colombia	Michael Lim, MD, Stanford University School of Medicine, Stanford, CA, United States	Claudio Gustavo Yampolsky, MD, Hospital Italiano de Buenos Aires, Buenos Aires, Argentina
Method of resection	Biopsy frame, navigation-guided biopsy, LITT bolt, insertion of laser catheter and attachment of driver, intraoperative MRI, ablation, removal of catheter and bolt	Right craniotomy first guided by navigation, U-shaped dural opening, expose STG and avoid vein of Labbe and MCA branches, corticectomy in STG, capsulotomy and internal debulking with ultrasonic aspirator, find gliotic plane to achieve gross total resection, watertight dural closure; redrape for left temporal craniotomy with navigation, U-shaped dural openings, corticectomy in MTG, same resection strategy as right lesion, watertight dural closure	Navigation-guided craniotomy, cruciate dural opening, intraoperative excisional biopsy, if biopsy consistent with treatment effect then resect lesion, if active tumor place radiation seeds	Right craniotomy first, fronto-temporal Penfield incision, temporal craniotomy, expose Sylvian fissure, have Sylvian fissure be top boundary and ITS inferior boundary, corticectomy in STG and dissect to reach tumor, en bloc removal. After 2 weeks of healing, left temporal incision, left temporal 4 x 4 cm craniotomy, cruciate dural opening, corticectomy in MTG based on navigation, supramarginal en bloc tumor removal
Complication avoidance	LITT with intraoperative MRI	Identify vasculature and avoid, internal debulking, address larger tumor first	Intraoperative biopsy, resection of lesion if radiation necrosis and tumor seeds if active tumor	Surgeries separated by 2 weeks, en bloc resection
Postoperative				
Admission	Floor	ICU	ICU	ICU
Postoperative complications feared	Field cut, venous infarct, pseudomeningocele	Cerebral edema	Field cut	Seizures, visual field deficit
Follow-up testing	MRI within 24 hours after surgery	MRI within 72 hours after surgery	MRI within 48 hours after surgery	MRI within 48 hours after surgery
Follow-up visits	14 days after surgery	7 days after surgery	14 days after surgery	7 days after surgery
Adjuvant therapies recommended	Observation	Observation, chemotherapy per oncology	Observation	Chemotherapy per oncology

LITT, laser interstitial thermal therapy; *ICU*, intensive care unit; *IOM*, intraoperative monitoring; *ITS*, inferior temporal sulcus; *MCA*, middle cerebral artery; *MRI*, magnetic resonance imaging; *MRS*, magnetic resonance spectroscopy; *MTG*, middle temporal gyrus; *PET*, positron emission tomography; *SSEP*, somatosensory evoked potential; *STG*, superior temporal gyrus.

Differential diagnosis and actual diagnosis

- Radiation necrosis
- Recurrent metastatic brain cancer
- High-grade glioma

Important anatomic and preoperative considerations

The recursive partitioning analysis classification system is the most commonly used classification system to prognosticate outcomes for patients with metastatic brain tumors (Chapter 32, Fig. 32.2).[10] The patient in this case is a recursive partitioning analysis class 2 because of her older age (>65 years), but has good functioning status (Karnofsky performance score ≥70), primary tumor control, and no systemic disease. She has bilateral lesions, with the larger lesion in the right middle superior temporal gyrus and left anterior middle temporal gyrus. For a full description of temporal lobe anatomy, see Chapters 10 and 11.

Approaches to this lesion

The ability to reliably distinguish between radiation necrosis and local tumor recurrence is limited.[7–9] Radiation necrosis in an inflammatory reaction that typically occurs 6 to 24 months after radiation therapy, in which radiographically it appears

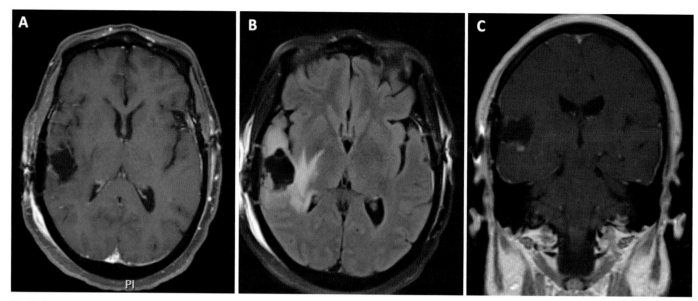

Fig. 39.2 Postoperative magnetic resonance imaging. (A) T1 axial image with gadolinium contrast; **(B)** T2 axial fluid attenuation inversion recovery image; **(C)** T1 coronal image with gadolinium contrast demonstrating gross total resection of the contrast-enhancing component of the lesion within the right superior temporal gyrus and left middle temporal gyrus.

similar to metastatic brain tumors with contrast enhancement and perilesional edema.[7–9] The risk factors for radiation necrosis include target dose and volume, previous radiation therapy, and concurrent use of systemic therapies, namely targeted therapies and immunotherapies.[7–9] The diagnosis is important because an erroneous diagnosis of recurrent tumor can lead to unnecessary open surgery or further SRS, which would worsen the radiation necrosis.[7–9] The most widely used imaging modalities for attempting to determine the differences between recurrent tumor and radiation necrosis include magnetic resonance imaging (MRI), MR perfusion (recurrent tumor has more perfusion than necrotic tissue), MR spectroscopy (increased choline:creatinine or choline:N-acetyl aspartate in tumor recurrence), and positron emission tomography-computed tomography (high amino acid uptake in tumors).[7–9] Despite these modalities, the sensitivity ranges from 80% to 95%.[7–9] It should be noted that lesions treated with SRS can have increase in lesional size 6 weeks to 15 months post-SRS before regression occurs.[7–9]

The management of radiation necrosis is dependent on the presence of symptoms.[7–9] Patients with symptomatic radiation necrosis include symptoms of mass effect (headaches, nausea, vomiting), seizures, or focal deficits depending on tumor location.[7–9] Lesions that are small or asymptomatic can be treated with observation with serial imaging, whereas symptomatic lesions can be tried on steroid therapy with serial imaging (4–8 week intervals).[7–9] Prolonged steroid therapy, however, can lead to steroid-toxicity, including myopathy, Cushing syndrome, gastric ulcers, cataracts, and others.[7–9] If patients continue to be symptomatic or cannot be weaned off of steroids, treatments include bevacizumab (humanized monoclonal antibody against vascular endothelial growth factor) that has been shown to reduce steroid doses and a radiographic response rate of 97% but often with persistent symptoms; hyperbaric oxygen therapy to promote perfusion and angiogenesis but its efficacy is controversial and is relatively expensive with significant time commitments (20–40

sessions); laser interstitial therapy that facilitates ablation of tumor and vascular endothelial growth factor–producing glial cells but its efficacy is limited and delayed; and surgical resection.[7–9] The advantages of surgical resection is that it provides immediate relief of mass effect, tissue for histological confirmation, and allows sooner weaning of steroids.[7–9] Surgical resection, however, does subject the patient to surgical risks, including neurologic deficits, infections, and wound dehiscence, among others.[7–9]

What was actually done

The patient was taken for bilateral craniotomies for the right and left temporal lesions with general anesthesia without intraoperative monitoring. Both lesions were targeted because they both had serial growth and increasing edema on serial imaging. The patient was induced and intubated per routine. The head was fixed in neutral position, with two pins centered over the inion and one pin on the forehead in the midline. The left lesion was targeted first because it was the smaller lesion and more sensitive to brain shifts. The head was turned 90 degrees to the right, and a linear incision was planned based on surgical navigation over the center of the lesion. The patient was draped in the usual standard fashion and given dexamethasone, levetiracetam, and cefazolin. The incision was made, and the skin and temporalis muscle were retracted with a Weitlaner retractor. A keyhole craniotomy was made over the left middle temporal gyrus lesion. The dura was opened in a cruciate fashion and tacked up. Ultrasound was used to confirm the lesion. A corticectomy was made over the middle temporal gyrus, the lesion was identified, and removed en bloc. Preliminary pathology was radiation necrosis. The dura, bone, and skin were closed in standard fashion. The patient was undraped, and the pins were rotated 180 degrees. The head was turned 90 degrees to the left, and a linear incision was planned based on surgical navigation over the center of the lesion. The patient was draped in the usual standard fashion and given an additional dose of cefazolin. The incision was made, and the skin and temporalis muscle were retracted with a Weitlaner retractor. A keyhole craniotomy was made over the right superior temporal gyrus lesion. The dura was opened in a cruciate fashion and tacked up. Ultrasound was used to confirm the lesion. A corticectomy was made over the superior temporal gyrus, the lesion was identified, and removed en bloc. Preliminary pathology was radiation necrosis. The dura, bone, and skin were closed in standard fashion.

The patient awoke at her neurologic baseline with full strength and was taken to the intensive care unit for recovery. An MRI was done within 48 hours after surgery and showed gross total resection of both temporal lesions (Fig. 39.2). The patient participated with physical and occupational therapy. The patient was discharged to home on postoperative day 2 with an intact neurologic examination. The patient was prescribed levetiracetam for 3 months, and dexamethasone was tapered to off over 14 days. The patient was seen at 2 weeks postoperatively for staple removal and remained neurologically intact without headaches. Pathology was radiation necrosis with no viable tumor cells. The lesion was observed with serial MRI examinations at 3- to 6-month intervals and had been stable for 18 months.

Commonalities among the experts

Half of the surgeons opted for the patient to undergo MR spectroscopy to better characterize the lesion prior to pursuing surgery. Half of the surgeons elected for resection of both lesions, one for resection of the right temporal lesion, and one for laser interstitial therapy of the right temporal lesion. The general goal was to achieve maximal safe resection. The majority of surgeons were concerned about the vein of Labbe and middle cerebral artery branches. The most feared complications were venous infarct and visual field deficits. Surgery was generally pursued with surgical navigation with perioperative steroids and antiepileptics. Most surgeons advocated for resecting the right temporal, larger lesion first before pursuing potential treatment of the contralateral lesion. Following surgery, all patients were admitted to the intensive care unit, and most surgeons requested imaging within 48 hours after surgery to assess for extent of resection and/or potential complications. Most surgeons advocated for observation of the lesion for potential recurrence.

SUMMARY OF QUALITY OF EVIDENCE TO GUIDE SPECIFIC INTERVENTIONS FOR THIS CASE

- MR perfusion for diagnosis of radiation necrosis—Class III.
- Surgical resection of radiation necrosis—Class III.

REFERENCES

1. Eichler AF, Loeffler JS. Multidisciplinary management of brain metastases. *Oncologist*. 2007;12:884–898.
2. Ewend MG, Morris DE, Carey LA, Ladha AM, Brem S. Guidelines for the initial management of metastatic brain tumors: role of surgery, radiosurgery, and radiation therapy. *J Natl Compr Canc Netw*. 2008;6:505–513; quiz 514.
3. Auslands K, Apskalne D, Bicans K, Ozols R, Ozolins H. Postoperative survival in patients with multiple brain metastases. *Medicina (Kaunas)*. 2012;48:281–285.
4. Baker CM, Glenn CA, Briggs RG, et al. Simultaneous resection of multiple metastatic brain tumors with multiple keyhole craniotomies. *World Neurosurg*. 2017;106:359–367.
5. Bindal RK, Sawaya R, Leavens ME, Lee JJ. Surgical treatment of multiple brain metastases. *J Neurosurg*. 1993;79:210–216.
6. Keohane D, Fitzgerald GP. The changing face of cancer treatments. *BMJ Case Rep*. 2018;2018:bcr-2018-224784.
7. Ahluwalia M, Barnett GH, Deng D, et al. Laser ablation after stereotactic radiosurgery: a multicenter prospective study in patients with metastatic brain tumors and radiation necrosis. *J Neurosurg*. 2018;130:804–811.
8. Detsky JS, Keith J, Conklin J, et al. Differentiating radiation necrosis from tumor progression in brain metastases treated with stereotactic radiotherapy: utility of intravoxel incoherent motion perfusion MRI and correlation with histopathology. *J Neurooncol*. 2017;134:433–441.
9. Kim JM, Miller JA, Kotecha R, et al. The risk of radiation necrosis following stereotactic radiosurgery with concurrent systemic therapies. *J Neurooncol*. 2017;133:357–368.
10. Gaspar L, Scott C, Rotman M, et al. Recursive partitioning analysis (RPA) of prognostic factors in three Radiation Therapy Oncology Group (RTOG) brain metastases trials. *Int J Radiat Oncol Biol Phys*. 1997;37:745–751.

40

Cerebellar metastatic brain cancer

Case reviewed by Omar Arnaout, Fernando Hakim, Diego Gomez, Fredric B. Meyer, Claudio Gustavo Yampolsky

Introduction

The brain is a common metastatic site for a variety of primary cancers.[1-6] The majority of metastatic brain cancers occur in the supratentorial space, but approximately 10% to 20% metastasize to the posterior fossa.[4,7,8] Cerebellar metastases, unlike most of their supratentorial counterparts, are associated with poorer survival, more distal recurrence, and higher risk of leptomeningeal disease.[4,7,8] Moreover, tumors in the posterior fossa can cause significant symptoms out of proportion to their size, in which lesions can cause obstructive hydrocephalus, brainstem compression, and herniation with acute neurologic decline faster than similar sized supratentorial lesions.[9,10] In this chapter, we present a case of a patient with a cerebellar metastasis.

Example case

Chief complaint: headaches and lethargy

History of present illness

A 78-year-old, right-handed woman with a history of hypertension presented with headaches and lethargy. Over the past 2 weeks, she complained of progressive bifrontal headaches and lethargy in which she sleeps more than she typically does. She denies any nausea or vomiting (Fig. 40.1).

Medications: Lisinopril.

Allergies: No known drug allergies.

Past medical and surgical history: Hypertension, negative breast biopsy 20 years prior.

Family history: No history of intracranial malignancies.

Social history: Retired school teacher, 30 pack per year smoking history, and occasional alcohol.

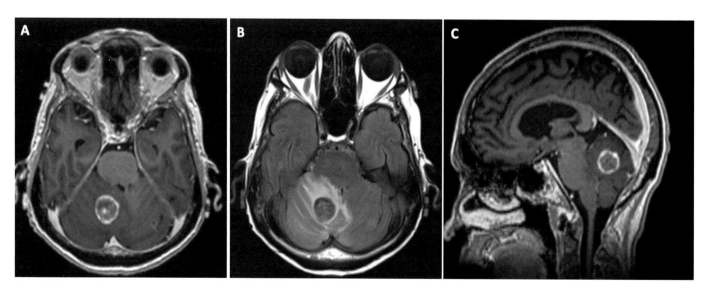

Fig. 40.1 Preoperative magnetic resonance imaging. (A) T1 axial image with gadolinium contrast; **(B)** T2 axial fluid attenuation inversion recovery image; **(C)** T1 sagittal image with gadolinium contrast magnetic resonance imaging scan demonstrating a heterogeneously enhancing lesion with peritumoral edema within the superior cerebellar hemisphere.

Physical examination: Awake, alert, oriented to person, place, and time; Cranial nerves II to XII intact; No drift, moves all extremities with full strength; Cerebellar: right > left finger-to-nose dysmetria.

Computed tomography chest/abdomen/pelvis: Enlarged mediastinal lymph nodes.

	Omar Arnaout, MD, Brigham and Women's Hospital, Boston, MA, United States	Fernando Hakim, MD, Diego Gomez, MD, Hospital Universitario Fundacion Santafe de Bogota, Bogota, Colombia	Fredric B. Meyer, MD, Mayo Clinic, Rochester, MN, United States	Claudio Gustavo Yampolsky, MD, Hospital Italiano de Buenos Aires, Buenos Aires, Argentina
Preoperative				
Additional tests requested	Chest, abdomen, pelvis CT	Oncology evaluation Thoracic surgery evaluation	Mediastinal lymph node biopsy evaluation Oncology evaluation	PET Oncology evaluation Mammogram
Surgical approach selected	Right suboccipital keyhole craniotomy	Midline suboccipital craniotomy	Midline suboccipital craniotomy	Midline suboccipital craniotomy
Anatomic corridor	Right infratentorial supracerebellar	Right transcerebellar hemisphere	Right transvermian	Right infratentorial supracerebellar
Goal of surgery	Gross total resection, relief of mass effect	Gross total resection, diagnosis, avoid obstructive hydrocephalus	Gross total resection, avoid obstructive hydrocephalus	Total resection without affecting function
Perioperative				
Positioning	Right three-quarters prone	Prone Concorde	Prone	Prone Concorde
Surgical equipment	Surgical navigation Surgical microscope	Surgical navigation Surgical microscope Ultrasonic aspirator	Surgical navigation Surgical microscope	Surgical navigation Surgical microscope
Medications	Steroids	Steroids Mannitol	Steroids	Steroids
Anatomic considerations	Transverse sinus, bridging veins, tentorium	Vermis, occipital and transverse sinuses	Torcula and transverse sinus	Transverse sinus, tentorium, cerebellum, PCA, SCA, precentral vein
Complications feared with approach chosen	Cerebellar herniation, cerebellar dysfunction, pain	Truncal ataxia with vermian injury, obstructive hydrocephalus	Injury to venous sinuses	Air embolism, retraction of cerebellar peduncles
Intraoperative				
Anesthesia	General	General	General	General
Skin incision	Paramedian linear from above sinus to above bottom of hairline	Midline linear	Midline linear from inion to C2	Midline linear from inion to C2
Bone opening	Right suboccipital	Right suboccipital over lesion	Midline suboccipital	Midline suboccipital
Brain exposure	Right cerebellar hemisphere	Right cerebellar hemisphere over lesion	Right cerebellar hemisphere over lesion	Bilateral cerebellar hemispheres

(continued on next page)

	Omar Arnaout, MD, Brigham and Women's Hospital, Boston, MA, United States	Fernando Hakim, MD, Diego Gomez, MD, Hospital Universitario Fundacion Santafe de Bogota, Bogota, Colombia	Fredric B. Meyer, MD, Mayo Clinic, Rochester, MN, United States	Claudio Gustavo Yampolsky, MD, Hospital Italiano de Buenos Aires, Buenos Aires, Argentina
Method of resection	Linear incision, subperiosteal dissection, acorn drill bit to make suboccipital craniectomy with inferior aspect of transverse sinus exposed, V-shaped dural opening based on transverse sinus, gentle retraction on superior cerebellar surface to allow egress of CSF, sacrifice small bridging veins along superior cerebellar surface, microsurgical dissection until quadrigeminal cistern reached, allow more egress of CSF to avoid retraction, corticectomy along superior cerebellar surface until tumor identified, perilesional dissection with central debulking if necessary, inspect for residual tumor, watertight dural closure, cranioplasty with bone cement	Midline muscle dissection, right suboccipital craniotomy below transverse sinus based on navigation, Y-shaped dural opening, coagulate cerebellar surface, navigation-guided white matter dissection, dissect and remove lesion en bloc until gliotic plane seen, occipital burr hole and ETV if edema seen, watertight dural closure	Midline muscle dissection, craniotomy up to torcula and transverse sinus on side of tumor, dura opened in Y-shaped pattern, drain CSF from cisterna magna to provide relaxation, work along top of vermis to identify entry point, 1-cm vertical incision, tumor entered and debulked, infold the capsule, inspect for retained capsule, watertight dural closure	Linear incision, suboccipital craniotomy exposing inferior border of transverse sinus and 4 cm to the right and 2 cm to the left, V-shaped dural opening based on transverse sinus, expose cisterna magna, open cisterna magna and release CSF to allow cerebellar relaxation, create working space between tentorium and superior cerebellar surface with minimal retraction, minimal corticectomy over tumor, gross total en bloc and supramarginal resection of tumor
Complication avoidance	Open cisterns to allow brain relaxation, avoid retraction, perilesional dissection	Craniotomy over tumor below sinus, en bloc resection, ETV if edema seen	Large craniotomy up to sinuses, dissect above vermis, small opening, internal debulking	Drain CSF from cisterna magna, small corticectomy, en bloc resection
Postoperative				
Admission	ICU	ICU	ICU	ICU
Postoperative complications feared	Cerebral edema, venous infarction, venous sinus thrombosis, stroke, hydrocephalus, CSF leak	Cerebral edema, hydrocephalus	Wound healing	CSF leak, swelling, nausea, vomiting, ataxia, headaches, nystagmus
Follow-up testing	MRI within 48 hours after surgery	CT within 72 hours after surgery	MRI within 24 hours after surgery	MRI within 48 hours after surgery
Follow-up visits	7–10 days after surgery	7 days after surgery	6 weeks after surgery with neurosurgery 2 weeks after surgery with oncology and radiation oncology	7 days after surgery with oncology and radiation oncology
Adjuvant therapies recommended	Consultation with oncology and radiation oncology	SRS to tumor cavity Chemotherapy per oncology	Radiation per radiation oncology	Radiation per radiation oncology Chemotherapy per oncology

CT, computed tomography; CSF, cerebrospinal fluid; ETV, endoscopic third ventriculostomy; ICU, intensive care unit; MRI, magnetic resonance imaging; PCA, posterior cerebral artery; PET, positron emission tomography; SCA, superior cerebellar artery; SRS, stereotactic radiosurgery.

Differential diagnosis and actual diagnosis

- Metastatic brain cancer
- Lymphoma
- High-grade glioma
- Cerebral abscess

Important anatomic and preoperative considerations

The recursive partitioning analysis classification system is the most commonly used classification system to prognosticate outcomes for patients with metastatic brain tumors (Chapter 32, Fig. 32.2).[11] The patient in this case is a recursive partitioning analysis class 2 because of good functioning status (Karnofsky performance score ≥70), despite having systemic disease and older age (>65 years). The primary lesion is unknown but assumed to be a metastatic brain tumor. The patient has a solitary lesion in the right superior cerebellar hemisphere.

For a full discussion of cerebellar anatomy, see Chapter 31. This lesion lies in the white matter of right cerebellar hemisphere, which houses the deep cerebellar nuclei (dentate, emboliform, globose, and fastigii).[12] Injury to this area can cause appendicular ataxia.[12]

Approaches to this lesion

To access lesions within the white matter of the cerebellar hemisphere, the cerebellar cortex and white matter must be transgressed. The conventional approach is to perform a large suboccipital craniotomy or craniectomy with large dural opening to allow the placement of bladed retractors. These retractors will allow visualization and access for resecting these deep-seated lesions by parting the superficial cortex and white matter.[13] The disadvantage of this larger approach is that it may increase the risk of complications, including pseudomeningocele, cerebrospinal fluid leak, blood loss, and pain.[13] The retractors themselves can induce tissue ischemia with parenchymal pressure, shearing of white matter tracts with inequivalent retraction forces, and areas that lack protection between the retractor blades.[13] An alternative to this approach is the use of tubular retactors.[14–17] The tubular retractors are placed through the brain parenchyma thus displacing the tissue.[14–17] It provides a protected corridor for accessing and resecting the lesion and provides circumferential equivalent retraction of the surrounding tissue to minimize shear forces.[14–17] However, the corridor is limited, and thus visualization can be challenging, as well as maneuverability for adequate access, resection, and hemostasis.[14–17]

What was actually done

The patient first underwent a lymph node biopsy that was consistent with non–small cell lung cancer. The patient was taken to surgery for a right suboccipital craniectomy for transcerebellar approach for brain tumor with general anesthesia without intraoperative monitoring. The patient was induced and intubated per routine. The head was fixed in neutral position, with two pins centered over the left external auditory meatus and one pin over the right external auditory meatus.

The patient was then placed prone onto chest rolls with the neck flexed and reduced. A right paramedian incision was planned based on surgical navigation. The patient was draped in the usual standard fashion and given dexamethasone and cefazolin. The right paramedian incision was made, and the skin and muscles were retracted with a Weitlaner retractor. A burr hole was made with a high-speed perforating drill and expanded with a cutting drill. The dura was opened in a cruciate fashion and tacked up. The pia was cauterized in line with the folia. The 50-mm tubular retractor was placed under navigation guidance superficially into the lesion. At intermittent intervals, an ultrasound probe was used to confirm trajectory prior to docking on the tumor. Once the retractor was docked on the lesion, the obturator was removed and the exoscope was brought in for visualization. The tumor was debulked internally, making sure that the retractor was locked onto the tumor to prevent tumor cell spread. The edges were then mobilized and then removed after internal debulking. The retractor was withdrawn once white matter was seen on all the edges. The dura was closed in standard fashion, and a burr hole cover was used to cover the 1.5-cm opening. The skin was closed in standard fashion.

The patient awoke at their neurologic baseline with full strength bilaterally and was taken to the intensive care unit for recovery. Magnetic resonance imaging was done within 48 hours after surgery and showed gross total resection (Fig. 40.2). The patient participated with physical and occupational therapy and was discharged to home on postoperative day 3 with an intact neurologic examination without dysmetria. The patient was prescribed dexamethasone that was tapered to off over 7 days after surgery. The patient was seen at 2 weeks postoperatively for suture removal and remained neurologically intact. Pathology was consistent with lung adenocarcinoma. The patient underwent postoperative stereotactic radiosurgery 2 weeks after surgery. The lesion was observed with serial magnetic resonance imaging examinations at 3 months, followed by 6-month intervals, and has been without local or distal recurrence for 18 months.

Commonalities among the experts

The majority of the surgeons opted for the patient to undergo oncology evaluation for prognostic information and systemic imaging to assess for disease burden. All surgeons elected for surgery of the cerebellar lesion, with the majority using a midline suboccipital craniotomy. Half of the surgeons chose a supracerebellar infratentorial approach, whereas the others chose a transvermian or transhemispheric approach. The general goal was gross total resection of the lesion to avoid obstructive hydrocephalus. The majority of surgeons were concerned about the venous sinuses, and the most feared complications were cerebellar damage, venous infract, and/or air emboli. Surgery was generally pursued with surgical navigation and a surgical microscope with perioperative steroids. Most surgeons advocated for drainage of cerebrospinal fluid early to decompress the brain, en bloc resection of the lesion, and limiting the corticectomy. Following surgery, all patients were admitted to the intensive care unit, and most surgeons requested imaging within 72 hours after surgery to assess for extent of resection and/or potential complications. Most surgeons advocated for radiation oncology evaluation for need of radiation therapy after surgery.

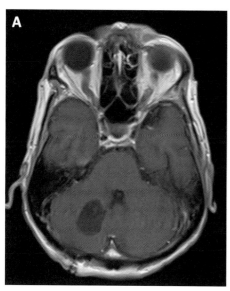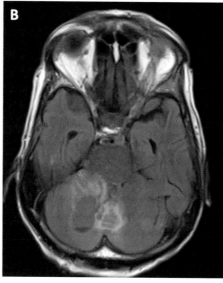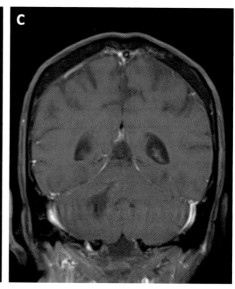

Fig. 40.2 Postoperative magnetic resonance imaging. (A) T1 axial image with gadolinium contrast; **(B)** T2 fluid attenuation inversion recovery axial image; **(C)** T1 coronal image with gadolinium contrast magnetic resonance imaging scan demonstrating gross total resection of the cerebellar hemisphere tumor.

SUMMARY OF QUALITY OF EVIDENCE TO GUIDE SPECIFIC INTERVENTIONS FOR THIS CASE

- Surgical resection plus radiation therapy versus radiation therapy alone for metastatic brain tumors—Class I.
- En bloc versus piecemeal resection of metastatic brain tumors—Class II-3.
- Use of tubular retractors for deep-seated metastatic brain tumors—Class III.
- Postoperative stereotactic radiation therapy after metastatic tumor resection—Class I.

REFERENCES

1. Chaichana KL, Acharya S, Flores M, et al. Identifying better surgical candidates among recursive partitioning analysis class 2 patients who underwent surgery for intracranial metastases. *World Neurosurg.* 2014;82:e267–e275.
2. Chaichana KL, Flores M, Acharya S, et al. Survival and recurrence for patients undergoing surgery of skull base intracranial metastases. *J Neurol Surg B Skull Base.* 2013;74:228–235.
3. Chaichana KL, Gadkaree S, Rao K, et al. Patients undergoing surgery of intracranial metastases have different outcomes based on their primary pathology. *Neurol Res.* 2013;35:1059–1069.
4. Chaichana KL, Rao K, Gadkaree S, et al. Factors associated with survival and recurrence for patients undergoing surgery of cerebellar metastases. *Neurol Res.* 2014;36:13–25.
5. Marchan EM, Peterson J, Sio TT, et al. Postoperative cavity stereotactic radiosurgery for brain metastases. *Front Oncol.* 2018;8:342.
6. Routman DM, Yan E, Vora S, et al. Preoperative stereotactic radiosurgery for brain metastases. *Front Neurol.* 2018;9:959.
7. Bender ET, Tome WA. Distribution of brain metastases: implications for non-uniform dose prescriptions. *Br J Radiol.* 2011;84:649–658.
8. Ghia A, Tome WA, Thomas S, et al. Distribution of brain metastases in relation to the hippocampus: implications for neurocognitive functional preservation. *Int J Radiat Oncol Biol Phys.* 2007;68:971–977.
9. Delattre JY, Krol G, Thaler HT, Posner JB. Distribution of brain metastases. *Arch Neurol.* 1988;45:741–744.
10. Yawn BP, Wollan PC, Schroeder C, Gazzuola L, Mehta M. Temporal and gender-related trends in brain metastases from lung and breast cancer. *Minn Med.* 2003;86:32–37.
11. Gaspar L, Scott C, Rotman M, et al. Recursive partitioning analysis (RPA) of prognostic factors in three Radiation Therapy Oncology Group (RTOG) brain metastases trials. *Int J Radiat Oncol Biol Phys.* 1997;37:745–751.
12. Ribas EC. Yagmurlu K, de Oliveira E, Ribas GC, Rhoton A Jr. Microsurgical anatomy of the central core of the brain. *J Neurosurg.* 2018;129:752–769.
13. Chaichana KL, Vivas-Buitrago T, Jackson C, et al. The radiographic effects of surgical approach and use of retractors on the brain after anterior cranial fossa meningioma resection. *World Neurosurg.* 2018;112:e505–e513.
14. Bakhsheshian J, Strickland BA, Jackson C, et al. Multicenter investigation of channel-based subcortical trans-sulcal exoscopic resection of metastatic brain tumors: a retrospective case series. *Oper Neurosurg (Hagerstown).* 2019;16:159–166.
15. Gassie K, Wijesekera O, Chaichana KL. Minimally invasive tubular retractor-assisted biopsy and resection of subcortical intra-axial gliomas and other neoplasms. *J Neurosurg Sci.* 2018;62:682–689.
16. Iyer R, Chaichana KL. Minimally invasive resection of deep-seated high-grade gliomas using tubular retractors and exoscopic visualization. *J Neurol Surg A Cent Eur Neurosurg.* 2018;79:330–336.
17. Jackson C, Gallia GL, Chaichana KL. Minimally invasive biopsies of deep-seated brain lesions using tubular retractors under exoscopic visualization. *J Neurol Surg A Cent Eur Neurosurg.* 2017;78:588–594.

41

Olfactory groove meningioma

Case reviewed by Francesco DiMeco, Massimiliano Del Bene, Ricardo J. Komotar, Daniel M. Prevedello, Hirofumi Nakatomi

Introduction

The most common tumors along the anterior skull base are meningiomas.[1] Among midline anterior skull base tumors, the most common locations in order of frequency are the olfactory groove, planum sphenoidale, and tuberculum sellae.[1] Olfactory groove meningiomas account for 5% to 15% of intracranial meningiomas, and typically arise from arachnoid cells of the cribriform plate of the ethmoid bone or the frontoethmoidal suture.[1] These lesions often frequently invade the bone and generate an osteoblastic resection.[1] In this chapter, we present a case of a patient with an olfactory groove meningioma.

Example case

Chief complaint: malodorous sensations with decreased smell
History of present illness
A 50-year-old, right-handed woman with a history of hypertension presented with malodorous sensations with decreased smell. For the past several years, she has noted decreased smells with intermittent periods in which she sensed malodorous sensations. She was seen by an ear, nose, and throat doctor who recommended imaging. A brain lesion was seen, and this was followed with a follow-up imaging that showed progressive growth and edema over 6 months (Fig. 41.1). She was referred for evaluation and management.

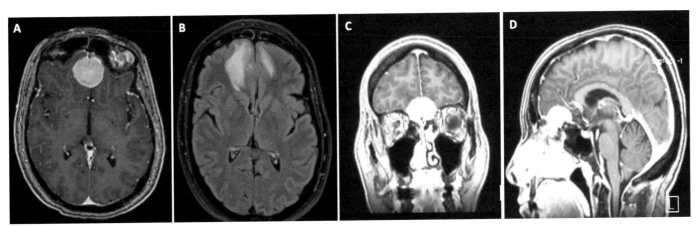

Fig. 41.1 Preoperative magnetic resonance imaging. (A) T1 axial image with gadolinium contrast; **(B)** T2 axial fluid attenuation inversion recovery image; **(C)** T1 coronal image with gadolinium contrast; **(D)** T1 sagittal image with gadolinium contrast magnetic resonance imaging scan demonstrating an enhancing lesion with peritumoral edema involving the olfactory groove.

Medications: Lisinopril.
Allergies: No known drug allergies.
Past medical and surgical history: Hypertension.
Family history: No history of intracranial malignancies.
Social history: Business owner, no smoking or alcohol.

Physical examination: Awake, alert, oriented to person, place, and time; Cranial nerves II to XII intact; No drift, moves all extremities with full strength; Absence of smell to camphor and alcohol.

	Francesco DiMeco, MD, Massimiliano Del Bene, MD, Carlo Besta Neurological Institute, Milan, Italy	Ricardo J. Komotar, MD, University of Miami, Miami, FL, United States	Daniel M. Prevedello, MD, Ohio State University, Columbus, OH, United States	Hirofumi Nakatomi, MD, PhD, University of Tokyo, Tokyo, Japan
Preoperative				
Additional tests requested	Head CT to evaluate bony involvement and lesion density/calcifications	Head CT to evaluate frontal sinuses	CT angiography University of Pennsylvania smell test Neuropsychological assessment	Cerebral angiogram ENT evaluation for possible biopsy DWI for sinusitis Alinamin test for smell detection Neuropsychological assessment
Surgical approach selected	Right fronto-temporal craniotomy	Right transpalpebral supraorbital craniotomy	Endoscope endonasal transcribriform	Bifrontal craniotomy
Anatomic corridor	Right subfrontal	Right subfrontal	Transcribriform	Basal interhemispheric/subfrontal
Goal of surgery	Near total resection with residual in ethmoid, Simpson grade 4	Gross total resection, Simpson grade I	Gross total resection, Simpson grade I	Near total resection, Simpson grade 2, SRS of nasal component
Perioperative				
Positioning	Right supine with 30-degree left rotation	Right supine slight left rotation	Supine, right head turn and left tilt in pins	Supine neutral
Surgical equipment	Surgical navigation Chisel Surgical microscope Ultrasound Ultrasonic aspiration	Surgical navigation Surgical microscope Ultrasonic aspirator	Surgical navigation Ultrasonic aspirator Tissue cutting device Endoscopes	Lumbar drain Surgical navigation IOM (VEP, SSEP) Surgical microscope Ultrasonic aspirator Weck and AVM clips Microanastamosis set
Medications	Mannitol Steroids Antiepileptics	Mannitol Steroids	Mannitol Steroids Antiepileptics	Steroids Antiepileptics
Anatomic considerations	Orbital roof, frontal sinus, inferior frontal gyrus, orbital gyrus, gyrus rectus, ACA and branches, olfactory groove, falx, basal cisterns	ACA, optic nerves, frontal sinus	ACA/ICA, optic nerves, orbits, frontal lobes	Olfactory nerves, ACA and branches
Complications feared with approach chosen	CSF leak, rhinorrhea	CSF leak, frontal sinus violation	Brain retraction, tumor recurrence	Olfactory nerve and ACA injury
Intraoperative				
Anesthesia	General	General	General	General
Skin incision	Right fronto-temporal curvilinear	Right eyebrow	None	Bicoronal

	Francesco DiMeco, MD, Massimiliano Del Bene, MD, Carlo Besta Neurological Institute, Milan, Italy	Ricardo J. Komotar, MD, University of Miami, Miami, FL, United States	Daniel M. Prevedello, MD, Ohio State University, Columbus, OH, United States	Hirofumi Nakatomi, MD, PhD, University of Tokyo, Tokyo, Japan
Bone opening	Right frontal	Supraorbital, lateral to frontal sinus	Bilateral middle turbinectomies/ anterior and posterior ethmoidectomies, sella/tuberculum/ planum/bilateral fovea ethmoidalis, crista galli and cribriform	Bifrontal
Brain exposure	Right frontal pole, temporal lobe, sylvian fissure	Right frontal pole	Anterior cranial fossa	Bilateral frontal
Method of resection	Right fronto-temporal craniotomy eccentric to the frontal side avoiding frontal sinus and paralleling orbital roof, craniotomy without burr hole, drill down lesser sphenoid wing, S-shaped dural opening with first limb paralleling orbit, as well as paralleling middle fossa floor, open basal cisterns, frontal lobe retraction with fixed brain retractor, interrupt blood supply from dural attachment, intralesional debulking, dissection of dome from pia, identification and preservation of olfactory nerves, leave ethmoidal portion alone to prevent CSF leak, skull base reconstruction with dural substitutes and autologous material if needed (pericranium, fat), watertight dural closure	Incision over right eyebrow, right supraorbital craniotomy lateral to the sinus based on navigation, dural opening, microscopic visualization and opening of opticocarotid cistern to allow brain relaxation, devascularize tumor from skull base, debulk tumor, dissect margins, remove dural and bone origin as needed, dural replacement, watertight dural closure	Bilateral middle turbinectomies/ anterior and posterior ethmoidectomies, right nasal flap raised and kept in lateral aspect of sinonasal cavity, Draf III frontal sinus, removal of sella/tuberculum/ planum/bilateral fovea ethmoidalis, removal of hyperostotic bone, ligation and severing of anterior and posterior ethmoidal arteries, removal of crista galli and cribriform plate, dura opened, falx cut anteriorly, tumor debulked, extracapsular dissection is performed and separated from ACAs and optic nerves, reconstruction with dural substitute/fat graft/nasoseptal flap	Lumbar drain, right thigh muscle fascial preparation, bicoronal incision with preservation of pericranium, bifrontal craniotomy with drilling of crista galli, W-shaped low dural opening, devascularize tumor at skull base along olfactory groove dura to planum sphenoidale until prechiasmatic cistern identified, debulk tumor in all four quadrants, after enough debulking then capsule dissection from frontal lobes, identify pial and dural feeders, microanastamosis if vascular injury encountered, repair dura with pericranium and thigh fascia, subgaleal drain
Complication avoidance	Navigation to stay lateral to frontal sinus, early devascularization, internal debulking, leaving ethmoidal content alone	Navigation to stay lateral to frontal sinus, internally debulk	Large bony opening, coagulation of dura and ethmoidal arteries, internal debulking before extracapsular dissection	IOM, devascularizing tumor early, debulking prior to capsule manipulation
Postoperative				
Admission	Floor	ICU	ICU	ICU
Postoperative complications feared	CSF leak, rhinorrhea	CSF leak, pseudomeningocele	CSF leak, seizures	Loss of smell, CSF leak, seizures, neurocognitive decline
Follow-up testing	CT within 24 hours after surgery MRI 3 months after surgery	MRI within 24 hours after surgery	Head CT immediately after surgery MRI within 24 hours after surgery	MRI/MRA/MRV within 72 hours after surgery

(continued on next page)

	Francesco DiMeco, MD, Massimiliano Del Bene, MD, Carlo Besta Neurological Institute, Milan, Italy	Ricardo J. Komotar, MD, University of Miami, Miami, FL, United States	Daniel M. Prevedello, MD, Ohio State University, Columbus, OH, United States	Hirofumi Nakatomi, MD, PhD, University of Tokyo, Tokyo, Japan
Follow-up visits	3 months after surgery	14 days after surgery	7 days after surgery with ENT	1 month after surgery
Adjuvant therapies recommended for WHO grade	Grade I–observation, radiation with recurrence Grade II–radiation Grade III–radiation	Grade I–observation Grade II–radiation Grade III–radiation/ chemotherapy	Grade I–observation Grade II–observation Grade III–radiation	Grade I–observation Grade II–SRS Grade III–radiation

ACA, anterior cerebral artery; *AVM,* arteriovenous malformation; *CSF,* cerebrospinal fluid; *CT,* computed tomography; *DWI,* diffusion-weighted imaging; *ENT,* ear, nose, and throat; *ICA,* internal carotid artery; *ICU,* intensive care unit; *IOM,* intraoperative monitoring; *MRA,* magnetic resonance angiography; *MRI,* magnetic resonance imaging; *MRV,* magnetic resonance venography; *SRS,* stereotactic radiosurgery; *SSEP,* somatosensory evoked potential; *VEP,* visual evoked potential.

Differential diagnosis and actual diagnosis

- Meningioma
- Hemangiopericytoma
- Esthesioneuroblastoma
- Metastatic brain cancer

Important anatomic and preoperative considerations

For anterior cranial fossa meningiomas, the distinction between olfactory groove, planum sphenoidale, and tuberculum sellae meningiomas is important because it dictates potential approaches, as well as potential risk of morbidity of adjacent structures.[1-3] Olfactory groove meningiomas arise from the cribriform plate anterior to the frontosphenoidal suture, planum sphenoidale meningiomas arise posterior to the frontosphenoidal suture and anterior to the chiasmatic sulcus, and tuberculum sellae meningiomas arise posterior to the chiasmatic sulcus.[1-3] Because of these anatomic distinctions, the symptomatology for each of these lesions is relatively unique.[1-3] Planum sphenoidale and tuberculum sellae meningiomas typically present earlier because of visual impairment, whereas olfactory groove meningiomas present later with more subacute symptoms, including anosmia, behavioral changes, and/or seizures.[1-3] Olfactory groove meningiomas typically derive their blood supply from the anterior and posterior ethmoidal arteries, which have connections with the ophthalmic artery and are therefore not frequently embolized.[1-3]

Approaches to this lesion

There are a variety of different approaches to olfactory groove meningiomas (Fig. 41.2).[1-4] These can be divided into cranial and endonasal approaches.[1-4] Cranial approaches can be unilateral and bilateral, in which the unilateral approaches include frontotemporal (pterional) and orbitolateral (supraorbital, modified orbitozygomatic, orbitozygomatic) craniotomies, whereas the bilateral approaches include bifrontal and bifrontal with orbital osteotomy (fronto-orbito-basal approach) craniotomies.[1-4] The

advantages of a unilateral cranial approach are that it minimizes potential bifrontal injury and allows an opportunity to avoid accessing the frontal sinus, whereas the disadvantages are difficulty identifying structures on the contralateral side of the tumor and longer working distance.[1-4] The bilateral approach has the shortest working distance and best visualization of the approaches; however, its disadvantages include potential for bifrontal injury and are usually associated with frontal sinus violations.[1-4] An alternative to cranial approaches are endoscopic endonasal transethmoidal and transsphenoidal approaches.[4,5] The advantages of these approaches are that they are easiest to achieve Simpson grade I resections by removing involved dura and bone (Table 41.1), minimizes frontal lobe manipulation, and addresses tumor blood supply early.[4-6] The disadvantages of the endonasal approach are need for and difficulty with skull base reconstruction, high risk of cerebrospinal fluid leak (approximately 25% in most series), increased rate of anosmia, and difficulty in tumor/blood vessel/neural manipulation.[4,5,7,8]

What was actually done

The patient was taken to surgery for an endoscopic endonasal transethmoidal and transsphenoidal resection of an olfactory groove meningioma, with right fascia lata graft, and lumbar drain placement under general anesthesia without intraoperative monitoring. The patient was induced and intubated per routine. The patient was set in the park bench position for placement of a lumbar drain at the L5-S1 interspace and remained clamped throughout the procedure. The patient was placed supine with the head in a horseshoe. The electromagnetic navigation was used to avoid the need for head fixation. The patient was draped in the usual standard fashion and given dexamethasone, levetiracetam, and cefazolin. A right fascia lata graft was obtained. Otolaryngology performed the approach by lateralizing the inferior turbinates bilaterally and removing the right middle turbinate. A maxillary antrostomy was done on the right side followed by anterior and posterior ethmoidectomies. A right nasoseptal flap was harvested and placed into the nasopharynx. The sphenoid sinus was entered, and the intersinus septations were removed. A posterior septectomy was done to allow bilateral naral

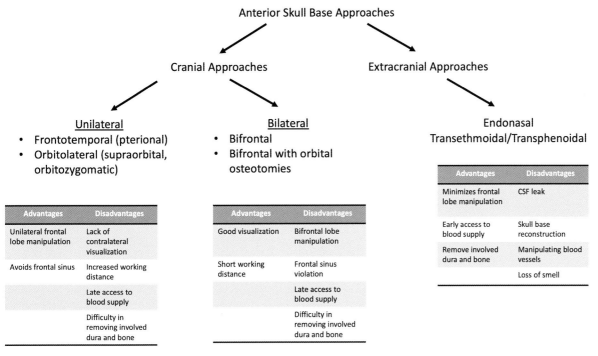

Fig. 41.2 Advantages and disadvantages for the different anterior skull base approaches. *CSF,* cerebrospinal fluid.

access. Using a three-handed technique with bilateral naral access, ethmoidal arteries were identified and coagulated. The hyperostotic bone of the cribriform plate was drilled with a high-speed coarse diamond drill to expose the dura of the anterior cranial fossa. The dura was cauterized further to minimize tumor blood supply. The dura was opened with an 11-blade knife, and the tumor was debulked internally with a combination of ultrasonic aspiration and a tissue-cutting device (NICO Myriad, NICO Corporation, Indianapolis, IN). Once the tumor was sufficiently debulked, the capsule was dissected from the surrounding parenchyma and removed. Preliminary pathology was a

meningioma. The brain was lined with Surgicel Fibrillar (Johnson & Johnson, New Brunswick, NJ) and gelfoam. The dura was reconstituted with a dural substitute in the subdural plane, followed by an absorbable plate and fascia lata in the epidural plane. The nasoseptal flap was mobilized to the anterior cranial fossa and bolstered with Merocel nasal packs (Medtronic Inc., Minneapolis, MN, USA).

The patient awoke at their neurologic baseline with full strength bilaterally and was taken to the intensive care unit for recovery. The lumbar drain was emptied at 5 to 10 cc per hour for 3 days and then removed. Magnetic resonance imaging was done within 48 hours after surgery and showed gross total resection with Simpson grade I resection (Fig. 41.3). The patient participated with physical and occupational therapy and was discharged to home on postoperative day 4 with an intact neurologic examination, except for expected anosmia. The patient was prescribed dexamethasone that was tapered to off over 5 days after surgery and levetiracetam for 3 months. The patient was seen at 2 weeks postoperatively and remained neurologically intact. Pathology was a World Health Organization (WHO) grade I meningioma. The lesion was observed with serial magnetic resonance imaging examinations at 3- and 6-month intervals and has been without recurrence for 12 months.

Commonalities among the experts

Half of the surgeons opted for the patient to undergo a head computed tomography scan to evaluate the extent of the frontal sinuses, a smell test to evaluate for anosmia, and neuropsychological evaluation to obtain baseline neurocognitive functioning prior to surgery. All surgeons elected for surgery of this lesion, in which the majority elected for a craniotomy (two unilateral subfrontal and one bifrontal)

Simpson Grade	Surgical Resection Characteristics	Symptomatic Percent Recurrence at 10 years
I	Complete removal, including resection of underlying bone and associated dura	9%
II	Complete removal and coagulation of dural attachment	19%
III	Complete removal without resection of dura or coagulation	29%
IV	Subtotal resection	44%
V	Simple decompression or biopsy	100%

Table 41.1 Simpson grade criteria used to assess extent of resection and risk of symptomatic recurrence

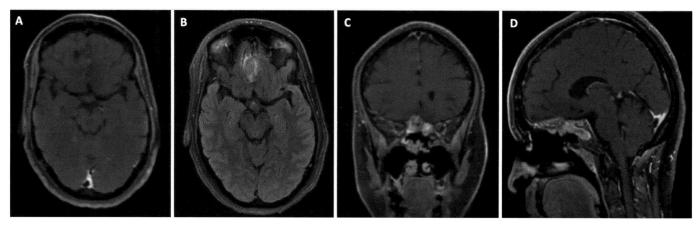

Fig. 41.3 Postoperative 3-month magnetic resonance imaging. (A) T1 axial image with gadolinium contrast; **(B)** T2 axial fluid attenuation inversion recovery image; **(C)** T1 coronal image with gadolinium contrast; **(D)** T1 sagittal image with gadolinium contrast magnetic resonance imaging scan demonstrating gross total resection of the olfactory groove meningioma.

of this lesion. Half of the surgeons also aimed for a Simpson grade I resection. The majority of surgeons were concerned about the extent of the frontal sinuses, the olfactory nerves, the anterior cerebral arteries, and their branches. The most feared complication by half of the surgeons was a cerebrospinal fluid leak. Surgery was generally pursued with surgical navigation, surgical microscope, and ultrasonic aspirator with perioperative steroids, antiepileptics, and mannitol. Most surgeons advocated for early coagulation of dural feeders, internal debulking before capsular manipulation, and avoiding the frontal sinus for unilateral approaches. Following surgery, most patients were admitted to the intensive care unit (one to the floor), and most surgeons requested imaging within 72 hours after surgery to assess for extent of resection and/or potential complications. Most surgeons advocated for observation for residual WHO grade I meningiomas, radiation for residual WHO grade II meningiomas, and radiation for all WHO grade III meningiomas regardless of extent of resection.

SUMMARY OF QUALITY OF EVIDENCE TO GUIDE SPECIFIC INTERVENTIONS FOR THIS CASE

- Endoscopic versus transcranial resection of anterior cranial fossa meningioma—Class II-2.
- Removal of involved dura and bone for meningiomas—Class II-3.

REFERENCES

1. Pallini R, Fernandez E, Lauretti L, et al. Olfactory groove meningioma: report of 99 cases surgically treated at the Catholic University School of Medicine. *World Neurosurg.* 2015;83:219–231. e1–e3.
2. Chaichana KL, Jackson C, Patel A, et al. Predictors of visual outcome following surgical resection of medial sphenoid wing meningiomas. *J Neurol Surg B Skull Base.* 2012;73:321–326.
3. Chaichana KL, Vivas-Buitrago T, Jackson C, et al. The radiographic effects of surgical approach and use of retractors on the brain after anterior cranial fossa meningioma resection. *World Neurosurg.* 2018;112:e505–e513.
4. Bander ED, Singh H, Ogilvie CB, et al. Endoscopic endonasal versus transcranial approach to tuberculum sellae and planum sphenoidale meningiomas in a similar cohort of patients. *J Neurosurg.* 2018;128:40–48.
5. Banu MA, Mehta A, Ottenhausen M, et al. Endoscope-assisted endonasal versus supraorbital keyhole resection of olfactory groove meningiomas: comparison and combination of 2 minimally invasive approaches. *J Neurosurg.* 2016;124:605–620.
6. Ehresman JS, Garzon-Muvdi T, Rogers D, et al. The relevance of Simpson grade resections in modern neurosurgical treatment of World Health Organization grade I, II, and III meningiomas. *World Neurosurg.* 2018;109:e588–e593.
7. de Divitiis E, Esposito F, Cappabianca P, Cavallo LM, de Divitiis O, Esposito I. Endoscopic transnasal resection of anterior cranial fossa meningiomas. *Neurosurg Focus.* 2008;25:E8.
8. Shetty SR, Ruiz-Trevino AS, Omay SB, et al. Limitations of the endonasal endoscopic approach in treating olfactory groove meningiomas. A systematic review. *Acta Neurochir (Wien).* 2017;159:1875–1885.

42

Planum meningioma

Case reviewed by Henry Brem, Basant K. Misra, Rodrigo Ramos-Zúñiga, Theodore H. Schwartz

Introduction

Anterior skull base meningiomas include olfactory groove, planum sphenoidale, and tuberculum sellae meningiomas.[1] Planum sphenoidale meningiomas account for 5% to 10% of intracranial meningiomas, and typically arise from arachnoid cells between the frontosphenoidal suture and the chiasmatic sulcus.[1] These lesions often invade the bone and generate an osteoblastic resection, as well as displace critical neurovascular structures, including the optic nerve and chiasm, as well as anterior cerebral artery vessels.[1] In this chapter, we present a case of a patient with planum sphenoidale meningioma.

Example case

Chief complaint: headaches
History of present illness
A 57-year-old, right-handed woman with a history of diabetes, hypertension, and hypercholesterolemia presented with

recurrent headaches. She has baseline headaches, but over the past 2 to 3 months complained of worsening bifrontal headaches that worsened with activity and improved with pain medication and rest. She denied any vision problems, loss of smell, nausea, or vomiting. Her primary care physician ordered brain imaging and referred her for evaluation and management (Fig. 42.1).

Medications: Irbesartan, metformin, lovastatin.
Allergies: No known drug allergies.
Past medical and surgical history: Diabetes, hypertension, hypercholesterolemia; cholecystectomy, appendectomy, tonsillectomy.
Family history: No history of intracranial malignancies.
Social history: Business owner, no smoking or alcohol.
Physical examination: Awake, alert, oriented to person, place, and time; Cranial nerves II to XII intact; No drift, moves all extremities with full strength.

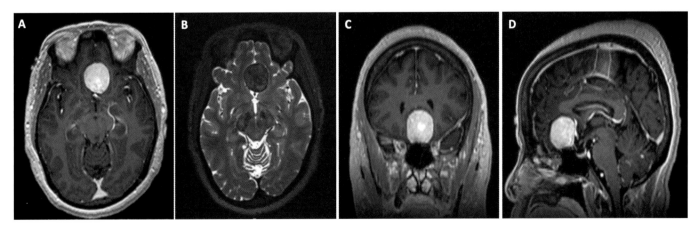

Fig. 42.1 Preoperative magnetic resonance imaging. (A) T1 axial image with gadolinium contrast; **(B)** T2 axial image; **(C)** T1 coronal image with gadolinium contrast; (D) T1 sagittal image with gadolinium contrast magnetic resonance imaging scan demonstrating an enhancing lesion involving the planum sphenoidale.

	Henry Brem, MD, Johns Hopkins University, Baltimore, MD, United States	Basant K. Misra, MBBS, MS, Hinduja National Hospital, V.S. Marg, Mahim, Mumbia, India	Rodrigo Ramos-Zúñiga, MD, PhD, University of Guadalajara, Guadalajara, Jalisco, Mexico	Theodore H. Schwartz, MD, Cornell University, New York, NY, United States
Preoperative				
Additional tests requested	MR angiography	Head CT Neuropsychological assessment Neuroophthalmology (visual fields) Pituitary hormone evaluation	MR angiography Neuroophthalmology (visual fields) Endocrinology evaluation	Head CT Smell test with ENT Neuroophthalmology evaluation with visual fields
Surgical approach selected	Bifrontal bicoronal craniotomy	Right frontotemporal craniotomy	Right supraorbital	Right supraorbital
Anatomic corridor	Left subfrontal	Right lateral subfrontal	Right supraorbital	Right supraorbital
Goal of surgery	Simpson grade I	Simpson grade I	Simpson grade I	Simpson grade I
Perioperative				
Positioning	Supine neutral	Spine with 30-degree left rotation	Supine neutral	Right supine with 30-degree left rotation
Surgical equipment	Surgical navigation IOM (MEP/SSEP/EEG) Surgical microscope Ultrasonic aspirator	Surgical microscope Ultrasonic aspirator	Surgical microscope Ultrasonic aspirator	Surgical microscope Endoscope
Medications	Mannitol Steroids Antiepileptics	Steroids Antiepileptics	Steroids	Mannitol Steroids Antiepileptics
Anatomic considerations	Frontal sinus, olfactory nerves, ACA, ICA, optic nerves and chiasm, infundibulum, anterior clinoid	Olfactory nerves, ACA, optic nerves	Frontal sinus, frontal lobe, olfactory nerves, ACOM/A1/A2 and perforators	Frontal sinus, supraorbital nerve, olfactory nerves, ACOM, optic chiasm, A2
Complications feared with approach chosen	Frontal sinusitis, anosmia, visual field deficit, stroke, CSF leak	Bilateral frontal lone injury, venous injury, anosmia	Anosmia, vision loss	Anosmia, CSF leak, vision loss, stroke
Intraoperative				
Anesthesia	General	General	General	General
Skin incision	Bicoronal	Right pterional	Eyebrow, ciliary edge	Eyebrow
Bone opening	Bifrontal craniotomy above frontal sinus	Right frontotemporal	Right supraorbital	Right supraorbital
Brain exposure	Left frontal lobe	Right frontal-temporal lobes	Right frontal lobe	Right frontal lobe

	Henry Brem, MD, Johns Hopkins University, Baltimore, MD, United States	Basant K. Misra, MBBS, MS, Hinduja National Hospital, V.S. Marg, Mahim, Mumbia, India	Rodrigo Ramos-Zúñiga, MD, PhD, University of Guadalajara, Guadalajara, Jalisco, Mexico	Theodore H. Schwartz, MD, Cornell University, New York, NY, United States
Method of resection	Bicoronal craniotomy above frontal sinus, dural opening on left, left subfrontal approach. Internal debulking of tumor on left then bilaterally, dissect capsule free from olfactory and optic nerves with preservation of ACA branches, decompress optic nerves and ICA, watertight dural closure, bone flap rinsed in Betadine	Frontotemporal incision, frontotemporal scalp flap, frontotemporal craniotomy with 3-cm subfrontal extension, semicircular dural opening based anteriorly, release CSF from Sylvian fissure, coagulation of tumor dural attachment, piecemeal excision, dissection of tumor from surrounding brain, watertight dural closure, reinforce suture line with galea and fibrin glue, placement of a subgaleal drain	Ciliary incision, supraorbital craniotomy lateral to frontal sinus, dural opening, drain cisterns under microscopic visualization, intratumoral decompression and biopsy, microvascular disconnection, capsular resection, resection and coagulation of cranial base, watertight dural closure	Ciliary incision from beyond superior temporal line to lateral edge of supraorbital notch, expose keyhole and zygoma, dissect periorbita, one piece craniotomy with removal of orbital rim, drill down skull base, open dura, open cisterns with microscopic visualization, minimize retractor use, devascularize tumor from skull base, decompress tumor, dissect from olfactory nerves/frontal lobe/optic chiasm/A2, endoscope and removal of any residual along cribriform, cement for bony defects
Complication avoidance	Craniotomy above frontal sinus, unilateral approach	Relax CSF from Sylvian fissure, coagulate tumor dural attachment	Tumor debulking, capsular disconnection	CT to evaluate sinuses, removal of orbital rim, limit use of retractor, decompress CSF early, debulk tumor before dissecting from critical structures
Postoperative				
Admission	ICU	ICU	Floor	Intermediate care
Postoperative complications feared	Anosmia, visual field deficit, motor weakness	Seizures, anosmia, venous infarct, contusion, CSF leak	Visual decline, olfactory deterioration, psychomotor agitation, CSF leak	CSF leak, anosmia, stroke
Follow-up testing	MRI within 24 hours after surgery	CT with contrast within 24 hours after surgery Hormonal assay Visual field evaluation MRI 3 months after surgery	CT immediately after surgery MRI within 48 hours after surgery	MRI within 48 hours after surgery
Follow-up visits	14 days after surgery 3 months, every 6 months after surgery	8 days after surgery	1 month after surgery	5 days after surgery 3 months after surgery with MRI
Adjuvant therapies recommended for WHO grade	Grade I–observation Grade II–observation and re-resect and radiate if recurs Grade III–radiation	Grade I–observation, repeat resection for recurrence Grade II–radiation if residual Grade III–radiation	Grade I–observation Grade II–observation Grade III–radiation	Grade I–observation Grade II–radiation if not Simpson grade I resection Grade III–radiation

ACA, anterior cerebral artery; *ACOM*, anterior communicating artery; *CSF*, cerebrospinal fluid; *CT*, computed tomography; *EEG*, electroencephalogram; *ENT*, ear, nose, and throat; *ICA*, internal carotid artery; *ICU*, intensive care unit; *IOM*, intraoperative monitoring; *MEP*; motor evoked potential; *MR*, magnetic resonance; *MRI*, magnetic resonance imaging; *SSEP*, somatosensory evoked potential.

Differential diagnosis and actual diagnosis

- Meningioma
- Hemangiopericytoma
- Metastatic brain cancer
- Lymphoma

Important anatomic and preoperative considerations

Anterior cranial fossa meningiomas include olfactory groove, planum sphenoidale, and tuberculum sellae meningiomas.[1–3] Although these tumors are in the same general location, it is important to distinguish between them prior to surgery, as their origin will dictate the location of adjacent structures and may dictate approach.[1–3] Olfactory groove meningiomas arise from the cribriform plate anterior to the frontosphenoidal suture, planum sphenoidale meningiomas arise posterior to the frontosphenoidal suture and anterior to the chiasmatic sulcus, and tuberculum sellae meningiomas arise posterior to the chiasmatic sulcus or limbus sphenoidale.[1–3] Because of these anatomic distinctions, the symptomatology for each of these lesions is relatively unique.[1–3] Planum sphenoidale and tuberculum sellae meningiomas typically present earlier because of visual impairment, whereas olfactory groove meningiomas present later with more subacute symptoms, including anosmia, behavioral changes, and/or seizures.[1–3] Planum sphenoidal meningiomas arise anterior to the optic chiasm, and therefore displace the chiasm posteriorly and often inferiorly.[1–3] Tuberculum sellae meningiomas rise posterior to the chiasmatic sulcus, and therefore displace the optic chiasm posteriorly and often superiorly.[1–3]

Approaches to this lesion

There are a variety of different approaches to planum sphenoidale meningiomas (Chapter 41, Fig. 41.2).[1–4] As with other anterior cranial fossa meningiomas, these approaches can be done through cranial and endonasal routes.[1–4] The cranial approaches can be unilateral and bilateral. The unilateral approaches include frontotemporal (pterional) and orbitolateral (supraorbital, modified orbitozygomatic, orbitozygomatic), whereas the bilateral approaches include bifrontal with or without orbital osteotomies (fronto-orbito-basal approach).[1–4] The advantages and disadvantages of these approaches are summarized in Chapter 41, Fig. 41.2. Unilateral approaches avoid bifrontal manipulation and can be placed laterally to avoid breaching the frontal sinus. In addition, the unilateral approaches can be supplemented with removal of the orbital roof to decrease potential brain retraction with increased superior-inferior visualization.[5] The disadvantages of the unilateral approach include increased working distance and potential difficulty with visualization, especially on the contralateral side of the tumor. The bilateral approach has the shortest working distance and best visualization of the approaches; however, its disadvantages include potential for bifrontal injury and are usually associated with frontal sinus violations.[1–4] As with the unilateral approach, it can be supplemented with orbital osteotomies to minimize brain retraction and to increase superior-inferior visualization.[5] Endonasal approaches are alternatives to cranial approaches.[4,6] The advantages of these approaches are that they avoid brain manipulation, address the blood supply to the tumor early, and provide the best means of removing involved dura and bone for improved Simpson grade resection (Chapter 41, Fig. 41.3); however, skull base reconstruction can be challenging and associated with cerebrospinal fluid leaks, increased risk of anosmia, and difficulty in tumor/blood vessel/neural manipulation.[4,6–9]

What was actually done

The patient was taken to surgery for a right modified orbitozygomatic craniotomy for resection of a planum sphenoidale meningioma with intraoperative somatosensory evoked potentials and electroencephalogram. The patient was induced and intubated per routine. The head was fixed in pins, with two pins centered on the inion, and one pin over the left forehead in the midpupillary line. The head was extended and turned 30 degrees to the right. A pterional incision was planned from the root of the zygoma to the vertex. The patient was draped in the usual standard fashion and given dexamethasone, levetiracetam, and cefazolin. The pterional incision was made making sure to stay above the temporalis fascia. After the fat pad was encountered, the temporalis fascia was incised, and a subfascial dissection was done to expose the orbital rim and frontal-zygomatic process and protecting the frontalis nerve. The temporalis muscle was then dissected anteriorly in the subperiosteal plane, and the flap was held in place with fishhooks attached to a retractor arm. A pterional flap was made that stayed lateral to the frontal sinus based on surgical navigation. The periorbita was dissected from the orbital rim, and the inferior orbital fissure was identified. An ultrasonic bone cutter was used to make cuts at the level of the frontozygomatic suture laterally, and lateral to the supraorbital nerve medially. These cuts were carried as posteriorly over the orbital roof as possible. The dura was then opened in a semicircular fashion and tacked up with sutures. The microscope was brought in for visualization. The frontal lobe was dissected off of the anterior cranial fossa, where the olfactory nerve was followed to the optic nerve. The brain was protected with cottonoids, and dynamic retraction was used with the sucker. The tumor was cauterized from the skull base to eliminate its blood supply. The tumor was debulked internally with an ultrasonic aspirator, and the edges of the tumor were mobilized inward until removed. Preliminary pathology was a meningioma. The dura, bone, and skin were closed in standard fashion with a subgaleal drain.

The patient awoke at their neurologic baseline with full strength bilaterally and intact vision and was taken to the intensive care unit for recovery. Magnetic resonance imaging was done within 48 hours after surgery and showed gross total resection with Simpson grade II resection, in which the anterior cranial fossa dura was cauterized but left in place (Fig. 42.2). The patient participated with physical and occupational therapy and was discharged to home on postoperative day 2 with an intact neurologic examination after subgaleal drain removal. The patient was prescribed dexamethasone that was tapered to off over 5 days after surgery, and levetiracetam for 7 days. The patient was seen at 2 weeks postoperatively for staple removal and remained neurologically intact. Pathology was a World Health Organization (WHO) grade

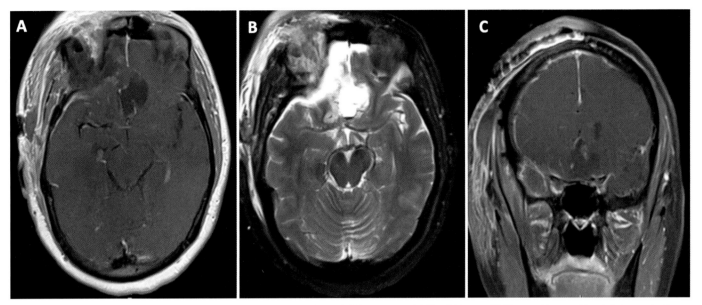

Fig. 42.2 Postoperative magnetic resonance imaging. (A) T1 axial image with gadolinium contrast; **(B)** T2 axial image; **(C)** T1 coronal image with gadolinium contrast magnetic resonance imaging scan demonstrating gross total resection of the planum sphenoidale meningioma.

I meningioma. The lesion was observed with serial magnetic resonance imaging examinations at 3- and 6-month intervals and has been without recurrence for 24 months.

Commonalities among the experts

The majority of the surgeons opted for the patient to undergo formal visual field evaluation, half-head computed tomography scan to evaluate tumor density and frontal sinus location, and half vascular imaging to better characterize vascular anatomy prior to surgery. All surgeons elected for craniotomy of this lesion, in which the majority elected for unilateral approach (two supraorbital and one frontotemporal). All surgeons aimed for a Simpson grade I resection. The majority of surgeons were concerned about the extent of the frontal sinuses, olfactory nerves, and the anterior cerebral arteries and their branches. The most feared complication was anosmia and vision loss. Surgery was generally pursued with surgical microscope and ultrasonic aspirator (with only one surgeon using surgical navigation) with perioperative steroids, antiepileptics, and mannitol. Most surgeons advocated for minimizing brain retraction, early drainage of cerebrospinal fluid, and internal debulking of tumor prior to capsule manipulation. Following surgery, half of the surgeons admitted their patients to the intensive care unit, and most surgeons requested imaging within 48 hours after surgery to assess for extent of resection and/or potential complications. Most surgeons advocated for observation for residual WHO grade I meningiomas, radiation for residual WHO grade II meningiomas, and radiation for all WHO grade III meningiomas.

SUMMARY OF QUALITY OF EVIDENCE TO GUIDE SPECIFIC INTERVENTIONS FOR THIS CASE

- Orbitozygomatic craniotomy for anterior cranial fossa meningiomas—Class III.

- Cauterizing dura instead of removal for anterior cranial fossa meningioma—Class II-3.

REFERENCES

1. Pallini R, Fernandez E, Lauretti L, et al. Olfactory groove meningioma: report of 99 cases surgically treated at the Catholic University School of Medicine, Rome. *World Neurosurg.* 2015;83:219–231.e1–e3.
2. Chaichana KL, Jackson C, Patel A, et al. Predictors of visual outcome following surgical resection of medial sphenoid wing meningiomas. *J Neurol Surg B Skull Base.* 2012;73:321–326.
3. Chaichana KL, Vivas-Buitrago T, Jackson C, et al. The radiographic effects of surgical approach and use of retractors on the brain after anterior cranial fossa meningioma resection. *World Neurosurg.* 2018;112:e505–e513.
4. Bander ED, Singh H, Ogilvie CB, et al. Endoscopic endonasal versus transcranial approach to tuberculum sellae and planum sphenoidale meningiomas in a similar cohort of patients. *J Neurosurg.* 2018;128:40–48.
5. Ruzevick J, Raza SM, Recinos PF, et al. Technical note: orbitozygomatic craniotomy using an ultrasonic osteotome for precise osteotomies. *Clin Neurol Neurosurg.* 2015;134:24–27.
6. Banu MA, Mehta A, Ottenhausen M, et al. Endoscope-assisted endonasal versus supraorbital keyhole resection of olfactory groove meningiomas: comparison and combination of 2 minimally invasive approaches. *J Neurosurg.* 2016;124:605–620.
7. de Divitiis E, Esposito F, Cappabianca P, Cavallo LM, de Divitiis O, Esposito I. Endoscopic transnasal resection of anterior cranial fossa meningiomas. *Neurosurg Focus.* 2008;25:E8.
8. Shetty SR, Ruiz-Trevino AS, Omay SB, et al. Limitations of the endonasal endoscopic approach in treating olfactory groove meningiomas. A systematic review. *Acta Neurochir (Wien).* 2017;159:1875–1885.
9. Ehresman JS, Garzon-Muvdi T, Rogers D, et al. The relevance of Simpson grade resections in modern neurosurgical treatment of World Health Organization grade I, II, and III meningiomas. *World Neurosurg.* 2018;109:e588–e593.

43

Tuberculum sellae meningioma

Case reviewed by Pablo Augusto Rubino, Román Pablo Arévalo, James J. Evans,
Tomas Garzon-Muvdi, Ricardo J. Komotar, Jorge Navarro-Bonnet

Introduction

Tuberculum sellae meningiomas are often grouped with the midline anterior skull base meningiomas.[1] These lesions account for 3% to 10% of intracranial meningiomas, and typically arise from arachnoid cells at the limbus sphenoidale, chiasmatic sulcus, and/or tuberculum.[1] These lesions often invade the bone and generate an osteoblastic resection, as well as displace critical neurovascular structures, including the optic nerve and chiasm, infundibulum, and anterior cerebral artery vessels.[1] Surgery for these lesions is associated with significant morbidity that ranges from 10% to 25% in several series, and can include vision loss, hormonal dysfunction, and cerebrospinal fluid leak, among others.[2,3] In this chapter, we present a case of a patient with a tuberculum sellae meningioma.

Example case

Chief complaint: vision loss

History of present illness

A 42-year-old, right-handed woman with a history of hypertension presented with vision loss. She noticed that over the past several months she had an increasing difficulty with seeing things in her peripheral fields. She noticed this especially at intersections when driving. Visual field testing showed optic nerve atrophy and right greater than left superior and inferior temporal field cuts (Fig. 43.1).

Medications: Lisinopril.

Allergies: No known drug allergies.

Past medical and surgical history: Hypertension, appendectomy, tonsillectomy.

Family history: No history of intracranial malignancies.

Social history: Lawyer, no smoking or alcohol.

Physical examination: Awake, alert, oriented to person, place, and time; Cranial nerves II to XII intact, except bitemporal field cuts to confrontation; No drift, moves all extremities with full strength.

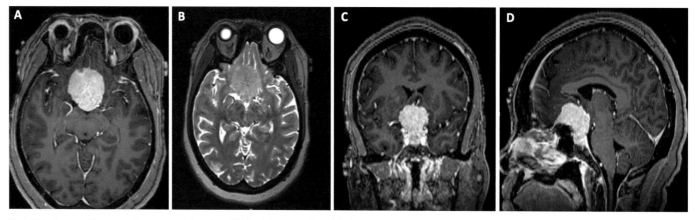

Fig. 43.1 Preoperative magnetic resonance imaging. (A) T1 axial image with gadolinium contrast; **(B)** T2 axial image; **(C)** T1 coronal image with gadolinium contrast; **(D)** T1 sagittal image with gadolinium contrast magnetic resonance imaging scan demonstrating an enhancing lesion involving the tuberculum sellae.

	Pablo Augusto Rubino, MD, Román Pablo Arévalo, MD, Hospital El Cruce, Buenos Aires, Argentina	James J. Evans, MD, Tomas Garzon-Muvdi, MD, Thomas Jefferson University, Philadelphia, PA, United States	Ricardo J. Komotar, MD, University of Miami, Miami, FL, United States	Jorge Navarro-Bonnet, MD, Oncologic Neurosurgery, Medica Sur, Mexico City, Mexico
Preoperative				
Additional tests requested	Neuropsychological assessment Pituitary hormone panel MRA	CT CT angiography	Endocrinology evaluation Ophthalmology evaluation	CT of the paranasal sinuses ENT evaluation Endocrinology evaluation Ophthalmology evaluation (visual fields)
Surgical approach selected	Right pterional craniotomy and anterior clinoidectomy	Endoscopic endonasal transplanum transtubercular	Right frontotemporal craniotomy	Extended endoscopic endonasal transsphenoidal
Anatomic corridor	Subfrontal, trans-Sylvian	Endonasal	Trans-Sylvian	Endonasal
Goal of surgery	Preservation of vision Simpson grade II	Maximal debulking, preservation of visual function, Simpson grade II–III	Simpson grade II	Simpson grade I
Perioperative				
Positioning	Supine neutral with slight rotation	Supine no pins	Right supine with slight rotation	Supine in pins
Surgical equipment	Surgical microscope Doppler Ultrasonic aspirator	Surgical navigation Endoscope Ultrasonic aspirator	Surgical navigation Surgical microscope Ultrasonic aspirator	Lumbar drain Surgical navigation Endoscope Ultrasonic aspirator
Medications	Mannitol Antiepileptics	None	Mannitol Steroids	None
Anatomic considerations	Bilateral ICAs, bilateral optic nerves, pituitary stalk	Bilateral ICAs, ACAs, superior hypophyseal arteries, optic nerves/chiasm, cavernous sinuses, basilar artery, pituitary gland	Bilateral ICAs and ACAs, bilateral optic nerves, pituitary stalk	Olfactory nerves, ICA, ACA, optic chiasm
Complications feared with approach chosen	ICA and optic nerve injury	Brain retraction	ICA, ACA, optic nerve, infundibulum injuries	Vascular injury, optic chiasm injury
Intraoperative				
Anesthesia	General	General	General	General
Skin incision	Right pterional	Fascia lata	Right pterional	None
Bone opening	Right frontal/temporal	Sphenoid bone, sella, tuberculum sellae, planum sphenoidale	Right frontal/temporal	Sphenoid bone, tuberculum sellae
Brain exposure	Right frontal/temporal	Anterior skull base	Right frontal/temporal	Tuberculum sellae

(continued on next page)

	Pablo Augusto Rubino, MD, Román Pablo Arévalo, MD, Hospital El Cruce, Buenos Aires, Argentina	James J. Evans, MD, Tomas Garzon-Muvdi, MD, Thomas Jefferson University, Philadelphia, PA, United States	Ricardo J. Komotar, MD, University of Miami, Miami, FL, United States	Jorge Navarro-Bonnet, MD, Oncologic Neurosurgery, Medica Sur, Mexico City, Mexico
Method of resection	Craniotomy on side with worse optic nerve functioning, drilling lesser sphenoid wing and supraorbital region parallel to orbital roof, dura opening, Sylvian fissure is split along the anterior limb, subfrontal approach with early identification of optic nerve/chiasm/ICA, wide dissection of arachnoid and opening of opticocarotid cistern, intradural anterior clinoidectomy, decompression of optic canal, tumor devascularization and debulking along the paramedian plane to avoid injuring contralateral optic nerve, identification of contralateral optic nerve once tumor is debulked sufficiently, continue debulking tumor with ultrasonic aspirator, mobilize capsule sharply from critical structures including ICA/ACA/ infundibulum through interoptic and opticocarotid cisterns, attempt to dissect from optic nerves but if cannot leave small remnant attached, inspect both optic canals	Obtain fascia lata graft for dural repair, ENT to assist, nasoseptal flap harvest, lateralization of bilateral middle turbinates, partial removal of posterior ethmoids, removal of skull base spanning tumor from planum to clivus, coagulation of dura, dura opened in midline and tumor debulked with ultrasonic aspirator or sharp/ dull dissection, extracapsular dissection sharply, margin of dura removed, fascia lata button graft used to reconstruct dura, nasoseptal flap applied, dural sealant, medialization of middle turbinates, no lumbar drain	Craniotomy, drill lesser sphenoid wing, open dura, open Sylvian fissure under microscopic visualization, wide arachnoid dissection with accessing the opticocarotid cistern, CSF drainage with brain relaxation, send off pathology, early identification of optic nerves/ICAs, tumor debulking with ultrasonic aspirator, dissect capsule from brain, protect critical structures (optic nerves, ICA, ACA, infundibulum), complete resection, dural closure with dural substitute	ENT to assist, harvest nasoseptal flap, removal of sphenoid bone and tuberculum sellae, coagulation of dura, dural opening, debulking with ultrasonic aspirator, sharp dissection to adherent structures, reconstruction using dural substitute as inlay and onlay with gasket seal, nasoseptal flap, lumbar drain for 3 days
Complication avoidance	Early identification of critical structures, wide arachnoid opening, sharp dissection from critical structures	Fascia lata button graft, coagulation of dura, debulk tumor prior to manipulation, nasoseptal flap	Early identification of critical structures, wide arachnoid and Sylvian fissure opening	Nasoseptal flap, gasket seal closure, lumbar drain, coagulation of dura
Postoperative				
Admission	ICU	ICU	ICU	Intermediate care
Postoperative complications feared	CSF leak, visual decline	CSF leak, visual decline, pituitary dysfunction	Visual decline, stroke, pituitary dysfunction	Anosmia, vasospasm, diabetes insipidus, CSF leak
Follow-up testing	MRI within 48 hours after surgery	MRI within 3 months after surgery	MRI within 24 hours after surgery Endocrine evaluation	Head CT immediately after surgery MRI within 48 hours after surgery Neuroophthalmology and endocrinology evaluation
Follow-up visits	1 month, 3 months, 6 months after surgery	1 week after surgery with ENT 3 weeks after surgery with neurosurgery	14 days after surgery	10 days after surgery
Adjuvant therapies recommended for WHO grade	Grade I–observation Grade II–observation Grade III–radiation	Grade I–observation Grade II–clinical trial Grade III–clinical trial	Grade I–observation Grade II–radiation Grade III–radiation/ chemotherapy	Grade I–radiation Grade II–radiation Grade III–radiation

ACA, anterior cerebral artery; CSF, cerebrospinal fluid; CT, computed tomography; ENT, ear, nose, and throat; ICA, internal carotid artery; ICU, intensive care unit; MRA, magnetic resonance angiography; MRI, magnetic resonance imaging.

Differential diagnosis and actual diagnosis

- Meningioma
- Hemangiopericytoma
- Metastatic brain cancer
- Lymphoma

Important anatomic and preoperative considerations

Anterior cranial fossa meningiomas include olfactory groove, planum sphenoidale, and tuberculum sellae meningiomas.[1,4,5] Tuberculum sellae meningiomas arise posterior to the origin of planum sphenoidale meningiomas at the limbus sphenoidale, chiasmatic sulcus, or tuberculum sellae.[1,4,5] This origin causes the optic chiasm to be displaced posteriorly and superiorly, as compared with planum sphenoidale meningiomas that typically cause posterior and inferior displacement of the optic chiasm.[1,4,5] Moreover, tuberculum sellae lesions can extend more inferiorly into the sellae, making extensive resection difficult based on surgical angle, visualization, and incorporation of critical structures, such as the infundibulum.[2,3] Tuberculum sellae meningiomas can also be further subdivided into tuberculum sellae and diaphragma sellae meningiomas, in which the latter are rarer and involves only the diaphragma.[2,3]

Approaches to This Lesion

There are a variety of approaches to tuberculum sellae meningiomas, which include cranial and endonasal routes (Chapter 41, Fig. 41.2).[1,4–6] The advantages and disadvantages of each are described in Chapter 41, Fig. 41.2. Cranial approaches can either be unilateral (frontotemporal) or bilateral (bifrontal).[1,4–6] Each of these approaches can be augmented with orbital osteotomies, which decrease the obstruction of bone overlying the orbit, thus increasing visualization in the superior/inferior dimension to improve working angles.[1,4–6] The alternative to a cranial approach is via an endonasal route.[6–9] As with other approaches, this can be expanded laterally by opening and/or removing the turbinates and/or the medial wall of the maxillary sinuses to increase the lateral working corridor.[6–9] Simpson grade I resections are difficult from a cranial approach for these lesions as compared with endonasal approaches (Chapter 41, Fig. 41.3).[10,11]

What was actually done

The patient was taken to surgery for a right modified orbitozygomatic craniotomy for resection of a tuberculum sellae meningioma with intraoperative somatosensory evoked potentials and electroencephalogram. The patient was induced and intubated per routine. The head was fixed in pins, with two pins centered on the inion and one pin over the left forehead in the midpupillary line. The head was extended and turned 30 degrees to the right. A pterional incision was planned from the root of the zygoma to the vertex. The patient was draped in the usual standard fashion and given dexamethasone, levetiracetam, and cefazolin. The pterional incision was made making sure to stay above the temporalis

fascia. After the fat pad was encountered, the temporalis fascia was incised, and a subfascial dissection was done to expose the orbital rim and frontal-zygomatic process and protecting the frontalis nerve. The temporalis muscle was then dissected anteriorly in the subperiosteal plane, and the flap was held in place with fishhooks attached to a retractor arm. A pterional flap was made that stayed lateral to the frontal sinus based on surgical navigation. The periorbita was dissected from the orbital rim, and the inferior orbital fissure was identified. An ultrasonic bone cutter was used to make cuts at the level of the frontozygomatic suture laterally and lateral to the supraorbital nerve medially. These cuts were carried as posteriorly over the orbital roof as possible. The dura was then opened in a semicircular fashion and tacked up with sutures. The microscope was brought in for visualization. The frontal lobe was dissected off of the anterior cranial fossa, where the olfactory nerve was identified and followed to the optic nerve. The brain was protected with cottonoids, and dynamic retraction was used with the sucker. The tumor was cauterized from the skull base to eliminate its bloody supply. The tumor was debulked internally with an ultrasonic aspirator, and the edges of the tumor were mobilized inward until removed, making sure to identify critical neurovascular structures. The tumor that extended into the sellae was dissected superiorly with pituitary rongeurs after identifying and preserving the infundibulum. Preliminary pathology was a meningioma. The dura, bone, and skin were closed in standard fashion with a subgaleal drain.

The patient awoke at their neurologic baseline with full strength bilaterally and intact vision and was taken to the intensive care unit for recovery. Magnetic resonance imaging was done within 48 hours after surgery and showed gross total resection with Simpson grade II resection, in which the anterior cranial fossa dura was cauterized but left in place (Fig. 43.2). The patient participated with physical and occupational therapy and was discharged to home on postoperative day 2 with an intact neurologic examination after subgaleal drain removal. The patient was prescribed dexamethasone that was tapered to off over 7 days after surgery, and levetiracetam for 7 days. The patient was seen at 2 weeks postoperatively for staple removal and remained neurologically intact. Pathology was a World Health Organization (WHO) grade I meningioma. The lesion was observed with serial magnetic resonance imaging examinations at 3- and 6-month intervals and has been without recurrence for 36 months.

Commonalities among the experts

The majority of the surgeons opted for the patient to undergo endocrinology and ophthalmology evaluations, and half requested a head computed tomography to evaluate tumor density and frontal sinus location prior to surgery. Half of the surgeons approached the lesion through an endoscopic endonasal route, whereas the other half preferred a right frontotemporal craniotomy (one trans-Sylvian and one subfrontal). Most surgeons aimed for a Simpson grade II resection. The majority were concerned about the bilateral internal carotid arteries, anterior cerebral arteries, optic nerves, and pituitary stalk. The most feared complication by surgeons was internal carotid artery injury and visual decline. Surgery was generally pursued with surgical navigation and ultrasonic aspirator (microscope in those

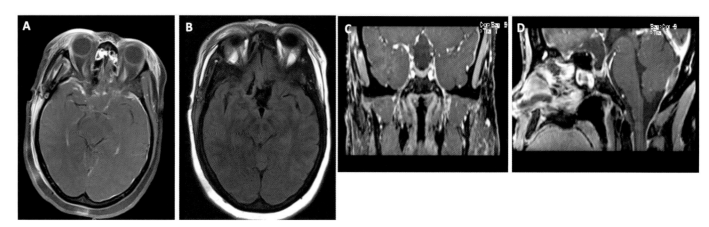

Fig. 43.2 Postoperative magnetic resonance imaging. (A) T1 axial image with gadolinium contrast; **(B)** T2 axial fluid attenuation inversion recovery image; **(C)** T1 coronal image with gadolinium contrast; **(D)** T1 sagittal image with gadolinium contrast magnetic resonance imaging scan demonstrating gross total resection of the tuberculum sellae meningioma.

pursuing craniotomies and endoscope in those pursuing endonasal) with perioperative mannitol in half of the surgeries. Most surgeons advocated for early identification of critical structures and internal debulking of tumor prior to capsule manipulation. Following surgery, most surgeons admitted their patients to the intensive care unit, and most surgeons requested imaging within 48 hours after surgery to assess for extent of resection and/or potential complications. Most surgeons advocated for observation for residual WHO grade I meningiomas, radiation for residual WHO grade II meningiomas, and radiation for all WHO grade III meningiomas.

SUMMARY OF QUALITY OF EVIDENCE TO GUIDE SPECIFIC INTERVENTIONS FOR THIS CASE

- Orbitozygomatic craniotomy for anterior cranial fossa meningiomas—Class III.
- Cauterizing dura instead of removal for anterior cranial fossa meningioma—Class II-3.

REFERENCES

1. Pallini R, Fernandez E, Lauretti L, et al. Olfactory groove meningioma: report of 99 cases surgically treated at the Catholic University School of Medicine, Rome. *World Neurosurg.* 2015;83:219–231.e1–e3.
2. Ajlan AM, Choudhri O, Hwang P, Harsh G. Meningiomas of the tuberculum and diaphragma sellae. *J Neurol Surg B Skull Base.* 2015;76:74–79.
3. Magill ST, Morshed RA, Lucas CG, et al. Tuberculum sellae meningiomas: grading scale to assess surgical outcomes using the transcranial versus transsphenoidal approach. *Neurosurg Focus.* 2018;44:E9.
4. Chaichana KL, Jackson C, Patel A, et al. Predictors of visual outcome following surgical resection of medial sphenoid wing meningiomas. *J Neurol Surg B Skull Base.* 2012;73:321–326.
5. Chaichana KL, Vivas-Buitrago T, Jackson C, et al. The radiographic effects of surgical approach and use of retractors on the brain after anterior cranial fossa meningioma resection. *World Neurosurg.* 2018;112:e505–e513.
6. Bander ED, Singh H, Ogilvie CB, et al. Endoscopic endonasal versus transcranial approach to tuberculum sellae and planum sphenoidale meningiomas in a similar cohort of patients. *J Neurosurg.* 2018;128:40–48.
7. Banu MA, Mehta A, Ottenhausen M, et al. Endoscope-assisted endonasal versus supraorbital keyhole resection of olfactory groove meningiomas: comparison and combination of 2 minimally invasive approaches. *J Neurosurg.* 2016;124:605–620.
8. de Divitiis E, Esposito F, Cappabianca P, Cavallo LM, de Divitiis O, Esposito I. Endoscopic transnasal resection of anterior cranial fossa meningiomas. *Neurosurg Focus.* 2008;25:E8.
9. Shetty SR, Ruiz-Trevino AS, Omay SB, et al. Limitations of the endonasal endoscopic approach in treating olfactory groove meningiomas. A systematic review. *Acta Neurochir (Wien).* 2017;159:1875–1885.
10. Ehresman JS, Garzon-Muvdi T, Rogers D, et al. The relevance of Simpson grade resections in modern neurosurgical treatment of World Health Organization grade I, II, and III meningiomas. *World Neurosurg.* 2018;109:e588–e593.
11. Simpson D. The recurrence of intracranial meningiomas after surgical treatment. *J Neurol Neurosurg Psychiatry.* 1957;20:22–39.

44

Convexity meningioma

Case reviewed by Arturo Ayala-Arcipreste, Carlos E. Briceno, Ricardo J. Komotar, Michael W. McDermott

Introduction

Meningiomas are among the most common primary brain tumor in adults, with an incidence that ranges from 1 to 8 per 100,000 people.[1] One of the most common locations for these lesions is along the cerebral convexity, in which they account for 20% to 30% of the lesions.[1–3] Even though convexity meningiomas are considered to be among the most surgically accessible brain tumors, these lesions can be associated with significant morbidity in which complications occur in about 10% of cases in most series.[2–5] In this chapter, we present a case of a patient with a convexity meningioma.

Example case

Chief complaint: left arm and leg weakness
History of present illness
A 39-year-old, right-handed woman with a history of bipolar disorder presented with left arm and leg weakness. Over the past several months, she had lost a lot of her hand strength and coordination in which she is unable to button her shirt with her left hand. She has also noticed that it feels like her left leg is weaker than her right and that she has to drag it to move (Fig. 44.1).
Medications: Lithium.
Allergies: No known drug allergies.

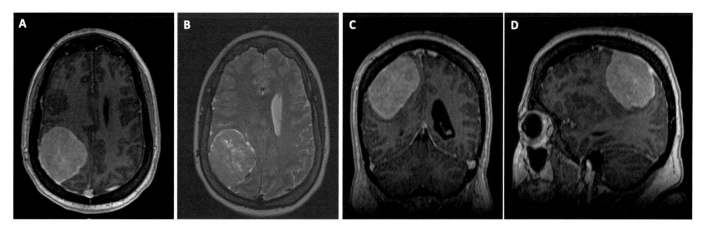

Fig. 44.1 Preoperative magnetic resonance imaging. (A) T1 axial image with gadolinium contrast; **(B)** T2 axial image; **(C)** T1 coronal image with gadolinium contrast; **(D)** T1 sagittal image with gadolinium contrast magnetic resonance imaging scan demonstrating an enhancing lesion involving the right parietal convexity.

Past medical and surgical history: Bipolar disorder.
Family history: No history of intracranial malignancies.
Social history: Lawyer, no smoking or alcohol.
Physical examination: Awake, alert, oriented to person, place, and time; Cranial nerves II to XII intact; Left drift, left upper extremity 4+/5 except hand 3/5, left lower extremity 4+/5, right upper extremity/right lower extremity 5/5.

	Arturo Ayala-Arcipreste, MD, Hospital Juarez de Mexico, Mexico City, Mexico	Carlos E. Briceno, MD, Paitilla Medical Center, Panama City, Panama	Ricardo J. Komotar, MD, University of Miami, Miami, FL, United States	Michael W. McDermott, MD, Herbert Wertheim College of Medicine, Florida International University, Miami, FL, United States
Preoperative				
Additional tests requested	Angiogram (venous and arterial) EEG Neuropsychological assessment Psychiatry evaluation Neuroanesthesia evaluation	DTI fMRI MRA/MRV Neuropsychological assessment EEG	Psychiatry evaluation Angiogram with possible embolization	Cerebral angiogram with embolization
Surgical approach selected	Right parieto-occipital craniotomy	Right parietal craniotomy	Right parietal craniotomy	Right frontoparietal craniotomy
Anatomic corridor	Right parieto-occipital	Right parietal	Right parietal	Right frontoparietal
Goal of surgery	Simpson grade I	Simpson grade I	Simpson grade I	Simpson grade I
Perioperative				
Positioning	Right three-quarters prone with left head rotation	Left dorsal decubitus with left head rotation	Right supine with left rotation	Right lateral
Surgical equipment	Surgical microscope Ultrasonic aspirator	Surgical navigation Surgical microscope Ultrasonic aspirator	Surgical navigation IOM (MEP) Ultrasonic aspirator	Surgical navigation Ultrasonic aspirator
Medications	Steroids Antiepileptics	Steroids Antiepileptics Mannitol, hypertonic saline	Steroids Mannitol	Steroids Antiepileptics Mannitol
Anatomic considerations	Vein of Trolard, SSS, branches of MCA and PCA	Motor and somatosensory cortices	Motor cortex, vein of Labbe and Trolard, SSS	Vein at posterior margin, SSS, primary motor and sensory cortices
Complications feared with approach chosen	Venous infarct	Venous infarct, motor deficit, sensory deficit, residual tumor	Motor deficit, venous infarct	Venous infarct
Intraoperative				
Anesthesia	General	General	General	General
Skin incision	Linear	Lazy S-shaped incision	Linear	Inverted U-shaped crossing midline
Bone opening	Right parieto-occipital	Right parietal	Right parietal	Right frontoparietal
Brain exposure	Right parieto-occipital	Right parietal	Right parietal	Right frontoparietal

	Arturo Ayala-Arcipreste, MD, Hospital Juarez de Mexico, Mexico City, Mexico	Carlos E. Briceno, MD, Paitilla Medical Center, Panama City, Panama	Ricardo J. Komotar, MD, University of Miami, Miami, FL, United States	Michael W. McDermott, MD, Herbert Wertheim College of Medicine, Florida International University, Miami, FL, United States
Method of resection	Linear incision calculated transversely with navigation, scalp flap preserving superficial temporal artery, craniotomy wide enough to cover the entire tumor and extra margin, dural tack up sutures, dural opening adjacent to tumor, devascularize tumor early on dural surface, protect brain surface with cottonoids, attempt to identify tumor-arachnoid interface, debulk center of tumor, once tumor volume has decreased sufficiently then sharp dissection of arachnoid from the tumor capsule, identify and protect venous structure at bottom of tumor, copious irrigation to allow hydrodissection, continue dissection until tumor completely removed, periosteum as dural substitute, insertion of subgaleal drain	Right parietal incision guided by navigation, harvest pericranium, parietal craniotomy guided by navigation, meticulous coagulation of dura, dural tack up sutures circumferentially incise dura and coagulate dural vessels leaving a wide margin (1–2 cm) of tumor-free dura, preservation of transdural veins, folding of involved dura over tumor to assist with tumor retraction, identify subarachnoid planes at tumor-brain interface, sharply opening planes avoiding pial violation, protect extracapsular en passage vessels, attempt en bloc resection with circumferentially dissecting tumor from brain with tumor coagulation, internal debulking if cannot be removed en bloc, protect brain with cottonoids, dissect deeper until tumor can be removed, inspect for dural tails and residual tumor nests, repair dural defect with pericranium or dural substitute, epidural drain	Right parietal craniotomy guided by navigation, open and resect involved dura, devascularize tumor early from dural feeders, protect veins (vein of Labbe and Trolard) and superior sagittal sinus if exposed, internal debulking with ultrasonic aspirator, dissect margins from brain, protect exposed critical structures, complete resection, dural substitute over dural defect	Subgaleal flap opening, pericranium raised separately, burr holes placed anteriorly and posteriorly 1.5 cm from midline and another laterally, right frontoparietal craniotomy guided by navigation, epidural space is dissected across midline, secondary flap is elevated across midline, sagittal sinus controlled with bipolar cautery and gelfoam, tack up sutures, tension of dura is palpated and measures to lower ICP are used if needed, margins of tumor marked on dura, cruciate dural opening over center of tumor and tumor debulked, after enough debulking dura is opened around tumor, brain-tumor interface developed, pericranium used for dural reconstruction, gaps in bone filled with bone cement
Complication avoidance	Devascularize tumor early, internal debulking of tumor, sharp dissection of tumor from arachnoid and critical structures, hydrodissection with irrigation	Devascularize tumor early, circumferentially remove dura, preservation of transdural veins, using dura for retraction, protect cortex, identify arachnoid planes, attempt en bloc resection	Devascularize tumor early, identify and protect critical venous structures, internal debulking prior to capsular manipulation	Pericranial harvest, bone flap in two separate pieces, internal debulking of tumor before developing interface
Postoperative				
Admission	ICU	ICU	ICU	ICU
Postoperative complications feared	Cerebral edema, seizures, venous infarct, CSF leak	Cerebral edema, seizures, motor and sensory deficit, CSF leak, cognitive deficit	Motor deficit, venous infarct	Seizures, venous infarct
Follow-up testing	CT within 24 hours after surgery MRI 1 month and 4 months after surgery	MRI within 72 hours after surgery MRI 2 months after surgery	MRI within 24 hours after surgery	MRI within 48 hours after surgery
Follow-up visits	10 days after surgery Physical therapy evaluation	14 days after surgery	14 days after surgery	2 weeks after surgery 6–8 weeks after surgery

(continued on next page)

	Arturo Ayala-Arcipreste, MD, Hospital Juarez de Mexico, Mexico City, Mexico	Carlos E. Briceno, MD, Paitilla Medical Center, Panama City, Panama	Ricardo J. Komotar, MD, University of Miami, Miami, FL, United States	Michael W. McDermott, MD, Herbert Wertheim College of Medicine, Florida International University, Miami, FL, United States
Adjuvant therapies recommended for WHO grade	Grade I–observation, surgery for residual Grade II–oncology/radiation oncology evaluation Grade III–oncology/radiation oncology evaluation	Grade I–observation Grade II–observation vs. radiation Grade III–radiation	Grade I–observation Grade II–radiation Grade III–radiation/chemotherapy	Grade I–observation Grade II–observation if Simpson grade I resection with MiB-1 <7% C, radiation if >7% Grade III–radiation

CSF, cerebrospinal fluid; *CT*, computed tomography; *DTI*, diffusion tensor imaging; *EEG*, electroencephalogram; *fMRI*, functional magnetic resonance imaging; *ICP*, intracranial pressure; *ICU*, intensive care unit; *IOM*, intraoperative monitoring; *MCA*, middle cerebral artery; *MEP*, motor evoked potentials; *MiB*, Mindbomb Homolog-1; *MRA*, magnetic resonance angiography; *MRI*, magnetic resonance imaging; *MRV*, magnetic resonance venogram; *PCA*, posterior cerebral artery; *SSS*, superior sagittal sinus.

Differential diagnosis and actual diagnosis

- Meningioma
- Hemangiopericytoma
- Metastatic brain cancer
- Lymphoma

Important anatomic and preoperative considerations

The convexity is generally defined as the superolateral surfaces of the brain in contact with the calvarium, and includes the areas covering the frontal, parietal, temporal, and occipital lobes.[2–5] Separate from these convexity meningiomas are parasagittal meningiomas that are in direct contact with the sagittal sinus.[2–5] Therefore convexity meningiomas include the subset of meningiomas that involve the superolateral surface of the frontal, parietal, temporal, and/or occipital lobes without direct contact of the sagittal sinus.[2–5] The frontal (Chapter 1), parietal (Chapter 9), temporal (Chapter 10), and occipital (Chapter 25) lobes have been previously discussed in detail. The lesion in this chapter involves the convexity overlying the right precentral, postcentral, and superior parietal lobule.

Approaches to this lesion

The general approaches for all brain tumors include observation with serial imaging, radiation therapy, and/or surgical therapy. In this case, the lesion is large with symptomatic mass effect with contralateral arm and leg weakness. Radiation therapy is not ideal because of the large size of the lesion, young age of the patient, and symptomatic mass effect.

What was actually done

The patient was taken to surgery for a right parietal craniotomy for resection of a parietal convexity meningioma with intraoperative somatosensory evoked potentials, motor evoked potentials, and electroencephalogram. The patient was induced and intubated per routine. The head was fixed in pins, with two pins over the left superior nuchal line and one pin over the right forehead in the midpupillary line. The patient was positioned into the three-quarters prone position. A miter or inverted U-incision was planned with the aid of surgical navigation, making sure to stay anterior and posterior from the lesion boundaries. The patient was draped in the usual standard fashion and given dexamethasone, levetiracetam, and cefazolin. The incision was made, and the flap was retracted inferiorly with fishhooks attached to the drapes. The surgical navigation was used to confirm the tumor boundaries, one burr hole was made ipsilateral to the sagittal sinus, and the craniotomy was used to create a flap that encompassed the lesion and approximately 1 cm more in each dimension. The dura was cauterized extensively to minimize the tumor's vascular supply. The dura was opened circumferentially around the tumor, making sure to stay at the interface between the tumor and the uninvolved brain. The dura was tacked up with sutures to provide counter tension, the center of the tumor was debulked with an ultrasonic aspirator, and the tumor was dissected from the surrounding pia. There was constant alternation between tumor debulking and capsule dissection until the tumor was removed. Preliminary pathology was a meningioma. The cavity was lined with Surgicel (Ethicon US, Somerville, NJ). Synthetic dural substitute was used to reconstitute the dura that was removed. The bone and skin were closed in standard fashion.

The patient awoke at their neurologic baseline with left-sided weakness and was taken to the intensive care unit for recovery. Magnetic resonance imaging was done within 48 hours after surgery and showed gross total resection with Simpson grade I resection (Chapter 41, Fig. 41.2) in which the involved dura was removed (Fig. 44.2). The patient participated with physical and occupational therapy and was discharged to home on postoperative day 2 with improved left-sided strength (4+/5 in the left upper extremity and 5/5 in the left lower extremity). The patient was prescribed dexamethasone that was tapered to off over 7 days after surgery, and levetiracetam for 7 days. The patient was seen at 2 weeks postoperatively and was neurologically intact. Pathology was a World Health Organization (WHO) grade I meningioma. The lesion was observed with serial magnetic resonance imaging examinations at 3- and 6-month intervals and has been without recurrence for 36 months.

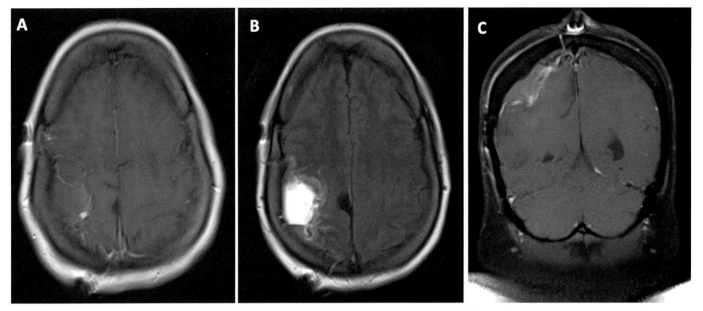

Fig. 44.2 Postoperative magnetic resonance imaging. (A) T1 axial image with gadolinium contrast; **(B)** T2 axial fluid attenuation inversion recovery image; **(C)** T1 coronal image with gadolinium contrast magnetic resonance imaging scan demonstrating gross total resection of the convexity meningioma.

Commonalities among the experts

The majority of the surgeons opted for the patient to undergo cerebral angiogram with possible embolization, as well as psychiatry evaluation prior to surgery. All surgeons approached the lesion through a right parietal-based craniotomy with an aim of a Simpson grade I resection. The majority of surgeons were concerned about the primary motor and sensory cortex, as well as venous anatomy, namely the vein of Trolard. The most feared complications were venous infract and motor deficit. Surgery was generally pursued with surgical navigation, surgical microscope, and ultrasonic aspirator with perioperative mannitol, steroids, and antiepileptics. Most surgeons advocated for early devascularity of the lesion, internal debulking, and sharp dissection of the tumor from the arachnoid. Following surgery, all surgeons admitted their patients to the ICU, and most surgeons requested imaging within 72 hours after surgery to assess for extent of resection and/or potential complications. Most surgeons advocated for observation for residual WHO grade I meningiomas, radiation versus observation for residual WHO grade II meningiomas, and radiation for all WHO grade III meningiomas.

SUMMARY OF QUALITY OF EVIDENCE TO GUIDE SPECIFIC INTERVENTIONS FOR THIS CASE

- Removal of involved dura to achieve Simpson grade I resection—Class II-3.

REFERENCES

1. Baldi I, Engelhardt J, Bonnet C, et al. Epidemiology of meningiomas. *Neurochirurgie.* 2018;64:5–14.
2. Morokoff AP, Zauberman J, Black PM. Surgery for convexity meningiomas. *Neurosurgery.* 2008;63:427–433; discussion 433–434.
3. Sanai N, Sughrue ME, Shangari G, Chung K, Berger MS, McDermott MW. Risk profile associated with convexity meningioma resection in the modern neurosurgical era. *J Neurosurg.* 2010;112:913–919.
4. Ehresman JS, Garzon-Muvdi T, Rogers D, et al. The relevance of Simpson grade resections in modern neurosurgical treatment of World Health Organization grade I, II, and III meningiomas. *World Neurosurg.* 2018;109:e588–e593.
5. Quinones-Hinojosa A, Kaprealian T, Chaichana KL, et al. Pre-operative factors affecting resectability of giant intracranial meningiomas. *Can J Neurol Sci.* 2009;36:623–630.

45

Parasagittal meningiomas without sinus invasion

Case reviewed by Henry Brem, Ricardo Díez Valle, Jacques J. Morcos, Tetsuro Sameshima

Introduction

Meningiomas are among the most common primary brain tumor in adults, and the most common locations are parasagittal/parafalcine lesions, which account for 25% of meningiomas.[1-5] These meningiomas arise from the arachnoid in or next to the falx, and therefore involve critical cortical draining veins and the sagittal sinus.[1-5] Surgical resection of these lesions, especially when they involve the middle and/or posterior third of the sagittal sinus, can be associated with significant morbidity.[6-9] The morbidity ranges from 10% to 30%, and mortality rates range from 5% to 15% in several series, and is significantly higher with sinus invasion.[10] In this chapter, we present a case of a patient with a parasagittal meningioma without sinus invasion.

Example case

Chief complaint: left leg weakness

History of present illness

A 55-year-old, right-handed woman with no significant past medical history who presented with left leg weakness. She stated that over the past several months, she had developed increasing difficult with strength in her left leg, but more specifically her left foot. A spine magnetic resonance imaging (MRI) scan was done and was negative for pathology to explain left foot weakness. She saw a neurologist who ordered a brain MRI (Fig. 45.1).

Medications: None.

Allergies: No known drug allergies.

Past medical and surgical history: None.

Family history: No history of intracranial malignancies.

Social history: Homemaker, no smoking or alcohol.

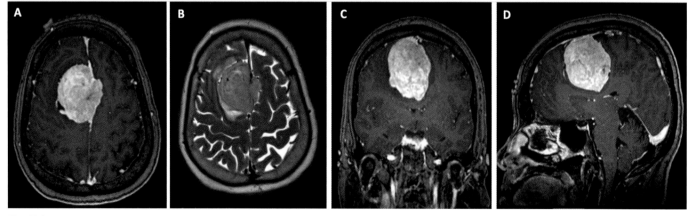

Fig. 45.1 Preoperative magnetic resonance imaging. (A) T1 axial image with gadolinium contrast; **(B)** T2 axial image; **(C)** T1 coronal image with gadolinium contrast; **(D)** T1 sagittal image with gadolinium contrast magnetic resonance imaging scan demonstrating an enhancing lesion of the right posterior frontal lobe with abutment of the sagittal sinus without obvious invasion.

Physical examination: Awake, alert, oriented to person, place, and time; Cranial nerves II to XII intact; No drift, moves all extremities with full strength, except left dorsiflexion/plantar-flexion 3/5.

Magnetic resonance venography: No sagittal sinus narrowing or obstruction.

	Henry Brem, MD, Johns Hopkins University, Baltimore, MD, United States	Ricardo Díez Valle, MD, PhD, Fundación Jimenez Diaz University Clinic, Madrid, Spain	Jacques J. Morcos, MD, University of Miami, Miami, FL, United States	Tetsuro Sameshima, MD, PhD, Hamamatsu University, Shizuoka, Japan
Preoperative				
Additional tests requested	MR angiography and venography	None	None	ASL MRI CT Cerebral angiogram
Surgical approach selected	Bifrontoparietal craniotomy	Bifrontoparietal craniotomy	Modified bicoronal craniotomy	Right frontal craniotomy
Anatomic corridor	Right interhemispheric	Right interhemispheric with falx excision	Right interhemispheric with falx excision	Right interhemispheric
Goal of surgery	Simpson grade I	Simpson grade I, likely grade II, without resection of the wall of the sagittal sinus	Simpson grade I, including SSS reconstruction	Simpson grade II
Perioperative				
Positioning	Supine neutral	Supine neutral	Left supine with 30-degree right rotation (SSS horizontal)	Supine neutral
Surgical equipment	Surgical navigation IOM (MEP/SSEP/EEG) Surgical microscope Ultrasonic aspirator Ultrasound Vascular clips	Surgical navigation Surgical microscope Ultrasonic aspirator	Surgical navigation Lumbar drain Surgical microscope Ultrasonic aspirator Vascular clips 5-0 Prolene to repair SSS	Surgical navigation Surgical microscope Ultrasonic aspirator
Medications	Steroids Mannitol Antiepileptics	Steroids	Steroids Mannitol Antiepileptics	None
Anatomic considerations	SSS, cortical veins, ACA/MCA branches	SSS, cortical veins, distal ACA, supplementary motor cortex	SSS, ACA and branches, premotor cortex, bridging veins	Bridging veins
Complications feared with approach chosen	Cerebral edema, SSS injury	SSS injury, retraction injury	Retraction injury	Venous infarct
Intraoperative				
Anesthesia	General	General	General	General
Skin incision	Linear bicoronal	Linear bicoronal	Linear bicoronal eccentric to the right	Inverted U incision
Bone opening	Bifrontal eccentric to right (burr holes off the sinus)	Bifrontal eccentric to right (burr holes over the sinus)	Bifrontal eccentric to right (burr holes off the sinus)	Right frontal craniotomy exposing superior sagittal sinus
Brain exposure	Right frontal	Right frontal	Bifrontal	Right frontal

(continued on next page)

	Henry Brem, MD, Johns Hopkins University, Baltimore, MD, United States	Ricardo Díez Valle, MD, PhD, Fundación Jimenez Diaz University Clinic, Madrid, Spain	Jacques J. Morcos, MD, University of Miami, Miami, FL, United States	Tetsuro Sameshima, MD, PhD, Hamamatsu University, Shizuoka, Japan
Method of resection	Bifrontal craniotomy eccentric to the right but extending at least 3 cm to the left, tenting sutures, dural opening at tumor-brain interface so only tumor pushes outward, U-shaped dural opening on right based on sagittal sinus, bipolar surface of tumor, internally debulk and remove, dissect capsule and preserve all host arteries and collateral veins, open dura on left and inspect for tumor involvement, remove falx from right side to visualize left side and confirm GTR, inspect SSS under microscopic visualization and attempt to remove remaining tumor if not adherent, leave small residual if tumor adherent to SSS, duraplasty, rinse bone flap in Betadine, subgaleal drain placement	Bifrontal craniotomy eccentric to the right with burr holes over sinus at the anterior and posterior limits, hemostasis over SSS with compression, coagulation of arterial meningeal branches, dural opening on right, dissection of arachnoid plane over the tumor, debulking with ultrasonic aspirator if hard, leave dissection of ACA branches until the end, leave superior medial border of SSS for end, attempt at resecting all without compromising SSS, for deeper part of the tumor care with pericallosal arteries, cross falx and dissect remaining deep tumor from contralateral brain, removal of dura and falx but not from SSS, closure with dural substitute	Bifrontal craniotomy eccentric to the right, U-shaped dural opening on right avoiding bridging veins and modify dural opening as necessary, drain 30 cc of CSF from lumbar drain, interhemispheric approach anterior to tumor and devascularize falx and proceed posteriorly, debulk tumor with ultrasonic aspirator and bipolar, identify ACA and branches before deepest portion of tumor removed, leave small portion on SSS for last part of surgery, remove from SSS with or without reconstruction with native dura, watertight dural closure, avoid use of retractors	Right frontal craniotomy with superior sagittal sinus exposure, dural incision to expose interhemispheric fissure with preservation of bridging veins, detachment of tumor from sagittal sinus and falx and internal tumor debulking, separate tumor from brain surface for gross total removal, remove convexity dura and dural reconstruction with periosteum
Complication avoidance	Control of SSS with bifrontal opening, open dura only tumor, leave SSS for last, leave component adherent to SSS alone	Control of SSS with right frontal opening, dissect in arachnoid plane, no retraction needed, decompress tumor from inside, leave SSS for last, remove dura from falx but leave dura along superior sagittal sinus	Right hemisphere down, devascularize early from falx, save SSS for last, avoid fixed retractors with positioning and lumbar drain, separate ACAs meticulously	Expose SSS, limit craniotomy to one side, spare bridging veins, separate from sagittal sinus, remove dural origin
Sinus reconstruction if necessary	Compression, muscle or fascia compression, primary closure, patch graft	Compression, suture, or synthetic patch	Compression and repair with native dura	Suture close or dural patch
Postoperative				
Admission	ICU	ICU	ICU	ICU
Postoperative complications feared	Cerebral edema, sinus thrombosis, venous infarct	Cerebral edema due to venous infarct, injury to arterial branches, SSS injury, left lower extremity weakness	SSS occlusion, bridging vein thrombosis, seizures, CSF leak, SMA syndrome, DVT	SSS thrombosis, cerebral venous occlusion
Follow-up testing	MRI/MRV within 24 hours after surgery	MRI within 24 hours after surgery	MRI within 48 hours after surgery 5% albumin for 3 days Physical and occupational therapy	CT immediately after and 1 day after surgery MRI within 7 days after surgery

	Henry Brem, MD, Johns Hopkins University, Baltimore, MD, United States	Ricardo Díez Valle, MD, PhD, Fundación Jimenez Diaz University Clinic, Madrid, Spain	Jacques J. Morcos, MD, University of Miami, Miami, FL, United States	Tetsuro Sameshima, MD, PhD, Hamamatsu University, Shizuoka, Japan
Follow-up visits	14 days after surgery 3 months, then every 6 months after surgery	7 days after surgery	10 days after surgery 6 weeks after surgery	3 months after surgery
Adjuvant therapies recommended for WHO grade	Grade I–observation Grade II–observation Grade III–observation for GTR, radiation if STR or recurs	Grade I–observation Grade II–radiation Grade III–radiation	Grade I–observation Grade II–radiation Grade III–radiation	Grade I–observation Grade II–observation Grade III–radiation

ACA, anterior cerebral artery; *ASL*, arterial spin labeling; *CSF*, cerebrospinal fluid; *CT*, computed tomography; *DVT*, deep vein thrombosis; *EEG*, electroencephalogram; *GTR*, gross total resection; *ICU*, intensive care unit; *IOM*, intraoperative monitoring; *MCA*, middle cerebral artery; *MEP*, motor evoked potential; *MR*, magnetic resonance; *MRI*, magnetic resonance imaging; *MRV*, magnetic resonance venography; *SMA*, supplementary motor area; *SSEP*, somatosensory evoked potential; *SSS*, superior sagittal sinus; *STR*, subtotal resection.

Differential diagnosis and actual diagnosis

- Meningioma
- Hemangiopericytoma
- Metastatic brain cancer
- Lymphoma

Important anatomic and preoperative considerations

The superior sagittal sinus is located in the midline along the attached margin of the falx.[11] It typically occurs within 1 cm of the midline, in which some studies have a predilection for the right side, whereas others show the left side.[11,12] It typically begins at or posterior to the foramen cecum, possesses draining veins that drain into the sagittal sinus in which the largest is located at or near the central sulcus, and predominantly drains into the right transverse sinus.[11] The anterior-most draining veins enter the sinus typically almost at right angles or in a slightly anterior direction, whereas the posterior draining veins turn more anteriorly to enter the sinus more obliquely.[11] The superior sagittal sinus can be divided into thirds based on length or as anterior to the bregma, middle between the bregma and lambda, and the posterior to the lambda.[11,12] In most surgical studies, it is considered that the anterior third of the superior sagittal sinus can be ligated; however, some patients will still develop significant morbidity, including cerebral edema, frontal lobe infarction, personality changes, memory loss, akinetic mutism, and death.[13] Patients with significant draining veins in terms of size, caliber, tributaries, and acute angles are more reliant on the anterior segment of the sagittal sinus for drainage.[13]

Approaches to this lesion

The general approaches for all brain tumors include observation with serial imaging, radiation therapy, and/or surgical therapy. In this case, the lesion is large with symptomatic mass effect with contralateral weakness and involved the middle third segment of the sagittal sinus. Radiation therapy is not ideal because of the large size of the lesion, young age of the patient, and symptomatic mass effect. When lesions involve the sagittal sinus, it is important to determine if the lesion abuts, invades, or obstructs the sagittal sinus. The Sindou grading classification system is used to characterize the degree of invasion and recommended interventions (Table 45.1).[10,14] In these studies, the morbidity was 11% and the mortality was 8%, in which the majority of these complications were due to venous sinus infarcts involving major draining veins.[10,14] However, these studies predated studies on stereotactic radiosurgery, and therefore the aggressiveness of tumors invading the sagittal sinus has

Table 45.1 Sindou classification and recommended treatment options for meningiomas involving the superior sagittal sinus

Sindou Classification	Characteristics	Recommended Procedure
Type I	Attached to outer surface of sinus wall	Removing outer layer of sinus wall with coagulation of dural attachment
Type II	Lateral recess involved	Resection of lateral recess component and suture of the recess defect
Type III	Lateral wall invaded	Resection of invaded wall and repair of lateral wall
Type IV	Entire lateral wall and roof of sinus both invaded	Resection of invaded wall, peeling with coagulation of attachment if possible, or subtotal resection of the roof
Type V	Sinus totally invaded with one wall being free	Resection of both invaded walls with or without reconstruction
Type VI	Sinus totally invaded without any free walls	Removal of the entire involved portion without venous bypass

been tempered.[1,5] For cases without complete obstruction, another option besides complete removal to obtain Simpson grade I resection (Chapter 41, Fig. 41.2) is to leave the tumor within the sinus and observe for growth, followed by possible stereotactic radiosurgery.[1,5]

What was actually done

The patient was taken to surgery for a bifrontal craniotomy for resection of a bilateral parasagittal meningioma with intraoperative somatosensory evoked potentials, motor evoked potentials, and electroencephalogram. The patient was induced and intubated per routine. The head was fixed in pins, with two pins over the left external auditory meatus and one pin over the right external auditory meatus. The head was flexed and kept neutral. A bifrontal incision in the coronal plane was planned over the middle part of the tumor based on surgical navigation, and the incision extended to the right superior temporal line and to the midpupillary line on the left. The patient was draped in the usual standard fashion and given dexamethasone, levetiracetam, and cefazolin. The incision was made, and the flap was retracted with cerebellar retractors. The location of the sagittal sinus was confirmed with navigation and was 5 mm to the right of the sagittal suture. Two burr holes were placed on the ipsilateral side at the anterior and posterior margin of the right side of the tumor, and two burr holes were placed on the left side of the sagittal sinus just posterior to the anterior burr hole and just anterior to the posterior burr hole to allow access to dissect the sagittal sinus from the overlying calvarium. The craniotome was used to perform a bifrontal bone flap that encompassed the lesion plus at least 1 cm on each margin. Gelfoam was placed over the sagittal sinus. The dura was cauterized extensively to minimize the tumor's vascular supply. The dura was opened in a semicircular fashion on the right, making sure to stay at the brain-tumor interface and tacked up over the sinus. The tumor was cauterized and debulked internally with an ultrasonic aspirator. Alternating between tumor debulking and capsule dissection, the tumor was then removed from the right side, and the falx was encountered. Under microscopic visualization, the falx was opened, and the tumor was removed from the contralateral side, preserving the sagittal sinus superiorly. Preliminary pathology was a meningioma. The attachment

appeared to be from the falx, and the falx was removed at all points of tumor attachment. The attachment of the tumor on the ipsilateral side of the sinus wall was identified, and the outer leaflet was removed. The cavity was lined with Surgicel (Ethicon US, Somerville, NJ). The dura, bone, and skin were closed in standard fashion.

The patient awoke at their neurologic baseline with left-sided foot weakness and was taken to the intensive care unit for recovery. An MRI was done within 48 hours after surgery and showed gross total resection with Simpson grade I resection (Chapter 41, Fig. 41.2) in which the involved falx and the outer leaflet of the sagittal sinus were removed (Fig. 45.2). The patient participated with physical and occupational therapy and was discharged to home on postoperative day 2 with intact strength. The patient was prescribed dexamethasone that was tapered to off over 7 days after surgery, and levetiracetam for 7 days. The patient was seen at 2 weeks postoperatively for staple removal and was neurologically intact. Pathology was a World Health Organization (WHO) grade I meningioma. The lesion was observed with serial MRI examinations at 3- and 6-month intervals and has been without recurrence for 24 months.

Commonalities among the experts

Half of the surgeons opted for the patient to undergo vascular imaging to better characterize the patency of the sinus and vascular feeders prior to surgery. All surgeons elected for surgery, in which the majority chose a bilateral craniotomy and all proceeding with a right interhemispheric approach. The general goal was a Simpson grade I resection in which half of the surgeons identified the need for falx resection. All surgeons were concerned about the superior sagittal sinus and draining veins, and most were concerned about the anterior cerebral arteries and their branches. The most feared complications were venous infarct from injury to the superior sagittal sinus and/or draining veins. Surgery was generally pursued with surgical navigation, surgical microscope, and ultrasonic aspirator with perioperative mannitol, steroids, and antiepileptics. Most surgeons advocated for control of the superior sagittal sinus with bifrontal opening, early devascularity of the lesion along the falx, and leaving the component along the superior sagittal sinus for

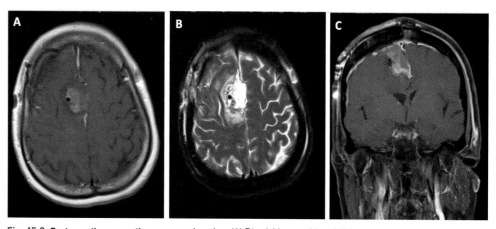

Fig. 45.2 Postoperative magnetic resonance imaging. (A) T1 axial image with gadolinium contrast; **(B)** T2 axial image; **(C)** T1 coronal image with gadolinium contrast magnetic resonance imaging scan demonstrating gross total resection of the right posterior frontal parasagittal meningioma.

the last. If venous injury occurred, the treatment algorithm was first compression, followed by direct suture repair, and then a patch as the last resort. Following surgery, all surgeons admitted their patients to the intensive care unit, and most surgeons requested imaging within 48 hours after surgery to assess for extent of resection and/or potential complications. Most surgeons advocated for observation for residual WHO grade I meningiomas, radiation versus observation for residual WHO grade II meningiomas, and radiation for all WHO grade III meningiomas.

SUMMARY OF QUALITY OF EVIDENCE TO GUIDE SPECIFIC INTERVENTIONS FOR THIS CASE

- Removal of involved falx and sinus wall to achieve Simpson grade I resection—Class II-3.

REFERENCES

1. Ehresman JS, Mampre D, Rogers D, Olivi A, Quinones-Hinojosa A, Chaichana KL. Volumetric tumor growth rates of meningiomas involving the intracranial venous sinuses. *Acta Neurochir (Wien)*. 2018;160:1531–1538.
2. DiMeco F, Li KW, Casali C, et al. Meningiomas invading the superior sagittal sinus: surgical experience in 108 cases. *Neurosurgery*. 2004;55:1263–1272; discussion 1272–1264.
3. Jusue-Torres I, Navarro-Ramirez R, Gallego MP, Chaichana KL, Quinones-Hinojosa A. Indocyanine green for vessel identification and preservation before dural opening for parasagittal lesions. *Neurosurgery*. 2013;73 ons145; discussion ons145.
4. Ricci A, Di Vitantonio H, De Paulis D, et al. Parasagittal meningiomas: our surgical experience and the reconstruction technique of the superior sagittal sinus. *Surg Neurol Int*. 2017;8:1
5. Kondziolka D, Flickinger JC, Perez B. Judicious resection and/or radiosurgery for parasagittal meningiomas: outcomes from a multicenter review. Gamma Knife Meningioma Study Group. *Neurosurgery*. 1998;43:405–413; discussion 413–404.
6. Ehresman JS, Garzon-Muvdi T, Rogers D, et al. The relevance of Simpson grade resections in modern neurosurgical treatment of World Health Organization grade I, II, and III meningiomas. *World Neurosurg*. 2018;109:e588–e593.
7. Morokoff AP, Zauberman J, Black PM. Surgery for convexity meningiomas. *Neurosurgery*. 2008;63:427–433; discussion 433–434.
8. Quinones-Hinojosa A, Kaprealian T, Chaichana KL, et al. Pre-operative factors affecting resectability of giant intracranial meningiomas. *Can J Neurol Sci*. 2009;36:623–630.
9. Sanai N, Sughrue ME, Shangari G, Chung K, Berger MS, McDermott MW. Risk profile associated with convexity meningioma resection in the modern neurosurgical era. *J Neurosurg*. 2010;112:913–919.
10. Sindou M. Meningiomas invading the sagittal or transverse sinuses, resection with venous reconstruction. *J Clin Neurosci*. 2001;8(Suppl 1):8–11.
11. Bruno-Mascarenhas MA, Ramesh VG, Venkatraman S, Mahendran JV, Sundaram S. Microsurgical anatomy of the superior sagittal sinus and draining veins. *Neurol India*. 2017;65:794–800.
12. Tubbs RS, Salter G, Elton S, Grabb PA, Oakes WJ. Sagittal suture as an external landmark for the superior sagittal sinus. *J Neurosurg*. 2001;94:985–987.
13. Sahoo SK, Ghuman MS, Salunke P, Vyas S, Bhar R, Khandelwal NK. Evaluation of anterior third of superior sagittal sinus in normal population: identifying the subgroup with dominant drainage. *J Neurosci Rural Pract*. 2016;7:257–261.
14. Sindou M, Hallacq P. Venous reconstruction in surgery of meningiomas invading the sagittal and transverse sinuses. *Skull Base Surg*. 1998;8:57–64.

46

Parasagittal meningioma with sinus obstruction

Case reviewed by Clark C. Chen, Mohamed El-Fiki, Gerardo Guinto, Michael W. McDermott

Introduction

Meningiomas make up approximately 36% of all intracranial tumors, where the most common location for these lesions is abutting the sagittal sinus or falx.[1-5] This location inevitably makes these tumors involve major venous sinuses and critical cortical draining veins.[1-5] As a result, meningiomas that involve the sagittal sinus or falx have a two- to threefold increase in complications as compared with their convexity counterparts.[1-6] Among parasagittal meningiomas, the ones that invade the sagittal sinus have varied management from subtotal resection with avoidance of the venous sinus to gross total resection with sinus reconstruction.[6-10] In this chapter, we present a case of a parasagittal meningioma with sinus invasion.

Example case

Chief complaint: seizures
History of present illness
A 47-year-old, right-handed woman with no significant past medical history presented after a seizure. She was at work and developed acute onset of loss of consciousness with eye rolling backward, right arm and leg shaking, followed by generalized tonic-clonic activity. She had not been sleeping very much because of tax deadlines. She was taken to the emergency room, where she became more coherent and was at her neurologic baseline. Imaging showed a brain lesion (Fig. 46.1).
Medications: None.
Allergies: No known drug allergies.

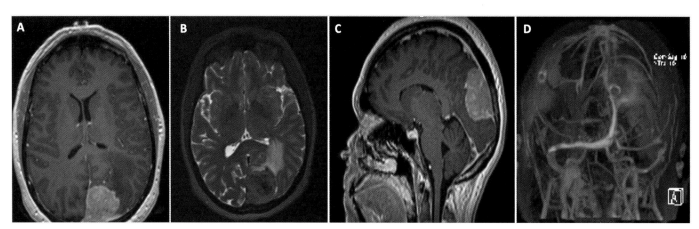

Fig. 46.1 Preoperative magnetic resonance imaging. (A) T1 axial image with gadolinium contrast; **(B)** T2 axial image; **(C)** T1 sagittal image with gadolinium contrast; **(D)** venogram magnetic resonance imaging scan demonstrating an enhancing lesion of the left parasagittal region with complete obstruction of the posterior third segment of the sagittal sinus.

Past medical and surgical history: None.
Family history: No history of intracranial malignancies.
Social history: Accountant, no smoking or alcohol.
Physical examination: Awake, alert, oriented to person, place, and time; Cranial nerves II to XII intact and full vision to confrontation; No drift, moves all extremities with full strength.
Magnetic resonance venography: Complete obstruction of the sagittal sinus at the posterior third segment.

	Clark C. Chen, MD, PhD, University of Minnesota, Minneapolis, MN, United States	Mohamed El-Fiki, MBBCh, MS, MD, Alexandria University, Alexandria, Egypt	Gerardo Guinto, MD, Centro Neurologico ABC, Mexico City, Mexico	Michael W. McDermott, MD, Herbert Wertheim College of Medicine, Florida International University, Miami, FL, United States
Preoperative				
Additional tests requested	DTI CTA for potential preop embolization CT chest, abdomen, pelvis Medical workup Ophthalmology evaluation	fMRI DTI Venogram Ophthalmology evaluation (visual fields)	fMRI DTI Neuropsychological assessment EEG	DTI Cerebral angiogram Ophthalmology evaluation (visual fields)
Surgical approach selected	Left occipital craniotomy with lumbar drain	Left parieto-occipital craniotomy and SSS repair	Left parieto-occipital craniotomy	Left parieto-occipital craniotomy crossing midline
Anatomic corridor	Left occipital	Left parietal	Left parietal	Left parietal
Goal of surgery	Gross total resection	Simpson grade II or III, maximal safe resection	Simpson grade I	Simpson grade II
Perioperative				
Positioning	Right lateral (left-side down)	Sitting position	Prone with head rotated 30–40 degrees to the left	Right three-quarters prone (left side down)
Surgical equipment	Lumbar drain Surgical navigation Surgical microscope IOM Ultrasonic aspirator	Surgical microscope Ultrasonic aspirator, Gore-Tex arterial graft	Surgical navigation Surgical microscope Ultrasonic aspirator	Surgical navigation Ultrasonic aspirator Doppler
Medications	Mannitol Steroids Antiepileptics	Mannitol, furosemide Steroids Antiepileptics	Steroids Antiepileptics	Mannitol Steroids Antiepileptics
Anatomic considerations	SSS, cortical drain veins, optic radiations, primary visual cortex	SSS, draining veins into the sinus, superior parietal lobe, superior optic radiations	SSS (posterior third), falx, parietal and occipital lobes	Parasagittal draining veins
Complications feared with approach chosen	Injury to SSS and cortical draining veins, visual deficit	SSS thrombosis, venous infarct, venous hypertension, visual field deficit	SSS bleeding, venous embolism and infarction, motor deficit, visual deficit	Venous infarct
Intraoperative				
Anesthesia	General	General	General	General
Skin incision	Inverted U	Linear bicoronal	Inverted U	Inverted U

(continued on next page)

	Clark C. Chen, MD, PhD, University of Minnesota, Minneapolis, MN, United States	Mohamed El-Fiki, MBBCh, MS, MD, Alexandria University, Alexandria, Egypt	Gerardo Guinto, MD, Centro Neurologico ABC, Mexico City, Mexico	Michael W. McDermott, MD, Herbert Wertheim College of Medicine, Florida International University, Miami, FL, United States
Bone opening	Left parieto-occipital craniotomy ipsilateral to SSS	Left parieto-occipital passing middles, burr holes on both sides of sinus	Left parieto-occipital passing midline, burr holes on both sides of sinus	Left parieto-occipital crossing midline
Brain exposure	Left parieto-occipital	Left parieto-occipital	Left parieto-occipital	Left parieto-occipital
Method of resection	Lumbar drain, precordial Doppler, tumor side down, craniotomy ipsilateral to SSS, U-shaped dural opening based on SSS making sure to preserve cortical veins, unclamp lumbar drain allowing free drainage at level of external auditory meatus, debulk tumor with ultrasonic aspirator under microscopic visualization, define plane between tumor and brain, removal of tumor inside SSS and dural reconstruction, resect falx, watertight dural closure with pericranium	Craniotomy on both sides of the sinus, opening dura on left, identify brain interface with microscopic visualization, preserve cortical veins draining into the sinus, open pia arachnoid and dissect veins away from surgical field, use minimal or no retraction, debulk tumor piecemeal or with ultrasonic aspirator, dissect away from falx preserving right side brain, leave SSS component until end, try to safely peel tumor away from sinus wall, if not possible may need removal of occluded SSS segment with venous anastomosis, closure with insertion of subgaleal drain	Myocutaneous flap, craniotomy on both sides of sinus with 3- to 4-cm margin of tumor and burr holes adjacent to sinus, U-shaped dural opening that is 2.5 cm surrounding tumor, dura in contact with the tumor is removed, tumor internally debulked with ultrasonic aspirator and bipolar coagulation, mobilization of capsule and preserving pia as much as possible, removal of tumor implant on falx with 1- to 1.5-cm margin, removal of tumor inside SSS until bleeding seen in front and behind tumor, transient compression of SSS and reconstruction, pericranium for dural reconstruction, drilling of inner side of involved calvarium	Mark midline and borders with navigation, inverted U-shaped incision based inferiorly crossing midline to the right, preserve pericranium for dural graft, left parietal-occipital bone flap 1.5-cm lateral to midline with superior and inferior burr holes, dissect bone from sagittal sinus with direct visualization, second bone flap to the right crossing midline, control midline bleeding with bipolar and gelfoam, peripheral dural tack ups, mark tumor margins on dura with marking pen, navigation and Doppler to define SSS, U-shaped dural opening based on SSS, detach tumor from dura to open dura medially, debulk tumor centrally and define brain-tumor interface, detach from midline if bleeding is an issue, confirm margins of closed/open SSS after superior/inferior/anteromedial margins defined with Doppler and navigation, open dural roof of SSS in midpoint and remove tumor within SSS leaving right wall intact, remove lesion until bleeding occurs and sew closed lumen, excise falx where attached to tumor, excise convexity dura and falx, dural closure with pericranium, resect involved inner table of involved bone, fill defects with bone cement and sand down bone, irrigate with Betadine and place vancomycin powder in subgaleal space, closure with subgaleal drain
Complication avoidance	Lumbar drain, precordial Doppler, ipsilateral craniotomy, internal debulking, resect falx, pericranial closure	Craniotomy on both sides, identify draining veins, leave SSS until the end	Craniotomy on both sides, removal of tumor along falx with margin, drilling of calvarium	Two-piece craniotomy crossing midline, central debulking, detach from falx if bleeding, remove tumor from lumen until bleeding in SSS occurs, remove involved bone

	Clark C. Chen, MD, PhD, University of Minnesota, Minneapolis, MN, United States	Mohamed El-Fiki, MBBCh, MS, MD, Alexandria University, Alexandria, Egypt	Gerardo Guinto, MD, Centro Neurologico ABC, Mexico City, Mexico	Michael W. McDermott, MD, Herbert Wertheim College of Medicine, Florida International University, Miami, FL, United States
Sinus reconstruction if needed	Apply pressure over tear with gelfoam/Surgicel, tension suture gelfoam/Surgicel with adjacent bone, direct repair	Dural patch graft if away from tumor site	Local compression for small defect, pericranium for large defect	Remain calm, expect injury as trying to find proximal and distal ends, assistant to grasp opening closed with nontoothed forceps, primary closure
Postoperative				
Admission	ICU	ICU	Floor	ICU
Postoperative complications feared	Air embolus, venous infarct, visual field deficit, seizures, Gerstmann syndrome	Venous hypertension, visual field deficit, calculation and spatial orientation problems	CSF leak, venous infarction	Visual field cut, venous infarct, seizures
Follow-up testing	MRI and MRV within 48 hours after surgery Physical and occupational therapy Ophthalmology evaluation as outpatient	CT immediately after surgery MRI 3 months after surgery	CT within 6–8 hours after surgery MRI 6 weeks after surgery EEG 2 years after surgery Neuropsychological assessment	MRI within 48 hours after surgery
Follow-up visits	2 weeks after surgery	1 month and every 3 months after surgery	6 weeks after surgery	10–14 days after surgery 6–8 weeks after surgery
Adjuvant therapies recommended for WHO grade	Grade I–observation, possible additional resection pending residual Grade II–observation vs. radiation Grade III–radiation	Grade I–observation Grade II–radiation Grade III–radiation	Grade I–observation Grade II–observation Grade III–radiosurgery	Grade I–observation Grade II–radiation Grade III–radiation

CSF, cerebrospinal fluid; *CT*, computed tomography; *CTA*, computed tomography angiography; *DTI*, diffusion tensor imaging; *EEG*, electroencephalogram; *fMRI*, functional magnetic resonance imaging; *ICU*, intensive care unit; *IOM*, intraoperative monitoring; *MRI*, magnetic resonance imaging; *MRV*, magnetic resonance venography; *SSS*, superior sagittal sinus.

Differential diagnosis and actual diagnosis

- Meningioma
- Hemangiopericytoma
- Metastatic brain cancer
- Lymphoma

Important anatomic and preoperative considerations

For a full detailed description of the sagittal sinus, see Chapter 45. The superior sagittal sinus is located in the midline along the attached margin of the falx.[11] It is often arbitrarily divided into thirds based on length or the location relative to the cranial sutures.[11,12] Based on its relationship to the sutures, the anterior segment is anterior to bregma, the middle segment is between bregma and lambda, and the posterior segment is posterior to lambda.[11,12] Conventionally,

in most surgical studies, it is considered that the anterior third of the superior sagittal sinus can be ligated, whereas the posterior two-thirds need to be preserved.[13] However, even ligation of the anterior segment of the sagittal sinus can cause significant morbidity, and therefore the draining veins need to be critically evaluated in terms of their size, caliber, tributaries, and acute angles to evaluate if the anterior segment can be ligated without significant morbidity.[13]

Approaches to this lesion

The options for meningiomas involving the sagittal sinus include observation, radiation therapy, and/or surgical resection. In this case, the lesion is large with symptomatic mass effect with seizures and involves the posterior third segment of the sagittal sinus. For small, asymptomatic tumors, these lesions can be watched with serial imaging. The sinus component of these meningiomas typically grow slowly and then plateau over time.[1] Radiation, including fractioned radiation and stereotactic radiosurgery, has typically been reserved for recurrent or partially resected lesions, in which some studies have shown that radiation therapy of partially resected tumors have less recurrence than nonradiated lesions.[5,6,14] The use of upfront radiation therapy is typically reserved for smaller tumors that are asymptomatic without mass effect, in difficult-to-access regions, or in patients who are poor surgical candidates.[5,6,14] For surgical resection, the management is controversial and ranges from subtotal resection with the goal of removing the extrasinus component and leaving the sinus component behind to aggressive resection with reconstruction of the sinus (Chapter 45, Fig. 45.2).[1-5] Modern series show no difference in tumor recurrence between gross total resection and subtotal resection with radiation therapy after documented growth.[6]

What was actually done

The patient was taken to surgery for a prone bioccipital craniotomy for resection of a bilateral parasagittal meningioma with resection of the occluded portion of the sinus with intraoperative somatosensory evoked potentials and electroencephalogram. The patient was induced and intubated per routine, as well as underwent placement of a right internal jugular vein central line and precordial Doppler to monitor for air emboli. The head was fixed in pins, with two pins over the right external auditory meatus and one pin over the left external auditory meatus. The patient was then placed prone onto chest rolls, and the head was flexed, reduced, and kept neutral. A linear incision was then made over the midline and extended inferiorly between the avascular plane between the suboccipital muscles. The patient was draped in the usual standard fashion and given dexamethasone, levetiracetam, and cefazolin. The incision was made, and the flap was retracted with cerebellar retractors. The location of the sagittal sinus was confirmed with navigation and was 5 mm to the right of the sagittal suture. Two burr holes were placed on the ipsilateral side at the anterior and posterior margin of the tumor, and two burr holes were placed on the contralateral side of the sagittal sinus just posterior to the anterior burr hole and just anterior to the posterior burr hole to allow access for dissecting the sagittal sinus from the overlying calvarium. The craniotome was used to perform a bilateral occipital bone flap that encompassed the lesion plus at least 1 cm on each margin. A Doppler was placed over the occluded portion of the sinus to confirm where the sinus was occluded and patent. In addition, indocyanine green was used to confirm occlusion. The dura was cauterized extensively to minimize the tumor's vascular supply. The dura was opened in a semicircular fashion, making sure to stay at the brain-tumor interface, and tacked up over the sinus. The tumor was cauterized and debulked internally with an ultrasonic aspirator. Alternating between tumor debulking and capsule dissection, the tumor was then removed until the only remnant was the sinus. Suture was used to occlude the sinus proximal and distal to the occlusion, and the sinus was removed where obstructed with scissors. Preliminary pathology was a meningioma. The convexity dura that involved the tumor was also removed. The dura was reconstituted with synthetic dura. The inner surface of the bone was drilled where the tumor was involved. The bone and skin were closed in standard fashion.

The patient awoke at their neurologic baseline with intact strength and full visual fields to confrontation and was taken to the intensive care unit for recovery. The patient was kept on intravenous fluid for 3 days. Magnetic resonance imaging was done within 48 hours after surgery and showed gross total resection with Simpson grade I resection (Chapter 41, Fig. 41.2) in which the involved dura and sinus were removed (Fig. 46.2). The patient participated with physical and occupational therapy and was discharged to home on postoperative day 4 with intact strength. The patient was prescribed dexamethasone that was tapered to off over 7 days after surgery, and levetiracetam for 7 days. The patient was seen at 2 weeks postoperatively for staple removal and was neurologically intact. Pathology was a World Health Organization (WHO) grade I meningioma. The lesion was observed with serial magnetic resonance imaging examinations at 3- and 6-month intervals and has been without recurrence for 18 months.

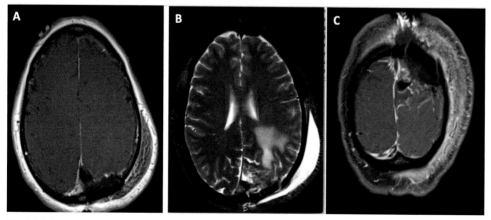

Fig. 46.2 Postoperative magnetic resonance imaging. (A) T1 axial image with gadolinium contrast; **(B)** T2 axial image; **(C)** T1 coronal image with gadolinium contrast magnetic resonance imaging scan demonstrating gross total resection of the left parasagittal meningioma with removal of the obstructed portion of the sinus.

Commonalities among the experts

All of the surgeons opted for the patient to undergo diffusion tensor imaging to evaluate for optic radiations, whereas half opted for vascular imaging to better characterize the patency of the sinus and vascular feeders, as well as formal visual field examination prior to surgery. All surgeons elected for surgery, in which the majority would perform a bilateral parieto-occipital craniotomy to have more control of the superior sagittal sinus. The general goal varied from Simpson grade I to III resection. All surgeons were concerned about the superior sagittal sinus and draining veins, and most were concerned about the visual cortex and optic radiations. The most feared complications were venous infarct from injury to the superior sagittal sinus and/or draining veins, as well as a visual field deficit. Surgery was generally pursued with surgical navigation, surgical microscope, and ultrasonic aspirator with perioperative mannitol, steroids, and antiepileptics. Most surgeons advocated for control of the superior sagittal sinus with bilateral opening, early devascularization of the lesion, and leaving the component along the superior sagittal sinus for last. If venous injury occurred, the treatment algorithm was first compression, followed by direct suture repair, and then a patch with pericranium as the last resort. Following surgery, most surgeons admitted their patients to the intensive care unit (one to the floor), and most surgeons requested imaging within 48 hours after surgery to assess for extent of resection and/or potential complications. Most surgeons advocated for observation for residual WHO grade I meningiomas, radiation versus observation for residual WHO grade II meningiomas, and radiation for all WHO grade III meningiomas.

SUMMARY OF QUALITY OF EVIDENCE TO GUIDE SPECIFIC INTERVENTIONS FOR THIS CASE

- Removal of involved dura and sinus to achieve Simpson grade I resection—Class II-3.

REFERENCES

1. Ehresman JS, Mampre D, Rogers D, Olivi A, Quinones-Hinojosa A, Chaichana KL. Volumetric tumor growth rates of meningiomas involving the intracranial venous sinuses. *Acta Neurochir (Wien)*. 2018;160:1531–1538.
2. DiMeco F, Li KW, Casali C, et al. Meningiomas invading the superior sagittal sinus: surgical experience in 108 cases. *Neurosurgery*. 2004;55:1263–1272; discussion 1272–1264.
3. Jusue-Torres I, Navarro-Ramirez R, Gallego MP, Chaichana KL, Quinones-Hinojosa A. Indocyanine green for vessel identification and preservation before dural opening for parasagittal lesions. *Neurosurgery*. 2013;73:ons145; discussion ons145.
4. Ricci A, Di Vitantonio H, De Paulis D, et al. Parasagittal meningiomas: our surgical experience and the reconstruction technique of the superior sagittal sinus. *Surg Neurol Int*. 2017;8:1.
5. Kondziolka D, Flickinger JC, Perez B. Judicious resection and/or radiosurgery for parasagittal meningiomas: outcomes from a multicenter review. Gamma Knife Meningioma Study Group. *Neurosurgery*. 1998;43:405–413; discussion 413–414.
6. Sughrue ME, Rutkowski MJ, Shangari G, Parsa AT, Berger MS, McDermott MW. Results with judicious modern neurosurgical management of parasagittal and falcine meningiomas. Clinical article. *J Neurosurg*. 2011;114:731–737.
7. Ehresman JS, Garzon-Muvdi T, Rogers D, et al. The relevance of Simpson grade resections in modern neurosurgical treatment of World Health Organization grade I, II, and III meningiomas. *World Neurosurg*. 2018;109:e588–e593.
8. Morokoff AP, Zauberman J, Black PM. Surgery for convexity meningiomas. *Neurosurgery*. 2008;63:427–433; discussion 433–434.
9. Quinones-Hinojosa A, Kaprealian T, Chaichana KL, et al. Preoperative factors affecting resectability of giant intracranial meningiomas. *Can J Neurol Sci*. 2009;36:623–630.
10. Sanai N, Sughrue ME, Shangari G, Chung K, Berger MS, McDermott MW. Risk profile associated with convexity meningioma resection in the modern neurosurgical era. *J Neurosurg*. 2010;112:913–919.
11. Bruno-Mascarenhas MA, Ramesh VG, Venkatraman S, Mahendran JV, Sundaram S. Microsurgical anatomy of the superior sagittal sinus and draining veins. *Neurol India*. 2017;65:794–800.
12. Tubbs RS, Salter G, Elton S, Grabb PA, Oakes WJ. Sagittal suture as an external landmark for the superior sagittal sinus. *J Neurosurg*. 2001;94:985–987.
13. Sahoo SK, Ghuman MS, Salunke P, Vyas S, Bhar R, Khandelwal NK. Evaluation of anterior third of superior sagittal sinus in normal population: identifying the subgroup with dominant drainage. *J Neurosci Rural Pract*. 2016;7:257–261.
14. Barbaro NM, Gutin PH, Wilson CB, Sheline GE, Boldrey EB, Wara WM. Radiation therapy in the treatment of partially resected meningiomas. *Neurosurgery*. 1987;20:525–528.

47

Parafalcine meningiomas

Case reviewed by Victor Garcia-Navarro, Michael W. McDermott, Peter Nakaji, Tony Van Havenbergh

Introduction

Parafalcine meningiomas are among the most common locations for meningiomas, in which they account for 25% of meningiomas along with parasagittal meningiomas.[1–5] Although they are in the same general vicinity as parasagittal meningiomas, parafalcine meningiomas are a different surgical entity, as they do not present themselves along the convexity surface.[6,7] This lack of convexity involvement means that superficial draining veins and the sagittal sinus must be traversed to reach the lesion.[6,7] In fact, there is a 10% to 20% complication rate among parafalcine meningiomas, which makes this location the third-highest rate of morbidity among all meningiomas after convexity and parasagittal meningiomas.[6,7] In this chapter, we present a case of a right parafalcine meningioma.

Example case

Chief complaint: left leg weakness
History of present illness
An 81-year-old, right-handed woman with hypertension, hypercholesterolemia, and dementia presented with progressive left leg weakness. For the past 5 to 6 months, she developed progressive difficulty with walking with left leg weakness. She underwent spine imaging that was negative. She, however, had scans of her brain done for dementia 4 years prior that revealed a small right parafalcine lesion. Repeat imaging showed significant growth of this lesion (Fig. 47.1).
Medications: Aspirin, lisinopril, hydrochlorothiazide, and atorvastatin.
Allergies: No known drug allergies.

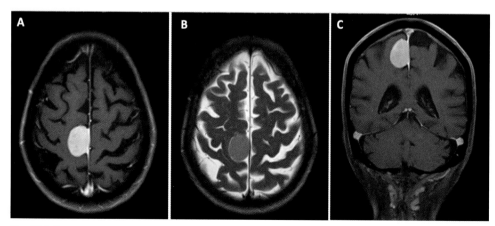

Fig. 47.1 Preoperative magnetic resonance imaging. (A) T1 axial image with gadolinium contrast; **(B)** T2 axial image; **(C)** T1 coronal image with gadolinium contrast magnetic resonance imaging scan demonstrating an enhancing lesion of the right parafalcine region underlying the precentral and postcentral gyri.

Past medical and surgical history: hypertension, hypercholesterolemia, dementia, hysterectomy, bladder surgery.
Family history: No history of intracranial malignancies.
Social history: Retired, independent with activities of daily living, no smoking or alcohol.

Physical examination: Awake, alert, oriented to person, place, and time; Cranial nerves II to XII intact and full vision to confrontation; No drift, moves all extremities with full strength except left lower extremity 4+/5.

	Victor Garcia-Navarro, MD, Tec de Monterrey Institute, Campus Guadalajara, Mexico	Michael W. McDermott, MD, Herbert Wertheim College of Medicine, Florida International University, Miami, FL, United States	Peter Nakaji, MD, Barrow Neurological Institute, Phoenix, AZ, United States	Tony Van Havenbergh, MD, PhD, GasthuisZusters Antwerpen, Antwerpen, Belgium
Preoperative				
Additional tests requested	Cardiology evaluation	Cardiology evaluation	Medical evaluation Physical therapy evaluation	MRV DTI Neuropsychological assessment
Surgical approach selected	Right frontoparietal craniotomy	Right parietal craniotomy	Left frontoparietal craniotomy	Right frontal craniotomy
Anatomic corridor	Right interhemispheric	Right interhemispheric	Left interhemispheric	Right interhemispheric
Goal of surgery	Simpson grade II	Simpson grade I	Simpson grade I	Simpson grade II
Perioperative				
Positioning	Semilateral (right head rotation)	Supine neutral	Right supine with left rotation (left-side down)	Supine with head 20-degree right rotation and right-side down
Surgical equipment	IOM Navigation Surgical microscope Ultrasonic aspirator	Surgical navigation Ultrasonic aspirator Surgical microscope	Surgical navigation IOM (MEP, SSEP) Surgical microscope Endoscope	Surgical navigation IOM (MEP, SSEP) Surgical microscope Ultrasonic aspirator
Medications	Steroids Antiepileptic	Mannitol Steroids Antiepileptic	Steroids	Antiepileptic
Anatomic considerations	SSS, draining veins	Draining veins, motor cortex, medial surface of left hemisphere	SSS	SSS, draining veins, motor cortex
Complications feared with approach chosen	Dural sinus injury, brain retraction injury	Venous infarct, cortical injury	Brain retraction injury, SSS injury	Venous injury
Intraoperative				
Anesthesia	General	General	General	General
Skin incision	Bicoronal linear/ sinusoidal	C-shaped	Bicoronal linear	Bicoronal curvilinear
Bone opening	Bilateral frontoparietal eccentric to right	Bilateral frontoparietal eccentric to right	Left frontoparietal adjacent to SSS	Right frontal craniotomy just ipsilateral to sagittal sinus
Brain exposure	Right frontoparietal with 3 cm of normal brain exposed	Right frontoparietal	Left frontoparietal	Right frontal lobe

(continued on next page)

	Victor Garcia-Navarro, MD, Tec de Monterrey Institute, Campus Guadalajara, Mexico	Michael W. McDermott, MD, Herbert Wertheim College of Medicine, Florida International University, Miami, FL, United States	Peter Nakaji, MD, Barrow Neurological Institute, Phoenix, AZ, United States	Tony Van Havenbergh, MD, PhD, GasthuisZusters Antwerpen, Antwerpen, Belgium
Method of resection	Bilateral frontoparietal craniotomy, burr holes on both sides of the sinus, craniotomy 3 cm larger than tumor. C-shaped dural opening, flap based on SSS, interhemispheric approach preserve cortical veins, devascularize tumor along falx and tumor surface, divide falx anterior and posterior to lesion, central debulking with ultrasonic aspirator, total resection with minimal brain retraction, dural coagulation if total removal not possible.	C-shaped incision based anteriorly, save pericranium for dural graft, mark midline, two right parasagittal burr holes 1.5-cm lateral to midline, remove bone flap and dissect across midline under direct visualization, second bone flap crossing midline to left, hemostasis of SSS with bipolar cauterization and gelfoam, tack up dural stitches, U-shaped dural opening based on SSS, detach tumor from falx, debulk tumor medially, identify lateral brain-tumor interface with microscope, incise falx after tumor removal beyond inferior attachment point, dural closure with pericranium and collagen sponge or fibrin glue, bone cement to fill in gaps and sand bone, irrigate with Betadine and place vancomycin in subgaleal space, closure with subgaleal drain	Meticulous positioning, coronal incision, burr hole on left edge of SSS, clear dura off of bone, rectangular craniotomy that is longer anterior to posterior as compared to laterally (approximately 2 cm width), dural opening based on SSS with preservation of veins, dissect down falx, open falx circumferentially around tumor, meticulous microscopic and endoscopic dissection, remove tumor	Right frontal craniotomy up to sagittal sinus, dural flap based on midline, approach the falx with preservation of draining veins, coagulation and cutting of dural base of tumor, debulk with ultrasonic aspirator
Complication avoidance	Preservation of draining veins, devascularize tumor early, avoid fixed retractors	Two piece craniotomy to cross SSS, detach early from falx, resect falx after tumor removal	Work from contralateral side, open falx circumferentially around tumor, microscope and endoscopic dissection and resection	Craniotomy up to sagittal sinus, preservation of draining veins, early coagulation of arterial feeders
Sinus repair if necessary	Compression, then muscle, then dural or periosteal flap position	Should not happen, direct pressure if roof of SSS, sutured closing if bleeding from lateral recess	Avoid craniotomy over sinus, otherwise tack up or cover with dural flap	Gelfoam and fibrin glue, periosteal patch, fascial patch, direct reconstruction
Postoperative				
Admission	ICU	ICU	ICU	ICU
Postoperative complications feared	Vascular injury to superior sagittal sinus, cortical veins or cortex, venous stroke	Seizures, SMA syndrome, venous infarct	Right cortical injury, delirium	Venous injury, increasing motor deficit

	Victor Garcia-Navarro, MD, Tec de Monterrey Institute, Campus Guadalajara, Mexico	Michael W. McDermott, MD, Herbert Wertheim College of Medicine, Florida International University, Miami, FL, United States	Peter Nakaji, MD, Barrow Neurological Institute, Phoenix, AZ, United States	Tony Van Havenbergh, MD, PhD, GasthuisZusters Antwerpen, Antwerpen, Belgium
Follow-up testing	CTA within 24 hours after surgery MRI within 72 hours after surgery	MRI within 48 hours after surgery	MRI within 48 hours after surgery Physical, occupational, speech therapy	CT within 24 hours after surgery MRI within 3 days after surgery
Follow-up visits	7–10 days after surgery	10–14 days after surgery 6–8 weeks after surgery	10–14 days after surgery	4 weeks after surgery
Adjuvant therapies recommended for WHO grade	Grade I–observation Grade II–observation Grade III–radiation	Grade I–observation Grade II–radiation Grade III–radiation	Grade I–observation Grade II–observation Grade III–radiation	Grade I–observation Grade II–radiation Grade III–radiation

ACA, anterior cerebral artery; CT, computed tomography; CTA, computed tomography angiography; DTI, diffusion tensor imaging; ICU, intensive care unit; IOM, intraoperative monitoring; MEP, motor evoked potential; MRI, magnetic resonance imaging; MRV, magnetic resonance venography; SMA, supplementary motor area; SSEP, somatosensory evoked potential; SSS, superior sagittal sinus.

Differential diagnosis and actual diagnosis

- Meningioma
- Hemangiopericytoma
- Metastatic brain cancer
- Lymphoma

Important anatomic and preoperative considerations

For a full detailed description of the sagittal sinus see Chapter 45. The falx cerebri is the largest structure of the intracranial dura that separates the cerebral hemispheres.[8] It is actually a double-fold of dura that resides in the interhemispheric fissure between the two hemispheres.[8] It attaches to the crista galli anteriorly and inferiorly, the midline of the cranium superiorly, and the superior surface of the tentorium cerebelli posteriorly and inferiorly.[8] The superior margin of the falx contacts the superior sagittal sinus, and the inferior margin contacts the inferior sagittal sinus and the superior surface of the corpus callosum.[8] The straight sinus resides between the attachment between the falx and the tentorium.[8] The structure of the falx is typically conserved with the rare exception of congenital disorders, such as holoprosencephaly.[8]

Approaches to this lesion

The options for meningiomas include observation, radiation therapy, and/or surgical resection. In this case, the lesion is large with symptomatic mass effect with left lower extremity weakness and has had progressive growth on serial imaging. For small, asymptomatic tumors, these lesions can be watched with serial imaging to evaluate if there is progressive growth, as many lesions will not display progressive growth.[9] Although the use of radiation therapy, including fractioned radiation and stereotactic radiosurgery, has typically been reserved for recurrent or partially resected lesions,[5,10,11] radiation therapy can also

be used in lieu of surgery for smaller tumors in difficult to access regions that demonstrate progressive growth and/or patients who are poor surgical candidates.[5,10,11] When surgical resection is pursued, the goal is to achieve a Simpson grade I resection, with gross total resection of the tumor and removal of the involved dura and bone (Chapter 45, Fig. 45.2).[1–5]

What was actually done

The patient was taken to surgery for a right parietal craniotomy for resection of the right paracentral parafalcine meningioma with intraoperative motor evoked potentials, somatosensory evoked potentials, and electroencephalogram. The patient was induced and intubated per routine. The head was fixed in pins, with two pins over the left external auditory meatus and one pin over the right external auditory meatus. The patient was placed supine with the neck flexed in neutral position. A linear incision was then made over the center of the lesion in the coronal plane that was eccentric to the right. The patient was draped in the usual standard fashion and given dexamethasone, levetiracetam, and cefazolin. The incision was made, and the flap was retracted with a cerebellar retractor. The location of the sagittal sinus was confirmed with navigation and was 5 mm to the left of the sagittal suture. Two burr holes were placed on the ipsilateral side of the tumor at the anterior and posterior tumor margins, and two burr holes beyond the lateral margin of the tumor. The excess burr holes were used because of the poor quality of the dura. The craniotome was used to perform a right parietal bone flap that remained just ipsilateral to the sagittal sinus. The dura overlying the sagittal sinus was dissected from the overlying bone, and the bone was removed with a high-speed drill to expose the right half of the sagittal sinus to facilitate dural opening. The dura was opened in a semicircular fashion with the base along the sagittal sinus. A large draining vein was identified over the center of the tumor and was preserved. The surgical microscope was brought in for the remainder of the case. The interhemispheric fissure was dissected anterior

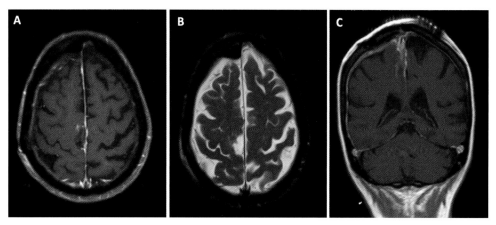

Fig. 47.2 **Postoperative magnetic resonance imaging. (A)** T1 axial image with gadolinium contrast; **(B)** T2 axial image; **(C)** T1 coronal image with gadolinium contrast magnetic resonance imaging scan demonstrating gross total resection of the right parafalcine meningioma with removal of the involved falx.

and posterior to the vein. The superficial aspect of the tumor was dissected from the cortex and protected with cottonoids. The tumor was cauterized and separated from the falx. The tumor was removed by alternating between tumor debulking with the ultrasonic aspirator and capsule dissection. Preliminary pathology was a meningioma. Both leaves of the falx where the tumor was attached to were removed to expose the contralateral side. The dura, bone, and skin were closed in standard fashion.

The patient awoke at their neurologic baseline with intact strength with improved left lower extremity strength and was taken to the intensive care unit for recovery. Magnetic resonance imaging was done within 48 hours after surgery and showed gross total resection with Simpson grade I resection (Chapter 41, Fig. 41.2) in which the falx was removed (Fig. 47.2). The patient participated with physical and occupational therapy and was discharged to home on postoperative day 3 with intact strength. The patient was prescribed dexamethasone that was tapered to off over 3 days after surgery, and levetiracetam for 7 days. The patient was seen at 2 weeks postoperatively for staple removal and was neurologically intact. Pathology was a World Health Organization (WHO) grade I meningioma. The lesion was observed with serial magnetic resonance imaging examinations at 3- and 6-month intervals and has been without recurrence for 36 months.

Commonalities among the experts

Half of the surgeons opted for cardiology evaluation for preoperative risk assessment prior to surgery. All surgeons elected for surgery, in which the majority would perform a right frontoparietal craniotomy for an ipsilateral interhemispheric approach, whereas the remaining would perform a left frontoparietal craniotomy for a contralateral interhemispheric approach. The general goal varied from Simpson grade I to II resection. All surgeons were concerned about the superior sagittal sinus and draining veins, and half were concerned about the motor cortex. The most feared complications were venous infarct from injury to the superior sagittal sinus and/or draining veins, as well as brain retraction injury. Surgery was generally

pursued with surgical navigation, surgical microscope, and ultrasonic aspirator with perioperative mannitol, steroids, and antiepileptics. Most surgeons advocated for control of the superior sagittal sinus with bilateral opening and early devascularity of the lesion. If venous injury occurred, the treatment algorithm included compression, direct suture repair, and/or patch with pericranium or folding the dura over. Following surgery, all surgeons admitted their patients to the intensive care unit, and most surgeons requested imaging within 72 hours after surgery to assess for extent of resection and/or potential complications. Most surgeons advocated for observation for residual WHO grade I meningiomas, radiation versus observation for residual WHO grade II meningiomas, and radiation for all WHO grade III meningiomas.

SUMMARY OF QUALITY OF EVIDENCE TO GUIDE SPECIFIC INTERVENTIONS FOR THIS CASE

- Removal of involved falx to achieve Simpson grade I resection—Class II-3.

REFERENCES

1. Ehresman JS, Mampre D, Rogers D, Olivi A, Quinones-Hinojosa A, Chaichana KL. Volumetric tumor growth rates of meningiomas involving the intracranial venous sinuses. *Acta Neurochir (Wien)*. 2018;160:1531–1538.
2. DiMeco F, Li KW, Casali C, et al. Meningiomas invading the superior sagittal sinus: surgical experience in 108 cases. *Neurosurgery*. 2004;55:1263–1272; discussion 1272–1274.
3. Jusue-Torres I, Navarro-Ramirez R, Gallego MP, Chaichana KL, Quinones-Hinojosa A. Indocyanine green for vessel identification and preservation before dural opening for parasagittal lesions. *Neurosurgery*. 2013;73; ons145; discussion ons145.
4. Ricci A, Di Vitantonio H, De Paulis D, et al. Parasagittal meningiomas: our surgical experience and the reconstruction technique of the superior sagittal sinus. *Surg Neurol Int*. 2017;8:1.
5. Kondziolka D, Flickinger JC, Perez B. Judicious resection and/or radiosurgery for parasagittal meningiomas: outcomes from a multicenter review. Gamma Knife Meningioma Study Group. *Neurosurgery*. 1998;43:405–413; discussion 413–414.

6. Bi WL, Zhang M, Wu WW, Mei Y, Dunn IF. Meningioma genomics: diagnostic, prognostic, and therapeutic applications. *Front Surg*. 2016;3:40.
7. Kong X, Gong S, Lee IT, Yang Y. Microsurgical treatment of parafalcine meningiomas: a retrospective study of 126 cases. *Onco Targets Ther*. 2018;11:5279–5285.
8. Rhoton AL Jr. The cerebrum. Anatomy. *Neurosurgery*. 2007;61:37–118; discussion 118–119.
9. Fountain DM, Soon WC, Matys T, Guilfoyle MR, Kirollos R, Santarius T. Volumetric growth rates of meningioma and its correlation with histological diagnosis and clinical outcome: a systematic review. *Acta Neurochir (Wien)*. 2017;159:435–445.
10. Barbaro NM, Gutin PH, Wilson CB, Sheline GE, Boldrey EB, Wara WM. Radiation therapy in the treatment of partially resected meningiomas. *Neurosurgery*. 1987;20:525–528.
11. Sughrue ME, Rutkowski MJ, Shangari G, Parsa AT, Berger MS, McDermott MW. Results with judicious modern neurosurgical management of parasagittal and falcine meningiomas. Clinical article. *J Neurosurg*. 2011;114:731–737.

48

Medial sphenoid wing meningioma

Case reviewed by Gerardo Guinto, Rodrigo Ramos-Zúñiga, Shaan M. Raza, Harry Van Loveren

Introduction

Meningiomas are relatively common neoplasms that arise from arachnoid cap cells and account for approximately 20% to 30% of all primary intracranial tumors.[1-3] Of all meningiomas, approximately 15% to 20% occur along the sphenoid wing that places them at a complex anatomic location, involving the optic nerve, cavernous sinus, and internal carotid and middle cerebral arteries.[4,5] Medial, as compared with middle and lateral, sphenoid wing meningiomas are closer to critical parasellar neurovascular structures, including the optic nerve, internal carotid artery (ICA), middle cerebral artery, and cavernous sinus, and surgery in these regions is associated with significant morbidity including vision loss, cerebral ischemia, and diplopia, among others.[5-8] Complication rates range from 20% to 40% (vision loss varies from 20%–30%), with gross total resections as low as 60% in several series.[6-8] In this chapter, we present a case of a dominant hemisphere medial sphenoid wing meningioma.

Example case

Chief complaint: left eye vision loss
History of present illness
A 33-year-old, right-handed woman with no significant past medical history presented with progressive left eye vision loss. For the past 5 to 6 months, she developed difficulty with seeing and has tried different glasses without improvement. She saw her optometrist who noted left optic nerve atrophy, and visual field testing revealed diminished vision in all quadrants in her left eye. Imaging was done (Fig. 48.1).
Medications: None.
Allergies: No known drug allergies.
Past medical and surgical history: C-section.
Family history: No history of intracranial malignancies.
Social history: Secretary, no smoking or alcohol.
Physical examination: Awake, alert, oriented to person, place, and time; Cranial nerves II to XII intact except only counting fingers in left eye; No drift, moves all extremities with full strength.

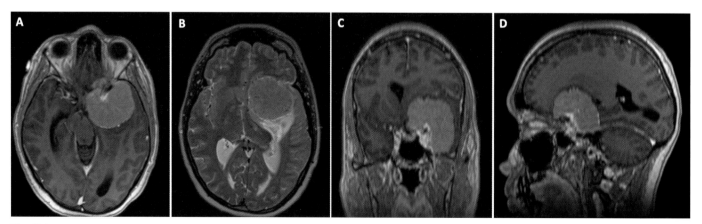

Fig. 48.1 Preoperative magnetic resonance imaging. (A) T1 axial image with gadolinium contrast; **(B)** T2 axial image; **(C)** T1 coronal image with gadolinium contrast; **(D)** T1 sagittal image with gadolinium contrast magnetic resonance imaging scan demonstrating an enhancing lesion involving the left medial sphenoid wing with encasement of the internal carotid artery.

	Gerardo Guinto, MD, Centro Neurologico ABC, Mexico City, Mexico	Rodrigo Ramos-Zúñiga, MD, PhD, University of Guadalajara, Guadalajara, Jalisco, Mexico	Shaan M. Raza, MD, Anderson Cancer Center, Houston, TX, United States	Harry Van Loveren, MD, University of South Florida, Tampa, FL, United States
Preoperative				
Additional tests requested	CT and CTA Neuropsychological assessment	MR angiography DTI Neuropsychological assessment	Neuroophthalmology evaluation MRA or CTA	Cerebral angiogram Neuroophthalmology evaluation
Surgical approach selected	Left pterional orbitozygomatic craniotomy	Left pterional orbitozygomatic craniotomy, anterior clinoidectomy	Left modified orbitozygomatic craniotomy, anterior clinoidectomy	Left frontotemporal craniotomy, orbitozygomatic osteotomy, posterior orbitotomy, anterior clinoidectomy
Anatomic corridor	Left trans-Sylvian	Left frontotemporal	Left trans-Sylvian	Left trans-Sylvian
Goal of surgery	Simpson grade II	Simpson grade II, decompression of optic apparatus, restoration of ICA flow	Simpson grade II because of being type I clinoidal meningioma, decompression of optic apparatus	Simpson grade I pending intraoperative evaluation
Perioperative				
Positioning	Left supine with 35 degree rotation to right	Left supine with slight right rotation	Left supine and right 30 degree rotation	Supine with right rotation
Surgical equipment	Surgical navigation Ultrasonic aspirator Reciprocating saw	Surgical microscope Ultrasonic aspirator	IOM (SSEP/EEG) Reciprocating saw Surgical microscope Ultrasonic aspirator	Surgical navigation Surgical microscope Micro Doppler Ultrasonic aspirator
Medications	Steroids Antiepileptics	Steroids Antiepileptics	Steroids Mannitol Antiepileptics	Steroids Antiepileptics Mannitol
Anatomic considerations	Orbit, anterior clinoid, cavernous sinus, ICA, MCA, frontal and temporal lobes	Optic canal, sphenoid wing, anterior clinoid, optic nerve and chiasm, cavernous sinus, ICA/ACA/ACOM and perforators	ICA, ophthalmic artery, PCOM, AChA, A1, M1, left optic nerve, optic chiasm, optic tract	ICA, MCA, ophthalmic artery, optic nerve and chiasms, hypothalamus, pituitary stalk, midbrain and cerebral peduncle, cranial nerves III/IV/VI, lateral cavernous sinus, superior orbital fissure
Complications feared with approach chosen	Injury to ICA and MCA, cavernous sinus, cerebral edema, seizures	Cranial neuropathy, optic nerve damage, neuroendocrine dysfunction	Injury to optic apparatus and vasculature	Retraction injury, stroke, brainstem injury, visual compromise
Intraoperative				
Anesthesia	General	General	General	General
Skin incision	Left pterional	Left pterional	Left pterional	Left frontotemporal
Bone opening	Left frontotemporal and orbit	Left frontotemporal and orbit	Left frontotemporal and orbit	Left frontotemporal and orbit, anterior clinoid, optic roof
Brain exposure	Left frontotemporal	Left frontotemporal	Left frontotemporal	Left frontotemporal

(continued on next page)

	Gerardo Guinto, MD, Centro Neurologico ABC, Mexico City, Mexico	Rodrigo Ramos-Zúñiga, MD, PhD, University of Guadalajara, Guadalajara, Jalisco, Mexico	Shaan M. Raza, MD, Anderson Cancer Center, Houston, TX, United States	Harry Van Loveren, MD, University of South Florida, Tampa, FL, United States
Method of resection	Frontotemporal skin flap with preservation of anterior branch of STA, subfascial temporalis opening to preserve frontalis nerve, frontotemporal craniotomy, orbitozygomatic osteotomy from supraorbital notch to posterior roof of orbit to lateral wall reaching inferior orbital fissure with an osteotomy in an inverted V-shape of the malar bone and osteotomy of zygoma, drilling of sphenoid ridge and anterior clinoidectomy to completely expose optic nerve, open dura, Sylvian fissure opening, begin tumor debulking, identify ICA and MCA and optic nerve early, dissect these areas from the tumor, if tumor stuck to these critical structures leave small fragments behind, make sure optic nerve completely free of tumor, debulk tumor until lateral cavernous sinus wall exposed with low voltage bipolar coagulation, removal of dura in contact with tumor and pericranium reconstruction	Left frontotemporal flap with preservation of STA, frontotemporal craniotomy, orbitozygomatic extension, extradural anterior clinoidectomy, open dura, intratumoral decompression, decompression of optic canal and nerve, leave cavernous sinus component alone, coagulation of skull base dura, closure with subgaleal drain	Left pterional incision to contralateral midpupillary line, preservation of pericranium, subfascial dissection to expose frontozygomatic process, pericranium and superficial temporalis fascia reflected anteriorly, temporalis reflected toward zygomatic arch, MacCarty keyhole, one-piece modified orbitozygomatic craniotomy, orbital osteotomy superior to IOF, drill sphenoid wing down to SOF, extradural clinoidectomy to unroof cavernous sinus and gain proximal control of ICA, unroof optic canal 270 degrees, open dura posterior to anterior along Sylvian fissure with T with one limb along SOF and other along optic canal, Sylvian fissure opening distal to where tumor involves vasculature, identify A1/AChA/ACOM, open dura of optic canal, trace optic nerve to chiasm and optic tract, resect tumor until plane until arachnoidal plane disappears likely near distal dural ring, papaverine soaked gelfoam laid over exposed vasculature, inspect anterior clinoid for communication with sphenoid sinus, close dura and use temporalis fascia to create subdural-epidural inlay-onlay along dural defect along optic canal and anterior clinoid followed by free pericranial graft along skull base, bolster closure with fibrin flue, titanium mesh to reconstruct sphenoid wing	Left frontotemporal flap, subfascial dissection to preserve frontalis nerve, MacCarty burr hole, frontotemporal craniotomy, zygomatic root cut anteriorly and posteriorly and left attached to masseter fascia, supraorbital nerve mobilized, orbitozygomatic osteotomy with mallet and chisel in one-piece with cut across medial supraorbital ridge/zygomaticofacial process near foramen/along the sphenoid from the burr hole to the IOF/across orbital roof with osteotome and mallet, sphenoid ridge is reduced, posterior orbitotomy with partial resection of the lateral orbital wall under microscopic visualization, optic canal is unroofed, extradural anterior clinoidectomy, Dolenc dural opening along Sylvian fissure, Sylvian fissure is opened, tumor debulked internally with ultrasonic aspirator, capsule mobilized from brain interface, circumferentially remove dura around lesion if possible to devascularize tumor, identify ipsilateral optic nerve then chiasm then contralateral optic nerve, tumor dissection to follow posteriorly to identify MCA and branches, once enough tumor is removed then dissect from cavernous sinus from front to back from SOF and bottom to top from foramen rotundum and ovale, dura cut along oculomotor nerve and removed along lateral wall of cavernous sinus, area inspected for residual, leave small remnants if cannot be dissected safely from neurovascular structures, fat graft if anterior clinoid cannot be repaired, synthetic orbital roof if necessary

	Gerardo Guinto, MD, Centro Neurologico ABC, Mexico City, Mexico	Rodrigo Ramos-Zúñiga, MD, PhD, University of Guadalajara, Guadalajara, Jalisco, Mexico	Shaan M. Raza, MD, Anderson Cancer Center, Houston, TX, United States	Harry Van Loveren, MD, University of South Florida, Tampa, FL, United States
Complication avoidance	Orbitozygomatic craniotomy, Sylvian fissure opening, identification of ICA/MCA/optic nerve early, leave small amounts of tumor if adherent to vessels	Orbitozygomatic craniotomy, extradural clinoidectomy, intratumoral decompression, optic canal decompression	Modified orbitozygomatic craniotomy, extradural anterior clinoidectomy, optic canal decompression, trace vasculature, recognition that the arachnoid plane between the tumor and the ICA may disappear near the clinoidal ring and limit the resection	Orbitozygomatic craniotomy, extradural clinoidectomy, intratumoral decompression, early identification of vessels, synthetic orbital roof to minimize enophthalmos
Postoperative				
Admission	ICU	ICU	Intermediate care	ICU
Postoperative complications feared	MCA stroke, CSF leak, inadvertent opening of paranasal sinuses	Optic nerve injury, cavernous cranial nerve injury, vascular damage, cerebral edema	Optic apparatus injury, vasospasm, CSF leak, seizures	Retraction injury, cerebral edema, stroke, visual loss, CSF leak
Follow-up testing	CT within 6–8 hours after surgery MRI 6 weeks after surgery EEG 2 years after surgery Neuropsychological	CT within 12 hours after surgery MRI within 24 hours after surgery	MRI within 48 hours after surgery Neuroophthalmology evaluation 2–4 weeks after surgery	CT same day after surgery MRI within 24 hours after surgery
Follow-up visits	6 weeks after surgery	1 month after surgery	10–14 days after surgery	10–14 days after surgery 6 weeks after surgery
Adjuvant therapies recommended for WHO grade	Grade I–observation Grade II–observation Grade III–radiation	Grade I–observation Grade II–observation Grade III–radiation	Grade I–observation Grade II–radiation if residual Grade III–radiation	Grade I–observation Grade II–radiation for residual Grade III–radiation

ACA, anterior cerebral artery; AChA, anterior choroidal artery; ACOM, anterior communicating artery; CSF, cerebrospinal fluid; CT, computed tomography; CTA, computed tomography angiography; DTI, diffusion tensor imaging; EEG, electroencephalogram; ICA, internal carotid artery; ICU, intensive care unit; IOF, inferior orbital fissure; IOM, intraoperative monitoring; MCA, middle cerebral artery; MR, magnetic resonance; MRA, magnetic resonance angiography; MRI, magnetic resonance imaging; PCOM, posterior communicating artery; SOF, superior orbital fissure; SSEP, somatosensory evoked potential; STA, superficial temporal artery.

Differential diagnosis and actual diagnosis

- Meningioma
- Hemangiopericytoma
- Metastatic brain cancer
- Lymphoma

Important anatomic and preoperative considerations

The sphenoid bone appears as bat wings when looked at anteriorly or posteriorly.[9,10] It can be divided into a middle portion consisting of the sphenoid body that contains the sella turcica and the sphenoid sinus; lateral portion consisting of greater and lesser sphenoid wings that are lateral to and anterior to the middle sphenoid portion, respectively; and an inferior portion consisting of pterygoid processes that project downward from the junction of the sphenoid body and greater sphenoid wings.[9,10] The greater sphenoid wing forms the anterior and lateral surface of the middle cranial fossa and possesses the foramen rotundum, foramen ovale, and foramen spinosum, as well as the posterior wall of the orbit.[9,10] The lesser sphenoid wing is triangular in shape that projects laterally from the anterosuperior part of the sphenoid body and consists of a base forming the medial end of the wing, a tip forming the lateral end of the wing, a superior surface forming the floor of the anterior cranial fossa, an inferior surface forming the upper boundary of the superior orbital fissure, a posterior surface that projects into the Sylvian fissure, and a medial surface that terminates in the anterior clinoid process.[9,10] The foramina and fissures within the greater and lesser sphenoid wings include the superior orbital fissure (oculomotor nerve, trochlear nerve, lacrimal/frontal/nasociliary branches of the ophthalmic, abducens, superior and inferior ophthalmic veins, sympathetic fibers of the cavernous plexus), foramen rotundum (maxillary nerve), foramen ovale (mandibular nerve), and foramen spinosum (middle meningeal artery).[9,10]

Sphenoid wing meningiomas can be divided into three groups based on the site of origin: medial third (or clinoidal), middle third, and lateral third.[11] Clinoidal meningiomas can be further divided into three subgroups based on its relationship with the ICA as it emerges from the cavernous sinus inferior and medial to the anterior clinoid process and passes between the inner and outer dural rings.[11] Group 1 clinoidal meningiomas arise from around the point where the carotid exits the distal dural ring, and therefore these tumors typically engulf the ICA, grow distally toward the ICA bifurcation, and encase the proximal middle cerebral artery.[11] In addition, because this area lacks arachnoid, these tumors typically are densely adherent to the ICA, invade the cavernous sinus, and also typically involve the optic nerve and chiasm.[11] Group 2 clinoidal meningiomas arise from the superior and lateral aspects of the anterior clinoid dura.[11] Unlike group 1 meningiomas, group 2 meningiomas typically have arachnoidal planes even though they also engulf the ICA, involve the optic nerve and chiasm, and invade the cavernous sinus.[11] Group 3 clinoidal meningiomas arise from the optic foramen and extend into the optic canal.[11] Middle and lateral sphenoid wing meningiomas are farther away from critical neurovascular structures, and therefore can reach large sizes before being diagnosed.[11]

Approaches to this lesion

As discussed in Chapter 41, options for meningiomas include observation, radiation therapy, and/or surgical resection. In this case, the lesion is large with symptomatic mass effect with progressive vision loss. Observation and radiation would not be recommended because of the progressive symptoms, involvement of the optic nerve, and large size of the tumor.[12–14] There are a variety of surgical approaches for clinoidal meningiomas, and include frontotemporal/pterional, frontotemporal-orbitozygomatic, and supra-orbital-pterional approaches, among others.[15] The frontotemporal or pterional approach is the conventional approach, whereas the orbitozygomatic involves removing the orbital rim and roof, thereby increasing the superior/inferior working angle.[15] The potential benefit of this is potentially less brain retraction, but is associated with periorbital swelling and possible enophthalmos.[15] In regard to approaching the tumor, the options include subfrontal, trans-Sylvian, and/or subtemporal approaches. The subfrontal approach will allow early identification of the optic nerve and ICA, but has a longer working corridor, as well as difficulty in visualizing the lateral portion of the tumor in the middle fossa and the portion of the tumor in the Sylvian fissure. The trans-Sylvian approach allows for early identification of critical vessels, but could potentially lead to vascular injury of the middle cerebral artery (MCA) and its branches, as well as Sylvian veins. The subtemporal approach allows for a shorter working distance to the superficial aspect of the tumor but makes it challenging to visualize the medial part of the tumor around the parasellar region.

What was actually done

The patient was taken to surgery for a left pterional craniotomy for trans-Sylvian resection of the medial sphenoid wing/clinoidal meningioma with intraoperative motor evoked potentials, somatosensory evoked potentials, and

electroencephalogram. The patient was induced and intubated per routine. The head was fixed in pins, with two pins over the inion and one pin over the right forehead in the midpupillary line. The patient's head was turned 15 degrees to the right, and the head was extended to allow the frontal lobe to retract from the anterior cranial fossa with gravity. A pterional incision was planned based on surgical navigation. The patient was draped in the usual standard fashion and given dexamethasone, levetiracetam, and cefazolin. The incision was made, and the myocutaneous flap was retracted anteriorly with fishhooks attached to a retractor arm. Two burr holes were placed (one at the temporal floor and one at the pterion), and a pterional bone flap that extended medially over the orbit up to the lateral edge of the frontal sinus was made. The sphenoid wing was drilled down so that the anterior and middle fossa were continuous. The anterior clinoid was removed extradurally, and the optic strut was drilled down to provide 270 degree of optic nerve decompression. The dura was then opened in a semicircular fashion and tacked up with sutures. The microscope was brought in for the remainder of the intradural portion of the case. The Sylvian fissure was opened with sharp dissection to identify the MCA and its branches, ICA terminus, and optic nerve. The tumor was removed with several alternating rounds of internal debulking and capsular dissection. At the most medial aspect of the tumor, it was adherent to the ICA, as well as the lateral lenticulostriate vessels of the MCA. Therefore this tumor was left behind. Preliminary pathology was a meningioma. The dura, bone, and skin were closed in standard fashion.

The patient awoke at their neurologic baseline with intact strength with improved left eye vision and was taken to the intensive care unit for recovery. Magnetic resonance imaging was done within 48 hours after surgery and showed near total resection (Simpson grade IV) (Chapter 41, Fig. 41.2) with expected residual medially near the ICA terminus (Fig. 48.2). The patient participated with physical and occupational therapy and was discharged to home on postoperative day 3 with intact strength and improved left eye vision. The patient was prescribed dexamethasone that was tapered to off over 7 days after surgery, and levetiracetam for 7 days. The patient was seen at 2 weeks postoperatively for staple removal and was neurologically intact with improved left eye vision in which she was able to read. Pathology was a World Health Organization (WHO) grade I meningioma. The lesion was observed with serial magnetic resonance imaging examinations at 3- and 6-month intervals and has been without recurrence for 18 months with nearly intact left eye vision.

Commonalities among the experts

All surgeons opted for the patient to undergo vascular imaging to better characterize the vessels within and around the lesion, and half opted for neuropsychological evaluation and formal ophthalmology evaluation prior to surgery. All surgeons elected for surgery, in which all would perform a left orbitozygomatic craniotomy and a frontotemporal or trans-Sylvian approach. The majority of surgeons also elected to perform an extradural anterior clinoidectomy. The majority aimed for a Simpson grade II resection. All surgeons were concerned about the optic nerve/chiasm/tract and major intracranial arteries, including the ICA, ACA, anterior communicating,

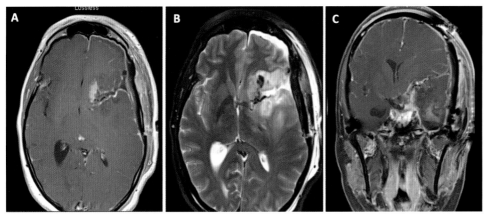

Fig. 48.2 **Postoperative magnetic resonance imaging. (A)** T1 axial image with gadolinium contrast; **(B)** T2 axial image; **(C)** T1 coronal image with gadolinium contrast magnetic resonance imaging scan demonstrating near total resection of the left medial sphenoid wing meningioma with small residual along the internal carotid artery.

posterior communicating, and perforating vessels. The majority of surgeons feared visual compromise, cranial neuropathy, and arterial vascular injury. Surgery was generally pursued with surgical navigation, surgical microscope, and ultrasonic aspirator with perioperative steroids and antiepileptics. All surgeons advocated for orbitozygomatic craniotomy to minimize brain manipulation, and most advocated for an anterior clinoidectomy and optic nerve decompression, internal debulking, and leaving remnants on critical vessels and nerves if adherent. Following surgery, all surgeons admitted their patients to the intensive care unit and requested imaging within 48 hours after surgery to assess for extent of resection and/or potential complications. Most surgeons advocated for observation for residual WHO grade I meningiomas, radiation versus observation for residual WHO grade II meningiomas, and radiation for all WHO grade III meningiomas.

SUMMARY OF QUALITY OF EVIDENCE TO GUIDE SPECIFIC INTERVENTIONS FOR THIS CASE

- Meningioma resection with visual decline as compared with radiation therapy—Class III.

REFERENCES

1. Bondy M, Ligon BL. Epidemiology and etiology of intracranial meningiomas: a review. *J Neurooncol.* 1996;29:197–205.
2. Claus EB, Bondy ML, Schildkraut JM, Wiemels JL, Wrensch M, Black PM. Epidemiology of intracranial meningioma. *Neurosurgery.* 2005;57:1088–1095.
3. Surawicz TS, McCarthy BJ, Kupelian V, Jukich PJ, Bruner JM, Davis FG. Descriptive epidemiology of primary brain and CNS tumors: results from the Central Brain Tumor Registry of the United States, 1990-1994. *Neuro Oncol.* 1999;1:14–25.
4. Cushing H, Eisenhardt L. *Meningiomas: Their Classification, Regional Behaviour, Life, History, and Surgical End Results.* Springfield, IL: Charles C. Thomas; 1938.
5. Chaichana KL, Jackson C, Patel A, et al. Predictors of visual outcome following surgical resection of medial sphenoid wing meningiomas. *J Neurol Surg B Skull Base.* 2012;73:321–326.
6. Nakamura M, Roser F, Jacobs C, Vorkapic P, Samii M. Medial sphenoid wing meningiomas: clinical outcome and recurrence rate. *Neurosurgery.* 2006;58:626–639.
7. Sughrue ME, Rutkowski MJ, Chen CJ, et al. Modern surgical outcomes following surgery for sphenoid wing meningiomas. *J Neurosurg.* 2013;119:86–93.
8. Verma SK, Sinha S, Sawarkar DP, et al. Medial sphenoid wing meningiomas: experience with microsurgical resection over 5 years and a review of literature. *Neurol India.* 2016;64:465–475.
9. Costea C, Turliuc S, Cucu A, et al. The "polymorphous" history of a polymorphous skull bone: the sphenoid. *Anat Sci Int.* 2018;93:14–22.
10. Jacquesson T, Mertens P, Berhouma M, Jouanneau E, Simon E. The 360 photography: a new anatomical insight of the sphenoid bone. Interest for anatomy teaching and skull base surgery. *Surg Radiol Anat.* 2017;39:17–22.
11. Al-Mefty O. Clinoidal meningiomas. *J Neurosurg.* 1990;73:840–849.
12. Barbaro NM, Gutin PH, Wilson CB, Sheline GE, Boldrey EB, Wara WM. Radiation therapy in the treatment of partially resected meningiomas. *Neurosurgery.* 1987;20:525–528.
13. Kondziolka D, Flickinger JC, Perez B. Judicious resection and/or radiosurgery for parasagittal meningiomas: outcomes from a multicenter review. Gamma Knife Meningioma Study Group. *Neurosurgery.* 1998;43:405–413; discussion 413–414.
14. Sughrue ME, Rutkowski MJ, Shangari G, Parsa AT, Berger MS, McDermott MW. Results with judicious modern neurosurgical management of parasagittal and falcine meningiomas. Clinical article. *J Neurosurg.* 2011;114:731–737.
15. Ruzevick J, Raza SM, Recinos PF, et al. Technical note: orbitozygomatic craniotomy using an ultrasonic osteotome for precise osteotomies. *Clin Neurol Neurosurg.* 2015;134:24–27.

49

Lateral sphenoid wing meningiomas

Case reviewed by Peter Nakaji, Kenji Ohata, Daniel M. Prevedello, Tony Van Havenbergh

Introduction

A common location (~20%) for meningiomas to occur is along the sphenoid wing.[1,2] The sphenoid wing extends from the anterior clinoid process medially to the pterional laterally, and can be divided into thirds in which meningiomas involving the medial third are referred to as clinoidal meningiomas, the middle third are referred to as middle sphenoid wing meningiomas, and the lateral third are referred to as lateral sphenoid wing meningiomas.[2-5] The distinction is important because even though these lesions all involve the sphenoid wing, they involve different neurovascular structures, and therefore have different potential morbidities.[2-5] Regardless, complication rates range from 20% to 40% for lesions with

sphenoid wing involvement.[3-5] In this chapter, we present a case of a dominant hemisphere lateral sphenoid wing meningioma.

Example case

Chief complaint: headaches

History of present illness

A 51-year-old, right-handed man with a history of hypertension, asthma, and diabetes presented with progressive headaches. For the past 3 to 4 months, he developed increasing frequency and severity of headaches that became unresponsive to pain medications. He denied any speaking problems, weakness, or visual difficulties. His primary care physician ordered a brain magnetic resonance imaging (MRI) scan (Fig. 49.1).

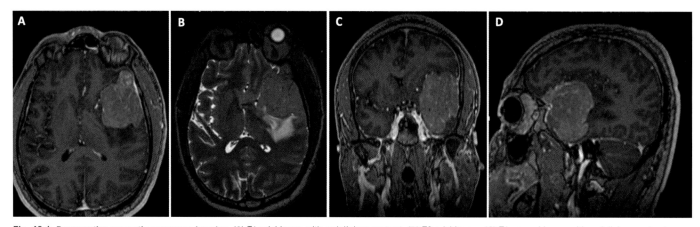

Fig. 49.1 Preoperative magnetic resonance imaging. (A) T1 axial image with gadolinium contrast; **(B)** T2 axial image; **(C)** T1 coronal image with gadolinium contrast; **(D)** T1 sagittal image with gadolinium contrast magnetic resonance imaging scan demonstrating an enhancing lesion involving the left lateral sphenoid wing.

Medications: Metoprolol, metformin, valsartan, budesonide.
Allergies: No known drug allergies.
Past medical and surgical history: Hypertension, asthma, and diabetes; femur and hand fracture.
Family history: No history of intracranial malignancies.

Social history: Insurance agent, no smoking, occasional alcohol.
Physical examination: Awake, alert, oriented to person, place, and time; Cranial nerves II to XII intact; No drift, moves all extremities with full strength.

	Peter Nakaji, MD, Barrow Neurological Institute, Phoenix, AZ, United States	Kenji Ohata, MD, PhD, Osaka City University, Osaka, Japan	Daniel M. Prevedello, MD, Ohio State University, Columbus, OH, United States	Tony Van Havenbergh, MD, PhD, GasthuisZusters Antwerpen, Antwerpen, Belgium
Preoperative				
Additional tests requested	Medicine evaluation	CT, CTA, CTB Angiogram	CTA Neuropsychological assessment Ophthalmology evaluation	Neuropsychological assessment
Surgical approach selected	Left mini-pterional craniotomy	Left frontotemporal craniotomy	Left frontotemporal craniotomy	Left frontotemporal craniotomy
Anatomic corridor	Left frontotemporal	Trans-Sylvian	Left frontotemporal	Left frontotemporal
Goal of surgery	Simpson grade I	Simpson grade I	Simpson grade I	Simpson grade I
Perioperative				
Positioning	Left supine with 45-degree right rotation	Left supine with 15-degree right rotation	Left supine with right head rotation	Left supine with 30-degree right rotation
Surgical equipment	Surgical navigation Surgical microscope Endoscope	Surgical navigation Surgical microscope Ultrasonic aspirator	Surgical navigation IOM (SSEP) Surgical microscope Ultrasonic aspirator	Surgical navigation IOM (EEG) Ultrasonic aspirator
Medications	Steroids	Antiepileptics	Steroids Antiepileptics Mannitol	Steroids Antiepileptics
Anatomic considerations	MCA, temporal and frontal cortex, Sylvian veins	MCA, Sylvian veins, superior orbital fissure	Orbit, MCA and branches, ICA, optic nerves, Broca area	Insular arteries, temporal cortex
Complications feared with approach chosen	MCA injury, damage to frontotemporal cortex, injury to Sylvian veins	Stroke, venous congestion	Language dysfunction, recurrence	Vascular injury, temporal cortex
Intraoperative				
Anesthesia	General	General	General	General
Skin incision	Pterional	Pterional	Pterional	Pterional
Bone opening	Left frontotemporal	Left frontotemporal	Left frontotemporal	Left frontotemporal
Brain exposure	Left frontotemporal	Left frontotemporal	Left frontotemporal	Left frontotemporal

(continued on next page)

	Peter Nakaji, MD, Barrow Neurological Institute, Phoenix, AZ, United States	Kenji Ohata, MD, PhD, Osaka City University, Osaka, Japan	Daniel M. Prevedello, MD, Ohio State University, Columbus, OH, United States	Tony Van Havenbergh, MD, PhD, GasthuisZusters Antwerpen, Antwerpen, Belgium
Method of resection	Incision centered over sphenoid wing with navigation, preserve STA and facial nerve branches, elevate galea, incise fascia, separate fascia from underlying muscle, split temporalis muscle along its fibers preserving innervation and blood supply, small craniotomy, drill sphenoid wing and frontotemporal bone flat past base of tumor, coagulate MMA and dura under tumor, open dura, internally debulk, microdissect tumor at all of its edges with frequent bed manipulation to allow surgeon visualization, endoscope visualization and resection for any difficult areas, resect involved dura, dural repair with dural substitute	Interfascial temporalis dissection, temporalis fascia pericranial vascularized flap, temporalis muscle turned posteroinferiorly, frontotemporal craniotomy, drill out sphenoid ridge to superior orbital fissure, coagulate MMA at foramen spinosum, dura peeled from SOF, U-shaped dural opening with incision in dura parallel to Sylvian fissure, removal of tumor around sphenoid ridge and caudal portion first, after debulking then dissect from brain surface, dissect tumor from MCA, remove dura from middle fossa as much as possible, reconstruct with pericranium	Left pterional incision, skin flap rotated anteriorly without muscle incision, subfascial incision and flap rotated anteriorly protecting frontal branch of facial nerve, left temporalis detached and rotated inferiorly, craniotomy based on navigation and exposing entire tumor base, MMA coagulated, dura is opened in the center of the tumor and tumor debulked, dura is opened around the lesion, Sylvian fissure is opened and ICA and MCA and branches are identified and protected under microscopic visualization, complete resection achieved, dura closed with allograft, insertion of subgaleal drain	Left frontotemporal craniotomy up to temporal base, dural incision around insertion zone of the tumor, dissection of arachnoidal plane at the surface of the tumor and cortex, internal debulking of tumor, dissect around tumor capsule, dural replacement with dural synthetic, drill out areas of hyperostosis if present
Complication avoidance	Bony opening past base of tumor, coagulate MMA and dural blood supply early, rolling/tilting patient to optimize visualization, endoscope to facilitate resection	Large bone opening, remove tumor from sphenoid ridge to allow tumor mobilization, dissect from MCA	Internal debulking of tumor early, Sylvian fissure opening to protect ICA and MCA	Dural incision around tumor edge, internal debulking, remove areas of bony involvement
Postoperative				
Admission	ICU	ICU	ICU	ICU
Postoperative complications feared	Speech dysfunction, motor deficit	Seizures, venous congestion, stroke	Pseudomeningocele, CSF leak, seizures, aphasia	Vascular injury, seizures, cerebral edema
Follow-up testing	MRI within 48 hours after surgery	CT immediately after surgery MRI 1 week after surgery	CT immediately after surgery MRI with DWI within 24 hours after surgery	MRI within 24 hours and 2 months after the surgery
Follow-up visits	10–14 days after surgery	3–6 months after surgery	14 days after surgery for staples 6 weeks after surgery for pathology	
Adjuvant therapies recommended for WHO grade	Grade I–observation Grade II–possible radiation Grade III–radiation	Grade I–observation Grade II–radiation Grade III–radiation	Grade I–observation Grade II–radiation if residual Grade III–radiation	Grade I–observation Grade II–radiation Grade III–radiation

CSF, cerebrospinal fluid; *CT*, computed tomography; *CTA*, computed tomography angiography; *CTB*, computed tomography of the brain; *DWI*, diffusion-weighted imaging; *EEG*, electroencephalogram; *ICA*, internal carotid artery; *ICU*, intensive care unit; *IOM*, intraoperative monitoring; *MCA*, middle cerebral artery; *MMA*, middle meningeal artery; *MRI*, magnetic resonance imaging; *SOF*, superior orbital fissure; *SSEP*, somatosensory evoked potentials; *STA*, superficial temporal artery.

Differential diagnosis and actual diagnosis

- Meningioma
- Hemangiopericytoma
- Metastatic brain cancer
- Lymphoma

Important anatomic and preoperative considerations

For a full description of the sphenoid bone, see Chapter 48. The greater sphenoid wing forms the anterior and lateral surface of the middle cranial fossa, as well as the posterior wall of the orbit.[6,7] The lesser sphenoid wing is triangular in shape that projects laterally from the anterosuperior part of the sphenoid body and consists of a medial surface that terminates in the anterior clinoid process.[6,7] The lateral sphenoid wing is the lateral third of the greater wing that is in proximity with the pterion, which makes lesions in this area come to the convexity surface.[6,7] Lateral and middle sphenoid wing meningiomas are generally considered more accessible than medial or clinoidal meningiomas because they are typically farther away from the parasellar structures, including the optic nerve, internal carotid artery, and cavernous sinus.[6,7] These lesions, however, may still extend to the clinoidal region and involve these structures, but are also associated with frequent bone involvement making Simpson grade I (Chapter 41, Fig. 41.2) resections challenging.

Approaches to this lesion

As discussed in Chapter 41, options for meningiomas include observation, radiation therapy, and/or surgical resection. In this case, the lesion is large with symptomatic mass effect with headaches. Observation and radiation would not be recommended because of the progressive symptoms and large size of the tumor.[8-10] There are a variety of surgical approaches for lateral sphenoid meningiomas, and include frontotemporal/pterional and frontotemporal-transzygomatic approaches, among others.[11] The frontotemporal or pterional approach is the conventional approach, whereas the transzygomatic approach involves performing osteotomies on the zygoma, thereby increasing the superior/inferior working angle from the temporal side.[11] The probable benefit of this is potentially less brain retraction, but can be associated with temporalis atrophy, temporomandibular joint pain, frontalis nerve injury, and double vision, among others.[11,12]

What was actually done

The patient was taken to surgery for a left pterional craniotomy for resection of the lateral sphenoid wing meningioma, with intraoperative motor evoked potentials, somatosensory evoked potentials, and electroencephalogram. The patient was induced and intubated per routine. The head was fixed in pins, with two pins over the inion and one pin over the right forehead in the midpupillary line. The patient's head was turned 60 degrees to the right, and a bump was placed under the left shoulder to facilitate turning. A pterional incision was planned based on surgical navigation. The patient was draped in the usual standard fashion and given dexamethasone, levetiracetam, and cefazolin. The incision was made, and the myocutaneous flap was retracted anteriorly with fishhooks attached to a retractor arm. Two burr holes were placed (one at the temporal floor and one at the pterion), and a pterional bone flap that extended medially over the orbit up to the lateral edge of the frontal sinus was made. The dura was then opened in a semicircular fashion, making sure to stay at the brain-tumor interface and tacked up with sutures. The tumor was cauterized and debulked internally to allow movement of the capsule. Alternating rounds of tumor debulking and capsular dissection was done until the tumor was removed. Preliminary pathology was a meningioma. The convexity dura was removed and replaced with a synthetic dural substitute. The dura, bone, and skin were closed in standard fashion.

The patient awoke at their neurologic baseline with intact strength and was taken to the intensive care unit for recovery. An MRI done within 48 hours after surgery showed gross total resection (Simpson grade I) (Fig. 49.2). The patient participated with physical and occupational therapy and was discharged to home on postoperative day 2 with

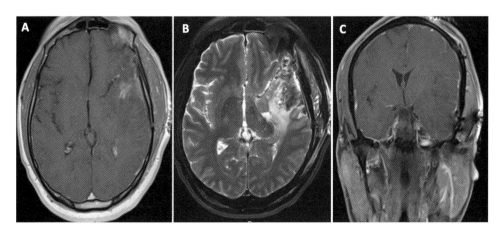

Fig. 49.2 Postoperative magnetic resonance imaging. (A) T1 axial image with gadolinium contrast; **(B)** T2 axial image; **(C)** T1 coronal image with gadolinium contrast magnetic resonance imaging scan demonstrating gross total resection of the left lateral sphenoid wing meningioma.

intact strength. The patient was prescribed dexamethasone that was tapered to off over 7 days after surgery, and levetiracetam for 7 days. The patient was seen at 2 weeks postoperatively for staple removal and was neurologically intact. Pathology was a World Health Organization (WHO) grade II atypical meningioma, and the patient underwent radiation therapy 1 month after surgery. The lesion was observed with serial MRI examinations at 3- and 6-months intervals and has been without recurrence for 36 months with an intact neurologic examination.

Commonalities among the experts

Half of the surgeons opted for the patient to undergo vascular imaging to better characterize the vessels within and around the lesion, and half opted for neuropsychological evaluation to determine baseline neurocognitive function prior to surgery. All surgeons elected for surgery, in which all would perform a left frontotemporal craniotomy and a frontotemporal approach. All surgeons aimed for a Simpson grade I resection. All surgeons were concerned about the middle cerebral artery (MCA) and its branches, and most were concerned about Sylvian veins. The majority of surgeons feared vascular injury to the MCA. Surgery was generally pursued with surgical navigation, surgical microscope, and ultrasonic aspirator with perioperative steroids and antiepileptics. The majority of surgeons advocated for large boney openings for exposure, early devascularization with coagulation of the dura and the middle meningeal artery, and internal debulking prior to dissecting from the MCA and its branches. Following surgery, all surgeons admitted their patients to the intensive care unit, and surgeons requested imaging within 48 hours after surgery to assess for extent of resection and/or potential complications. Most surgeons advocated for observation for residual WHO grade I meningiomas, radiation for residual WHO grade II meningiomas, and radiation for all WHO grade III meningiomas.

SUMMARY OF QUALITY OF EVIDENCE TO GUIDE SPECIFIC INTERVENTIONS FOR THIS CASE

- Meningioma resection with removal of dural attachment—Class III.
- Radiation therapy after atypical meningioma resection—Class III.

REFERENCES

1. Cushing H, Eisenhardt L. *Meningiomas: Their Classification, Regional Behaviour, Life, History, and Surgical End Results*. Springfield, IL: Charles C. Thomas; 1938.
2. Chaichana KL, Jackson C, Patel A, et al. Predictors of visual outcome following surgical resection of medial sphenoid wing meningiomas. *J Neurol Surg B Skull Base*. 2012;73:321–326.
3. Nakamura M, Roser F, Jacobs C, Vorkapic P, Samii M. Medial sphenoid wing meningiomas: clinical outcome and recurrence rate. *Neurosurgery*. 2006;58:626–639; discussion 626–639.
4. Sughrue ME, Rutkowski MJ, Chen CJ, et al. Modern surgical outcomes following surgery for sphenoid wing meningiomas. *J Neurosurg*. 2013;119:86–93.
5. Verma SK, Sinha S, Sawarkar DP, et al. Medial sphenoid wing meningiomas: experience with microsurgical resection over 5 years and a review of literature. *Neurol India*. 2016;64:465–475.
6. Costea C, Turliuc S, Cucu A, et al. The "polymorphous" history of a polymorphous skull bone: the sphenoid. *Anat Sci Int*. 2018;93:14–22.
7. Jacquesson T, Mertens P, Berhouma M, Jouanneau E, Simon E. The 360 photography: a new anatomical insight of the sphenoid bone. Interest for anatomy teaching and skull base surgery. *Surg Radiol Anat*. 2017;39:17–22.
8. Barbaro NM, Gutin PH, Wilson CB, Sheline GE, Boldrey EB, Wara WM. Radiation therapy in the treatment of partially resected meningiomas. *Neurosurgery*. 1987;20:525–528.
9. Kondziolka D, Flickinger JC, Perez B. Judicious resection and/or radiosurgery for parasagittal meningiomas: outcomes from a multicenter review. Gamma Knife Meningioma Study Group. *Neurosurgery*. 1998;43:405–413; discussion 413–404.
10. Sughrue ME, Rutkowski MJ, Shangari G, Parsa AT, Berger MS, McDermott MW. Results with judicious modern neurosurgical management of parasagittal and falcine meningiomas. Clinical article. *J Neurosurg*. 2011;114:731–737.
11. Ruzevick J, Raza SM, Recinos PF, et al. Technical note: orbitozygomatic craniotomy using an ultrasonic osteotome for precise osteotomies. *Clin Neurol Neurosurg*. 2015;134:24–27.
12. Langevin CJ, Hanasono MM, Riina HA, Stieg PE, Spinelli HM. Lateral transzygomatic approach to sphenoid wing meningiomas. *Neurosurgery*. 2010;67:377–384.

50

Cavernous sinus meningiomas

Case reviewed by Pablo Augusto Rubino, Román Pablo Arévalo, Chae-Yong Kim, Laligam N. Sekhar, Harry Van Loveren

Introduction

A relatively uncommon location for meningiomas is within the cavernous sinus.[1,2] Surgery within the cavernous sinus has undergone constant change from observation to aggressive surgical resection to stereotactic radiosurgery.[3–5] Surgery within this region has been tempered by the risk of uncontrollable bleeding and damage to the cranial nerves.[3–5] Meningiomas can involve just the cavernous sinus but can also grow into the cavernous sinus from elsewhere, including the tuberculum sellae, medial sphenoid wing, and petroclival regions, among others.[3–5] In this chapter, we present a case of a left cavernous sinus meningioma.

Example case

Chief complaint: headaches and left eye vision loss

History of present illness

A 57-year-old, right-handed woman with rheumatoid arthritis presented with progressive headaches and left eye vision loss. For the past 5 to 6 months, she had increasing frequency and severity of headaches, and also complained of left eye vision loss. She saw an ophthalmologist who found left optic nerve atrophy and decreased visual fields in the left eye in all quadrants (Fig. 50.1).

Medications: Prednisone.

Allergies: No known drug allergies.

Past medical and surgical history: Rheumatoid arthritis, appendectomy, hysterectomy.

Family history: No history of intracranial malignancies.

Social history: Lawyer, no smoking, occasional alcohol.

Physical examination: Awake, alert, oriented to person, place, and time; Cranial nerves II to XII intact except decreased visual acuity in the left eye; No drift, moves all extremities with full strength.

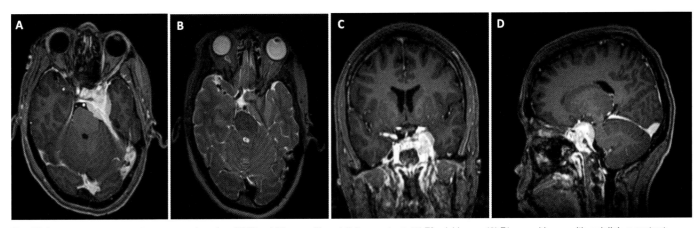

Fig. 50.1 Preoperative magnetic resonance imaging. (A) T1 axial image with gadolinium contrast; **(B)** T2 axial image; **(C)** T1 coronal image with gadolinium contrast; **(D)** T1 sagittal image with gadolinium contrast magnetic resonance imaging scan demonstrating an enhancing lesion involving the left cavernous sinus.

	Pablo Augusto Rubino, MD, Román Pablo Arévalo, MD, Hospital El Cruce, Buenos Aires, Argentina	Chae-Yong Kim, MD, PhD, Seoul National University Bundang Hospital, Seoul, South Korea	Laligam N. Sekhar, MD, Harborview Medical Center, University of Washington, Seattle, WA, United States	Harry Van Loveren, MD, University of South Florida, Tampa, FL, United States
Preoperative				
Additional tests requested	Pituitary hormone panel Neuropsychological assessment MR angiography OCT	Cerebral angiogram Neuroophthalmology evaluation	Cerebral angiogram with carotid compression to assess collaterals CT bone	MRA Neuroophthalmology
Surgical approach selected	Left pretemporal approach with anterior clinoidectomy and anterior petrosectomy	Left frontotemporal craniotomy	Left frontotemporal craniotomy, orbital osteotomy, optic nerve decompression, anterior clinoidectomy	Left frontotemporal orbitozygomatic, posterior orbitotomy, anterior clinoidectomy, anterior petrosectomy
Anatomic corridor	Left pretemporal	Left subfrontal	Left trans-Sylvian	Left trans-Sylvian
Goal of surgery	Extensive resection and visual preservation (Simpson grade II–IV)	Optic nerve decompression, expected subtotal resection	Optic nerve decompression, extensive resection without cranial nerve injury, Simpson grade II–III	Decompression of left optic nerve and brainstem in preparation for radiation, Simpson grade IV resection
Perioperative				
Positioning	Left supine	Left supine	Left supine with 45 degree right rotation, neck preparation	Supine with 45 degree right rotation
Surgical equipment	Doppler Ultrasonic aspirator Lumbar drain	Surgical navigation IOM Ultrasonic aspirator	Surgical navigation IOM (SSEP, MEP) Surgical microscope	Surgical navigation Surgical microscope Ultrasonic aspirator
Medications	Mannitol Antiepileptics	Steroids	Mannitol Steroids Antiepileptics	Mannitol Steroids Antiepileptics
Anatomic considerations	Left ICA, optic nerve, trigeminal nerve and its branches, lateral wall and roof of cavernous sinus, subarcuate eminence, Kawase triangle	Optic nerve, ICA, ACA, MCA	Left ICA, optic nerve, cavernous sinus cranial nerves	Optic nerve and chiasm, ICA, basilar artery, PCA, anterior choroidal, brainstem, cranial nerves III/IV/VI, SOF
Complications feared with approach chosen	ICA, optic nerve, oculomotor, cavernous sinus injuries	Left temporal lobe injury, arterial injury	Optic and cranial nerve, ICA injury	Brain retraction injury, optic nerve injury
Intraoperative				
Anesthesia	General	General	General	General
Skin incision	Left pterional	Left pterional	Left pterional	Left pterional
Bone opening	Left pretemporal	Left frontotemporal with limited posterolateral orbitotomy and extradural clinoidectomy	Left frontotemporal, orbital osteotomy	Left frontotemporal, orbital osteotomy, orbital roof, anterior clinoidectomy
Brain exposure	Left pretemporal	Left frontotemporal	Left frontotemporal	Left frontotemporal

	Pablo Augusto Rubino, MD, Román Pablo Arévalo, MD, Hospital El Cruce, Buenos Aires, Argentina	Chae-Yong Kim, MD, PhD, Seoul National University Bundang Hospital, Seoul, South Korea	Laligam N. Sekhar, MD, Harborview Medical Center, University of Washington, Seattle, WA, United States	Harry Van Loveren, MD, University of South Florida, Tampa, FL, United States
Method of resection	Lumbar drain placed, left pretemporal craniotomy, drilling of lesser sphenoid wing, drainage from lumbar drain, middle fossa peeling to separate dural sheaths from middle fossa dura, separation of the extra from intracavernous tumor portions, extradural portion removed, secure petrosal and intracavernous portions of the ICA, dura is opened to access the superior and external walls of the cavernous sinus, anterior clinoidectomy, removal of intracavernous portion of tumor, anterior petrosectomy by identifying limits of Kawase triangle (GSPN laterally, arcuate eminence posteriorly, posterior edge of Gasserian ganglion, petrous ridge medially), identify meatal plane (bisection of 120 degree angle between GSPN and arcuate eminence) and drilling of petrous ridge, removal of the bone (between V3 anteriorly, ICA/cochlea laterally, superior semicircular canal/IAC posteriorly until dura of posterior fossa reached, T-shaped posterior fossa dura opening with ligation and sectioning of superior petrosal sinus with care of trochlear and trigeminal nerves, removal of remaining posterior fossa tumor component, small sheets of tumor may be left if they are adherent to ICA or cranial nerves, lumbar drain for 48–72 hours	Left frontotemporal craniotomy, posterolateral orbitotomy, drill down sphenoid wing and extradural clinoidectomy and optic canal unroofing, open dura, subfrontal approach with early identification of optic nerve and ICA, unroof optic canal, opening of the falciform ligament and optic nerve sheath, follow these structures through tumor, internal debulking of tumor, extracapsular devascularization and dissection, removal of involved dura and bone	Left frontotemporal craniotomy with full orbitotomy, extradural optic nerve decompression under microscopic visualization consisting of anterior clinoidectomy and decompression of orbital roof, open dura, Sylvian fissure dissection, complete optic nerve decompression with opening of the falciform ligament and optic canal, remove tumor from optic nerve then subdural space, open cavernous sinus superiorly and laterally and remove tumor if soft, dura closure with graft	Left frontotemporal incision, subfascial dissection, MacCarty burr hole, one piece orbitozygomatic with orbital cuts done with mallet and osteotome, pterion is further reduced, complete posterior orbitotomy, optic canal unroofed, anterior clinoidectomy, dura opened in Dolenc fashion along Sylvian fissure, dura cut circumferentially around tumor, dissection around cavernous sinus by mobilizing temporal dura, opening of lateral wall of cavernous sinus, anterior petrosectomy using Kawase approach at the petrous apex on plane overlying predicted location of IAC and anterior to it, posterior fossa dura exposed, drill posteriorly to reveal dura of IAC, continue drilling posteriorly toward superior semicircular canal and laterally toward the cochlea, temporal lobe dura is cut perpendicular to superior petrosal sinus, posterior fossa dura opened, superior petrosal sinus ligated, dura retracted with sutures, posterior fossa component excavated with ultrasonic aspirator, capsule mobilized from brainstem and cranial nerves, removal of cavernous sinus component last, if tumor is soft can be removed but if hard leave attached to cranial nerves, reconstruction with dural substitute, fill dead space in clinoidal and subtemporal areas with fat

(continued on next page)

	Pablo Augusto Rubino, MD, Román Pablo Arévalo, MD, Hospital El Cruce, Buenos Aires, Argentina	Chae-Yong Kim, MD, PhD, Seoul National University Bundang Hospital, Seoul, South Korea	Laligam N. Sekhar, MD, Harborview Medical Center, University of Washington, Seattle, WA, United States	Harry Van Loveren, MD, University of South Florida, Tampa, FL, United States
Complication avoidance	Extradural removal of tumor first, securing of ICA for intracavernous tumor removal, leaving residual adherent to critical structures, anterior petrosectomy for wide posterior fossa exposure from middle fossa, lumbar drain for 48–72 hours	Extradural clinoidectomy and optic canal unroofing, early identification of optic nerve and ICA, opening falciform ligament, removal of involved dura and bone	Full orbitotomy, anterior clinoidectomy and optic nerve decompression, trans-Sylvian opening, remove tumor from optic nerve first and cavernous sinus portion last	Orbitozygomatic craniotomy, optic nerve decompression, anterior petrosectomy, leaving cavernous sinus portion for last
Postoperative				
Admission	ICU	ICU	ICU	ICU
Postoperative complications feared	Cranial nerve III palsy, visual decline	Left temporal lobe injury, arterial injury	ICA injury, seizures, cerebral edema, cranial nerve injuries, loss of work	Left optic nerve, cranial nerve III/IV/VI palsy, CSF leak
Follow-up testing	MRI within 48 hours after surgery	MRI within 48 hours after surgery Neuroophthalmology evaluation	CT or MRI immediately after surgery	CT day of surgery MRI within 24 hours after surgery
Follow-up visits	1 month after surgery	1 month after surgery	10 days after surgery	10 days after surgery 6 weeks after surgery
Adjuvant therapies recommended for WHO grade	Grade I–observation Grade II–observation Grade III–radiation	Grade I–observation Grade II–SRS Grade III–conventional radiotherapy	Grade I–radiation Grade II–radiation Grade III–radiation	Grade I–observation Grade II–radiation with residual Grade III–radiation

ACA, anterior cerebral artery; *CSF*, cerebrospinal fluid; *CT*, computed tomography; *GSPN*, greater superficial petrosal nerve; *IAC*, internal auditory canal; *ICA*, internal carotid artery; *ICU*, intensive care unit; *IOM*, intraoperative monitoring; *MCA*, middle cerebral artery; *MEP*, motor evoked potentials; *MR*, magnetic resonance; *MRA*, magnetic resonance angiography; *MRI*, magnetic resonance imaging; *OCT*, optical coherence tomography; *PCA*, posterior cerebral artery; *SOF*, superior orbital fissure; *SRS*, stereotactic radiosurgery; *SSEP*, somatosensory evoked potentials.

Differential diagnosis and actual diagnosis

- Meningioma
- Hemangiopericytoma
- Metastatic brain cancer
- Pituitary adenomas
- Chondrosarcoma

Important anatomic and preoperative considerations

The cavernous sinuses are paired venous structures located in the middle fossa in the parasellar region.[6] They are comprised of venous trabeculation with lateral, medial, anterior, posterior, and superior walls.[6] The lateral wall faces the temporal lobe, the medial wall faces the sella turcica and pituitary gland, the anterior wall faces the superior orbital fissure and near the inferior surface of the anterior clinoid process, the posterior wall is the anterior face of the posterior fossa and the apex of the petrous portion of the temporal bone, and the superior wall faces the basal cisterns.[6] The

cavernous sinus is surrounded by dura, in which the lateral dural wall is composed of two layers, with the outer dural layer and the inner membranous layer.[6] The outer layer faces the medial temporal lobe, and the membranous layer is in contact with the venous spaces and cranial nerves.[6] The vascular structures within the cavernous sinus include the cavernous segment of the internal carotid artery (ICA) and several venous tributaries, including the superior and inferior ophthalmic veins, the superficial middle cerebral vein, the inferior cerebral vein, and the sphenoparietal sinus.[6] The venous cavernous sinus exits include the superior and inferior petrosal sinuses, the emissary veins of the foramen ovale, the inferior ophthalmic vein, and the deep facial vein that connects with the pterygoid plexus.[6] The nervous structures within the lateral cavernous wall are the oculomotor, the trochlear, the ophthalmic branch of the trigeminal nerve, and the maxillary branch of the trigeminal nerve, whereas the abducens passes more medially on the lateral side of the ICA.[6] Cavernous sinus meningiomas can arise from the cavernous sinus dura itself, or can arise from adjacent dura, including the sphenoid wing, clinoid process, and petroclival regions, among others.[6]

Approaches to this lesion

As discussed in Chapter 41, options for meningiomas include observation, radiation therapy, and/or surgical resection. In this case, the lesion is large with symptomatic mass effect with vision loss. Observation and radiation would not be recommended because of the progressive symptoms and involvement of the optic canal.[7–9] As with other middle fossa meningiomas, there are a variety of surgical approaches, including frontotemporal/pterional, frontotemporal-orbitozygomatic, frontotemporal-transzygomatic, and supraorbital modified zygomatic approaches, among others.[10,11] The frontotemporal or pterional approach is the conventional approach, whereas the zygomatic approach involves performing osteotomies of either the superior and lateral orbital rims (orbitozygomatic), superior orbital rim (modified orbitozygomatic), and zygoma (transzygomatic).[10,11] These zygomatic extensions increase the visualization angles by removing bone, which can also minimize brain retraction.[12] However, these procedures can be associated with enophthalmos, double vision, temporalis atrophy, temporomandibular joint pain, and frontalis nerve injury, among others.[10,11]

What was actually done

The patient was taken to surgery for a left supraorbital craniotomy with circumferential decompression of the optic nerve and anterior clinoidectomy. The patient was induced and intubated per routine. The head was fixed in pins, with two pins over the inion and one pin over the right forehead in the midpupillary line. The patient's head was turned 15 degrees to the right and extended to allow the frontal lobe to retract from the anterior cranial fossa with gravity. A supraorbital incision was planned, making sure to stay lateral to the frontal sinus based on surgical navigation and extended laterally into the patient's eye wrinkle creases. The patient was draped in the usual standard fashion and given dexamethasone, levetiracetam, and cefazolin. The incision was made, and sharp dissection was used down to the periosteum. The flap was then retracted with fishhooks attached to the drapes. A high-speed drill was used to drill a burr hole at the MacCarty keyhole. The craniotome was used to make the superior cranial cut, and an ultrasonic bone scalpel was used to make the cuts in the orbital rim lateral to the frontal sinus and medially to the frontozygomatic suture, as well as along the orbital roof. Using an extradural dissection, the orbitotemporal fold was identified and cut under microscopic visualization. The clinoid was exposed, and the base was drilled and then fractured. The optic roof and strut were then drilled with continuous irrigation. The falciform ligament was identified and opened. The optic nerve was decompressed on its superior, medial, and lateral walls. The bone and skin were closed in standard fashion.

The patient awoke at their neurologic baseline with intact vision and was taken to the postoperative recovery unit. No postoperative imaging was done. The patient participated with physical and occupational therapy and was discharged to home on postoperative day 1 with intact vision. The patient was prescribed dexamethasone for 24 hours. The patient was seen at 1 week postoperatively for suture removal and was neurologically intact with intact vision. The patient was examined by neuroophthalmology at 3 months postoperatively

and had improved vision. The lesion was observed with serial magnetic resonance imaging examinations at 3- and 6-month intervals and has been without recurrence for 12 months with an intact neurologic examination.

Commonalities among the experts

All surgeons opted for the patient to undergo vascular imaging to better characterize the vessels within and around the lesion (half formal cerebral angiogram and the other half magnetic resonance angiography), and most opted for ophthalmologic evaluation for baseline visual function prior to surgery. All surgeons elected for surgery, in which all would perform a left frontotemporal craniotomy. The majority of surgeons would have the patient undergo an anterior clinoidectomy and optic nerve decompression, and half would pursue an anterior petrosectomy. Half of the surgeons would pursue a trans-Sylvian approach to the lesion. The majority of surgeons expected subtotal or Simpson grade IV resection. All surgeons were concerned about the left ICA and optic nerve. The majority of surgeons feared vascular injury to the ICA, optic nerve injury, and brain parenchyma injury. Surgery was generally pursued with surgical navigation, surgical microscope, ultrasonic aspirator, and intraoperative monitoring with perioperative steroids, antiepileptics, and mannitol. The majority of surgeons advocated for extradural clinoidectomy and optic nerve decompression, intradural identification and decompression of the optic nerve, and leaving the cavernous sinus component for the end. Following surgery, all surgeons admitted their patients to the intensive care unit, and surgeons requested imaging within 48 hours after surgery to assess for extent of resection and/or potential complications. Most surgeons advocated for observation for residual World Health Organization (WHO) grade I meningiomas, radiation for residual WHO grade II meningiomas, and radiation for all WHO grade III meningiomas.

SUMMARY OF QUALITY OF EVIDENCE TO GUIDE SPECIFIC INTERVENTIONS FOR THIS CASE

- Optic nerve decompression for cavernous sinus meningiomas with vision decline—Class III.

REFERENCES

1. Cushing H, Eisenhardt L. *Meningiomas: Their Classification, Regional Behaviour, Life, History, and Surgical End Results*. Springfield, IL: Charles C. Thomas; 1938.
2. Chaichana KL, Jackson C, Patel A, et al. Predictors of visual outcome following surgical resection of medial sphenoid wing meningiomas. *J Neurol Surg B Skull Base*. 2012;73:321–326.
3. Abdel-Aziz KM, Froelich SC, Dagnew E, et al. Large sphenoid wing meningiomas involving the cavernous sinus: conservative surgical strategies for better functional outcomes. *Neurosurgery*. 2004;54:1375–1383; discussion 1383–1384.
4. Kano H, Park KJ, Kondziolka D, et al. Does prior microsurgery improve or worsen the outcomes of stereotactic radiosurgery for cavernous sinus meningiomas? *Neurosurgery*. 2013;73:401–410.

5. Yasuda A, Campero A, Martins C, Rhoton AL Jr., de Oliveira E, Ribas GC. Microsurgical anatomy and approaches to the cavernous sinus. *Neurosurgery.* 2008;62:1240–1263.
6. Sindou M. Meningiomas invading the sagittal or transverse sinuses, resection with venous reconstruction. *J Clin Neurosci.* 2001;8(Suppl 1):8–11.
7. Barbaro NM, Gutin PH, Wilson CB, Sheline GE, Boldrey EB, Wara WM. Radiation therapy in the treatment of partially resected meningiomas. *Neurosurgery.* 1987;20:525–528.
8. Kondziolka D, Flickinger JC, Perez B. Judicious resection and/or radiosurgery for parasagittal meningiomas: outcomes from a multicenter review. Gamma Knife Meningioma Study Group. *Neurosurgery.* 1998;43:405–413; discussion 413–414.
9. Sughrue ME, Rutkowski MJ, Shangari G, Parsa AT, Berger MS, McDermott MW. Results with judicious modern neurosurgical management of parasagittal and falcine meningiomas. Clinical article. *J Neurosurg.* 2011;114:731–737.
10. Ruzevick J, Raza SM, Recinos PF, et al. Technical note: orbitozygomatic craniotomy using an ultrasonic osteotome for precise osteotomies. *Clin Neurol Neurosurg.* 2015;134:24–27.
11. Langevin CJ, Hanasono MM, Riina HA, Stieg PE, Spinelli HM. Lateral transzygomatic approach to sphenoid wing meningiomas. *Neurosurgery.* 2010;67:377–384.
12. Chaichana KL, Vivas-Buitrago T, Jackson C, et al. The radiographic effects of surgical approach and use of retractors on the brain after anterior cranial fossa meningioma resection. *World Neurosurg.* 2018;112:e505–e513.

51

Cerebellopontine angle meningioma

Case reviewed by Gordon Li, Hirofumi Nakatomi, Vicent Quilis-Quesada, Jamie J. Van Gompel

Introduction

Cerebellopontine angle (CPA) meningiomas account only for ~1% of meningiomas; however, among posterior fossa meningiomas; they account for 50% to 60% of these lesions.[1–4] Lesions in this region are typically slow-growing and reach large sizes before presenting with symptoms that include hearing loss/tinnitus, ataxia, headache, facial pain, facial numbness, and/or swallowing difficulties, among others.[1–4] Surgery in this region is associated with morbidity rates that range from 40% to 60% in several series, with subtotal resection rates of 15% to 60%.[1–4] As a result of these surgical risks, radiation therapy has also been offered not only postoperatively but also upfront for these lesions.[5] In this chapter, we present a case of a patient with a left CPA meningioma.

Example case

Chief complaint: left facial twitching and weakness
History of present illness
A 57-year-old, right-handed woman with known left CPA lesion presented with increased left facial twitching and weakness. She was diagnosed with this lesion approximately 10 years prior during workup for headaches. This was followed with serial imaging without significant change in tumor size (Fig. 51.1). However, she developed progressive left facial twitching and weakness over the past 2 to 3 months.
Medications: None.
Allergies: No known drug allergies.
Past medical and surgical history: Meningioma, right knee surgery.
Family history: No history of intracranial malignancies.
Social history: Nurse, no smoking, occasional alcohol.
Physical examination: Awake, alert, oriented to person, place, and time; Cranial nerves II to XII intact (including intact hearing) except left House-Brackmann 2/6; No drift, moves all extremities with full strength; Cerebellar: no finger-to-nose dysmetria.

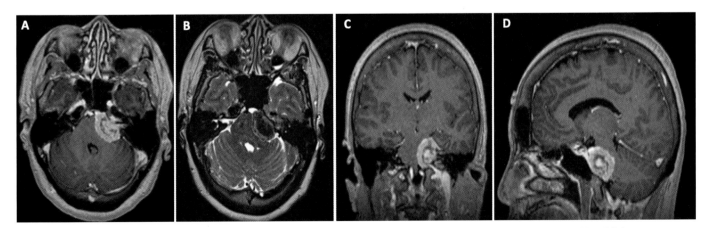

Fig. 51.1 Preoperative magnetic resonance imaging. (A) T1 axial image with gadolinium contrast; **(B)** T2 axial image; **(C)** T1 coronal image with gadolinium contrast; **(D)** T1 sagittal image with gadolinium contrast magnetic resonance imaging scan demonstrating an enhancing lesion in the left cerebellopontine angle.

	Gordon Li, MD, Stanford University, Palo Alto, CA, United States	Hirofumi Nakatomi, MD, PhD, University of Tokyo, Tokyo, Japan	Vicent Quilis-Quesada, MD, PhD, University of Valencia, Valencia, Spain	Jamie J. Van Gompel, MD, Mayo Clinic, Rochester, MN, United States
Preoperative				
Additional tests requested	Audiogram	Audiogram (PTA, SDS) BAERs/MR for facial spasm ENT evaluation (facial function, swallowing, phonics) Cerebral angiogram	CT angiogram CT	Audiogram
Surgical approach selected	Left retrosigmoid craniotomy	Left retrosigmoid craniotomy with IAC opening	Left retrosigmoid craniotomy, IAC opening, suprameatal petrosectomy	Left retrosigmoid craniotomy, suprameatal petrosectomy
Anatomic corridor	Left retrosigmoid	Left retrosigmoid	Left retrosigmoid	Left retrosigmoid
Goal of surgery	Extensive resection, decompress brainstem, avoid cranial nerve injury, Simpson grade III	Simpson grade II, with preservation of cranial nerves	Simpson grade I	Extensive resection without neurological compromise, decompress brainstem, Simpson grade III
Perioperative				
Positioning	Left supine with right rotation	Left lateral	Left park bench	Left lateral decubitus
Surgical equipment	Surgical navigation IOM (MEP, SSEP, cranial nerves) Surgical microscope Brain retractor Ultrasonic aspirator	Surgical navigation IOM (MEP, facial EMG, BAERs) Surgical microscope Ultrasonic aspirator Weck/AVM clips Microanastamosis set	IOM (MEP, SSEP, BAERs, cranial nerves V, VII–XII) Surgical microscope Ultrasonic aspirator	IOM (BAERs, cranial nerves V and VII) Surgical microscope
Medications	Steroids	Mannitol Steroids	None	Steroids
Anatomic considerations	Brainstem, cranial nerves V–XI	Cranial nerves V–XI	Sigmoid sinus, AICA, cranial nerves IV–V/VII–XII, SCA, superior petrosal vein, brainstem	Cranial nerves V, VII, and VIII
Complications feared with approach chosen	Cranial nerves, brainstem, cerebellum, sigmoid/transverse sinus injury, CSF leak	Hearing decline and facial palsy	Cranial neuropathy, vascular injury	Hearing loss, facial weakness, facial numbness
Intraoperative				
Anesthesia	General	General	General	General
Skin incision	Retrosigmoid linear	Retrosigmoid lazy S	Retroauricular U-shaped	Retrosigmoid curvilinear
Bone opening	Suboccipital up to transverse sinus, lateral to sigmoid, and inferior to foramen magnum	Suboccipital, retrosigmoid with exposure of transverse-sigmoid sinuses, removal of foramen magnum and condylar drilling	Suboccipital, retrosigmoid with exposure of transverse-sigmoid sinuses	Suboccipital, retrosigmoid
Brain exposure	Cerebellum and CPA	Cerebellum and CPA	Cerebellum and CPA	Cerebellum and CPA

	Gordon Li, MD, Stanford University, Palo Alto, CA, United States	Hirofumi Nakatomi, MD, PhD, University of Tokyo, Tokyo, Japan	Vicent Quilis-Quesada, MD, PhD, University of Valencia, Valencia, Spain	Jamie J. Van Gompel, MD, Mayo Clinic, Rochester, MN, United States
Method of resection	Retrosigmoid linear incision that is one-third above and two-thirds below transverse sinus extending to foramen magnum, burr hole at transverse/sigmoid sinus, suboccipital craniotomy down to foramen, dural opening, open cisterna magna and release CSF, brain retractor to move cerebellum away, identify tentorium and tumor, stimulate tumor to confirm nondorsal location of facial nerve, cut window into tumor and debulk with ultrasonic aspirator, once enough debulking find trigeminal nerve superiorly and lower cranial nerves inferiorly, continue to stimulate and debulk, peel tumor off of brainstem gently, attempt gross total resection, unless stuck to cranial nerves VII or VIII or brainstem, close dura with dural graft if necessary, cover bone defect with bone cement	Suboccipital craniotomy with foramen magnum opening and condylar drilling, Y-shaped dural opening, continuous epidural suction, dissect lateral cerebellomedullary fissure to identify foramen of Luschka and paratrigeminal cistern, electrodes to monitor cranial nerves VII and VIII, devascularize tumor from petrotentorial angle (often meningohypophyseal trunk/tentorial/ascending pharyngeal artery), debulk tumor in four quadrant division to identify cranial nerves, dissect from brainstem after enough debulking, open IAC with attention to the posterior semicircular canal and endolymphatic sac, remove IAC tumor component with curettes, secure IAC air cells with muscle and glue, dural closure, subgaleal drain insertion	Layer by layer dissection to facilitate closure, suboccipital craniotomy with exposure of transverse and sigmoid sinuses, dural opening, open cisterna magna for cerebellar relaxation, CPA and tumor exposure, tumor debulking, subarachnoid dissection, cranial nerve and vessel exposure and preservation, IAC drilling and tumor resection, suprameatal approach, tumor resection, dural removal and bone drilling, inferior part of the tumor resection from lower cranial nerves, watertight dural closure with dural graft if necessary	Suboccipital retrosigmoid craniotomy, dural opening, identify and stimulate for cranial nerves, remove as much tumor between cranial nerves as possible with ultrasonic aspirator or bipolar cautery, drill out suprameatal bone superior to the IAC to the Meckel cave to expose superior portion of tumor, remove more tumor, watertight dural closure
Complication avoidance	Decompress cisterna magna, identify superior and inferior poles, stimulate for CN VII, leave residual if adherent	Large bone opening with foramen magnum and condylar fossa, electrodes to monitor cranial nerves VII and VIII, debulking of tumor before dissecting	Large bone opening, decompress cisterna magna, debulk tumor, drilling out IAC and suprameatal approach, leave inferior tumor for last	Large bone opening, work in-between cranial nerves, suprameatal bone drilling

Postoperative

Admission	ICU	ICU	ICU	Intermediate care
Postoperative complications feared	Cranial nerve injury, CSF leak, brainstem stroke	Hearing loss, facial palsy, facial dysesthesias	Facial nerve injury, lower cranial neuropathy, vascular complications, CSF leak	Hearing loss, facial weakness, facial numbness, stroke
Follow-up testing	MRI 3–6 months after surgery	MRI/MRA/MRV within 72 hours after surgery	MRI within 48 hours after surgery	MRI within 3 months after surgery
Follow-up visits	10 days after surgery	1 month after surgery	4–6 weeks after surgery	3 months after surgery
Adjuvant therapies recommended for WHO grade	Grade I–observation Grade II–radiation Grade III–radiation	Grade I–observation Grade II–SRS Grade III–radiation	Grade I–observation Grade II–observation Grade III–observation	Grade I–observation Grade II–radiation Grade III–radiation

AICA, anterior inferior cerebellar artery; *AMR*, abnormal muscle response; *AVM*, arteriovenous malformation; *BAERs*, brainstem auditory evoked responses; *CPA*, cerebellopontine angle; *CSF*, cerebrospinal fluid; *CT*, computed tomography; *EMG*, electromyography; *ENT*, ear, nose, and throat; *IAC*, internal auditory canal; *ICU*, intensive care unit; *IOM*, intraoperative monitoring; *MEP*, motor evoked potentials; *MRA*, magnetic resonance angiography; *MRV*, magnetic resonance venography; *MRI*, magnetic resonance imaging; *PTA*, pure tone audiogram; *SCA*, superior cerebellar artery; *SDS*, speech discrimination scores; *SRS*, stereotactic radiosurgery; *SSEP*, somatosensory evoked potentials.

Differential diagnosis and actual diagnosis

- Meningioma
- Schwannoma
- Epidermoid
- Metastatic brain cancer

Important anatomic and preoperative considerations

CPA meningiomas are usually found to arise from cells lining the arachnoid villi, placing them in close proximity to various cranial nerve roots and their foramina.[1–4] Posterior fossa meningiomas are often grouped together because of their relative rarity.[4] Sekhar and Jannetta[4] proposed a classification scheme based on the site of dural attachment, in which type I involves the cerebellar convexity and lateral tentorial edge, type II the lateral petrous ridge and CPA, type III the jugular foramen, type IV the petroclival, type V the foramen magnum, and type VI unclassified. These type II meningiomas typically grow along the posterior aspect of the petrous bone posterior to the internal acoustic canal, but can extend elsewhere into the middle cranial fossa, internal auditory canal (IAC), and jugular foramen, among others.[1–4] Kunii et al.[6] subdivided posterior fossa meningiomas into petroclival in which the trigeminal nerve is displaced laterally, tentorial in which tumor attachment occurs at the medial tentorium, anterior petrous in which tumor attachment is anterior to the IAC, and posterior petrous in which the tumor is located posterior the IAC.

The CPA is the angle created by the cerebellum and the pons, and is formed by the cerebellopontine fissure.[7] This fissure is created when the cerebellum folds over to the pons, which creates a subarachnoid cistern in the CPA.[7] Within this angle lies the facial and vestibulocochlear nerves, the cerebellar flocculus and lateral recess of the fourth ventricle, and the anterior inferior cerebellar artery (AICA) and its branches.[7] The AICA follows the ventral surface of the pons, but within the CPA typically makes a long loop laterally to the IAC, and in 15% to 25% of cases, passes into the IAC before turning back on itself into the CPA.[7] The AICA typically passes below cranial nerves VII and VIII; however, 25% to 50% of the time it passes between the cranial nerves, and approximately 10% to 15% it passes above cranial nerves VII and VIII.[7] The petrosal vein, also known as the Dandy vein, drains the cerebellum and lateral brainstem to the superior or inferior petrosal sinus, whereas the vein of Labbe drains blood from the inferior and lateral surface of the temporal lobe to the superior petrosal sinus or transverse sinus.[7] The facial nerve arises 2 to 3 mm anterior to the root entry zone of the vestibulocochlear nerve, and the foramen of Luschka is located inferior and posterior to the root entry zone of the facial and vestibulocochlear nerves.[7] Inferior and anterior to the foramen of Luschka is the olive, and posterior to the olive lies the rootlets of cranial nerves IX, X, and XI.[7] Cranial nerve XII exits through the hypoglossal canal anterior to the olive.[7] The facial nerve leaves the brainstem anterior to the foramen of Luschka and passes through the CPA accompanied by the vestibulocochlear nerve and enters the IAC through the anterior superior margin of the porous.[7] The vestibulocochlear arises from the brainstem just posterior to the facial nerve.[7] The nervus intermedius leaves the brainstem with the vestibulocochlear nerve, and later crosses over to become associated with the facial nerve at variable distances.[7]

Approaches to this lesion

The most common approaches to CPA meningiomas are retrosigmoid, subtemporal, and transtemporal.[1–4] The choice of approach depends on the tumor characteristics (size, location, extension into surrounding structures), patient characteristics (age, functional status), and surgeon preference.[1–4] A retrosigmoid approach involves removing the occipital bone below the transverse sinus and medial to the sigmoid sinus, and the approach is lateral to the cerebellum. This approach can be extended by opening the bone past the transverse and/or sigmoid sinus in what is called an extended retrosigmoid approach, which facilitates dural opening by a few millimeters to increase working angles and visualization.[8] The advantages of the retrosigmoid approach are that it is the conventional approach, ease at decompression with opening the cisterna magna, and that it allows adequate access to the CPA, whereas its primary disadvantage includes difficulty to access supratentorial tumor components.[8] The subtemporal approach involves approaching the lesion from a supratentorial approach with opening the tentorium to access the infratentorial space.[9] The advantages of the subtemporal approach is access to the supra- and infratentorial space concomitantly, whereas the disadvantages include potential injury to the temporal lobe and vein of Labbe, trochlear nerve injury, and difficulty with accessing areas below the line of the interpeduncular fossa.[9] The transtemporal approach involves performing retromastoid and temporal craniotomies followed by removing the petrous and tympanic bone to expose the intratemporal parts of the facial nerve, petrous internal carotid artery, sigmoid sinus, and jugular bulb.[10] The advantages of this approach are that it minimizes temporal lobe retraction and provides early identification of the facial nerve, whereas its disadvantages include high risk of cerebrospinal fluid leak and loss of hearing.[10]

What was actually done

The patient underwent preoperative audiogram for baseline hearing and had diminished hearing on the left. She was taken to surgery for a left suboccipital retrosigmoid craniectomy for resection of the CPA meningioma with general anesthesia with intraoperative somatosensory evoked potentials, motor evoked potentials, and cranial nerves V, VII, VIII, and IX to XI monitoring. The patient was induced and intubated per routine. The head was fixed in neutral position, with two pins centered over the right external auditory meatus and one pin over the left external auditory meatus. The patient was then placed into the left park bench position. A lazy S-incision was planned in the suboccipital region that extended just above the transverse sinus to just below the foramen magnum. The patient was draped in the usual standard fashion and given dexamethasone and cefazolin. The incision was made, and a myocutaneous flap was made, and the skin and muscles were retracted with a cerebellar retractor. A

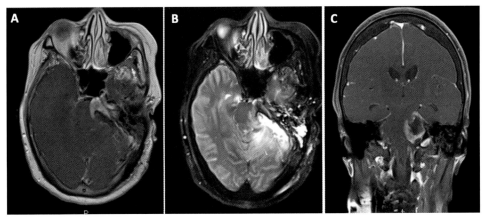

Fig. 51.2 Postoperative magnetic resonance imaging. (A) T1 axial image with gadolinium contrast; **(B)** T2 axial image; **(C)** T1 coronal image with gadolinium contrast magnetic resonance imaging scan demonstrating subtotal resection of the cerebellopontine angle tumor with residual along the brainstem.

high-speed drill was used to thin the bone overlying the left cerebellar hemisphere and transverse and sigmoid sinuses. The bone was removed with Kerrison and Leksell rongeurs so that the bottom of the transverse and lateral aspect of the sigmoid sinuses were exposed. In addition, the lip of the foramen magnum was removed. The dura was opened in a cruciate fashion, with one limb being at the transverse-sigmoid junction. The cisterna magna was opened to decompress the posterior fossa. The microscope was brought in for the remainder of the intradural portion of the case. The cerebellum was retracted medially with cottonoids and dynamic retraction. The jugular foramen cranial nerves were identified and dissected from the tumor margin. The petrosal veins were identified, coagulated, and ligated to identify the superior margin and tentorial edge. The facial nerve stimulator was used to stimulate the dorsal surface of the tumor. The tumor was then debulked internally with an ultrasonic aspirator, followed by capsular dissection. Preliminary pathology was meningioma. Alternating tumor debulking and capsular dissection was done until the trigeminal nerve was identified. The lateral spread response of the facial nerve stopped with the debulking. The tumor was noted to be adherent to the brainstem, middle cerebellar peduncle, and trigeminal nerve. The decision was to debulk the tumor and leave the capsule on the brainstem edge to minimize chance of injury. The dura, bone, and skin were closed in standard fashion.

The patient awoke at their neurologic baseline with full strength bilaterally, intact facial expression, and preserved hearing, and was taken to the intensive care unit for recovery. Magnetic resonance imaging was done within 48 hours after surgery and showed expected subtotal resection with residual along the brainstem (Fig. 51.2). The patient participated with physical and occupational therapy and was discharged to home on postoperative day 5 with an intact neurologic examination. The patient was prescribed dexamethasone that was tapered to off over 7 days after surgery. The patient was seen at 2 weeks postoperatively for suture removal and remained neurologically intact. Pathology was a World Health Organization (WHO) grade I meningioma. The patient was observed with serial magnetic resonance imaging examinations at 3 months, followed by 6-month intervals, and has been without tumor recurrence for 18 months.

Commonalities among the experts

Most of the surgeons opted for the patient to undergo an audiogram for baseline hearing evaluation, and half requested an angiogram to better characterize the vessels within and around the lesion prior to surgery. All surgeons elected for surgery through a retrosigmoid craniotomy, in which half supplemented this approach with a suprameatal petrosectomy. Half of the surgeons expected a Simpson grade III resection. All surgeons were concerned about the brainstem and the cranial nerves, namely cranial nerves V to XI. The majority of surgeons feared cranial neuropathy, namely facial weakness and hearing loss. Surgery was generally pursued with surgical navigation, surgical microscope, ultrasonic aspirator, and intraoperative monitoring with electromyography of the cranial nerves, as well as perioperative steroids. The majority of surgeons advocated for large boney opening, cerebrospinal fluid decompression, internal debulking, and leaving adherent tumor behind. Following surgery, most surgeons admitted their patients to the intensive care unit, and surgeons requested imaging within 72 hours after surgery to assess for extent of resection and/or potential complications. Most surgeons advocated for observation for residual WHO grade I meningiomas, radiation for residual WHO grade II meningiomas, and radiation for all WHO grade III meningiomas.

SUMMARY OF QUALITY OF EVIDENCE TO GUIDE SPECIFIC INTERVENTIONS FOR THIS CASE

- Subtotal resection for CPA meningiomas adherent to the brainstem—Class III.
- Cranial nerve monitoring for posterior fossa surgery—Class III.
- Postoperative radiation therapy for meningioma recurrence—Class II-3.

REFERENCES

1. He X, Liu W, Wang Y, Zhang J, Liang B, Huang JH. Surgical management and outcome experience of 53 cerebellopontine angle meningiomas. *Cureus.* 2017;9:e1538.
2. Matthies C, Carvalho G, Tatagiba M, Lima M, Samii M. Meningiomas of the cerebellopontine angle. *Acta Neurochir Suppl.* 1996;65:86–91.
3. Roberti F, Sekhar LN, Kalavakonda C, Wright DC. Posterior fossa meningiomas: surgical experience in 161 cases. *Surg Neurol.* 2001;56:8–20; discussion 20–21.
4. Sekhar LN, Jannetta PJ. Cerebellopontine angle meningiomas. Microsurgical excision and follow-up results. *J Neurosurg.* 1984;60:500–505.
5. Park SH, Kano H, Niranjan A, Flickinger JC, Lunsford LD. Stereotactic radiosurgery for cerebellopontine angle meningiomas. *J Neurosurg.* 2014;120:708–715.
6. Kunii N, Ota T, Kin T, et al. Angiographic classification of tumor attachment of meningiomas at the cerebellopontine angle. *World Neurosurg.* 2011;75:114–121.
7. Rhoton AL Jr. The cerebellopontine angle and posterior fossa cranial nerves by the retrosigmoid approach. *Neurosurgery.* 2000;47:S93–S129.
8. Liebelt BD, Huang M, Britz GW. A comparison of cerebellar retraction pressures in posterior fossa surgery: extended retrosigmoid versus traditional retrosigmoid approach. *World Neurosurg.* 2018;113:e88–e92.
9. Choque-Velasquez J, Hernesniemi J. One burr-hole craniotomy: subtemporal approach in helsinki neurosurgery. *Surg Neurol Int.* 2018;9:164.
10. Sekhar LN, Estonillo R. Transtemporal approach to the skull base: an anatomical study. *Neurosurgery.* 1986;19:799–808.

52

Petroclival meningioma

Case reviewed by Gerardo Guinto, José Hinojosa Mena-Bernal, Gustavo Pradilla, Laligam N. Sekhar, Isaac J. Abecassis

Introduction

Petroclival meningiomas are relatively rare among meningiomas (~1%) that arise from the upper two-thirds of the clivus at the petroclival junction.[1-4] As compared with clival meningiomas, they are located medial to the internal auditory meatus and posterior to the Gasserian ganglion, which causes them to displace the brainstem posteriorly and contralaterally and may extend into the cavernous and petrosal sinuses, parasellar region, and middle cranial fossa, among others.[4] As a result, these tumors displace and surround critical neurovascular structures, typically posteriorly, and invade several bony structures and multiple brain compartments, making surgery for these lesions associated with significant morbidity (10%–50%) and mortality (~10%).[4] These lesions were initially considered inoperable, but with advances in surgical techniques and equipment and radiosurgery, these lesions are now being treated more frequently with multiple treatment modalities.[1-4] In this chapter, we present a case of a patient with a right petroclival meningioma.

Example case

Chief complaint: right facial weakness, swallowing difficulties, and imbalance

History of present illness

A 48-year-old, right-handed man with diabetes and hypertension presented with right facial weakness, swallowing difficulties, and imbalance. For the past 6 to 9 months, he noted increasing asymmetry in his face. In addition, he has complained of 1 to 2 weeks of swallowing problems in which he could not swallow solid foods, and also complained of imbalance in which he feels as though he is drunk. He was seen in the emergency room where imaging revealed a brain lesion (Fig. 52.1).

Medications: Glipizide, candesartan.

Allergies: No known drug allergies.

Past medical and surgical history: Diabetes, hypertension.

Family history: No history of intracranial malignancies.

Social history: Landscaper, no smoking, occasional alcohol.

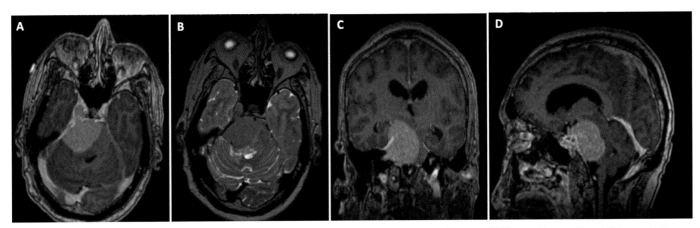

Fig. 52.1 Preoperative magnetic resonance imaging. (A) T1 axial image with gadolinium contrast; **(B)** T2 axial image; **(C)** T1 coronal image with gadolinium contrast; **(D)** T1 sagittal image with gadolinium contrast magnetic resonance imaging scan demonstrating an enhancing lesion in the right petroclival region.

Physical examination: Awake, alert, oriented to person, place, and time; Cranial nerves II to XII intact, except right House-Brackmann 2/6 and weakness in right palate elevation; No drift, moves all extremities with full strength; Cerebellar: no finger-to-nose dysmetria but with truncal ataxia.

	Gerardo Guinto, MD, Centro Neurologico ABC, Mexico City, Mexico	José Hinojosa Mena-Bernal, MD, PhD, Sant Joan de Deu, Barcelona, Spain	Gustavo Pradilla, MD, Emory University, Atlanta, GA, United States	Laligam N. Sekhar, MD, Isaac J. Abecassis, MD, University of Washington, Seattle, WA, United States
Preoperative				
Additional tests requested	Cerebral angiogram Audiogram Facial EMG Neuropsychological assessment	Audiogram	ENT evaluation CT temporal bones CT angiogram Audiogram Swallow evaluation	Cerebral angiogram, possible embolization Audiogram Medicine evaluation Swallowing evaluation
Surgical approach selected	Right posterior transpetrosal	Right extended retrosigmoid craniotomy with intradural suprameatal and transtentorial extension	Right combined transpetrosal and retrolabyrinthine transcrusal, anterior petrosectomy	Right frontal EVD, right temporo-occipital craniotomy with posterior petrosectomy, abdominal fat graft
Anatomic corridor	Right posterior transpetrosal	Right suboccipital	Right transpetrosal, retrolabyrinthine, anterior petrosectomy	Presigmoid with posterior petrosectomy
Goal of surgery	Simpson grade III with removal of posterior and supratentorial fossa components leaving cavernous sinus component behind	Simpson grade II or III, decompression of neural structures	Simpson grade III, maximal safe resection	Simpson grade II or III, maximal safe resection with preservation of neurologic function
Perioperative				
Positioning	Right supine with 40–45-degree left rotation	Right park bench	Right lateral park bench	Right lateral with head laterally flexed
Surgical equipment	IOM (CN V, VII, VIII, XI; SSEPs) Surgical microscope Ultrasonic aspirator	IOM (MEP, SSEP, BAERs) Surgical microscope Ultrasonic aspirator Endoscope	Surgical navigation IOM (MEP, SSEP, BAERs, CN VII EMG) Surgical microscope Ultrasonic aspirator Nerve simulator	Surgical navigation IOM (CN V–XII) Ultrasonic aspirator Endoscope Retractor system
Medications	Steroids Antiepileptics	Steroids	Steroids Antiepileptics Mannitol	Steroids Antiepileptics Mannitol
Anatomic considerations	Brainstem, CN IV–XII, basilar artery and its branches, temporal lobe, tentorium, petrous bone, superior petrosal sinus, vein of Labbe, lateral and sigmoid sinuses	Sigmoid sinus, mastoid air cells, brainstem, CN III–VIII, AICA, basilar and perforators, cavernous sinus, temporal lobe	Brainstem, CN III–X, greater superficial petrosal nerve, basilar artery, AICA, SCA, PCOM, ICA, eustachian tube, semicircular canals, cochlea, endolymphatic sac	Sigmoid sinus, labyrinth, brainstem, CN IV/V/VII, vein of Labbe
Complications feared with approach chosen	CN dysfunction, brainstem stroke, venous infarction, CSF leak, temporal lobe contusion	Facial nerve paralysis, injury to vein of Labbe, injury to sigmoid or transverse sinus	CN deficits, dysphagia, aspiration, pseudomeningocele, CSF leak	Brainstem injury, basilar artery perforator avulsion, cranial neuropathy, sigmoid sinus injury
Intraoperative				
Anesthesia	General	General	General	General
Skin incision	Question mark from mastoid tip, around ear to zygomatic root in front of tragus	Linear 2–3 cm behind mastoid process above transverse sinus to lateral rim of foramen magnum	Inverted U from root of zygoma over superior temporal line to mastoid	C-shaped 3–4 fingerbreadths behind ear just anterior to above the root of zygoma and down into neck

	Gerardo Guinto, MD, Centro Neurologico ABC, Mexico City, Mexico	José Hinojosa Mena-Bernal, MD, PhD, Sant Joan de Deu, Barcelona, Spain	Gustavo Pradilla, MD, Emory University, Atlanta, GA, United States	Laligam N. Sekhar, MD, Isaac J. Abecassis, MD, University of Washington, Seattle, WA, United States
Bone opening	Pre- and retrosigmoid area and posterior temporal	Right suboccipital	Mastoidectomy, temporal-occipital craniotomy, anterior petrosectomy	Mastoidectomy, temporal-occipital craniotomy, posterior petrosectomy
Brain exposure	Pre- and retrosigmoid area and posterior subtemporal	Right retrosigmoid	Temporal and presigmoid	Temporal and presigmoid
Method of resection	Skin incision with preservation of STA and fascia, bone exposed along spine of Henle and zygomatic root, drill along temporal line toward mastoid air cells with identification of transverse and sigmoid sinuses to expose sinodural angle, exposure of presigmoid dura, retrosigmoid craniectomy plus posterior temporal craniotomy, dural opening in the presigmoid space in a vertical line and horizontally along temporal dura with ligation and sectioning of superior petrosal sinus, transverse dural opening in, cutting of tentorium to identify trochlear, gentle retraction of temporal lobe, internal debulking of tumor, coagulating branches of meningohypophyseal trunk, removal of supratentorial component followed by posterior fossa along brainstem, leave adherent components behind, close dura except presigmoid area closed with grafts and fibrin adhesives	Linear skin incision, burr hole below asterion, approximate 3- x 3-cm craniotomy, exposure of transverse and sigmoid sinuses, dura opened in C- or Y-shaped based on sinuses, CSF slowly drained from cisterna magna, cerebellum retracted from CPA, arachnoid over cerebellomedullary cistern dissected, retractor advanced over surface facing petrous bone, tumor identified and debulked with ultrasonic aspirator, sharp dissection around inferior pole of tumor freeing from CN VII–VIII, dissection in caudal to cranial and from dorsal to ventral, identify CN V, identify and ligate superior petrosal vein, dissect tumor from basilar and perforators, transtentorial extension by incision tentorium, identify CN IV, debulk tumor in supratentorial and cavernous sinus components, suprameatal extension if tumor cannot be resected from the Meckel cave, drill laterally up to posterior and superior semicircular canals to facilitate opening of the Meckel cave, inspection with endoscope, watertight dural closure	Preparation for abdominal fat graft, inverted U incision, suprafascial dissection over temporalis muscle with preservation of pericranium, temporal and posterior cervical muscles dissected away from the skull and retracted inferiorly and laterally, mastoidectomy by ENT with skeletonization of sigmoid and transverse sinuses/semicircular canals/jugular bulb, seal off area with bone wax, temporal-occipital craniotomy, dural tack up sutures, anterior petrosectomy, middle meningeal artery is coagulated and cut, dura elevated to expose GSPN, expose middle fossa with intradural dissection, expose internal auditory canal/ICA/posterior fossa/petroclival junction with preservation of cochlea, tympanic cavity packed with muscle, dural opening in the presigmoid area and brought anteriorly to subtemporal area, division of superior petrosal sinus, resect portion of tentorium for increased exposure with protection of CN IV, debulk tumor with ultrasonic aspirator while cauterizing tumor capsule, identify and protect CN V (inferior, anterior, lateral aspect)/CN VI, CN III, basilar artery at deep medial portion, resect tumor in Meckel's cave, close dura, presigmoid dural defect closed with inlay of dural substitute/fat graft/Surgicel, dural sealant, vascularized pericranial graft reflected over dura	Place right frontal EVD, position lateral, C-shaped incision, elevate scalp with sternocleidomastoid and reflect anteriorly, dissect other muscles separately and retract downward, split temporalis, self-retaining retractor to move soft tissue, expose edge of EAC, burr holes above root of zygoma/temporal/straddling transverse sinus/straddling transverse-sigmoid sinus/bottom of retrosigmoid craniotomy, remove retrosigmoid and temporal craniotomies if sinus not adherent to bone, removal bone over sinus, mastoidectomy and skeletonize sigmoid sinus and presigmoid window up to antrum air cells, avoid semicircular canals, wax mastoid air cells, open retrosigmoid dura, drain lateral cerebellomedullary cistern, open supra- and infratentorial dura separately in linear fashion up to superior petrosal sinus, place rubber-dammed patties along cerebellum and temporal lobe, coagulate and ligate superior petrosal sinus, sequential bipolar cautery, and cut tentorium down with care to not injury CN 4 staying behind posterior clinoid process, open the Meckel cave to liberate CN 5, piecemeal tumor removal between CN IV/V/VII/VIII and minimize working near CN VII/VIII and III, dissect tumor away from brainstem maintaining arachnoid plane, dissection of basilar artery and perforators as needed, follow tumor into cavernous sinus if soft, remove dural base of tumor from petroclival area, minimize temporal lobe retraction and stretching vein of Labbe, close dura with dural graft and fibrin glue, rotation posterior portion of temporal with fascia to cover mastoid process and petrous bone, apply fat as needed

(continued on next page)

	Gerardo Guinto, MD, Centro Neurologico ABC, Mexico City, Mexico	José Hinojosa Mena-Bernal, MD, PhD, Sant Joan de Deu, Barcelona, Spain	Gustavo Pradilla, MD, Emory University, Atlanta, GA, United States	Laligam N. Sekhar, MD, Isaac J. Abecassis, MD, University of Washington, Seattle, WA, United States
Complication avoidance	Large bony opening, internal debulking, leave adherent tumor and cavernous sinus component behind	Large bony opening, internal debulking, transtentorial extension, intradural suprameatal extension if needed	Large bony opening, obstruction of potential CSF pathways, identify and preserve CNs, pericranial graft	Large bony opening, multiple craniotomies, obstruction of potential CSF pathways, identify and preserve CNs, minimize temporal lobe retraction, minimize stretch of vein of Labbe, maintain arachnoid over brainstem
Postoperative				
Admission	ICU	ICU	ICU, likely intubated	ICU
Postoperative complications feared	Motor deficit, CN deficits especially lower CNs, brainstem stroke, temporal lobe contusion, seizures	Hydrocephalus, seizures, CSF leak, stroke, cerebral edema, new neurologic deficit (CN deficit, ataxia, motor weakness, facial weakness)	CN deficits, dysphagia, aspiration, pseudomeningocele, CSF leak	CSF leak, hydrocephalus, trochlear nerve injury, swallowing difficulty, corneal sensory loss, facial weakness, hearing loss, seizures
Follow-up testing	CT within 6–8 hours after surgery MRI 6 weeks after surgery Radiation of tumor inside cavernous sinus and adherent to brainstem Facial EMG if there are facial deficits EEG for seizures	MRI within 24 hours after surgery ENT evaluation for swallowing and audiogram Ophthalmology evaluation	MRI within 24 hours after surgery Swallow evaluation Physical and occupational therapy	CT immediately after surgery MRI prior to discharge EVD overnight Swallow evaluation
Follow-up visits	6 weeks after surgery	15 days and 3 months after surgery	4 weeks after surgery	2 and 6 weeks after surgery
Adjuvant therapies recommended for WHO grade	Grade I–radiosurgery Grade II–radiosurgery Grade III–standard radiation	Grade I–observation, second look surgery Grade II–second look surgery vs. radiation Grade III–fractionated radiation or proton beam therapy	Grade I–observation Grade II–radiation Grade III–radiation	Grade I–observation vs. radiation depending on age Grade II–fractionated radiation or proton beam therapy Grade III–fractionated radiation or proton beam therapy

AICA, anterior inferior cerebellar artery; *BAERs*, brainstem auditory evoked responses; *CN*, cranial nerve; *CPA*, cerebellopontine angle; *CSF*, cerebrospinal fluid; *CT*, computed tomography; *EAC*, external auditory canal; *EEG*, electroencephalogram; *EMG*, electromyogram; *ENT*, ear, nose, and throat; *EVD*, external ventricular drain; *GSPN*, greater superficial petrosal nerve; *ICA*, internal carotid artery; *ICU*, intensive care unit; *IOM*, intraoperative monitoring; *MEP*, motor evoked potential; *MRI*, magnetic resonance imaging; *PCOM*, posterior communicating artery; *SCA*, superior cerebellar artery; *SSEP*, somatosensory evoked potential; *STA*, superficial temporal artery.

Differential diagnosis and actual diagnosis

- Meningioma
- Schwannoma
- Chondrosarcoma
- Chordoma

Important anatomic and preoperative considerations

The petroclival junction is defined as the upper clivus and the anterior third of the petrous apex anterior to the internal auditory canal (IAC) and medial to the trigeminal nerve.[5,6] This is different than lesions involving the cerebellopontine angle (see Chapter 51) or the posterior face of the petrous portion of the temporal bone, which have different surgical approaches and associated morbidities.[5,6] The dura within this region allows tumors to grow into adjacent structures and multiple compartments, including the cavernous sinus, the Meckel cave, parasellar regions including sphenoid sinus and sella, tentorium, and foramen magnum, among others.[5,6] This area opens superiorly into the supratentorial space and inferiorly into the cerebellopontine angle, and exposing this area requires exposing the dorsal clivus, vertical aspect of the posterior face of the temporal petrous bone, and ventral brainstem surface along with the critical neurovascular structures within this region.[5,6]

The temporal bone is a complex anatomic structure.[5,6] The petrous portion of the temporal bone is shaped like a pyramid and resides between the sphenoid and occipital bones, in which it has an upper surface that forms the posterior aspect of the middle cranial fossa and a medial surface that is part of the posterior fossa.[5,6] It houses the middle and inner ear cavities, the IAC, carotid canal, and jugular foramen.[5,6] The base of the petrous bone is fused with the internal surfaces of the squamous and mastoid parts of the temporal bone.[5,6] The apex resides at the angular interval between the posterior portion of the greater sphenoid wing and basilar part of the occipital bone, which is where the carotid canal exists and forms the posterolateral boundary of foramen lacerum.[5,6] In addition, the petrous bone has anterior, posterior, and inferior surfaces.[5,6] The anterior surface is connected with the inner surface of the temporal squamous portion via the petrosquamosal suture and forms the posterior part of the middle cranial fossa.[5,6] There are several ridges and depressions along the anterior surface of the petrous bone, including a groove anteriorly where the trigeminal ganglion resides (trigeminal depression), posterior to that groove is a ridge called the arcuate eminence indicating superior semicircular canal, and posterior and lateral is a groove of the tegmen tympani indicating the tympanic cavity.[5,6] Anterior to the trigeminal ganglion is the carotid canal.[5,6] The posterior surface of the petrous bone forms the anterior part of the posterior fossa, in which the center is demarcated by the IAC, which is where the facial and vestibulocochlear nerves exit.[5,6] Posterior to the IAC is the vestibular aqueduct that transmits the endolymphatic sac.[5,6] The inferior surface forms part of the exterior skull base, where near the apex is the attachment of the levator veli palatini and the cartilaginous portion of the auditory tube, and posterior to this is the carotid canal and posteromedially is the jugular foramen.[5,6] In addition to the three surfaces, there are also three angles: superior, posterior, and anterior.[5,6] The superior angle is where the tentorium is attached and where the superior petrosal vein runs.[5,6] The posterior angle is bounded medially by the channel of the inferior petrosal sinus and laterally by the jugular fossa.[5,6] The anterior angle consists of the petrosquamosal suture and the medial part that articulates with the sphenoid.[5,6]

Approaches to this lesion

There are a variety of different approaches to petroclival meningiomas, in which the approaches are dependent on the goals of surgery, site of attachment, and surgeon preference.[1–4] When the goal is gross total resection, most advocate for combined supra- and infratentorial approaches.[1–4] Hakuba et al.[7] recommended a combined subfrontal/subtemporal approach for upper clival meningiomas that extended toward the tuberculum sellae, transpetrosal-transtentorial approaches for upper and mid-clival meningiomas (see Chapter 51), and suboccipital/far-lateral approaches for mid and lower clival lesions (see Chapter 51). Couldwell et al.[8] published their combined series on petroclival meningiomas, and their approaches included retrosigmoid (also known as retromastoid, see Chapter 51), supra- and infratentorial transpetrosal (anterior petrosectomy involves removal of petrous apex anterior to the IAC, posterior petrosectomy involves removal of petrous pyramid posterior to the IAC), transtemporal (retrolabyrinthine, translabyrinthine, or transcochlear), subtemporal, and frontotemporal transcavernous. Samii and Tatagiba[9] also advocated for the use of combined retromastoid-subtemporal approaches with preservation of the sigmoid and transverse sinus via a presigmoid approach. Sekhar and Estonillo[3] promoted various approaches, including the retromastoid, anterior subtemporal with or without infratemporal extension, posterior subtemporal, and presigmoid transpetrous approaches. In general, the approaches have a variety of names but can be

divided into posterior (retrosigmoid or retromastoid), lateral (presigmoid, subtemporal, infratemporal), anterolateral (transpetrosal), and/or anterior (transcavernous) approaches, in which the approaches can be combined together to increase the number of working angles.[4]

What was actually done

Prior to the surgery, the patient underwent preoperative audiogram for assessing baseline hearing function and had diminished hearing on the right. The patient was taken to surgery for a right suboccipital extended retromastoid craniectomy for resection of the posterior fossa portion of the petroclival meningioma with general anesthesia with intraoperative somatosensory evoked potentials; motor evoked potentials; and cranial nerves V, VII, VIII, and IX to XI monitoring. This was chosen instead of a combined supra- and infratentorial approach because the patient was symptomatic from the posterior fossa component of the tumor, and the supratentorial tumor could be resected at a later stage. The patient was induced and intubated per routine. The head was fixed in neutral position, with two pins centered over the left external auditory meatus and one pin over the right external auditory meatus. The patient was then placed into the right park bench position. A lazy S-incision was planned in the suboccipital region that extended just above the transverse sinus to just below the foramen magnum. The patient was draped in the usual standard fashion and given dexamethasone and cefazolin. The incision was made, and a myocutaneous flap was made, and the skin and muscles were retracted with a cerebellar retractor. A high-speed drill was used to thin the bone overlying the left cerebellar hemisphere and transverse and sigmoid sinuses. The bone was removed with Kerrison punches and Leksell rongeurs so that the transverse and sigmoid sinuses were exposed. In addition, the lip of the foramen magnum was removed. The dura was opened in a cruciate fashion, with one limb being at the transverse-sigmoid junction. The cisterna magna was opened to decompress the posterior fossa. The microscope was brought in for the remainder of the intradural portion of the case. The cerebellum was retracted medially with cottonoids and dynamic retraction. The jugular foramen cranial nerves were identified and dissected from the tumor margin. The petrosal veins were identified, coagulated, and sectioned to identify the superior margin and tentorial edge. The facial nerve stimulator was used to stimulate the dorsal surface of the tumor. The tumor was then debulked internally with an ultrasonic aspirator, followed by capsular dissection. Preliminary pathology was meningioma. Alternating tumor debulking and capsular dissection was done until the trigeminal nerve, facial, and vestibulocochlear nerves were identified. The tentorium was left intact, and the supratentorial tumor was not addressed and reserved for a later stage. The dura, bone, and skin were closed in standard fashion.

The patient was kept intubated overnight because of the length of the procedure with blood pressure control and taken to the intensive care unit for recovery. The patient was extubated on postoperative day 1 moving all extremities with full strength but had worsened facial nerve function on the right but with full eye closure (House-Brackmann 3/6) and loss of hearing on the right. Magnetic resonance imaging was done within 48 hours after surgery and

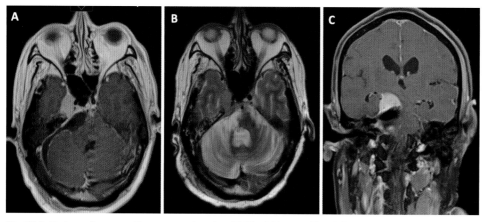

Fig. 52.2 Postoperative magnetic resonance imaging. (A) T1 axial image with gadolinium contrast; **(B)** T2 axial image; **(C)** T1 coronal image with gadolinium contrast magnetic resonance imaging scan demonstrating subtotal resection of the petroclival meningioma with residual in the supratentorial space.

showed expected subtotal resection with residual in the supratentorial space (Fig. 52.2). The patient developed postoperative pneumonia and had a prolonged hospital stay. The patient participated with physical, occupational, and speech therapy and was discharged to rehabilitation on postoperative day 8 with an intact examination, except right House-Brackmann 3/6 and loss of hearing on the right. In addition, he as eating without difficulty. The patient was prescribed dexamethasone that was tapered to off over 14 days after surgery. The patient was seen at 2 weeks postoperatively for suture removal and remained neurologically unchanged. Pathology was a World Health Organization (WHO) grade I meningioma. The patient was observed with serial magnetic resonance imaging examinations at 3 months, followed by 6-month intervals, and has been without tumor recurrence for 24 months. The supratentorial component of the tumor remains unchanged.

Commonalities among the experts

All surgeons opted for the patient to undergo an audiogram for baseline hearing evaluation, and the majority requested vascular imaging (two cerebral angiograms, one computed tomography angiography) to better characterize the vessels within and around the lesion prior to surgery, and half opted for swallowing evaluation. The majority of surgeons pursued transpetrosal approach (two posterior petrosectomies and one anterior petrosectomy). All surgeons expected a Simpson grade III resection. Most surgeons were concerned about the brainstem, cranial nerves (anywhere from cranial nerves III–XII), and the vein of Labbe. The majority of surgeons feared cranial neuropathy, brainstem injury, and venous infarct. Surgery was generally pursued with surgical navigation, surgical microscope, ultrasonic aspirator, and intraoperative monitoring with electromyography of the cranial nerves, as well as perioperative steroids and antiepileptics. The majority of surgeons advocated for large boney opening, cerebrospinal fluid decompression, internal debulking, and leaving adherent tumor behind. Following surgery, all surgeons admitted their patients to the intensive care unit, and requested imaging within 24 hours after surgery to

assess for extent of resection and/or potential complications. Most surgeons advocated for observation versus radiation for residual WHO grade I meningiomas, radiation for residual WHO grade II meningiomas, and radiation for all WHO grade III meningiomas.

SUMMARY OF QUALITY OF EVIDENCE TO GUIDE SPECIFIC INTERVENTIONS FOR THIS CASE

- Subtotal resection for petroclival meningiomas—Class III.
- Cranial nerve monitoring for posterior fossa surgery—Class III.

REFERENCES

1. Flannery TJ, Kano H, Lunsford LD, et al. Long-term control of petroclival meningiomas through radiosurgery. *J Neurosurg.* 2010;112:957–964.
2. Liebelt BD, Huang M, Britz GW. A comparison of cerebellar retraction pressures in posterior fossa surgery: extended retrosigmoid versus traditional retrosigmoid approach. *World Neurosurg.* 2018;113:e88–e92.
3. Sekhar LN, Estonillo R. Transtemporal approach to the skull base: an anatomical study. *Neurosurgery.* 1986;19:799–808.
4. Maurer AJ, Safavi-Abbasi S, Cheema AA, Glenn CA, Sughrue ME. Management of petroclival meningiomas: a review of the development of current therapy. *J Neurol Surg B Skull Base.* 2014;75:358–367.
5. Altieri R, Sameshima T, Pacca P, et al. Detailed anatomy knowledge: first step to approach petroclival meningiomas through the petrous apex. Anatomy lab experience and surgical series. *Neurosurg Rev.* 2017;40:231–239.
6. Rhoton Jr AL. The cerebellopontine angle and posterior fossa cranial nerves by the retrosigmoid approach. *Neurosurgery.* 2000;47:S93–S129.
7. Hakuba A, Nishimura S, Tanaka K, Kishi H, Nakamura T. Clivus meningioma: six cases of total removal. *Neurol Med Chir (Tokyo).* 1977;17:63–77.
8. Couldwell WT, Fukushima T, Giannotta SL, Weiss MH. Petroclival meningiomas: surgical experience in 109 cases. *J Neurosurg.* 1996;84:20–28.
9. Samii M, Tatagiba M. Experience with 36 surgical cases of petroclival meningiomas. *Acta Neurochir (Wien).* 1992;118:27–32.

53

Tentorial meningiomas

Case reviewed by Michael R. Chicoine, Guilherme C. Ribas, Jacques J. Morcos, Gelareh Zadeh, Farshad Nassiri

Introduction

Tentorial meningiomas account for 3% to 6% of intracranial meningiomas and arise from the tentorium.[1-3] They are characterized by multicompartmental growth and can involve the supra- and infratentorial space with involvement of several critical neurovascular structures, including the transverse and cavernous sinuses.[1-3] Because the tentorium is a vast structure, there are a variety of surgical approaches that have been devised for resecting these lesions.[1-3] Each of these different tentorial locations is associated with different Simpson-grade resections (Chapter 41, Fig. 41.2) and risks of morbidity.[1-4] In this chapter, we present a case of a patient with a left lateral tentorial meningioma involving the transverse sinus.

Example case

Chief complaint: confusion

History of present illness

A 54-year-old, right-handed man with a history of coronary artery disease with coronary stent, hypertension, and hypercholesterolemia presented with confusion. His family states that over the past 3 months he had become increasingly forgetful in which he forgets his keys, where things are in the house, and where he is supposed to be. He saw a neurologist, and imaging was done that revealed this brain lesion (Fig. 53.1).

Medications: Aspirin, clopidogrel, metoprolol, simvastatin.

Allergies: No known drug allergies.

Past medical and surgical history: Coronary artery disease with coronary stent 2 years prior, hypertension, hypercholesterolemia, cholecystectomy.

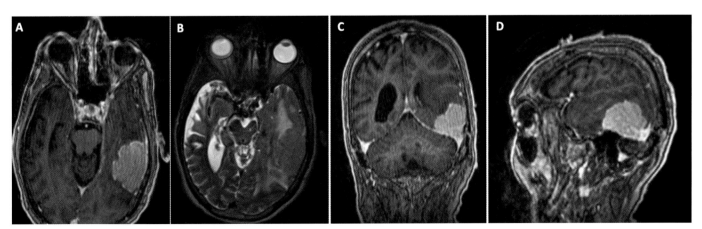

Fig. 53.1 Preoperative magnetic resonance imaging. (A) T1 axial image with gadolinium contrast; **(B)** T2 axial image; **(C)** T1 coronal image with gadolinium contrast; **(D)** T1 sagittal image with gadolinium contrast magnetic resonance imaging scan demonstrating an enhancing lesion involving the left posterolateral tentorium with invasion into the transverse sinus.

Family history: No history of intracranial malignancies.

Social history: Lawyer, no smoking, occasional alcohol.

Physical examination: Awake, alert, oriented to person, place, and time; Cranial nerves II to XII intact; No drift, moves all extremities with full strength.

Magnetic resonance venography: Stenosis of transverse-sigmoid junction but with flow.

	Michael R. Chicoine, MD, Washington University, St. Louis, MO, United States	Guilherme C. Ribas, MD, PhD, Hospital Israelita Albert Einstein, São Paulo, Brazil	Jacques J. Morcos, MD, University of Miami, Miami, FL, United States	Gelareh Zadeh, MD, PhD, Farshad Nassiri, MD, Toronto Western Hospital, Toronto, Canada
Preoperative				
Additional tests requested	CT head Cerebral angiogram	Cerebral angiogram +/− embolization	Cardiology evaluation including evaluation of PFO Neuropsychological assessment	Angiogram/venogram Neuropsychological assessment Anesthesiology evaluation
Surgical approach selected	Left middle fossa craniotomy, partial mastoidectomy, lumbar drain, and possible abdominal fat graft	Left suprapetrosal craniotomy with posterior extension	Left posterior temporal craniotomy with lumbar drain	Left posterior temporal craniotomy
Anatomic corridor	Left middle fossa	Left posterior temporal	Left posterior temporal	Left posterior temporal
Goal of surgery	Maximal tumor resection, Simpson grade III	Simpson grade II	Simpson grade II, but likely Simpson grade IV	Maximal tumor resection, Simpson grade I if sinus nondominant and Simpson grade III if dominant
Perioperative				
Positioning	Left three-quarter lateral/park bench	Left lateral park bench	Left supine with right rotation without compromising jugular veins	Left lateral
Surgical equipment	Lumbar drain Surgical navigation Surgical microscope Ultrasonic aspirator	Surgical navigation Ultrasonic aspirator	Lumbar drain Precordial Doppler Surgical navigation Surgical microscope Ultrasonic aspirator Bypass instruments	Surgical navigation Surgical microscope IOM (cranial nerve stimulator) Doppler Ultrasonic aspirator
Medications	Mannitol Steroids Antiepileptics	Antiepileptics	Mannitol Steroids Antiepileptics	Mannitol Steroids
Anatomic considerations	Vein of Labbe, transverse and sigmoid sinuses, facial nerve, temporal lobe	Local veins, transverse-sigmoid junction	Vein of Labbe, transverse-sigmoid junction, external ear canal	Vein of Labbe, transverse-sigmoid junction, pial-tumor interface
Complications feared with approach chosen	Venous sinus or vein of Labbe injury, cerebral edema, CSF leak, temporal lobe venous infarct	Venous injury, bleeding, cerebral edema	Venous injury, temporal lobe injury	Sinus thrombosis/injury, venous injury
Method of sinus repair	Avoid sinus injury by leaving tumor remnants; if small, occlude with muscle or gelfoam; for large, mobilize nearby dura to close or dura substitute; last resort is to occlude with preservation of vein of Labbe and collaterals	Attempt to coagulate site of bleeding, application of hemostatic agents, suture attempt with or without muscle plug, sinus ligation as last resort	Microsurgical repair with direct suturing, vein patch, or reimplantation of dural flap	Dominant sinus–tamponade with gelfoam, head down, primary repair; nondominant sinus–pack with thrombotic material if no tumor and reconstruction if tumor in sinus

	Michael R. Chicoine, MD, Washington University, St. Louis, MO, United States	Guilherme C. Ribas, MD, PhD, Hospital Israelita Albert Einstein, São Paulo, Brazil	Jacques J. Morcos, MD, University of Miami, Miami, FL, United States	Gelareh Zadeh, MD, PhD, Farshad Nassiri, MD, Toronto Western Hospital, Toronto, Canada
Intraoperative				
Anesthesia	General	General	General	General
Skin incision	C-shaped from anterior/superior aspect of tumor, curve to posterior aspect of tumor, and to left mastoid	Horseshoe	Question mark	Horseshoe
Bone opening	Left temporal, mastoid	Temporal	Left posterior temporal with removal of bone over transverse-sigmoid junction	Left posterior temporal
Brain exposure	Temporal lobe	Temporal lobe	Temporal lobe	Temporal lobe
Method of resection	Myocutaneous flap, temporal occipital craniotomy to expose superior aspect of transverse sinus, partial mastoidectomy to expose transverse and sigmoid sinuses, dura opened, internal debulking, establish plane between tumor and brain with telfa, remove tumor from venous structures if possible, reconstruct dura with dural substitute, mastoid defect filled with fat and cranioplasty with titanium mesh or bone cement	Left temporal horseshoe incision, left suprapetrosal craniotomy with posterior extension with basal burr holes anterior to tragus/superior to parietomastoid and squamous meeting points/superior to asterion with surgical navigation, drill inferior temporo-occipital bone margin, open dura with dural detachment from tumor from superior to inferior, special attention to identifying and preserving draining veins into transverse sinus, careful dissection of tumor superior/anterior/posterior surfaces from brain with aid of cottonoid patties, coagulation and division of basal aspect of tumor, removal of tumor with suction or ultrasonic aspiration depending on consistency ideally from outer surface to center, curettage and coagulation of residual tumor attached to basal dura	Posterior temporal craniotomy along skull base, drill bone around transverse-sigmoid junction, drain 30 cc of CSF from lumbar drain, open dura based on middle fossa floor paying attention to vein of Labbe, removal of tumor dural attachments, develop plane between tumor and pia, debulk tumor but leave tumor attached to Labbe and transverse-sigmoid junction until end, resection of residual component, chase tumor into sinus with sinus repair if needed with dural patch, pericranial duraplasty, wax air cells	Harvest pericranial graft for duroplasty, craniotomy based on navigation with 1-cm border with 2–3 burr holes along the middle cranial fossa with one on transverse-sigmoid sinus junction and two superiorly, bipolar dura to devascularize tumor from posterior middle meningeal artery, C-shaped dural opening with 1-cm margin based on tentorium, tumor removal with sequential tumor debulking and separation or arachnoid/pial surface with microscopic visualization, debulk tumor with ultrasonic aspirator and roll capsule inward until tentorium reached, sharp dissection from transverse-sigmoid sinus junction, coagulate sinus and tentorial edges, watertight dural closure with pericranium

(continued on next page)

	Michael R. Chicoine, MD, Washington University, St. Louis, MO, United States	Guilherme C. Ribas, MD, PhD, Hospital Israelita Albert Einstein, São Paulo, Brazil	Jacques J. Morcos, MD, University of Miami, Miami, FL, United States	Gelareh Zadeh, MD, PhD, Farshad Nassiri, MD, Toronto Western Hospital, Toronto, Canada
Complication avoidance	Mastoidectomy, debulk tumor before separating from brain, identify and preserve sinuses and vein of Labbe, fill mastoid defect with abdominal fat	Low access to tumor, subtemporal dural devascularization, identification and preservation of draining veins	Drilling out transverse-sigmoid junction, careful inspection of vein of Labbe, no self-retaining retractors, leave portion attached to venous structures until end, leave residual on Labbe if needed, wax air cells	Pericranial graft, craniotomy with margins, coagulate dura to devascularize tumor, sequential debulking and capsule manipulation, sharp dissection from venous structures
Postoperative				
Admission	ICU	ICU	ICU	ICU
Postoperative complications feared	Temporal lobe venous infarction, cerebral edema, CSF leak	Venous or sinus thrombosis, cerebral edema	Venous infarct, CSF leak, temporal lobe edema, seizures	Venous infarct, sinus injury
Follow-up testing	CT immediately after surgery MRI 3–4 months after surgery	MRI within 48 hours after surgery	Albumin 250 cc every 8 hours for 3–4 days MRI within 48 hours after surgery Lumbar drain clamped for 48 hours to monitor for CSF leak	MRI within 48 hours after surgery
Follow-up visits	7–14 days after surgery	2–3 months after surgery	10 days and 6 weeks after surgery	4–6 weeks after surgery
Adjuvant therapies recommended for WHO grade	Grade I–observation Grade II–radiation (SRS, hypofractionated, EBRT, or proton) Grade III–radiation (SRS, hypofractionated, EBRT, or proton)	Grade I–observation Grade II–radiation Grade III–radiation	Grade I–observation Grade II–radiosurgery Grade III–fractionated radiotherapy	Grade I–observation Grade II–radiation Grade III–possible re-resection if large, radiation, molecular analyses

CSF, cerebrospinal fluid; *CT*, computed tomography; *EBRT*, external beam radiation therapy; *ICU*, intensive care unit; *IOM*, intraoperative monitoring; *MRI*, magnetic resonance imaging; *PFO*, patent foramen ovale; *SRS*, stereotactic radiosurgery.

Differential diagnosis and actual diagnosis

- Meningioma
- Hemangiopericytoma
- Metastatic brain tumor
- Lymphoma

Important anatomic and preoperative considerations

The cerebellar tentorium, also known as the tentorium cerebelli, is a crescent-shaped extension of the dura that separates the cerebellum and brainstem from the occipital and temporal lobes.[5] The tentorium is attached to the superior borders of the temporal bone and posterior clinoid process via the anterior and posterior petroclinoidal folds, and along the transverse sinus and occipital bone posteriorly.[5] The free margin is along the anterior edge of the tentorium and is U-shaped and referred to as the tentorial incisura.[5] The midbrain comprises the anterior portion of the incisura, and the superior vermis and splenium of the corpus callosum occupy the posterior half of the opening.[5] The tentorium attaches anteriorly to the anterior clinoid process, which is superior to the cavernous sinus.[5] At this anterior margin, the oculomotor and trochlear cranial nerves enter the lateral wall of the cavernous sinus, and the trigeminal nerve and ganglion reside at the petrous apex (see Chapter 52) and the bottom layer of the tentorium, whereas above the incisura is the temporal hippocampal gyri and posterior cerebral artery.[5] The falx cerebri is attached to the tentorium superiorly, and the falx cerebelli is attached inferiorly.[5,6] There are several dural venous sinuses associated with the tentorium, and include the straight sinus (at the junction between the tentorium and falx) that is formed by the inferior sagittal sinus and vein of Galen and drains into the torcula; transverse sinus that drains blood from the torcula and adheres to the tentorium posteriorly; superior petrosal sinus drains the cavernous sinus and drains into the transverse sinus and travels in the attached part of the tentorium; and tentorial sinuses that collect both supra- and infratentorial bridging veins.[5,7]

Approaches to this lesion

Because the tentorium is such as vast structure, there are a variety of surgical approaches.[1-3] Yasargil classified tentorial meningiomas into medial incisural, falcotentorial, paramedian, peritorcular, and lateral tentorial lesions.[3] Nanda et al.[3] classified the approaches into posterior, posterolateral, and anterolateral approaches. The posterior approaches are best for lesions at the posterior aspect of the tentorium, including posterior medial incisural, falcotentorial, and peritorcular meningiomas, and the factors that are important to consider include whether the tumor involves the supra- and/or infratentorial compartments, angulation of the tentorium, and the location of deep draining veins.[3] These posterior approaches include occipital interhemispheric transtentorial for supratentorial tumors in the midline, infratentorial supracerebellar for midline and paramedian infratentorial tumors, and combined supra- and infratentorial approaches for torcular tumors and tumors that span both supra- and infratentorial compartments.[3] The posterolateral approaches are best for lesions along the anteromedial tentorial edge and along the attachment to the petrous bone.[3] These posterolateral approaches include retromastoid or retrosigmoid suboccipital for tumors involving the petrous bone in which a petrosectomy can be used to access the supratentorial tumor component, and presigmoid for lateral tentorial meningiomas with both supra- and infratentorial components.[3] The anterolateral approaches are best for lesions along the anterior tentorial incisura.[3] These anterolateral approaches include subtemporal for tumors anterior to the brainstem along the tentorial incisura, and trans-Sylvian (typically with orbitozygomatic osteotomies) for similar lesions but with less necessary brain retraction.[3]

What was actually done

The patient was taken to surgery for left temporal craniotomy for resection of the lateral tentorial meningioma with general anesthesia with intraoperative somatosensory evoked potentials and electroencephalogram monitoring. Because the transverse-sigmoid junction was patent on magnetic resonance venography, the plan was to resect the lesion up the sinus, leaving the sinus component alone. The patient was induced and intubated per routine. The head was fixed, with two pins over the right superior nuchal line and one pin over the left forehead in the midpupillary line. The patient was then placed into the left lateral position. A linear incision was made through the center of the lesion that extended below the transverse sinus based on surgical navigation. The patient was draped in the usual standard fashion and given levetiracetam, dexamethasone, and cefazolin. The incision was made, a myocutaneous flap was made, and the skin and muscles were retracted with a cerebellar retractor. A high-speed drill was used to make a burr hole anterior and posterior to the lesion adjacent to the transverse sinus. The craniotome was used to make a temporal bone flap to encompass the lesion with a couple centimeters of margin in the anterior, superior, and posterior dimensions, but making sure to stay above the transverse sinus. The dura was opened in a semicircular fashion with the base along the transverse sinus. The tumor was identified and coagulated and disconnected from the tentorium. The tumor was debulked internally with an ultrasonic aspirator, followed by capsular dissection. Preliminary pathology was meningioma. Alternating tumor debulking and capsular dissection was done until the tumor was removed. The sinus wall was inspected and was intact, and a Doppler was used to confirm patency. Because the sinus was patent, the tumor in the transverse sinus was left alone. The dura, bone, and skin were closed in standard fashion.

The patient awoke with an intact neurologic examination and was taken to the intensive care unit for recovery. Magnetic resonance imaging was done within 48 hours after surgery and showed expected subtotal resection with residual in the transverse sinus (Fig. 53.2). The patient participated with physical and occupational therapy and was discharged to home on postoperative day 2 with an intact neurologic examination. The patient was prescribed dexamethasone that was tapered to off over 7 days after surgery, and 1 week of levetiracetam. The patient was seen at 2 weeks postoperatively for staple removal and remained neurologically intact. Pathology was a World Health Organization (WHO) grade II meningioma. The patient underwent stereotactic radiosurgery 4 weeks after surgery. The patient was observed with serial magnetic resonance imaging examinations at 3 months, followed by 6-month intervals, and has been without tumor recurrence for 36 months. The sinus component of the tumor remains unchanged.

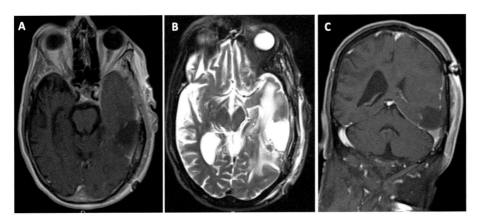

Fig. 53.2 Postoperative magnetic resonance imaging. (A) T1 axial image with gadolinium contrast; **(B)** T2 axial image; **(C)** T1 coronal image with gadolinium contrast magnetic resonance imaging scan demonstrating subtotal resection of the tentorial meningioma with residual in the transverse sinus.

Commonalities among the experts

Most surgeons opted for the patient to undergo a cerebral angiogram to better characterize the vessels within and around the lesion, as well as the status of the sinus prior to surgery. The majority of surgeons pursued a posterior temporal craniotomy. All surgeons expected a Simpson grade III or IV resection. Most were concerned about the vein of Labbe, as well as the transverse-sigmoid sinuses. All surgeons feared a venous infarct, and most feared injury to the temporal lobe. Surgery was generally pursued with surgical navigation, surgical microscope, and ultrasonic aspirator, with perioperative steroids, antiepileptics, and mannitol. The majority of surgeons advocated for early devascularization of the tumor, internal debulking, and leaving tumor adherent to the venous sinuses behind. Following surgery, all surgeons admitted their patients to the intensive care unit, and requested imaging within 48 hours after surgery to assess for extent of resection and/or potential complications. Most surgeons advocated for observation for residual WHO grade I meningiomas, radiation for residual WHO grade II meningiomas, and radiation for all WHO grade III meningiomas.

SUMMARY OF QUALITY OF EVIDENCE TO GUIDE SPECIFIC INTERVENTIONS FOR THIS CASE

- Subtotal resection for meningiomas invading the sinus—Class III.
- Radiation therapy for subtotal resection of grade II meningiomas—Class III.

REFERENCES

1. Biroli A, Talacchi A. Surgical management of lateral tentorial meningiomas. *World Neurosurg.* 2016;90:430–439.
2. Hashemi M, Schick U, Hassler W, Hefti M. Tentorial meningiomas with special aspect to the tentorial fold: management, surgical technique, and outcome. *Acta Neurochir (Wien).* 2010;152:827–834.
3. Nanda A, Patra DP, Savardekar A, et al. Tentorial meningiomas: reappraisal of surgical approaches and their outcomes. *World Neurosurg.* 2018;110:e177–e196.
4. Ehresman JS, Garzon-Muvdi T, Rogers D, et al. The relevance of Simpson grade resections in modern neurosurgical treatment of World Health Organization grade I, II, and III meningiomas. *World Neurosurg.* 2018;109:e588–e593.
5. Rai R, Iwanaga J, Shokouhi G, Oskouian RJ, Tubbs RS. The tentorium cerebelli: a comprehensive review including its anatomy, embryology, and surgical techniques. *Cureus.* 2018;10:e3079.
6. Quinones-Hinojosa A, Chang EF, Chaichana KL, McDermott MW. Surgical considerations in the management of falcotentorial meningiomas: advantages of the bilateral occipital transtentorial/transfalcine craniotomy for large tumors. *Neurosurgery.* 2009;64:260–268; discussion 268.
7. Ehresman JS, Mampre D, Rogers D, Olivi A, Quinones-Hinojosa A, Chaichana KL. Volumetric tumor growth rates of meningiomas involving the intracranial venous sinuses. *Acta Neurochir (Wien).* 2018;160:1531–1538.

54

Foramen magnum meningiomas

Case reviewed by Carlos E. Briceno, Nasser M. F. El-Ghandour, Gustavo Pradilla, Jacques J. Morcos

Introduction

Foramen magnum meningiomas are considered common tumors in rare locations, in which they account for approximately 3% of intracranial meningiomas.[1-4] They, however, account for approximately 70% of the benign lesions within the foramen magnum.[1-4] These lesions can present with headache, cervical pain, gait ataxia, and symptoms of cervical myelopathy.[1-4] Most of these lesions occur intradurally with involvement of several critical neurovasculature structures, including the vertebral artery, brainstem, and lower cranial nerves.[1-4] Because of the limited confines at the cervicomedullary junction, these lesions represent a surgical challenge because of access, minimizing brain manipulation, and possible spinal instability.[1-4] The rate of permanent morbidity in these cases ranges from 0% to 60% in several series.[1-4] In this chapter, we present a case of a patient with a foramen magnum meningioma.

Example case

Chief complaint: decreased hand function and imbalance
History of present illness
A 32-year-old, right-handed man with no significant past medical history presented with decreased hand function and imbalance. Over the past 6 to 12 months, he noticed decreasing dexterity in writing and fine motor skills, such as buttoning his shirt. He also had difficulties with balance in which he feels as though he is tripping more, and had difficulties feeling the ground. His primary care physician ordered imaging that showed a brain lesion (Fig. 54.1).
Medications: None.
Allergies: No known drug allergies.
Past medical and surgical history: Tonsillectomy.
Family history: No history of intracranial malignancies.
Social history: University professor, no smoking or alcohol.
Physical examination: Awake, alert, oriented to person, place, and time; Cranial nerves II to XII intact; No drift, moves all extremities with full strength; Reflexes: 3+ in upper and lower extremities, with positive Hoffman sign, no clonus.

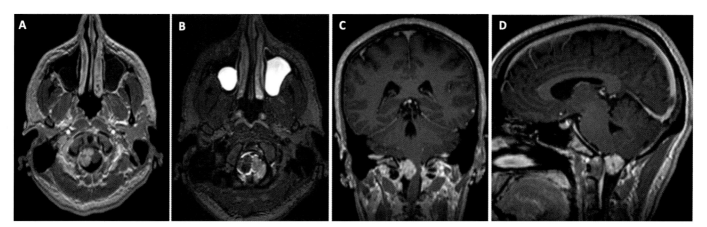

Fig. 54.1 Preoperative magnetic resonance imaging. (A) T1 axial image with gadolinium contrast; **(B)** T2 axial image; **(C)** T1 coronal image with gadolinium contrast; **(D)** T1 sagittal image with gadolinium contrast magnetic resonance imaging scan demonstrating an enhancing lesion involving the right foramen magnum region.

	Carlos E. Briceno, MD, Paitilla Medical Center, Panama City, Panama	Nasser M. F. El-Ghandour, MD, Cairo University, Cairo, Egypt	Gustavo Pradilla, MD, Emory University, Atlanta, GA, United States	Jacques J. Morcos, MD, University of Miami, Miami, FL, United States
Preoperative				
Additional tests requested	MRA MRV CT cervical spine Laryngeal endoscopy/ swallow evaluation	ENT for sinusitis CT bone windows MRA	CTA or angiogram CT cervical spine Swallow evaluation	MRA MRV
Surgical approach selected	Suboccipital craniotomy, C1 laminectomy	Right suboccipital craniotomy, C1 hemilaminectomy, partial removal of ipsilateral occipital condyle	Right far lateral craniotomy	Midline suboccipital craniotomy and C1 laminectomy
Anatomic corridor	Posterolateral suboccipital	Far lateral transcondylar	Far lateral transcondylar	Midline suboccipital
Goal of surgery	Simpson grade II, decompression of brainstem and upper cervical cord, possible grade III if engulfs vertebral artery or lower cranial nerves	Gross total resection, Simpson grade II	Simpson grade I or II, decompression of brainstem with preservation of cranial nerves	Gross total resection, Simpson grade II
Perioperative				
Positioning	Prone slight right rotation	Left lateral decubitus	Right lateral park bench	Prone
Surgical equipment	Surgical navigation Surgical microscope IOM (MEP, SSEP, BAERs) Brain stimulator Doppler Ultrasonic aspirator	Lumbar drain Surgical navigation IOM (cranial nerves, SSEP, BAERs) Surgical microscope Ultrasonic aspirator	Surgical navigation IOM (SSEP, MEP, BAERs) Ultrasonic aspirator Surgical microscope	Surgical navigation IOM (SSEP, MEP) Surgical microscope Aneurysm clips
Medications	Steroids Mannitol, hypertonic saline	Steroids	Steroids Mannitol	Steroids
Anatomic considerations	Cranial nerves IX–XII, medulla, upper cervical cord, V3/V4 and branches, spinal arteries, PICA, AICA, basilar artery, occipital condyle, fourth ventricle, cerebellar tonsils, inferior vermis	Mastoid and sigmoid sinuses, dentate ligament, C1 nerve root, cranial nerves V–VII, VA/AICA/PICA/ SCA, brainstem, spinal cord	Brainstem, lower cranial nerves (IX–XII), VA, PICA	Right VA/PICA, lower cranial nerves, medulla, upper cervical spinal cord
Complications feared with approach chosen	Transverse/sigmoid sinus injury, VA injury, craniospinal instability, cervicomedullary displacement	Cranial nerve dysfunction, motor deficit, craniocervical instability	Lower cranial nerve dysfunction, pseudomeningocele, CSF leak	Injury to arteries and nerves
Intraoperative				
Anesthesia	General	General	General	General
Skin incision	Inverted hockey stick	Inverted hockey stick	Inverted hockey stick	Midline linear
Bone opening	Midline small suboccipital, C1 lamina	Suboccipital, right occipital condyle, C1 lamina	Suboccipital, left occipital condyle, C1-2 hemilamina	Midline small suboccipital, C1 lamina
Brain exposure	Cerebellum, brainstem, upper cervical spinal cord	Cerebellum, brainstem, upper cervical spinal cord	Cerebellum, brainstem, upper cervical spinal cord	Cerebellum, brainstem, upper cervical spinal cord

	Carlos E. Briceno, MD, Paitilla Medical Center, Panama City, Panama	Nasser M. F. El-Ghandour, MD, Cairo University, Cairo, Egypt	Gustavo Pradilla, MD, Emory University, Atlanta, GA, United States	Jacques J. Morcos, MD, University of Miami, Miami, FL, United States
Method of resection	Suboccipital craniotomy with bone removal to level of condyle, identify dural entrance of VA, curvilinear dural opening and reflect laterally, dural sutures for retraction, mobilize vertebral artery, section C1 nerve rootlets, mobilize cranial nerve XI, coagulate tumor capsule and lateral dural attachment, centrally debulk with ultrasonic aspirator, vertebral artery localization with Doppler, retraction of tumor capsule into area of decompression, mobilize tumor laterally away from cervicomedullary junction, cut pial adhesions and divide small tumor feeders, inferior mobilization of upper tumor pole to dissect lower cranial nerves and PICA, piecemeal removal of tumor to expose anterolateral dural attachment, curette tumor remnants away and coagulate, subtotal resection is difficult to separate from cranial nerves or neurovasculature structures, watertight closure with dural graft	Incision from mastoid tip to superior nuchal line down toward C2 spinous process, detaching of muscles from C1 and C2, subperiosteal dissection to identify and protect VA, displace VA to see lateral mass of C1, C1 laminectomy, suboccipital craniotomy to expose medial edge of sigmoid sinus, drilling medial side of atlas and occipital condyle (20%), dura opened in curvilinear fashion from transverse-sigmoid junction to midline, identification and isolation of VA, division of upper dentate ligaments and C1 nerve root, resection through corridor between cranial nerves and brainstem, internal debulking, duraplasty for watertight closure, cranioplasty	Incision at level of superior nuchal line 3–4 cm above mastoid traversing posteriorly and right angle bend at midline down to C3 spinous process, suprafascial dissection, pericranium preserved for closure, T-shaped suboccipital muscle incision with muscle cuff made for reattachment, dissection down to C1-3 spinous process, flap retracted anteriorly and inferiorly, VA identified at sulcus arteriosus of C1, as well as at C2, suboccipital craniectomy posterior to transverse-sigmoid junction, C1 full hemilaminectomy posterior and medial to VA, C2 superior laminectomy, VA freed from foramen transversarium, 50% of posterior-medial aspect of occipital condyle drilled away, C-shaped dural opening with one limb anteriorly at sigmoid sinus and inferior limb at jugular bulb, dura retracted with sutures, achieve proximal and distal control of VA at superior and inferior aspects of mass, tumor pseudocapsule dissected sharply from surrounding cerebellum and cervicomedullary area, cranial nerves X–XII protected at superior aspect of exposure, ventral tumor attachment cauterized, internal debulking with ultrasonic aspirator with extracapsular dissection, dural attachments cauterized, dural closure with dural graft and sealant, pericranial graft to reinforce dural closure	Midline incision, C1 laminectomy and resection of right C1 lamina to lateral mass, identification of VA in sulcus arteriosus, suboccipital craniotomy, right paramedian dural opening, section right dentate ligaments, identify cranial nerve XI/VA/PICA, devascularize base of tumor at lateral dural wall, remove tumor in one piece if possible, possible separation of dural leaves from tumor origin, watertight dural closure

(continued on next page)

	Carlos E. Briceno, MD, Paitilla Medical Center, Panama City, Panama	Nasser M. F. El-Ghandour, MD, Cairo University, Cairo, Egypt	Gustavo Pradilla, MD, Emory University, Atlanta, GA, United States	Jacques J. Morcos, MD, University of Miami, Miami, FL, United States
Complication avoidance	Identify extradural VA, section C1 nerve rootlets, internal debulking, Doppler for vertebral artery localization, coagulate small tumor feeders, piecemeal removal from neurovasculature structures	Large bony opening, identification of VA both extra- and intradural, sectioning of dentate ligament, working between cranial nerves and brainstem, lumbar drain	Identification of extradural VA and mobilization, control of VA proximal and distal to tumor, protection of lower cranial nerves, sharp dissection from neurovascular structures, pericranial reinforcement	Early identification of VA and cranial nerves, IOM with cranial nerve stimulation, sectioning of dentate ligament
Postoperative				
Admission	ICU	ICU	ICU	ICU
Postoperative complications feared	Cerebellar/brainstem/upper cervical cord injury, hydrocephalus, lower cranial nerve injury, CSF leak, subdural hematoma, meningitis	Cranial nerve dysfunction, CSF leak, craniocervical instability	Lower cranial nerve dysfunction, pseudomeningocele, CSF leak	CSF leak, spinal accessory palsy, DVT
Follow-up testing	MRI within 24 hours after surgery MRI 2 months after surgery	MRI within 24 hours after surgery	MRI within 24 hours after surgery Physical and occupational therapy Swallow evaluation	MRI 4 within 8 hours after surgery
Follow-up visits	14 days after surgery	14 days after surgery	4 weeks after surgery	14 days after surgery
Adjuvant therapies recommended for WHO grade	Grade I–observation Grade II–radiation if Simpson grade IV Grade III–radiation	Grade I–observation Grade II–radiation Grade III–radiation	Grade I–observation Grade II–radiation Grade III–radiation	Grade I–observation Grade II–radiation Grade III–radiation

AICA, anterior inferior cerebellar artery; BAERs, brainstem auditory evoked responses; CSF, cerebrospinal fluid; CT, computed tomography; CTA, computed tomography angiography; DVT, deep vein thrombosis; ENT, ear, nose, and throat; ICU, intensive care unit; IOM, intraoperative monitoring; MEP, motor evoked potential; MRA, magnetic resonance angiography; MRI, magnetic resonance imaging; MRV, magnetic resonance venography; PICA, posterior inferior cerebellar artery; SCA, superior cerebellar artery; SSEP, somatosensory evoked potentials; VA, vertebral artery.

Differential diagnosis and actual diagnosis

- Meningioma
- Schwannoma
- Metastatic brain tumor

Important anatomic and preoperative considerations

Foramen magnum meningiomas are classified as intra- and/or extradural, in which the majority are intradural.[1-4] Among the intradural lesions, they can be anterior, posterior, or lateral, in which the most common locations are anterior, followed by anterolateral, and then posterolateral.[1-4] Although the classification is disparate, most classify foramen magnum meningiomas that are centrally located between the lower third of the clivus and the body of C2 anteriorly, jugular tubercles and C2 lamina laterally, and occipital bone and the C2 spinous process posteriorly.[2] These lesions are also intricately involved with the V3 (from C2 to the dura) and V4 (from the dura to the basilar artery) segments of the vertebral artery, in which the vertebral artery can be above, below, or encompassed by the lesion.[2] The vascular supply often originates from the anterior (arises from the vertebral artery at typically C2 or C3) and posterior (arises from the posterior arch of the atlas) vertebral artery meningeal branches, as well as the meningeal branches of the external carotid artery (ascending pharyngeal and occipital arteries).[2] The lower cranial nerves are typically in close association with these lesions.[2] The glossopharyngeal, vagus, and spinal accessory nerves arise in the postolivary sulcus to enter the jugular foramen after passing ventral to the choroid plexus within the foramen of Luschka and dorsal to the vertebral artery.[2] The ascending spinal accessory nerve ascends through the foramen magnum behind the dentate ligament (extends from the pia to the dura laterally) and unites with the upper medullary rootlets.[2] The hypoglossal nerve arises from the preolivary sulcus and runs behind the vertebral artery to reach the hypoglossal canal.[2]

Approaches to this lesion

The approaches to foramen magnum meningiomas are predicated by site of dural attachment, location of the vertebral artery, and surgeon preference.[1-4] These approaches can be categorized into posterior, posterolateral, anterolateral, and anterior approaches.[1–4] The most common posterior approach is a midline suboccipital craniotomy with or without cervical laminectomies.[1] The advantages of this posterior approach are that it is familiar to most surgeons, it minimizes pain by dissecting in the avascular plane, and is minimally destabilizing, whereas the disadvantages are limited access to the lateral and ventral aspects of the cervicomedullary junction, potential need for cervicomedullary manipulation, and potential difficulty in identifying the vertebral artery, especially where it enters the dura at the V2/V3 junction.[1] The most common posterolateral approach is the far lateral transcondylar approach, in which it is more of a paramedian approach that involves removing the occipital bone, unilateral C1 lamina, and occipital condyle.[5] The advantages of this posterolateral approach are that it provides more posterolateral access to the cervicomedullary junction with bone removal to minimize cervicomedullary manipulation, and identifies the V2/V3 segment of the vertebral artery early for vascular control, but can be associated with potential vertebral artery injury, spinal instability, and cervical pain from muscular dissection.[5] The anterolateral approach is called the extreme lateral transcondylar approach, which involves accessing the cervicomedullary junction behind the jugular vein in front of the vertebral artery with removing the occipital condyles, which places it more anterolateral than the far lateral approach.[6,7] The advantages of this approach is that it provides good lateral and anterolateral visualization of the cervicomedullary junction and minimizes the need for retraction and manipulation; however, the disadvantages include unfamiliar approach, potential vertebral artery injury especially with transposition, and spinal instability.[6,7] The anterior approach is the transoral-transclival approach that involves accessing ventral lesions through the oropharynx.[8] The advantages of this approach are that it obviates the need for brain retraction and keeps critical neural and vascular structures laterally and posteriorly, whereas its disadvantages include risk of wound dehiscence, cerebrospinal fluid leak, unfamiliarity, and small working corridors.[7]

What was actually done

The patient was taken to surgery for midline suboccipital craniotomy with right far lateral transcondylar extension for resection of the foramen magnum meningioma with general anesthesia and intraoperative motor evoked potentials, somatosensory evoked potentials, and cranial nerves IX, X, XI, and XII monitoring. The patient was induced and intubated per routine. The head was fixed, with two pins over the left external auditory meatus and one pin over the right external auditory meatus. The patient was then placed into the prone position on chest rolls. A midline linear incision was planned from the inion down to the C2 spinous process. The patient was draped in the usual standard fashion and given dexamethasone and cefazolin. The incision was made, and the suboccipital muscles were dissected in the avascular plane. The skin and muscles were retracted with a cerebellar retractor. A high-speed drill was used to create a suboccipital craniotomy incorporating the foramen magnum and a C1 laminectomy. A right far lateral transcondylar extension was done by identifying the vertebral artery at the sulcus arteriosus with Doppler ultrasound and drilling the occipital condyle until the bone was removed lateral to the lateral margin of the dura at the cervicomedullary junction. The dura was opened in the midline and angled to the right at the superior and inferior aspects of the opening to allow the dura to retract to the right. The microscope was brought in for the remainder of the intradural portion of the case. The nerve stimulator was used to identify cranial nerve XI, which was dorsal to the lesion. The dentate ligament and dorsal C1 nerve roots were identified and sectioned to allow access to the tumor. The tumor was debulked internally with an ultrasonic aspirator, followed by capsular dissection. Preliminary pathology was meningioma. Alternating tumor debulking and capsular dissection was done until the tumor was removed. The dura, bone, and skin were closed in standard fashion.

The patient awoke with an intact neurologic examination and was taken to the intensive care unit for recovery. Magnetic resonance imaging was done within 48 hours after surgery and showed gross total resection of the tumor (Fig. 54.2). The patient participated with physical, occupational, and speech therapy and was discharged to home on postoperative day 5 with an intact neurologic examination. The patient was prescribed dexamethasone that was tapered to off over 14 days after surgery. The patient was seen at 2 weeks postoperatively for suture removal and remained neurologically intact. Pathology was a World Health Organization (WHO) grade I meningioma. The patient was observed with serial magnetic resonance imaging examinations at 3 months, followed by 6-month intervals, and has been without tumor recurrence for 36 months.

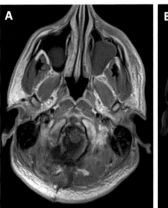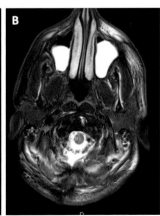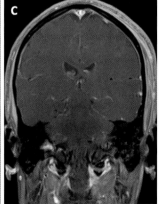

Fig. 54.2 Postoperative magnetic resonance imaging. (A) T1 axial image with gadolinium contrast; **(B)** T2 axial image; **(C)** T1 coronal image with gadolinium contrast magnetic resonance imaging scan demonstrating gross total resection of the foramen magnum meningioma.

Commonalities among the experts

All surgeons opted for the patient to undergo vascular imaging (three magnetic resonance angiography, one computed tomography [CT] angiography) to better characterize the vessels within and around the lesion; most surgeons opted for a CT head or CT cervical spine to evaluation tumor density; and half of the surgeons requested formal swallow evaluation prior to surgery. All surgeons pursued a suboccipital craniotomy and C1 laminectomy of the lesion, in which two surgeons supplemented their approach with partial occipital condylar resection. All surgeons expected a Simpson grade II resection. All surgeons were concerned about the lower cranial nerves, vertebral artery, and posterior inferior cerebellar artery, in which most were concerned about the brainstem and spinal cord. The majority of surgeons feared lower cranial neuropathy and vascular injury. Surgery was generally pursued with surgical navigation, surgical microscope, ultrasonic aspirator, and intraoperative monitoring with electromyography of the cranial nerves, as well as perioperative steroids and mannitol. The majority of surgeons advocated for early identification of the extradural portion of the vertebral artery, sectioning of the dentate ligament, internal debulking, and protection of lower cranial nerves. Following surgery, all surgeons admitted their patients to the intensive care unit and requested imaging within 48 hours after surgery to assess for extent of resection and/or potential complications. Most surgeons advocated for observation for residual WHO grade I meningiomas, radiation for residual WHO grade II meningiomas, and radiation for all WHO grade III meningiomas.

SUMMARY OF QUALITY OF EVIDENCE TO GUIDE SPECIFIC INTERVENTIONS FOR THIS CASE

- Far lateral transcondylar for foramen magnum meningiomas—Class III.

REFERENCES

1. Bernard F, Lemee JM, Delion M, Fournier HD. Lower third clivus and foramen magnum intradural tumor removal: the plea for a simple posterolateral approach. *Neurochirurgie*. 2016;62:86–93.
2. Bruneau M, George B. Foramen magnum meningiomas: detailed surgical approaches and technical aspects at Lariboisiere Hospital and review of the literature. *Neurosurg Rev*. 2008;31:19–32; discussion 32–33.
3. Leon-Ariza DS, Campero A, Romero Chaparro RJ, Prada DG, Vargas Grau G, Rhoton Jr AL. Key aspects in foramen magnum meningiomas: from old neuroanatomical conceptions to current far lateral neurosurgical intervention. *World Neurosurg*. 2017;106:477–483.
4. Flores BC, Boudreaux BP, Klinger DR, Mickey BE, Barnett SL. The far-lateral approach for foramen magnum meningiomas. *Neurosurg Focus*. 2013;35:E12.
5. Pai SB, Raghuram G, Keshav GC, Rodrigues E. Far-lateral transcondylar approach to anterior foramen magnum lesions: our experience. *Asian J Neurosurg*. 2018;13:651–655.
6. Liu JK. Extreme lateral transcondylar approach for resection of ventrally based meningioma of the craniovertebral junction and upper cervical spine. *Neurosurg Focus*. 2012;33:1.
7. Sen CN, Sekhar LN. An extreme lateral approach to intradural lesions of the cervical spine and foramen magnum. *Neurosurgery*. 1990;27:197–204.
8. Crockard HA, Sen CN. The transoral approach for the management of intradural lesions at the craniovertebral junction: review of 7 cases. *Neurosurgery*. 1991;28:88–97; discussion 97–98.

55

Falcotentorial meningiomas

Case reviewed by Sébastien Froelich, Pierre-Olivier Champagne, Javier Avendano Mendez-Padilla, Laligam N. Sekhar, Isaac J. Abecassis, Harry Van Loveren

Introduction

Meningiomas that arise along the tentorium account for 3% to 6% of intracranial meningiomas.[1-5] Because the tentorium is a large dural fold that separates the supra- and infratentorial spaces, tumors can occur in a variety of places.[1-5] Yasargil classified tentorial meningiomas into medial incisural, falcotentorial, paramedian, peritorcular, and lateral tentorial lesions.[6] Falcotentorial meningiomas are generally those tumors that occupy the area where the falx attaches to the tentorium with involvement of the straight sinus; however, some also include those tumors along the posteromedial tentorial incisura.[1-5] In this chapter, we present a case of a patient with a falcotentorial meningioma.

Example case

Chief complaint: headaches and lethargy

History of present illness

A 44-year-old, right-handed woman with no significant past medical history who presented with increasing headaches and lethargy. Over the past 2 to 3 weeks, she complained of worsening headaches and increasing fatigue. This had interfered with her work. She denied any nausea or vomiting, double vision, or focal weakness (Fig. 55.1).

Medications: None.

Allergies: No known drug allergies.

Past medical and surgical history: None.

Family history: No history of intracranial malignancies.

Social history: Baker, no smoking or alcohol.

Physical examination: Awake, alert, oriented to person, place, and time; Cranial nerves II to XII intact; No drift, moves all extremities with full strength.

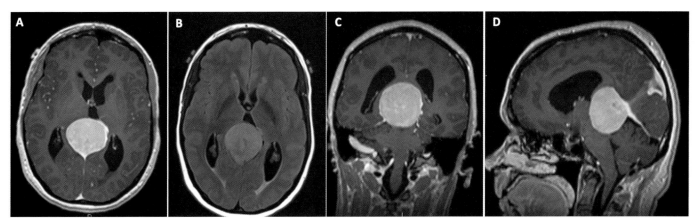

Fig. 55.1 Preoperative magnetic resonance imaging. (A) T1 axial image with gadolinium contrast; **(B)** T2 axial fluid attenuation inversion recovery image; **(C)** T1 coronal image with gadolinium contrast; **(D)** T1 sagittal image with gadolinium contrast magnetic resonance imaging scan demonstrating an enhancing lesion involving the falcotentorial region.

	Sébastien Froelich, MD, Pierre-Olivier Champagne, MD, PhD, Neurosurgery Hospital, Lariboisiere, Paris, France	Javier Avendano Mendez-Padilla, MD, National Institute of Neurology and Neurosurgery, Tlalpan, Mexico	Laligam N. Sekhar, MD, Isaac J. Abecassis, MD, University of Washington, Seattle, WA, United States	Harry Van Loveren, MD, University of South Florida, Tampa, FL, United States
Preoperative				
Additional tests requested	CT MRI with CISS/FIESTA MRV CT angiogram	Cerebral angiogram/ venogram	Cerebral angiogram/ venogram with possible embolization	Cerebral angiogram
Surgical approach selected	Right occipital transtentorial craniotomy	Right parieto-occipital craniotomy	Right frontal EVD, bilateral occipital and suboccipital craniotomy	Bilateral occipital/ suboccipital craniotomy, supra- and infratentorial approach with EVD
Anatomic corridor	Occipital transtentorial	Posterior interhemispheric	Occipital transtentorial with possible supracerebellar infratentorial	Supracerebellar infratentorial
Goal of surgery	Simpson grade II or III	Simpson I resection, preserve vascularity	Simpson grade II or III because of possible straight sinus invasion	Simpson grade I pending venous occlusion by tumor
Perioperative				
Positioning	Prone with 5- to 10-degree left rotation	Semi-sitting	Semiprone, right-side down	Prone
Surgical equipment	Surgical navigation Surgical microscope with ICG Doppler Ultrasonic aspirator	IOM (SSEP, cranial nerves) Surgical navigation Surgical microscope Ultrasonic aspirator	EVD Surgical navigation IOM (SSEP, MEP, BAERs) Surgical microscope Ultrasonic aspirator Endoscope Retractor system	EVD Surgical navigation IOM (SSEP/MEP) Surgical microscope Ultrasonic aspirator
Medications	Steroids Antiepileptics	Steroids Mannitol	Steroids Antiepileptics Mannitol	Steroids Antiepileptics Mannitol
Anatomic considerations	Straight sinus, cortical draining veins, tentorium, internal cerebral veins, vein of Galen, vein of Rosenthal, splenium, third ventricle, pineal gland, tectum, PCA, trochlear nerve	Venous sinuses, inferior longitudinal sinus, vein of Galen, brainstem injury	Venous sinuses, deep draining veins cortical veins on occipital lobe, brainstem	Brainstem, deep central veins (Galen, straight sinus, ICV, Rosenthal)
Complications feared with approach chosen	Venous infarct	Superior sagittal sinus injury, venous injury or infarction, intratumoral hemorrhage	Venous injury, cortical retraction injury of visual cortex	Retraction injury, venous injury, brainstem injury, inability to resect tumor
Intraoperative				
Anesthesia	General	General	General	General
Skin incision	Right paramedian linear	Right linear perpendicular to sagittal sinus	Inverted U-shaped over occipital and suboccipital regions	Linear from above inion to C2 spinous process
Bone opening	Right occipital	Right parieto-occipital	Bilateral occipital/suboccipital	Bilateral occipital/ suboccipital
Brain exposure	Right occipital lobe	Right parietal lobe, interhemispheric fissure	Bilateral occipital and cerebellar hemispheres	Bilateral occipital and cerebellar hemispheres

	Sébastien Froelich, MD, Pierre-Olivier Champagne, MD, PhD, Neurosurgery Hospital, Lariboisiere, Paris, France	Javier Avendano Mendez-Padilla, MD, National Institute of Neurology and Neurosurgery, Tlalpan, Mexico	Laligam N. Sekhar, MD, Isaac J. Abecassis, MD, University of Washington, Seattle, WA, United States	Harry Van Loveren, MD, University of South Florida, Tampa, FL, United States
Method of resection	Linear incision 1 cm right parasagittal, cruciate incision in pericranium, retraction of skin using pericranium to avoid self-retaining retractors, two burr holes on the SSS and one on the transverse sinus using cutting and diamond burrs, drill over torcula if needed, occipital craniotomy encompassing sinuses, shave midline border of craniotomy, preparation for EVD is needed using surgical navigation, dural opening 1 cm away and parallel to the SSS and transverse sinus with counter incision toward torcula, evaluate venous flow with Doppler, expose falx and tentorium, EVD if necessary to avoid brain retraction, identify straight sinus using observation/ navigation/Doppler, incise tentorium 1 cm away from sinus, coagulate dural margin to enlarge dural opening, debulk tumor with ultrasonic aspirator, peel away arachnoid from tumor after sufficient debulking, venous preservation leaving tumor remnant if needed, watertight dural closure, remove EVD, tack up sutures	Lumbar drain linear incision crossing sagittal sinus burr holes across sinus, craniotomy that exposes sagittal sinus, dura opened based on sagittal sinus, drain CSF from EVD, occipital lobe minimally retracted to expose interhemispheric fissure, retract falx upward, divide small bridging veins from occipital lobe to falx, identify and preserve deep basal veins, devascualrize tumor as much as possible, centrally debulk tumor with ultrasonic aspirator, mobilize tumor, remove supratentorial component, if necessary divide falcotentorial dura and tentorium 1 cm parallel to straight sinus watching for fourth cranial nerve, resect infratentorial compoent, watertight dural closure, EVD for at least 1 day	Right frontal EVD, inverted U-shaped incision, burr holes straddling sagittal sinus (4)/right lateral (2), 3 piece craniotomy (right occipital up to sinus, left occipital after dissecting SSS, suboccipital craniotomy down through foramen magnum), open suboccipital dura, drain cisterna magna, L-shaped dural opening in right occipital area, dural opening in supracerebellar area avoiding large veins, expose tumor by right parasagittal approach, divide tentorium lateral to straight sinus, expose tumor by supracerebellar approach if needed, debulk tumor and dissect from surrounding structures, maintain arachnoid plane over brainstem and only dissect after sufficient tumor debulked, leave tumor if adherent to vein of Galen/ anterior tentorial notch/ straight sinus, protect deep veins, confirm resection with endoscope, watertight dural closure with graft as needed, dural tack up sutures	Right frontal EVD placed in supine position, positioned prone, occipital craniotomy with exposure of torcula/transverse/ sagittal sinuses, suboccipital dura opened and reflected toward torcula, tumor exposed and debulked, capsule mobilized, tentorium circumferential cut to allow supratentorial exposure and debulked, if necessary can open supratentorial dura toward sagittal sinus, retract occipital lobes laterally and access tumor between hemispheres
Complication avoidance	Possible EVD, expose sagittal and transverse sinuses, minimal occipital lobe retraction, open tentorium adjacent to straight sinus, debulk tumor prior to manipulating arachnoid, leave tumor remnant to preserve veins	Lumbar drain, expose sagittal and transverse sinuses, minimal occipital lobe retraction, identification of basal veins, divide falx and tentorium to access contralateral and infratentorial components, watertight dural closure	EVD, multiple craniotomies to protect sinus, drain CSF early, maintain arachnoid plane over brainstem, protect deep draining veins, use of endoscope to inspect cavity	EVD first, bilateral occipital/ suboccipital craniotomy, removal of tentorium to allow supratentorial access, possible occipital interhemispheric if debulking not adequate
Postoperative				
Admission	ICU	ICU	ICU	ICU
Postoperative complications feared	Venous thrombosis or infarct, diplopia, hemianopsia	Venous infarct, brainstem lesion, hydrocephalus	Venous infarct, occipital cortical injury, brainstem injury, injury to deep draining veins, hydrocephalus, seizures	Brainstem injury, venous infarct, CSF leak, hydrocephalus

(continued on next page)

	Sébastien Froelich, MD, Pierre-Olivier Champagne, MD, PhD, Neurosurgery Hospital, Lariboisiere, Paris, France	Javier Avendano Mendez-Padilla, MD, National Institute of Neurology and Neurosurgery, Tlalpan, Mexico	Laligam N. Sekhar, MD, Isaac J. Abecassis, MD, University of Washington, Seattle, WA, United States	Harry Van Loveren, MD, University of South Florida, Tampa, FL, United States
Follow-up testing	CT within 12 hours after surgery MRI/MRV within 48 hours after surgery	CT immediately after surgery and 1 day after surgery MRI within 72 hours after surgery	CT immediately after surgery MRI prior to discharge EVD 1 day after surgery	CT same day after surgery MRI within 24 hours after surgery
Follow-up visits	2 months after surgery	2 weeks and 1 month after surgery	2 and 6 weeks after surgery	10 days after surgery 6 weeks after surgery
Adjuvant therapies recommended for WHO grade	Grade I–observation Grade II–radiation if growth Grade III–radiation	Grade I–observation Grade II–radiation if residual Grade III–radiation if residual	Grade I–observation vs. radiation depending on age Grade II–fractionated radiation or proton beam therapy Grade III–fractionated radiation or proton beam therapy	Grade I–observation Grade II–radiation if residual Grade III–radiation

BAERs, brainstem auditory evoked responses; *CISS*, constructive interference steady state; *CSF*, cerebrospinal fluid; *CT*, computed tomography; *EVD*, external ventricular drain; *FIESTA*, fast imaging employing steady-state acquisition; *ICG*, indocyanine green; *ICU*, intensive care unit; *ICV*, internal cerebral vein; *IOM*, intraoperative monitoring; *MEP*, motor evoked potential; *MRI*, magnetic resonance imaging; *MRV*, magnetic resonance venography; *PCA*, posterior cerebral artery; *SSEP*, somatosensory evoked potential; *SSS*, superior sagittal sinus.

Differential diagnosis and actual diagnosis

- Meningioma
- Hemangiopericytoma
- Metastatic brain tumor
- Lymphoma
- Pineocytoma
- Germ cell tumors

Important anatomic and preoperative considerations

For a full discussion of falcine and tentorial anatomy, see Chapters 47 and 53, respectively. The falx is a dural fold in the interhemispheric fissure that separates the cerebral hemispheres.[7] It attaches to the crista galli anteriorly and inferiorly, the midline of the cranium superiorly, and the superior surface of the tentorium cerebelli posteriorly and inferiorly.[7] The superior margin of the falx contacts the superior sagittal sinus, and the inferior margin contacts the inferior sagittal sinus and the superior surface of the corpus callosum.[7] The tentorium is another dural fold that separates the cerebellum and brainstem from the occipital and temporal lobes, where it attaches to the superior borders of the temporal bone and posterior clinoid process via the anterior and posterior petroclinoidal folds, and along the transverse sinus and occipital bone posteriorly.[8] The straight sinus resides between the attachment between the falx and the tentorium.[7] Falcotentorial meningiomas, despite involving the fixed structures of the falx and the tentorium, can be in the supratentorial, infratentorial, or both, and can incorporate other critical venous structures besides

the straight sinus, including the transverse sinus, torcula, petrosal sinuses, and deep draining veins, among others.[1–5] In addition, they can be supplied by branches of the internal carotid artery, choroidal arteries, meningohypophyseal trunk, and/or posterior cerebral artery.[1–5]

Approaches to this lesion

For a full description of surgical approaches for tentorial meningiomas, see Chapter 53. There are a variety of approaches that have been described for falcotentorial meningiomas, including occipital transtentorial for supratentorial tumors, infratentorial supracerebellar for midline and paramedian infratentorial tumors, and combined supra- and infratentorial approaches for tumors that span both supra- and infratentorial compartments.[2–6]

What was actually done

The patient was taken to surgery for midline suboccipital craniotomy for an infratentorial supracerebellar approach for a falcotentorial meningioma in the semisitting position (Concorde) with general anesthesia and intraoperative somatosensory evoked potentials and electroencephalogram monitoring. The patient was induced and intubated per routine. The head was fixed, with two pins over the left external auditory meatus and one pin over the right external auditory meatus. The patient was then placed into the prone semisitting position. A midline linear incision was planned from above the torcula down below the foramen magnum based on surgical navigation.

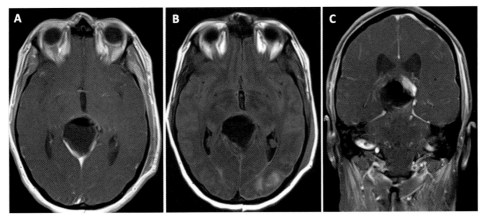

Fig. 55.2 Postoperative magnetic resonance imaging. (A) T1 axial image with gadolinium contrast; **(B)** T2 axial fluid attenuation inversion recovery image; **(C)** T1 coronal image with gadolinium contrast magnetic resonance imaging scan demonstrating subtotal resection of the falcotentorial meningioma with residual along the left cerebral vein of Galen.

The patient was draped in the usual standard fashion and given levetiracetam, dexamethasone, and cefazolin. The incision was made, and the suboccipital muscles were dissected in the avascular plane. The skin and muscles were retracted with a cerebellar retractor. A high-speed perforating drill was used to drill four burr holes, with one on each side of the sagittal sinus above the torcula and two burr holes below the transverse sinus laterally. The craniotome was then used to make a combined bioccipital and suboccipital craniotomy that exposed the sagittal sinus, torcula, and transverse sinuses. The dura was opened in a semicircular fashion with the base along the transverse sinus and torcula and tacked up. The microscope was brought in for the remainder of the intradural portion of the case. The arachnoid was dissected above the cerebellum in the infratentorial space, and all superficial veins were coagulated and cut. The tumor was then identified. The tumor was debulked internally with an ultrasonic aspirator, followed by capsular dissection. Preliminary pathology was meningioma. Alternating tumor debulking and capsular dissection was done until the tumor was removed. The inferior pole was resected first, followed by the superior pole. At the superior aspect, a portion of the tumor was adherent to the cerebral vein of Galen. This remaining tumor segment was left behind because of concern for injuring the vein. The dura, bone, and skin were closed in standard fashion.

The patient awoke with an intact neurologic examination and was taken to the intensive care unit for recovery. Magnetic resonance imaging was done within 48 hours after surgery and showed expected subtotal resection with residual near the left cerebral vein of Galen (Fig. 55.2). The patient participated with physical and occupational therapy and was discharged to home on postoperative day 4 with an intact neurologic examination. The patient was prescribed dexamethasone that was tapered to off over 7 days after surgery, and 1 week of levetiracetam. The patient was seen at 2 weeks postoperatively for suture removal and remained neurologically intact. Pathology was a World Health Organization (WHO) grade I meningioma. The patient was observed with serial magnetic resonance imaging

examinations at 3 months, followed by 6-month intervals, and has been without tumor recurrence for 36 months. The remaining tumor along the vein of Galen remains unchanged.

Commonalities among the experts

All surgeons opted for the patient to undergo vascular imaging (three cerebral angiogram, one computed tomography angiography) to better characterize the vessels within and around the lesion prior to surgery. Most of the surgeons pursued primarily an occipital transtentorial approach, in which one surgeon advocated for an occipital transtentorial with possible supracerebellar infratentorial. Most surgeons expected a Simpson grade II or III resection. All surgeons were concerned about the venous sinuses and deep draining veins (internal cerebral veins, vein of Galen), and most were concerned about the brainstem. All surgeons feared venous infarct, and half were concerned about retraction injury. Surgery was generally pursued with surgical navigation, external ventricular drain, surgical microscope, and ultrasonic aspirator, with perioperative steroids, mannitol, and antiepileptics. The majority of surgeons advocated for placement of an external ventricular drain at the beginning of the case, minimal retraction of the occipital lobe, opening of tentorium, and protection of deep draining veins. Following surgery, all surgeons admitted their patients to the intensive care unit, and requested imaging within 48 hours after surgery to assess for extent of resection and/or potential complications. Most surgeons advocated for observation for residual WHO grade I meningiomas, radiation for residual WHO grade II meningiomas, and radiation for all WHO grade III meningiomas.

SUMMARY OF QUALITY OF EVIDENCE TO GUIDE SPECIFIC INTERVENTIONS FOR THIS CASE

- Infratentorial supracerebellar approach for falcotentorial meningiomas—Class III.

REFERENCES

1. Talacchi A, Biroli A, Hasanbelliu A, Locatelli F. Surgical management of medial tentorial meningioma: falcotentorial and torcular. *World Neurosurg.* 2018;115:e437–e447.
2. Bassiouni H, Asgari S, Konig HJ, Stolke D. Meningiomas of the falcotentorial junction: selection of the surgical approach according to the tumor type. *Surg Neurol.* 2008;69:339–349; discussion 349.
3. Couldwell WT. Left occipital craniotomy for resection of falcotentorial meningioma. *Neurosurg Focus.* 2017;43:V9.
4. Hong CK, Hong JB, Park H, et al. Surgical treatment for falcotentorial meningiomas. *Yonsei Med J.* 2016;57:1022–1028.
5. Quinones-Hinojosa A, Chang EF, Chaichana KL, McDermott MW. Surgical considerations in the management of falcotentorial meningiomas: advantages of the bilateral occipital transtentorial/transfalcine craniotomy for large tumors. *Neurosurgery.* 2009; 64:260–268; discussion 268.
6. Nanda A, Patra DP, Savardekar A, et al. Tentorial meningiomas: reappraisal of surgical approaches and their outcomes. *World Neurosurg.* 2018;110:e177–e196.
7. Rhoton Jr AL. The cerebrum. Anatomy. *Neurosurgery.* 2007;61: 37–118; discussion 118–119.
8. Rai R, Iwanaga J, Shokouhi G, Oskouian RJ, Tubbs RS. The tentorium cerebelli: a comprehensive review including its anatomy, embryology, and surgical techniques. *Cureus.* 2018;10:e3079.

56

Nonfunctional pituitary adenoma with vision loss

Case reviewed by Peter Bullock, Paul A. Gardner, Nelson M. Oyesiku, Joseph Quillin, Rodrigo Ramos-Zúñiga

Introduction

Pituitary adenomas have an estimated prevalence of 10%, in which they are considered the fourth most common intracranial tumor after gliomas, meningiomas, and schwannomas.[1] It is estimated that approximately 50% of pituitary adenomas are clinically nonfunctional adenomas, in which they either secrete no hormones or clinically silent hormones.[1] These nonfunctional pituitary macroadenomas can either be incidental or cause significant hypothalamic or pituitary dysfunction, vision loss, ophthalmoplegia, and/or symptoms of mass effect (i.e., headaches).[2-5] The long-term control rate following surgery is 70% to 80% in several studies, in which smaller tumor size and lack of cavernous sinus invasion are associated with higher chances of tumor control.[2-5] In addition, surgery can lead to improvement in one or more hormonal abnormalities in 15% to 50% of patients, but can induce loss of one or more pituitary hormones in 2% to 15% of patients.[2-5] In this chapter, we present a case of a patient with a nonfunctional pituitary macroadenoma with bitemporal visual field loss.

Example case

Chief complaint: amenorrhea
History of present illness
A 36-year-old, right-handed woman with no significant past medical history presented with amenorrhea. She stated she had not had her menstrual cycle for almost 1 year. She was seen by her obstetrician who ordered a prolactin test and it was elevated. This led to imaging (Fig. 56.1).
Medications: None.
Allergies: No known drug allergies.

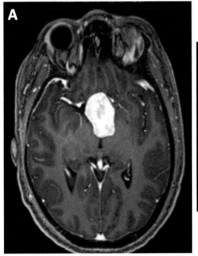
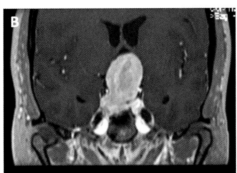
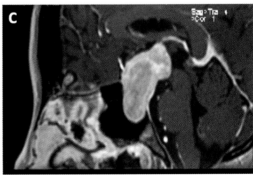

Fig. 56.1 Preoperative magnetic resonance imaging. (A) T1 axial image with gadolinium contrast; **(B)** T1 coronal image with gadolinium contrast; **(C)** T1 sagittal image with gadolinium contrast magnetic resonance imaging scan demonstrating an enhancing lesion involving the sellar and suprasellar space with elevation of the optic chiasm.

Past medical and surgical history: None.
Family history: No history of intracranial malignancies.
Social history: Accountant, no smoking or alcohol.
Physical examination: Awake, alert, oriented to person, place, and time; Cranial nerves II to XII intact, except bitemporal hemianopsia to confrontation; No drift, moves all extremities with full strength.
Pituitary labs: Prolactin 75 ng/ml (even after dilution), thyroid-stimulating hormone/T4, cortisol, insulin-like growth factor-1 all within normal limits.

	Peter Bullock, FRCS, MRCP, London Clinic, London, England	Paul A. Gardner, MD, University of Pittsburgh, Pittsburgh, PA, United States	Nelson M. Oyesiku, MD, PhD, Joseph Quillin, MD, Emory University, Atlanta, GA, United States	Rodrigo Ramos-Zúñiga, MD, PhD, University of Guadalajara, Guadalajara, Jalisco, Mexico
Preoperative				
Additional tests requested	MR angiography CT Neuroendocrinology evaluation Neuroophthalmology evaluation	CT angiogram Neuroendocrinology evaluation (a.m. cortisol) Neuroophthalmology evaluation (visual fields) ENT evaluation	High-resolution T2 MRI Neuroophthalmology evaluation (visual fields, OCT) Neuroendocrinology evaluation ENT evaluation Pregnancy test	MR angiography Neuroophthalmology evaluation (visual fields)
Surgical approach selected	Endoscopic endonasal transsphenoidal	Endoscopic endonasal transsphenoidal and transtubercular	Endoscopic endonasal transsphenoidal and transtubercular with lumbar drain	Microsurgical endonasal transsphenoidal
Other teams involved during surgery	ENT	ENT	ENT	ENT
Anatomic corridor	Endonasal transsphenoidal	Endonasal transsphenoidal and transtubercular	Endonasal transsphenoidal and transtubercular	Endonasal transsphenoidal
Goal of surgery	Extensive resection, preservation of pituitary function, visual improvement	Gross total resection, preservation of pituitary function, visual recovery	Gross total resection	Tumor decompression, decompression of optic apparatus, control of prolactin production
Perioperative				
Positioning	Supine with pins, 15 degree left rotation	Supine with skull pins, right rotation and slight extension with head/back elevated	Supine with skull pins, 10-degree right rotation	Supine with slight left rotation without skull pins
Surgical equipment	Surgical navigation Endoscopes	IOM (SSEP) Surgical navigation Endoscopes Cranial Doppler	Lumbar drain Surgical navigation 0- and 30-degree endoscopes Cranial Doppler Ultrasonic aspirator	Fluoroscopy Surgical microscope Sellar floor implant
Medications	Steroids Tranexamic acid	Steroids	None	Steroids
Anatomic considerations	Sella, optic nerves, ICA	Parasellar and paraclival ICA, opticocarotid recesses, sphenoid limbus, cavernous sinus walls, pituitary gland	Cavernous carotid arteries, optic nerves, ACOM, lamina terminalis, hypothalamus	Sphenoid sinus, sellar floor, ICA, diaphragma sella
Complications feared with approach chosen	Hypopituitarism, vision loss, CSF leak, ICA injury, meningitis	Hypopituitarism, vision loss, CSF leak, carotid injury	Retraction injury to frontal and temporal lobes, neurovascular injury to optic nerve, ICA, basilar artery, hypothalamus	Injury to ICA or pterygopalatine arteries, optic nerve injury, pituitary/pituitary stalk injury

	Peter Bullock, FRCS, MRCP, London Clinic, London, England	Paul A. Gardner, MD, University of Pittsburgh, Pittsburgh, PA, United States	Nelson M. Oyesiku, MD, PhD, Joseph Quillin, MD, Emory University, Atlanta, GA, United States	Rodrigo Ramos-Zúñiga, MD, PhD, University of Guadalajara, Guadalajara, Jalisco, Mexico
Intraoperative				
Anesthesia	General	General	General	General
Bone opening	Anterior wall of sphenoid sinus, sella	+/− right middle turbinate, partial right superior turbinate, anterior wall of sphenoid sinus, posterior ethmoidectomy, sella from cavernous to cavernous, tuberculum, medial and lateral opticocarotid recess	+/− right middle turbinate, wide sphenoid osteotomy, posterior ethmoidectomy, removal of sella from cavernous to cavernous sinus, tuberculum	Anterior wall of sphenoid sinus, sellar floor
Brain exposure	Sella	Sella complete right cavernous sinus and medial left cavernous sinus, tuberculum removal	Sella cavernous to cavernous sinus and tuberculum removal	Sella
Method of resection	ENT starts the approach, wide sphenoidotomy and mobilizing nasoseptal flap, bone removed from sellar face, identification of ICA/optic canals and confirmed with navigation, dura opened with diamond knife, develop plane of pseudocapsule with dissector starting at apex and working circumferentially around the tumor, deliver tumor likely in piecemeal given the size with large right-angle ring curette starting at floor and moving superiorly, remove lateral portions of tumor before diaphragm descends, observe for descent of diaphragma sella, inspection with 30-and 45-degree angled scopes, multi-layer closure with nasoseptal flap in gasket seal like fashion, place lumbar drain for 72 hours if there is a concern for CSF leak	Lateralize or resect right middle turbinate, partial resection of right superior turbinate to expose sphenoid ostium, harvest left nasoseptal flap, lateralize left middle turbinate, posterior ethmoidectomy, nasal protective sleeves, drill down sphenoid rostrum and expose lateral recess, strip sphenoid mucosa, remove bone over sella and expose entire right medial cavernous sinus and medial left cavernous sinus and up to sphenoid limbus and medial opticocarotid recesses, dura opened in an inverted V shape, tumor resected with two suctions and pituitary rongeur to peel tumor capsule, dissection continues laterally up the cavernous walls, resection superiorly with angled endoscopes into third ventricle, inspect cavity, if high flow leak use collagen inlay and nasoseptal flap, nasal packing	Lateralize inferior turbinates, +/− resection of right middle turbinate, partial resection of inferior aspect of superior turbinate, posterior septectomy, wide sphenoid sinus opening, resection of sphenoid rostrum/ bilateral posterior ethmoid air cells, raise large right Hadad nasoseptal flap, removal of sellar face from cavernous to cavernous sinus, drill out clival recess, thin sphenoid tuberculum past limbus dural fold and reflect bone away, open dura, extracapsular dissection, assessment for residual tumor nests and CSF leak, retrieval of nasoseptal flap, Nasopore	Local anesthetic and local vasopressors into nasal septum and turbinates, nasoseptal flap dissection, displacement of septum, location of sphenoid ostia, resection of anterior wall of sphenoid sinus, anatomic localization of sellar floor and carotid prominences with direction under microscopic vision and fluoroscopy, drilling of sellar floor and removal with rongeurs, tumor micropuncture to confirm absence of cavernous sinus bleeding, intratumoral debulking, tumor aspiration and curettage, capsular resection with preservation of diaphragma, repair of sellar floor with chitosan, fat graft in sphenoid sinus, nasoseptal flap placement, intranasal ventilation tubes

(continued on next page)

	Peter Bullock, FRCS, MRCP, London Clinic, London, England	Paul A. Gardner, MD, University of Pittsburgh, Pittsburgh, PA, United States	Nelson M. Oyesiku, MD, PhD, Joseph Quillin, MD, Emory University, Atlanta, GA, United States	Rodrigo Ramos-Zúñiga, MD, PhD, University of Guadalajara, Guadalajara, Jalisco, Mexico
Complication avoidance	Wide bony opening, removal of tumor floor and working upward, inspection with angled scopes, nasoseptal flap for dural reconstruction	Harvesting nasal septal flap, wide bony opening, exposure of right cavernous sinus, two suction technique, identify tumor capsule, inspection with angled scope	Harvesting nasal septal flap, wide sellar opening, extracapsular dissection, close attention to right cavernous sinus, inspection with various scopes for residual and CSF leaks	Harvesting nasal septal flap, fluoroscopy to guide localization, micropuncture, sphenoid sinus fat and nasoseptal flap, lumbar drain if needed for 24 hours
Postoperative				
Admission	High dependency unit	Intermediate care	Floor	ICU
Postoperative complications feared	CSF leak, hypopituitarism, diabetes insipidus	CSF leak, hypopituitarism, diabetes insipidus	HPA dysfunction (adrenal insufficiency, diabetes insipidus, SIADH), CSF leak	Injury to pterygopalatine and ICA, optic nerve damage, diabetes insipidus, adrenal insufficiency
Follow-up testing	Maintain strict fluid balance Vision checked every 4 hours MRI within 24 hours of surgery and 3 months after surgery	8 a.m. cortisol and prolactin 2 days after surgery Daily electrolytes and strict fluid assessment CT immediately after surgery if large CSF leak MRI 3 months after surgery	Daily BMP, postoperative day two 8 a.m. cortisol, LD for 3 days MRI 3 months after surgery	CT within 24 hours after surgery MRI within 72 hours after surgery Sodium checks and urine volumes Neuroendocrine evaluation 24 hours after surgery
Follow-up visits	3 months after surgery with neurosurgery 1 week after surgery with ENT 2 weeks after surgery with endocrinology	1 week after surgery for neurosurgery and ENT 2 weeks after surgery for endocrinology and ophthalmology	1 week after surgery for neuroendocrinology 2 weeks after surgery for ENT 6 weeks after surgery for neurosurgery	4 weeks after surgery

ACOM, anterior communicating artery; *BMP*, basic metabolic panel; *CSF*, cerebrospinal fluid; *CT*, computed tomography; *ENT*, ear, nose, and throat; *HPA*, hypothalamic-pituitary axis; *ICA*, internal carotid artery; *ICU*, intensive care unit; *IOM*, intraoperative monitoring; *LD*, lumbar drain; *MR*, magnetic resonance; *MRI*, magnetic resonance imaging; *OCT*, optic coherence tomography; *SIADH*, syndrome of inappropriate antidiuretic hormone; *SSEP*, somatosensory evoked potentials.

Differential diagnosis and actual diagnosis

- Pituitary adenoma
- Meningioma
- Metastatic brain tumor
- Craniopharyngioma
- Germinoma

Important anatomic and preoperative considerations

The sellar region has important bony, vascular, and neural anatomy.[6] The sella or pituitary fossa is a component of the body of sphenoid bone and is bounded anteriorly by the tuberculum sellae and posteriorly by the dorsum sellae.[6] Anteriorly to the tuberculum sellae is the chiasmatic sulcus, and the dorsum sellae is continuous with the clivus in which the upper portion is part of the sphenoid bone and the lower is part of the occipital bone.[6] The carotid sulcus extends along the lateral surface of the body of the sphenoid.[6] At the inferior aspect of the body of the sphenoid, the vomer attaches to the anterior half of the body of the sphenoid and separates the sphenoid ostia.[6] The sphenoid ostia are the openings to the sphenoid sinus, in which the pneumatization process starts in the presellar area, then extends below and behind the sella, and typically reaches their full size by adolescence.[6] The sphenoid sinus can take on a conchal, presellar, or sellar formation that can affect surgical strategy.[6] The conchal type (1%–2%) is when the area below the sella is composed of bone without an air cavity, the presellar type (15%–25%) is when the air cavity does not penetrate below the anterior tip of the sellar wall, and the sellar type (70%–85%) is where the air cavity extends below the sella and is the most common type.[6] The septations within the sphenoid sinus are often located off midline, and most commonly terminate near the carotid artery.[6] The carotid artery forms a prominence in the posterior sinus wall and along the anterior margin of the sella, and the optic canals protrude into the superolateral portion of the sinus, whereas the maxillary division of the trigeminal nerve protrudes into the inferolateral part of the sinus.[6] The diaphragma sellae forms the roof of the sella turcica, where it covers the pituitary gland except for the area that transmits the pituitary stalk.[6] The distance separating carotid artery and the pituitary gland ranges from 1 to 3 mm; however, in some cases the artery can protrude through the medial wall of the cavernous sinus.[6] As a result, injury can occur during transsphenoidal surgery, but injury can also occur from injury to the branches of the carotid artery, including the inferior hypophyseal artery or small capsular branches.[6] There are also anterior and posterior intercavernous sinuses that pass anterior and posterior to the hypophysis, respectively.[6] The cavernous sinus surrounds the horizontal portion of the carotid artery and the abducens nerve.[6] For a full detail of the cavernous sinus, see Chapter 50.

There are classification schemes that have been devised to described sellar changes, tumor extension, and cavernous sinus involvement.[7,8] The most commonly used classification system to describe sellar changes and pituitary tumor extension is the Hardy classification scheme, which is broken up into sellar changes (grades 0–5) and tumor extension (grades A–E) (Table 56.1). In addition, the Knosp classification scheme is used to describe invasion into the cavernous sinus (Table 56.2).[8] The tumor presented in this case is a Hardy grade 2C with sellar expansion but no focal destruction, and tumor extends into third ventricle up to the foramen of Monro, and a Knosp grade 1 in which the tumor extends into the cavernous sinus on the right past the medial internal carotid artery line but not past the median internal carotid artery line.

Table 56.1 Hardy classification scale for sellar changes and pituitary tumor extension

Sella turcica	
Grade 0	Size <10 mm, sella normal
Grade 1	Size <19 mm, sella expanded
Grade 2	Size >10 mm, sella expanded
Grade 3	Size >10 mm, focal destruction
Grade 4	Size >10 mm, diffuse destruction
Grade 5	Distant spread
Extrasellar extension	
Grade A	Bulges into chiasmatic cistern
Grade B	Reaches floor of the third ventricle
Grade C	Extension into the third ventricle up to the foramen of Monro
Grade D	Extends into the temporal and frontal fossa
Grade E	Extradural spread (extend into or out of the cavernous sinus)

Hardy classification scheme for pituitary adenomas in relation to sellar location and tumor extension.

Table 56.2 Knosp classification scheme for tumor cavernous sinus involvement

Grade 0	Tumor does not extend past the medial ICA line
Grade 1	Tumor crosses medial but does not extend past median ICA line
Grade 2	
Grade 3	Tumor extends beyond median line but does not extend past lateral ICA line
Grade 4	Tumor extends past lateral ICA line
	Circumferential

On coronal view of the sella, the medial line connects the medial walls of the ICAs, median line connects the center of the ICAs, and lateral line connects lateral walls of the ICAs.

ICA, internal carotid artery.

Approaches to this lesion

The approaches to sellar pathology can be divided into transsphenoidal and transcranial approaches (Fig. 56.2).[9–13] The transsphenoidal approaches include endonasal and sublabial, whereas transcranial approaches include pterional and supraorbital.[9,10] The most common approach is an endonasal transsphenoidal, whereby one or two nostrils are used to access the sphenoid sinus.[14] The corridor for this approach can be enlarged by performing an expanded endonasal approach, which can include unilateral or bilateral removal of the middle turbinates, maxillary antrostomy, and/or anterior and posterior ethmoidectomies.[9,10] This can be done endoscopically or microscopically (typically with a speculum), but currently endoscopically is the more common approach.[9–13] The advantages of the endonasal transsphenoidal approach are that it is minimally invasive, avoids need for brain retraction, provides an expanded view within the sella, and approaches the sella directly, whereas the disadvantages are sometimes needing skull base reconstruction, loss of smell, increased risk of cerebrospinal fluid (CSF) leak, and limited operating corridor.[9,10] The sublabial approach requires a gingival incision, subperiosteal dissection to the upper aspect of the rostrum of the maxilla, and submucosal dissection along the nasal cavity up along the nasal septum into the sphenoid sinus.[9] This approach is typically done with a microscope and a speculum.[9,11,13] The advantages of this approach, like the endonasal approach, are that is avoids the need for brain retraction and approaches the sella directly, whereas the disadvantages include mouth numbness and pain, increased risk of CSF leak, and limited operating corridor.[9–13] The most common cranial approach is a pterional approach, whereby a pterional craniotomy is done and the lesion is approached via a trans-Sylvian or subfrontal approach typically using the intraoptic or opticocarotid triangles for resection.[9,10] The advantages of the pterional transcranial approach are that it identifies the optic nerves and optic chiasm early for decompression, allows easy access to the suprasellar space, minimizes risk of CSF leak, and has a larger working corridor, whereas the disadvantages include brain manipulation, potential brain retraction, and difficulty with accessing the sella.[9,10] An alternative cranial approach is a supraorbital craniotomy, which can be achieved with a transpalpebral (eyebrow), transciliary (eyelid), or modified orbitozygomatic craniotomies.[15–17] The advantages and

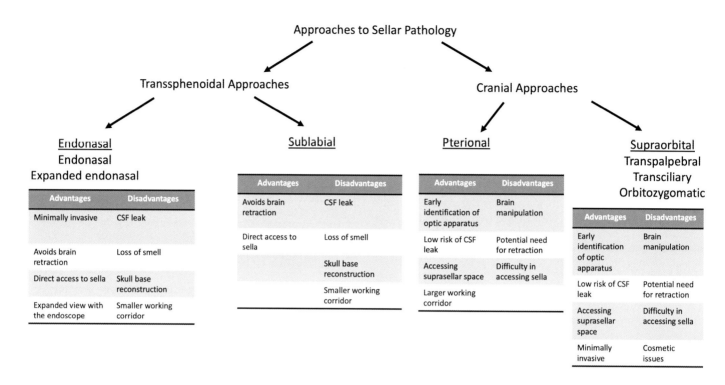

Fig. 56.2 Diagram of approaches to sellar pathology. *CSF*, cerebrospinal fluid.

disadvantages of the supraorbital approach are similar to the pterional approach.[15–17] The advantages of the supraorbital over the pterional is that it is minimally invasive and potentially minimizes brain retraction with removal of the orbital rim, whereas its disadvantages are potentially cosmetic issues and a smaller working corridor.[15–17]

What was actually done

The patient was taken to surgery for an endoscopic endonasal resection of a nonfunctional pituitary macroadenoma with otolaryngology with general anesthesia and no intraoperative monitoring. The patient was induced and intubated per routine. An electromagnetic navigation system with preoperative magnetic resonance imaging (MRI) and computed tomography were used to avoid the need for head pinning. The left lower abdominal quadrant was prepped in case a fat graft was needed. The patient was draped in the usual standard fashion and given cefazolin. With the assistance of a rhinologist, the right middle and inferior turbinates were displaced laterally. A right nasal septal flap was raised and placed into the nasopharynx. A posterior septectomy was done to allow bi-nasal access. The sphenoid ostia were opened bilaterally, and the intersinus septation was drilled flush with the sellar face. The bone overlying the sella was thinned with a diamond drill until the dura was identified. A nerve hook was used to dissect the dura in the epidural plane, and up- and down-going Kerrison punches were used to remove the bone until both cavernous sinuses, floor of the sella, and planum sphenoidale were identified. The tuberculum was removed. The dura was opened in a cruciate fashion with an arachnoid knife, and the dura was removed with a side-cutting tissue biting device (Myriad, NICO Corporation, Indianapolis, IN).

The tumor was debulked first at the inferior aspect by identifying the floor, followed by the bilateral cavernous sinuses, and moving upward until the diaphragma sellae fell into the sellar cavity. The tumor was debulked until no more tumor was visible. Preliminary pathology was pituitary adenoma. A couple of rounds of Valsalva were used to see if more tumor would fall into the cavity. A small CSF leak was encountered, and the sella was packed with gelfoam, followed by a dural substitute in the epidural plane, and tucked into the bone edges of the sella. The nasoseptal flap was used to reinforce the opening. Nasal packings were placed bilaterally. No lumbar drain or fat graft was used.

The patient awoke at their neurologic baseline and was taken to the intensive care unit for recovery. An MRI was done within 24 hours after surgery and showed subtotal resection with residual in the suprasellar space but with good decompression of the optic apparatus (Fig. 56.3). The sodium and urine specific gravity were checked every 4 to 6 hours, and she had one episode of diabetes insipidus requiring desmopressin. The morning cortisol was 12, and no hydrocortisone was given. The nasal packings were removed 24 hours after surgery. The patient participated with physical therapy and was discharged to home on postoperative day 2 with 7 days of cefdinir. The patient was seen in the ear, nose, and throat (ENT) clinic for endoscopic examination and cleaning on postoperative day 7. The patient was seen at 2 weeks postoperatively and reported full vision in all visual fields. Pathology was nonfunctional pituitary adenoma, and hormonal stains were negative. The patient underwent formal visual field examination at 3 months postoperatively and had full visual fields. The lesion was observed with serial MRI examinations at 3- to 6-month intervals, and the residual had been stable for 36 months.

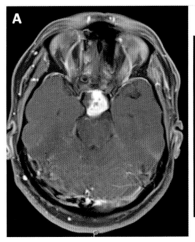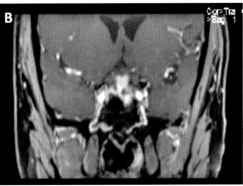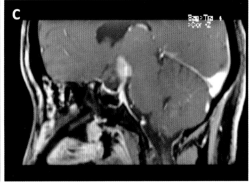

Fig. 56.3 Postoperative magnetic resonance imaging. (A) T1 axial image with gadolinium contrast; **(B)** T1 coronal image with gadolinium contrast; **(C)** T1 sagittal image with gadolinium contrast magnetic resonance imaging scan demonstrating subtotal resection with a small residual near the optic chiasm.

Commonalities among the experts

The majority of surgeons opted for the patient to undergo vascular imaging (half computed tomography angiography, one magnetic resonance angiography) to better delineate the location and course of the internal carotid arteries, endocrinology and ophthalmology evaluations, and ENT consultation. All surgeons pursued a transnasal transsphenoidal approach, in which the majority used an endoscope and half elected to remove the tuberculum. All surgeons performed the surgery in combination with otolaryngology. Most surgeons aimed for extensive resection with decompression of the optic apparatus, and half aimed for gross total resection. Most surgeons were cognizant of the paraclival and parasellar carotid arteries and the optic nerves. Most surgeons were concerned about visual decline and hypopituitarism. Surgery was generally pursued with surgical navigation, endoscope, and cranial Doppler, with perioperative steroids. The majority of surgeons advocated for a wide sellar opening, harvesting of a nasoseptal flap, and protection of the pituitary gland. Following surgery, patient admissions varied from floor to intensive care unit, and surgeons requested imaging 3 months after surgery to assess for extent of resection.

SUMMARY OF QUALITY OF EVIDENCE TO GUIDE SPECIFIC INTERVENTIONS FOR THIS CASE

- Endoscopic endonasal versus microscopic approach—Class II-2.
- Surgery for nonfunctional pituitary macroadenoma with visual deficits—Class II-3.
- Observation of residual pituitary adenoma—Class III.

REFERENCES

1. Molitch ME. Diagnosis and treatment of pituitary adenomas: a review. *JAMA*. 2017;317:516–524.
2. Anagnostis P, Adamidou F, Polyzos SA, Efstathiadou Z, Panagiotou A, Kita M. Non-functioning pituitary adenomas: a single center experience. *Exp Clin Endocrinol Diabetes*. 2011;119:314–319.
3. Ebersold MJ, Quast LM, Laws Jr ER. Scheithauer B, Randall RV. Long-term results in transsphenoidal removal of nonfunctioning pituitary adenomas. *J Neurosurg*. 1986;64:713–719.
4. Ezzat S, Asa SL, Couldwell WT, et al. The prevalence of pituitary adenomas: a systematic review. *Cancer*. 2004;101:613–619.
5. Sanai N, Quinones-Hinojosa A, Narvid J, Kunwar S. Safety and efficacy of the direct endonasal transsphenoidal approach for challenging sellar tumors. *J Neurooncol*. 2008;87:317–325.
6. Rhoton Jr AL. The sellar region. *Neurosurgery*. 2002;51:S335–S374.
7. Mooney MA, Hardesty DA, Sheehy JP, et al. Rater reliability of the hardy classification for pituitary adenomas in the magnetic resonance imaging era. *J Neurol Surg B Skull Base*. 2017;78:413–418.
8. Knosp E, Steiner E, Kitz K, Matula C. Pituitary adenomas with invasion of the cavernous sinus space: a magnetic resonance imaging classification compared with surgical findings. *Neurosurgery*. 1993;33:610–617; discussion 617–618.
9. Liu JK, Weiss MH, Couldwell WT. Surgical approaches to pituitary tumors. *Neurosurg Clin N Am*. 2003;14:93–107.
10. Couldwell WT. Transsphenoidal and transcranial surgery for pituitary adenomas. *J Neurooncol*. 2004;69:237–256.
11. Eseonu CI, ReFaey K, Garcia O, Salvatori R, Quinones-Hinojosa A. Comparative cost analysis of endoscopic versus microscopic endonasal transsphenoidal surgery for pituitary adenomas. *J Neurol Surg B Skull Base*. 2018;79:131–138.
12. Eseonu CI, ReFaey K, Pamias-Portalatin E, et al. Three-hand endoscopic endonasal transsphenoidal surgery: experience with an anatomy-preserving mononostril approach technique. *Oper Neurosurg (Hagerstown)*. 2018;14:158–165.
13. Eseonu CI, ReFaey K, Rincon-Torroella J, et al. Endoscopic versus microscopic transsphenoidal approach for pituitary adenomas: comparison of outcomes during the transition of methods of a single surgeon. *World Neurosurg*. 2017;97:317–325.
14. Frazier JL, Chaichana K, Jallo GI, Quinones-Hinojosa A. Combined endoscopic and microscopic management of pediatric pituitary region tumors through one nostril: technical note with case illustrations. *Childs Nerv Syst*. 2008;24:1469–1478.
15. Raza SM, Boahene KD, Quinones-Hinojosa A. The transpalpebral incision: its use in keyhole approaches to cranial base brain tumors. *Expert Rev Neurother*. 2010;10:1629–1632.
16. Raza SM, Garzon-Muvdi T, Boaehene K. et al: The supraorbital craniotomy for access to the skull base and intraaxial lesions: a technique in evolution. *Minim Invasive Neurosurg*. 2010;53:1–8.
17. Raza SM, Quinones-Hinojosa A, Lim M, Boahene KD. The transconjunctival transorbital approach: a keyhole approach to the midline anterior skull base. *World Neurosurg*. 2013;80:864–871.

57

Nonfunctional pituitary adenoma abutting chiasm

Case reviewed by Lucas Alverne Freitas de Albuquerque, Arturo Ayala-Arcipreste, Edward R. Laws, Daniel Donoho, Nelson M. Oyesiku, Joseph Quillin

Introduction

The incidence of pituitary adenomas varies in many studies, in which radiographic studies have ranged from 1% to 40%, and postmortem studies have ranged from 1% to 35%.[1] Based on a meta-analysis, the estimated prevalence of pituitary adenomas is 16.7%.[1] With the widespread availability of imaging, the percent of incidental pituitary adenomas appears to be increasing.[2–4] It is estimated that 30% of pituitary adenomas are discovered incidentally, in which the majority of these were macroadenomas that were clinically nonfunctional and extended into the suprasellar space with abutment of the optic chiasm.[2–4] Although some advocate surgery for these lesions with optic chiasm involvement, others have advocated conservative management as the risks of pituitary apoplexy (0.6/100 patient-years), visual field deficits

(0.6/100 patient-years), and endocrine dysfunction (0.8/100 patient-years) remain low.[2–4] In this chapter, we present a case of a patient with a nonfunctional pituitary macroadenoma that was incidentally discovered without symptoms.

Example case

Chief complaint: headaches
History of present illness
A 59-year-old, right-handed woman with a history of diabetes and hypertension presented with headaches. Over the past 9 to 12 months, she complained of worsening migraines in terms of frequency and intensity. She underwent magnetic resonance imaging (MRI) that showed a pituitary lesion (Fig. 57.1). Visual fields were full on formal visual field testing with ophthalmology.

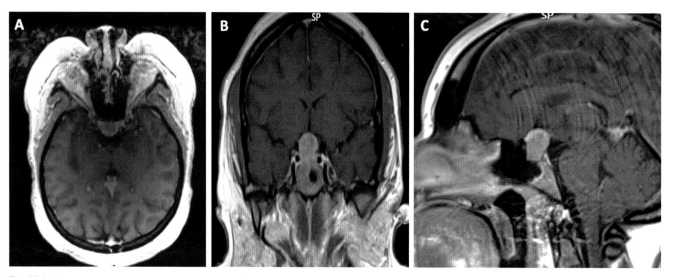

Fig. 57.1 Preoperative magnetic resonance imaging. (A) T1 axial image with gadolinium contrast; **(B)** T1 coronal image with gadolinium contrast; **(C)** T1 sagittal image with gadolinium contrast magnetic resonance imaging scan demonstrating an enhancing lesion involving the sellar and suprasellar space with involvement of the optic chiasm.

Medications: Irbesartan, metformin.
Allergies: No known drug allergies.
Past medical and surgical history: Diabetes, hypertension, cholecystectomy, appendectomy.
Family history: No history of intracranial malignancies.
Social history: Store owner, no smoking or alcohol.

Physical examination: Awake, alert, oriented to person, place, and time; Cranial nerves II to XII intact with full visual fields to confrontation; No drift, moves all extremities with full strength.
Pituitary labs: Prolactin, thyroid stimulating hormone/T4, cortisol, insulin-like growth factor-1 all within normal limits.

	Lucas Alverne Freitas de Albuquerque, MD, Hospital Geral de Fortaleza, Ceara, Brazil	Arturo Ayala-Arcipreste, MD, Hospital Juarez de Mexico, Mexico City, Mexico	Edward R. Laws, MD, Daniel Donoho, MD, Brigham and Women's Hospital, Boston, MA, United States	Nelson M. Oyesiku, MD, PhD, Joseph Quillin, MD, Emory University, Atlanta, GA, United States
Preoperative				
Additional tests requested	CT maxillofacial Anesthesiology evaluation Endocrinology evaluation ENT evaluation	CT paranasal sinuses Endocrinology evaluation Ophthalmology evaluation (visual fields) Cardiology evaluation	FSH, LH, calcium MRI Cardiology evaluation	High-resolution T2 MRI Neuroophthalmology evaluation (visual fields, OCT) Endocrinology evaluation ENT evaluation Pregnancy test
Surgical approach selected	Endoscopic transnasal transsphenoidal	Endoscopic transnasal transsphenoidal	Endoscopic transnasal transsphenoidal	Endoscopic transnasal transsphenoidal
Other teams involved during surgery	ENT	ENT	+/− ENT	ENT
Anatomic corridor	Transnasal transsphenoidal	Transnasal transsphenoidal	Transnasal transsphenoidal	Transnasal transsphenoidal
Goal of surgery	Gross total resection, optic apparatus decompression, avoid future vision loss, improve headaches	Gross total resection, optic apparatus decompression, preservation of infundibulum and pituitary gland	Gross total resection, optic apparatus decompression, preservation of normal gland	Gross total resection
Perioperative				
Positioning	Supine without pins	Supine without pins	Supine with skull clamps	Supine with skull clamps, 10-degree right rotation
Surgical equipment	Endoscope	Endoscope Surgical navigation Microdoppler	Endoscope Microdoppler Microdebrider	0-degree endoscope Surgical navigation Ultrasonic aspirator Nasopore
Medications	None	Steroids	None	None
Anatomic considerations	Pituitary gland, internal carotid arteries, optic apparatus	Nasal structures, sphenoid sinus, sellar and parasellar regions, ICA, optic nerves and chiasm	ICA, pituitary gland, diaphragma sellae	Cavernous carotid arteries, optic nerves, ACOM
Complications feared with approach chosen	CSF leak, vascular injury	ICA injury, pituitary/ infundibulum injury, vision loss, cavernous sinus injury	Visual loss, hypopituitarism, injury to infundibulum, CSF leak	ICA/ACA injury, diminished olfaction, optic nerve injury
Intraoperative				
Anesthesia	General	General	General	General
Skin incision	None	None	None	None

(continued on next page)

	Lucas Alverne Freitas de Albuquerque, MD, Hospital Geral de Fortaleza, Ceara, Brazil	Arturo Ayala-Arcipreste, MD, Hospital Juarez de Mexico, Mexico City, Mexico	Edward R. Laws, MD, Daniel Donoho, MD, Brigham and Women's Hospital, Boston, MA, United States	Nelson M. Oyesiku, MD, PhD, Joseph Quillin, MD, Emory University, Atlanta, GA, United States
Bone opening	Sphenoid osteotomy, removal of sellar bone	Sphenoid osteotomy and sphenoid sinus, floor of sella	Wide sphenoid osteotomy, removal of sellar bone	Right middle turbinate, wide sphenoid osteotomy, posterior ethmoidectomy, removal of sella from cavernous to cavernous sinus
Brain exposure	Sella	Sella	Sella	Sella cavernous sinus to cavernous sinus
Method of resection	Use of primarily 30-degree endoscope, lateralization of bilateral inferior and middle turbinates, nasoseptal flap on the left side, expose and open anterior wall of sphenoid sinus, large opening made in right posterior septum for binostril approach, identify sella, anterior wall of sella opened with high-speed drill or Kerrison rongeurs, open dura, tumor dissection, position nasoseptal flap, medialization and reposition of middle and inferior turbinates	Dislocation of bilateral middle and superior turbinates, identify sphenoid ostia and nasal septum, harvesting of nasoseptal flap bilaterally, expand both sphenoid ostum initially with Kerrison rongeur and drill, removal of mucosa in sphenoid sinus, removal of sellar bone, cauterize dura, open dura in cruciate fashion, use curettes to remove tumor in a clockwise fashion, use Doppler to localize ICA laterally, identify diaphragm, verify hemostasis using small pieces of gelfoam or Surgicel, use bone fragment to reconstruct sellar floor, use nasoseptal flap, apply fibrin glue, place nasal plugs	Lateralize bilateral middle turbinates, posterior septectomy with preservation of rescue flaps, exposure of sphenoid ostia, removal of sphenoid face out to lateral recesses and rostral aspect of sphenoid, removal of sphenoid sinus septations and mucosa, remove sellar face, open dura, resect tumor extracapsularly if possible, evaluate for CSF leak, abdominal fat if leak present, reconstruct sellar face with medpore/septal cartilage or bone, medialize middle turbinates	Lateralize inferior turbinates, right middle turbinate resection and free mucosal graft harvesting, partial resection of inferior aspect of superior turbinate, posterior septectomy, wide sphenoid sinusotomy and resection of rostrum, bilateral posterior ethmoidectomy, wide sphenoidotomy from cavernous to cavernous sinus, dural opening, extracapsular dissection of tumor, careful inspect for tumor and CSF leak, dural substitute inlay covered with free mucosal graft, Nasopore
Complication avoidance	Leave turbinates, binostril approach, nasoseptal flap	Unilateral nostril approach, systematic tumor resection, Doppler to localize ICA, bone for sellar floor reconstruction, nasoseptal flap for repair	Leave middle turbinates, wide sellar opening, extracapsular dissection, inspection for residual and CSF leaks	Wide sellar opening, extracapsular dissection, inspection for residual and CSF leaks
Postoperative				
Admission	ICU	Floor	Floor	Floor
Postoperative complications feared	CSF leak, pituitary dysfunction	CSF leak, diabetes insipidus	Hypopituitarism, hyponatremia, diabetes insipidus, visual loss, ICA/cavernous sinus injury	HPA dysfunction (adrenal insufficiency, diabetes insipidus, SIADH), CSF leak
Follow-up testing	MRI 3 months after surgery; Pituitary hormone evaluation 10 days and 3 months after surgery	Sodium and urine analyses for 72 hours after surgery; CT within 24 hours after surgery; MRI 5–6 weeks after surgery	Sodium and cortisol 7 days after surgery; Endocrine panel 6 weeks after surgery; MRI 3 months after surgery	Daily BMP, postoperative day two 8 a.m. cortisol; MRI 3 months after surgery

	Lucas Alverne Freitas de Albuquerque, MD, Hospital Geral de Fortaleza, Ceara, Brazil	Arturo Ayala-Arcipreste, MD, Hospital Juarez de Mexico, Mexico City, Mexico	Edward R. Laws, MD, Daniel Donoho, MD, Brigham and Women's Hospital, Boston, MA, United States	Nelson M. Oyesiku, MD, PhD, Joseph Quillin, MD, Emory University, Atlanta, GA, United States
Follow-up visits	7–10 days for hormonal evaluation 1, 3 months, 6 months, yearly after surgery	2 months after surgery 10 days after surgery with ENT and endocrinology	1 week after surgery for neuroendocrinology 3 months after surgery for neurosurgery	1 week after surgery for neuroendocrinology 2 weeks after surgery for ENT 6 weeks after surgery for neurosurgery

ACOM, anterior communicating artery; BMP, basic metabolic panel; CSF, cerebrospinal fluid; CT, computed tomography; ENT, ear, nose, and throat; FSH, follicle stimulating hormone; HPA, hypothalamic-pituitary axis; ICA, internal carotid artery; ICU, intensive care unit; LH, luteinizing hormone; MRI, magnetic resonance imaging; OCT, optic coherence tomography; SIADH, syndrome of inappropriate antidiuretic hormone.

Differential diagnosis and actual diagnosis

- Pituitary adenoma
- Meningioma
- Metastatic brain tumor
- Craniopharyngioma
- Germinoma

Important anatomic and preoperative considerations

For a full discussion of sellar anatomy in regard to the bony, vascular, and neural anatomy, see Chapter 56, and for the cavernous sinus, refer to Chapter 50. As pituitary lesions grow superiorly, they can displace the diaphragma sellae superiorly and/or enlarge or penetrate through the aperture of the infundibulum to involve the suprasellar space.[5] The third ventricle resides above the sella turcica, pituitary gland, and midbrain, and is surrounded laterally by the thalami and hypothalamus.[5] The floor of the third ventricle consists of the optic chiasm, infundibulum, tuber cinereum, mammillary bodies, posterior perforated substances, and tegmentum of the midbrain.[5] Pituitary macroadenomas that occupy the suprasellar space do so at the anterior incisural region in front of the midbrain, which is bounded by the optic chiasm superiorly, posteriorly by the cerebral peduncles and interpeduncular cistern, posterolaterally by the uncus, and laterally by the component of the Sylvian fissure below the anterior perforated substance.[5] The interpeduncular and chiasmatic cisterns are separated by the Liliequist membrane, which is an arachnoid sheet that extends from the dorsum sellae to the anterior edge of the mammillary bodies.[5] The optic chiasm typically overlies the diaphragma sellae and the pituitary gland (~70%), whereas the prefixed chiasm overlies the tuberculum sellae (~15%), and the postfixed chiasm overlies the dorsum sellae (~15%).[5] A cranial approach to the suprasellar space can therefore be limited by a prefixed chiasm and a superior protruding tuberculum sella, but does not affect a transsphenoidal approach.[5]

The Hardy and Knosp classification schemes are used to describe sellar changes and tumor extension and cavernous sinus involvement, respectively (Chapter 56, Figs. 56.3 and 56.4).[6,7] The tumor presented in this case is a Hardy grade 2B with sellar expansion but no focal destruction, and tumor extends to the floor of the third ventricle, and a Knosp grade 0 in which the tumor does not extend past the median internal carotid artery line.

Approaches to this lesion

The approaches to sellar pathology can be divided into transsphenoidal and transcranial approaches and are described in detail in Chapter 56, Fig. 56.2.[8–12] The modern conventional approach to sellar pathology is a transsphenoidal approach.[8–12] Transsphenoidal approaches include endonasal and sublabial approaches, and the most commonly used is an endoscopic endonasal approach.[13] The corridor for this approach can be enlarged by performing an expanded endonasal approach, which can include unilateral or bilateral removal of the middle turbinates, maxillary antrostomy, and/or anterior and posterior ethmoidectomies.[8,9] This is typically done for larger tumors with significant suprasellar extension and/or tumors with extension into the cavernous sinus.[8,9] The advantages of the endonasal transsphenoidal approach are that it is minimally invasive, avoids need for brain retraction, provides an expanded view within the sella, and approaches the sella directly, whereas the disadvantages are sometimes needing skull base reconstruction, loss of smell, increased risk of cerebrospinal fluid leak, and limited operating corridor.[8–12]

What was actually done

The patient was taken to surgery for an endoscopic endonasal resection of a nonfunctional pituitary macroadenoma with otolaryngology with general anesthesia and no intraoperative monitoring. The patient was induced and intubated per routine. An electromagnetic navigation system with preoperative MRI and computed tomography were used to avoid the need for head pinning. The patient was draped in the usual standard fashion and given cefazolin. With the assistance of a rhinologist, the right middle and inferior turbinates were displaced laterally. A right nasal septal flap was raised and placed into the nasopharynx. A posterior septectomy was done to allow bilateral nasal access. The sphenoid ostia were opened bilaterally, and the intersinus septation was drilled flush with the sellar face. The bone overlying the sella was thinned with a diamond drill until the dura was identified. A nerve hook was used to dissect the dura in the epidural plane, and up- and down-going Kerrison punches were used to remove the bone until both cavernous sinuses and the floor of the sella were identified. The tuberculum sellae was not removed. The dura was opened in a cruciate fashion with an arachnoid knife, and the dura was removed with a side-cutting tissue biting device (Myriad, NICO Corporation, Indianapolis, IN). The tumor was debulked first at the inferior aspect by identifying the floor, followed by the bilateral cavernous sinuses, and moving upward until the diaphragma sellae fell into the sellar cavity using a combination of suction, side-cutting tissue device, and ring curettes. The tumor was debulked until no more tumor was visible. Preliminary pathology was pituitary adenoma. The diaphragma was seen herniating into the cavity, and the gland was identified at the superior left quadrant. The nasoseptal flap was replaced and sutured in place because no cerebrospinal fluid leak was seen. Nasal packings were placed bilaterally. No lumbar drain or fat graft was used.

The patient awoke at their neurologic baseline and was taken to the postoperative recovery unit and the surgical floor for recovery. An MRI was done within 24 hours after surgery, which showed gross total resection (Fig. 57.2). The sodium and urine specific gravity were checked every 4 to 6 hours, and no episodes of diabetes insipidus occurred, postoperative a.m. cortisol was 13, and no hydrocortisone was given. The nasal packings were removed 24 hours after surgery. The patient participated with physical therapy and was discharged to home on postoperative day 2 with 7 days of cefdinir. The patient was seen in the ear, nose, and throat clinic for endoscopic examination and cleaning on postoperative day 7. The patient was seen at 2 weeks postoperatively and reported full vision in all visual fields. Pathology was nonfunctional pituitary adenoma, and hormonal stains were negative. The patient underwent formal visual field examination at 3 months postoperatively and had full visual fields. The lesion was observed with serial MRI examinations at 3- and 6-month intervals, and no recurrence has been noted for 48 months.

Commonalities among the experts

The majority of surgeons opted for the patient to undergo endocrinology evaluation; half opted for computed tomography for bony anatomy detail, and half opted for ophthalmology, cardiology, and endocrinology evaluation prior to surgery. All surgeons pursued an endoscopic endonasal transsphenoidal approach, and all aimed for gross total resection with decompression of the optic apparatus. Half of the surgeons also identified the need for preservation of the pituitary gland. All surgeons would likely perform the surgery in combination with otolaryngology. Most surgeons were cognizant about the parasellar carotid arteries and the optic nerves. Most were concerned about visual decline and vascular injury. Surgery was generally pursued with endoscopic equipment, with no special additional medications. The majority of surgeons advocated for preservation of the turbinates, extracapsular dissection, thorough inspection for cerebrospinal fluid leaks, and use of nasoseptal flaps if cerebrospinal fluid leaks are found. Following surgery, most surgeons admitted their patients to the floor, and requested imaging 3 months after surgery to assess for extent of resection.

SUMMARY OF QUALITY OF EVIDENCE TO GUIDE SPECIFIC INTERVENTIONS FOR THIS CASE

- Endoscopic endonasal versus microscopic approach—Class II-2.
- Surgery for nonfunctional pituitary macroadenoma with no visual deficits—Class III.

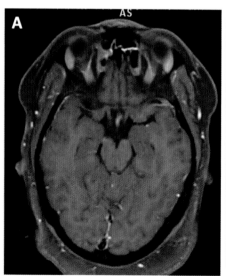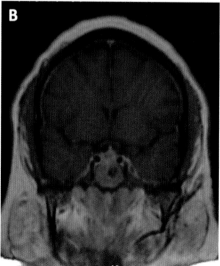

Fig. 57.2 Postoperative magnetic resonance imaging. (A) T1 axial image with gadolinium contrast; **(B)** T1 coronal image with gadolinium contrast magnetic resonance imaging scan demonstrating gross total resection of the lesion.

REFERENCES

1. Ezzat S, Asa SL, Couldwell WT, et al. The prevalence of pituitary adenomas: a systematic review. *Cancer*. 2004;101:613–619.
2. Iglesias P, Arcano K, Trivino V, et al. Prevalence, clinical features, and natural history of incidental clinically non-functioning pituitary adenomas. *Horm Metab Res*. 2017;49:654–659.
3. Sivakumar W, Chamoun R, Nguyen V, Couldwell WT. Incidental pituitary adenomas. *Neurosurg Focus*. 2011;31:E18.
4. Sanno N, Oyama K, Tahara S, Teramoto A, Kato Y. A survey of pituitary incidentaloma in Japan. *Eur J Endocrinol*. 2003;149:123–127.
5. Rhoton Jr AL. The sellar region. *Neurosurgery*. 2002;51:S335–S374.
6. Knosp E, Steiner E, Kitz K, Matula C. Pituitary adenomas with invasion of the cavernous sinus space: a magnetic resonance imaging classification compared with surgical findings. *Neurosurgery*. 1993;33:610–617; discussion 617–618.
7. Mooney MA, Hardesty DA, Sheehy JP, et al. Rater reliability of the hardy classification for pituitary adenomas in the magnetic resonance imaging era. *J Neurol Surg B Skull Base*. 2017;78:413–418.
8. Liu JK, Weiss MH, Couldwell WT. Surgical approaches to pituitary tumors. *Neurosurg Clin N Am*. 2003;14:93–107.
9. Couldwell WT. Transsphenoidal and transcranial surgery for pituitary adenomas. *J Neurooncol*. 2004;69:237–256.
10. Eseonu CI, ReFaey K, Garcia O, Salvatori R, Quinones-Hinojosa A. Comparative cost analysis of endoscopic versus microscopic endonasal transsphenoidal surgery for pituitary adenomas. *J Neurol Surg B Skull Base*. 2018;79:131–138.
11. Eseonu CI, ReFaey K, Pamias-Portalatin E, et al. Three-hand endoscopic endonasal transsphenoidal surgery: experience with an anatomy-preserving mononostril approach technique. *Oper Neurosurg (Hagerstown)*. 2018;14:158–165.
12. Eseonu CI, ReFaey K, Rincon-Torroella J, et al. Endoscopic versus microscopic transsphenoidal approach for pituitary adenomas: comparison of outcomes during the transition of methods of a single surgeon. *World Neurosurg*. 2017;97:317–325.
13. Frazier JL, Chaichana K, Jallo GI, Quinones-Hinojosa A. Combined endoscopic and microscopic management of pediatric pituitary region tumors through one nostril: technical note with case illustrations. *Childs Nerv Syst*. 2008;24:1469–1478.

58

Pituitary apoplexy

Case reviewed by James J. Evans, Tomas Garzon-Muvdi, Paul A. Gardner, Carl H. Snyderman, Chae-Yong Kim, Tetsuro Sameshima

Introduction

Pituitary apoplexy is a potentially life-threatening condition due to acute ischemia or hemorrhage within the pituitary gland, and typically occurs in the setting of a pituitary adenoma.[1,2] The incidence of pituitary apoplexy in patients with pituitary adenomas occurs in 1% to 26% of patients in some series, and can be the primary presentation of a pituitary tumor in up to 80% of patients.[1,2] The most common symptoms are sudden and severe headaches in 90% to 100%, nausea and vomiting in 40% to 80%, decreased visual acuity in 45% to 90%, visual field defect in 40% to 75%, ophthalmoplegia in 50% to 80%, and altered consciousness in 5% to 40%.[1,2] The majority of patients (up to 80%) will have a deficiency in one or more anterior pituitary hormones, in which adrenal insufficiency occurs in 60% to 75% of patients.[1,2] For patients with apoplexy who present with ophthalmoplegia without visual field deficits, the management can sometimes be controversial, as there are reports with resolution of ophthalmoplegia with both conservative and surgical management.[3,4] In this chapter, we present a case of a patient with a pituitary apoplexy.

Example case

Chief complaint: headaches, lethargy, and double vision
History of present illness
A 70-year-old, right-handed man with a history of diabetes, hypertension, and coronary artery disease presented with acute onset of headaches, lethargy, and double vision. He was in his usual state of health until this morning when he had acute onset of the worst headache of his life, double vision with inability to move right eye in all directions, and lethargy. He was taken to the emergency room, where brain imaging was done (Fig. 58.1).

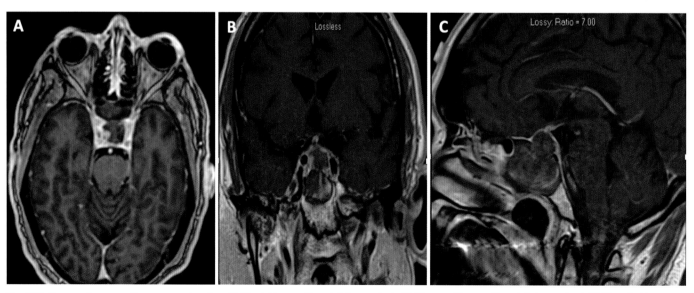

Fig. 58.1 Preoperative magnetic resonance imaging. (A) T1 axial image with gadolinium contrast; **(B)** T1 coronal image with gadolinium contrast; **(C)** T1 sagittal image with gadolinium contrast magnetic resonance imaging scan demonstrating a heterogeneously enhancing lesion involving the sellar and suprasellar space without optic chiasm compression but with involvement of the right cavernous sinus.

Medications: Irbesartan, metformin, aspirin, clopidogrel.
Allergies: No known drug allergies.
Past medical and surgical history: Diabetes, hypertension, coronary artery disease, cataracts, carpel tunnel, right knee replacement.
Family history: No history of intracranial malignancies.
Social history: Retired veteran, remote smoking history, no alcohol.

Physical examination: Awake, lethargic, oriented to person, place, and time; Cranial nerves II to XII intact, except right cranial nerve III palsy with ptosis, visual fields full to confrontation; No drift, moves all extremities with full strength.
Pituitary labs: Prolactin 0, random cortisol 3, thyroid stimulating hormone/T4, and insulin-like growth factor-1 within normal limits.

	James J. Evans, MD, Tomas Garzon-Muvdi, MD, Thomas Jefferson University, Philadelphia, PA, United States	Paul A. Gardner, MD, Carl H. Snyderman, MD, MBA, University of Pittsburgh, Pittsburgh, PA, United States	Chae-Yong Kim, MD, PhD, Seoul National University Bundang Hospital, Seoul, South Korea	Tetsuro Sameshima, MD, PhD, Hamamatsu University, Hamamatsu, Shizuoka, Japan
Preoperative				
Additional tests requested	Pituitary hormone evaluation Endocrinology evaluation Neuroophthalmology evaluation	CT angiogram Endocrinology evaluation Neuroophthalmology evaluation ENT evaluation 8 a.m. cortisol	CT maxillofacial Pituitary hormone evaluation Serum electrolytes and markers for infection Neuropsychological assessment Neuroophthalmology evaluation	CT head Pituitary hormone evaluation
Surgical approach selected	Endoscopic endonasal transsphenoidal	Endoscopic endonasal transsphenoidal, partial transclival	Endoscopic endonasal transsphenoidal	Endoscopic endonasal transsphenoidal
Other teams involved during surgery	ENT	ENT	ENT	None
Anatomic corridor	Transnasal transsphenoidal	Transnasal transsphenoidal/transclival	Transnasal transsphenoidal	Transnasal transsphenoidal
Goal of surgery	Maximal resection	Complete resection with preservation of pituitary function	Decompression, diagnosis	Decompression (except cavernous sinus component), diagnosis
Perioperative				
Positioning	Supine without pins	Supine with pins	Supine without pins	Supine with pins
Surgical equipment	Surgical navigation Endoscope	IOM (SSEP) Surgical navigation Endoscope Microdoppler	Surgical navigation Endoscope Intraoperative CT or MRI	Surgical navigation Endoscope Ultrasonic aspirator
Medications	Steroids	Steroids	Steroids Thyroid medication if low	None
Anatomic considerations	ICAs, optic nerves, diaphragma sellae, pituitary gland and stalk	Parasellar and paraclival ICAs, opticocarotid recesses, cavernous sinus walls, pituitary glands	Optic chiasm, cavernous sinus, ICA	Cavernous sinus
Complications feared with approach chosen	CSF leak, recurrent hemorrhage from residual tumor	CSF leak, hypopituitarism, vision loss	Anosmia	Cavernous sinus injury
Intraoperative				
Anesthesia	General	General	General	General
Skin incision	None	None	None	None

(continued on next page)

	James J. Evans, MD, Tomas Garzon-Muvdi, MD, Thomas Jefferson University, Philadelphia, PA, United States	Paul A. Gardner, MD, Carl H. Snyderman, MD, MBA, University of Pittsburgh, Pittsburgh, PA, United States	Chae-Yong Kim, MD, PhD, Seoul National University Bundang Hospital, Seoul, South Korea	Tetsuro Sameshima, MD, PhD, Hamamatsu University, Hamamatsu, Shizuoka, Japan
Bone opening	Right greater than left sphenoidotomy, removal of sellar face from tuberculum to floor and cavernous to cavernous	Right middle turbinate, bottom right superior turbinate, wide sphenoidotomy, upper clivus	Wide sphenoidotomy, removal of sellar bone, posterior planum sphenoidale, subchiasmatic groove, tuberculum, medial OCR, bilateral optic canals	
Brain exposure	Sella	Sella	Sella	Sella
Method of resection	Bilateral middle turbinates lateralized, identify right sphenoid ostium, wide right sphenoidotomy, preservation of mucosa, same procedure on left but limited sphenoidotomy, removal of sellar bone from tuberculum sella to sellar floor and cavernous to cavernous sinus, dura cauterized and opened in cruciate fashion, sellar mass debulked with ring curettes along floor to dorsum and then laterally to cavernous sinuses and then superiorly to decompress diaphragma, preserve normal gland, dura reconstructed with synthetic dura and sealant, middle turbinated medialized with Nasopore in middle meatus	Lateralization/resection of right middle turbinate, partial resection of right superior turbinate, lateralize left middle turbinate, disarticulate posterior septum from rostrum of sphenoid, preserve right nasoseptal flap, protect nasal corridor with sleeves, open into sphenoid, do not disrupt tumor, additional resection of posterior superior nasal septum if necessary, drill to floor and lateral recesses of sphenoid sinus, resect tumor out of lateral and clival recesses using two suckers, hemostasis before entering sella, remove remaining sella bone and expose right cavernous sinus, remove tumor with two suction tips with attention to right cavernous sinus, angled endoscope to inspect for residual, reconstruct with mucosa from right middle turbinate or nasoseptal flap if leak present	Nasal cavity packed with epinephrine soaked pledgets, bilateral middle and superior turbinates lateralized, right nasoseptal flap harvested and stored in choanae, posterior septum disarticulated, wide bilateral sphenoidotomy, septostomy, drill down of posterior planum sphenoidale/ subchiasmatic groove/ tuberculum/optic canals/medial OCR, expose superior intercavernous sinus, coagulate exposed dura, separate dural opening in planum and sella, tack up sutures, internal decompression, papaverine-soaked pledgets to optic nerves, nasoseptal flap if necessary for CSF leak	Right nasoseptal flap, enter sphenoid sinus, debulk as much tumor as possible using ultrasonic aspirator and curettes, spare right cavernous sinus
Complication avoidance	Nasoseptal flap, limited sphenoidotomy, debulk from floor to diaphragma	Nasoseptal flap, wide bony opening, two suction resection, attention to right cavernous sinus	Nasoseptal flap, wide bony opening, papaverine to optic nerves	Nasoseptal flap, do not compromise cavernous sinus
Postoperative				
Admission	ICU or intermediate care	ICU	Intermediate care	Floor
Postoperative complications feared	CSF leak, pituitary dysfunction, rehemorrhage	CSF leak, pituitary dysfunction, rehemorrhage	Decreasing olfaction, CSF leak	CSF leak, pituitary dysfunction, worsening cranial nerve palsy

	James J. Evans, MD, Tomas Garzon-Muvdi, MD, Thomas Jefferson University, Philadelphia, PA, United States	Paul A. Gardner, MD, Carl H. Snyderman, MD, MBA, University of Pittsburgh, Pittsburgh, PA, United States	Chae-Yong Kim, MD, PhD, Seoul National University Bundang Hospital, Seoul, South Korea	Tetsuro Sameshima, MD, PhD, Hamamatsu University, Hamamatsu, Shizuoka, Japan
Follow-up testing	MRI 3 months after surgery Pituitary panel 3 months after surgery a.m. cortisol after surgery Sodium/SG if UOP >250 cc/hr for 2 hours	8 a.m. cortisol level 48 hours after surgery if off of steroids Prolactin level 1 day after surgery Daily electrolytes, strict fluid assessment CT immediately after surgery only if large CSF leak MRI 3 months after surgery	MRI within 48 hours after surgery Pituitary hormonal analysis ENT evaluation MRI 3 months after surgery	CT immediately after and 1 day after surgery Pituitary hormonal analysis MRI within 7 days after surgery
Follow-up visits	1 week after surgery with ENT 2 weeks after surgery with neurosurgery	1 week after surgery with ENT 1 week after surgery with neurosurgery 2 weeks after surgery with endocrinology and ophthalmology	1 month after surgery	3 months after surgery

CSF, cerebrospinal fluid; *CT*, computed tomography; *ENT*, ear, nose, and throat; *ICA*, internal carotid artery; *ICU*, intensive care unit; *IOM*, intraoperative monitoring; *MRI*, magnetic resonance imaging; *OCR*, opticocarotid recess; *SG*, specific gravity; *SSEP*, somatosensory evoked potential; *UOP*, urine output.

Differential diagnosis and actual diagnosis

- Pituitary adenoma
- Metastatic brain tumor
- Craniopharyngioma

Important anatomic and preoperative considerations

For a full discussion of sellar anatomy in regard to the bony, vascular, and neural features, see Chapters 56 and 57, and for the cavernous sinus, refer to Chapter 50. The pituitary gland has a rich vascular supply, in which the anterior lobe is supplied by the superior hypophyseal artery and traverses along the pituitary stalk, as well as portal vessels that originate dorsally at capillaries from the median eminence, whereas the posterior pituitary is supplied by the inferior hypophyseal artery.[5] There are anastomoses between both hypophyseal arteries and the portal vessels.[5] This rich vascular supply makes the pituitary gland vulnerable to ischemia and/or hemorrhage.[5]

The Hardy and Knosp classification schemes are used to describe sellar changes and tumor extension and cavernous sinus involvement, respectively (Chapter 56, Figs. 56.3 and 56.4).[6,7] The tumor presented in this case is a Hardy grade 4B with focal destruction of the sellar floor, and the tumor bulges into the chiasmatic cistern, and a Knosp grade 2 in which the tumor does extend past the median line up to the lateral internal carotid artery line.

Approaches to this lesion

As discussed in Chapter 56, Fig. 56.2, the approaches to sellar pathology can be divided into transsphenoidal and transcranial approaches.[8,9] The modern conventional approach to sellar pathology is a transsphenoidal approach, in which the most common transsphenoidal approach is enodnasally.[8,9] The endonasal approach can be done with an endoscope or a microscope.[8–12] The endoscopic approach can be done with just neurosurgery or neurosurgery and otolaryngology combined.[8–12] The advantages of the endoscopic approach are that it is minimally invasive and provides angled views within the sella that allows visualization within the cavernous sinus, whereas its disadvantages include lack of stereoscopic or three-dimensional vision in most imaging modalities, need for skull base reconstruction, and potentially higher risk of cerebrospinal fluid (CSF) leak.[8–12] The endoscopic approach can also be done with a microscope and typically requires a speculum.[10–13] The advantages of this approach over the endoscope are that it provides stereoscopic vision and bimanual technique; however, its disadvantages include lack of panoramic visualization within the sella and cavernous sinuses, and limited working corridor.[10–13] It should be noted that the endoscopic approach also allows for bimanual techniques if the endoscope is held by an assistant surgeon or holding arm.[8,9]

What was actually done

The patient was started on stress-dose intravenous hydrocortisone (100 mg). The patient was taken to surgery for an urgent endoscopic endonasal resection for a pituitary apoplexy without otolaryngology with general anesthesia and no intraoperative monitoring. The patient was induced and intubated per routine. An electromagnetic navigation system with preoperative magnetic resonance imaging (MRI) was used to avoid the need for head pinning. The patient was draped in the usual standard fashion and given cefazolin and 50 mg hydrocortisone. Using just the right naris, the right middle and inferior turbinates were displaced laterally. A right nasal septal flap was raised and placed into

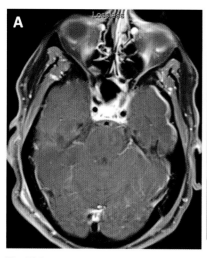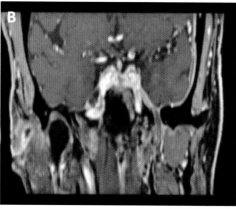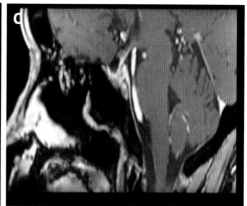

Fig. 58.2 Postoperative magnetic resonance imaging. (A) T1 axial image with gadolinium contrast; **(B)** T1 coronal image with gadolinium contrast; **(C)** T1 sagittal image with gadolinium contrast magnetic resonance imaging scan demonstrating gross total resection of the lesion.

the nasopharynx. The sphenoid ostia were identified and opened bilaterally, and the intersinus septation was drilled flush with the sellar face. The bone overlying the sella was thinned with a diamond drill until the dura was identified. A nerve hook was used to dissect the dura in the epidural plane, and up- and down-going Kerrison punches were used to remove the bone until both cavernous sinuses and the floor of the sella were identified. The tuberculum sellae was not removed. The dura was opened in a cruciate fashion with an arachnoid knife, and the dura was removed with a side-cutting tissue-biting device (Myriad, NICO Corporation, Indianapolis, IN). The tumor was debulked first at the inferior aspect by identifying the floor, followed by the bilateral cavernous sinuses, and moving upward until the diaphragma sellae fell into the sellar cavity using a combination of suction, side-cutting tissue device, and ring curettes. The right cavernous sinus was inspected with a 30-degree endoscope, and the tumor was removed from the cavernous sinus. Preliminary pathology was necrotic pituitary tissue. The diaphragma was seen herniating into the cavity, and the gland was identified at the superior right quadrant. The nasoseptal flap was replaced and sutured in place because no CSF leak was seen. No lumbar drain or fat graft was used.

The patient awoke at their neurologic baseline with persistent right cranial nerve III weakness with ptosis and ophthalmoplegia and was taken to the intensive care unit for recovery. An MRI was done within 24 hours after surgery that showed gross total resection (Fig. 58.2). The sodium and urine specific gravity were checked every 4 to 6 hours, and no episodes of diabetes insipidus occurred. He was kept on hydrocortisone (20 mg in the morning and 10 mg in the afternoon). The patient participated with physical therapy and was discharged to home on postoperative day 2 with 7 days of cefdinir and improved ptosis and ophthalmoplegia. The patient was seen at 2 weeks postoperatively and reported full vision in all visual fields and resolution of his cranial nerve III weakness with no ptosis and no ophthalmoplegia. Pathology was pituitary apoplexy with necrotic pituitary tissue. All hormonal stains were negative.

The patient underwent formal visual field examination at 3 months postoperatively and had full visual fields. The lesion was observed with serial MRI examinations at 3- to 6-month intervals, and no recurrence has been seen at 36 months postoperatively.

Commonalities among the experts

The majority of surgeons opted for the patient to undergo computed tomography for bony anatomic detail, hormonal and endocrinology evaluation to determine pituitary hormonal status, and ophthalmology evaluation for baseline visual functioning assessment prior to surgery. All surgeons pursued an endoscopic endonasal transsphenoidal approach (one would supplement with partial transclival), half aimed for decompression, and half aimed for maximal resection. All surgeons performed the surgery in combination with otolaryngology. Most surgeons were cognizant of the parasellar carotid arteries, cavernous sinus, and optic nerves. The most feared complication was a CSF leak. Surgery was generally pursued with surgical navigation and endoscopic equipment, with perioperative steroids. The majority of surgeons advocated for use of nasal septal flaps, wide sellar opening, and preservation of the cavernous sinus. Following surgery, most surgeons admitted their patients to the intensive care unit or intermediate care and requested imaging 3 months after surgery to assess for extent of resection.

SUMMARY OF QUALITY OF EVIDENCE TO GUIDE SPECIFIC INTERVENTIONS FOR THIS CASE

- Surgery for pituitary apoplexy with ophthalmoplegia and no visual field deficits—Class III.
- Endoscopic endonasal versus microscopic approach—Class II-2.
- One nostril versus two nostrils for endoscopic endonasal approaches—Class III.

REFERENCES

1. Briet C, Salenave S, Bonneville JF, Laws ER, Chanson P. Pituitary apoplexy. *Endocr Rev*. 2015;36:622–645.
2. Verrees M, Arafah BM, Selman WR. Pituitary tumor apoplexy: characteristics, treatment, and outcomes. *Neurosurg Focus*. 2004;16:E6.
3. Fan Y, Bao X, Wang R. Conservative treatment cures an elderly pituitary apoplexy patient with oculomotor paralysis and optic nerve compression: a case report and systematic review of the literature. *Clin Interv Aging*. 2018;13:1981–1985.
4. Maccagnan P, Macedo CL, Kayath MJ, Nogueira RG, Abucham J. Conservative management of pituitary apoplexy: a prospective study. *J Clin Endocrinol Metab*. 1995;80:2190–2197.
5. Rhoton Jr AL. The sellar region. *Neurosurgery*. 2002;51:S335–S374.
6. Knosp E, Steiner E, Kitz K, Matula C. Pituitary adenomas with invasion of the cavernous sinus space: a magnetic resonance imaging classification compared with surgical findings. *Neurosurgery*. 1993;33:610–617; discussion 617–618.
7. Mooney MA, Hardesty DA, Sheehy JP, et al. Rater reliability of the hardy classification for pituitary adenomas in the magnetic resonance imaging era. *J Neurol Surg B Skull Base*. 2017;78:413–418.
8. Liu JK, Weiss MH, Couldwell WT. Surgical approaches to pituitary tumors. *Neurosurg Clin N Am*. 2003;14:93–107.
9. Couldwell WT. Transsphenoidal and transcranial surgery for pituitary adenomas. *J Neurooncol*. 2004;69:237–256.
10. Eseonu CI, ReFaey K, Garcia O, Salvatori R, Quinones-Hinojosa A. Comparative cost analysis of endoscopic versus microscopic endonasal transsphenoidal surgery for pituitary adenomas. *J Neurol Surg B Skull Base*. 2018;79:131–138.
11. Eseonu CI, ReFaey K, Pamias-Portalatin E, et al. Three-hand endoscopic endonasal transsphenoidal surgery: experience with an anatomy-preserving mononostril approach technique. *Oper Neurosurg (Hagerstown)*. 2018;14:158–165.
12. Eseonu CI, ReFaey K, Rincon-Torroella J, et al. Endoscopic versus microscopic transsphenoidal approach for pituitary adenomas: comparison of outcomes during the transition of methods of a single surgeon. *World Neurosurg*. 2017;97:317–325.
13. Frazier JL, Chaichana K, Jallo GI, Quinones-Hinojosa A. Combined endoscopic and microscopic management of pediatric pituitary region tumors through one nostril: technical note with case illustrations. *Childs Nerv Syst*. 2008;24:1469–1478.

59

Cushing pituitary adenoma

Case reviewed by Nelson M. Oyesiku, Joseph Quillin, Henry W. S. Schroeder, Tony Van Havenbergh, Gabriel Zada

Introduction

Cushing syndrome is caused by excess cortisol, in which the most common cause of endogenous Cushing syndrome is Cushing disease.[1,2] Cushing syndrome can be diagnosed with late night salivary cortisol, 24-hour urine free cortisol, and/or low-dose dexamethasone suppression in which two of three are confirmatory.[1,2] Cushing disease is caused by a pituitary adenoma that secretes adrenocorticotropic hormone (ACTH), which stimulates secretion of cortisol by the adrenal glands and leads to hypertension, diabetes, obesity, osteoporosis, and peripheral vascular disease, among others.[1,2] Cushing disease has a prevalence of 39.1 per million people, with an annual incidence of 1.2 to 2.4 per 1 million people per year.[1,2] Untreated Cushing disease is associated with two- to fivefold increased mortality.[1,2] The majority (90%) of Cushing disease are diagnosed when they are microadenomas (< 1 cm), in which the median diameter is 6 mm at

discovery.[1,2] In this chapter, we present a case of a patient with a Cushing pituitary macroadenoma.

Example case

Chief complaint: headaches, weight gain
History of present illness
A 32-year-old, right-handed woman with no significant past medical history who presented with headaches and weight gain. For the past 2 years, she had gained 30 to 40 pounds, despite healthy diet and frequent exercise. She had noted that her face was fuller, as well as facial hair growth and acne. She saw her endocrinologist and had elevated urinary and salivary cortisol and failed a low-dose dexamethasone suppression test. A brain MRI was done and showed a pituitary lesion (Fig. 59.1).
Medications: None.
Allergies: No known drug allergies.
Past medical and surgical history: None.
Family history: No history of intracranial malignancies.

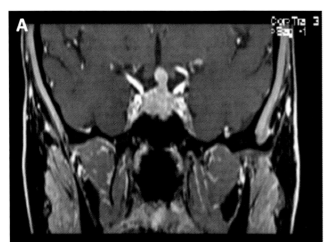
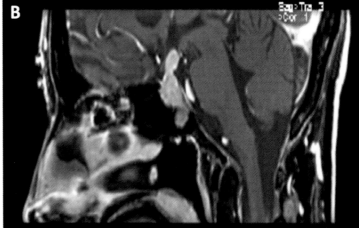

Fig. 59.1 Preoperative magnetic resonance imaging. (A) T1 coronal image with gadolinium contrast; **(B)** T1 sagittal image with gadolinium contrast magnetic resonance imaging scan demonstrating a nonenhancing lesion involving the sellar and suprasellar space without abutment of the optic chiasm.

Social history: Nurse, no smoking or alcohol.

Physical examination: Awake, alert, oriented to person, place, and time; Cranial nerves II to XII intact, visual fields full to confrontation; No drift, moves all extremities with full strength.

Pituitary labs: Elevated salivary and urinary cortisol and failed low-dose dexamethasone suppression test; prolactin, thyroid stimulating hormone/T4, insulin-like growth factor-1 all within normal limits.

	Nelson M. Oyesiku, MD, PhD, Joseph Quillin, MD, Emory University, Atlanta, GA, United States	Henry W. S. Schroeder, MD, PhD, University of Greifswald, Greifswald, M-V, Germany	Tony Van Havenbergh, MD, PhD, GasthuisZusters Antwerpen, Antwerpen, Belgium	Gabriel Zada, MD, University of Southern California, Los Angeles, CA, United States
Preoperative				
Additional tests requested	Neuroophthalmology evaluation (visual fields, OCT) Endocrinology evaluation ENT evaluation Pregnancy test High-resolution T2 MRI	Neuroophthalmology evaluation (visual fields) CT maxillofacial Anesthesiology evaluation	Neuroophthalmology evaluation (visual fields) Endocrinology evaluation	Neuroophthalmology evaluation (visual fields) Endocrinology evaluation with full pituitary panel High-resolution MRI
Surgical approach selected	Endoscopic transnasal transsphenoidal and transtubercular with lumbar drain	Endoscopic endonasal transsphenoidal and transtubercular	Endoscopic endonasal	Endoscopic endonasal transsphenoidal
Other teams involved during surgery	ENT	ENT	ENT	None
Anatomic corridor	Transnasal transsphenoidal and transtubercular	Transnasal transsphenoidal and transtubercular	Transnasal transsphenoidal	Transnasal transsphenoidal
Goal of surgery	Gross total resection, biochemical cure	Gross total resection, biochemical cure	Gross total resection, biochemical cure	Maximal safe tumor removal
Perioperative				
Positioning	Supine with pins, 10-degree right rotation	Supine with pins, right rotation and slight extension	Supine with slight right turn with pins	Supine no pins
Surgical equipment	Lumbar drain Surgical navigation 0- and 30-degree endoscopes Cranial Doppler Ultrasonic aspirator	Endoscopes	Surgical navigation Endoscopes Tissue shaver	Surgical navigation Endoscopes Microdoppler
Medications	None	Steroids	Steroids	None
Anatomic considerations	Cavernous carotid arteries, optic nerves, infundibulum, ACOM	Pituitary stalk, cavernous carotid arteries	ICA, pituitary stalk, optic structures, cavernous carotid artery	Carotid arteries, pituitary gland, optic apparatus
Complications feared with approach chosen	ICA/ACA injury, hypothalamic injury, diabetes insipidus, hypopituitarism, CSF leak	Damage to olfactory mucosa, injury to ICA and pituitary stalk, CSF leak	ICA injury, CSF leak, damage to pituitary gland	Vision loss, cerebral edema, neurologic deficits, seizures
Intraoperative				
Anesthesia	General	General	General	General
Skin incision	None	None	None	None

(continued on next page)

	Nelson M. Oyesiku, MD, PhD, Joseph Quillin, MD, Emory University, Atlanta, GA, United States	Henry W. S. Schroeder, MD, PhD, University of Greifswald, Greifswald, M-V, Germany	Tony Van Havenbergh, MD, PhD, GasthuisZusters Antwerpen, Antwerpen, Belgium	Gabriel Zada, MD, University of Southern California, Los Angeles, CA, United States
Bone opening	+/- right middle turbinate, wide sphenoid osteotomy, posterior ethmoidectomy, removal of sella from cavernous to cavernous sinus, removal of tuberculum	Sphenoid osteotomy, intersinus septations, sellar floor, tuberculum, adjacent planum	Posterior nasal septum, anterior wall of sphenoid sinus, sella	Wide sphenoid osteotomy
Brain exposure	Sella from cavernous to cavernous sinus and tuberculum removal	Sella, tuberculum, adjacent planum	Sella	Sella from cavernous to cavernous sinus
Method of resection	Lateralize inferior turbinates, +/- resection of right middle turbinate, partial resection of inferior aspect of superior turbinate, posterior septectomy, wide sphenoid sinus opening, resection of sphenoid rostrum/ bilateral posterior ethmoid air cells, raise large right Hadad nasoseptal flap, removal of sellar face from cavernous to cavernous sinus, drill out clival recess, thin sphenoid tuberculum past limbus dural fold and reflect bone away, open dura, extracapsular dissection, assessment for residual tumor nests and CSF leak, retrieval of nasoseptal flap, Nasopore	Lateralization of all turbinates, harvest right nasoseptal flap and storage in nasopharynx, reverse flap on left, open sphenoid sinus and drill all septi, removal sellar floor/ tuberculum/adjacent planum, incise dura, resect tumor with curettes and forceps, open suprasellar dura to access suprasellar component if no descent, inspect cavity with various angled scopes, pack fat in the sellar area, position nasoseptal flap with fibrin glue, nasal tamponades	Binostril approach, resection of posterior nasal septum, wide opening of anterior wall of sphenoid sinus, open the anterior bony part of the sella, H-shaped dural opening, sharp dissection of tumor from normal pituitary, dissect starting at lower part of the tumor allowing the diaphragm to descend downward, use curettes if necessary, endoscopic inspection of resection cavity for residual tumor, no tampons in nostrils	Lateralization of bilateral middle turbinates, widening of sphenoid ostium, harvesting of rescue nasal mucosal flaps, removal of sphenoid rostrum, removal of sphenoid sinus septations, verification of sellar floor, removal of sellar floor, microdoppler to confirm carotid arteries and navigation for tumor boundaries, dural opening, tumor debulking with curette, angled endoscopes to look into suprasellar cistern, Valsalva to evaluate for CSF leak, repair of CSF leak with autologous gat or fascia lata, alloderm, or nasoseptal flap, medialization of turbinates
Complication avoidance	Harvesting nasal septal flap, wide sellar opening, extracapsular dissection, close attention to right cavernous sinus, inspection with various scopes for residual and CSF leaks	Harvesting nasal septal flap, inverted flap on the contralateral side, wide bony opening of sella/tuberculum/ planum, inspection with various scopes	Sharp dissection of tumor from normal pituitary, start at lower part of tumor	Harvesting nasal septal flap, wide sellar opening, inspection with various scopes for residual and CSF leaks
Postoperative				
Admission	Floor	Intermediate care	ICU	ICU or floor
Postoperative complications feared	HPA dysfunction (adrenal insufficiency, diabetes insipidus, SIADH), CSF leak	Hyponatremia, CSF leak	CSF leak, diabetes insipidus	CSF leak, vision loss, hypopituitarism, adrenal insufficiency, diabetes insipidus

	Nelson M. Oyesiku, MD, PhD, Joseph Quillin, MD, Emory University, Atlanta, GA, United States	Henry W. S. Schroeder, MD, PhD, University of Greifswald, Greifswald, M-V, Germany	Tony Van Havenbergh, MD, PhD, GasthuisZusters Antwerpen, Antwerpen, Belgium	Gabriel Zada, MD, University of Southern California, Los Angeles, CA, United States
Follow-up testing	Daily BMP, daily 8 a.m. cortisols until nadir established, LD for 3 days MRI 3 months after surgery	Continue hydrocortisone for 3 months with endocrinology tapering, endocrinology testing 3 months after surgery MRI 24 hours after surgery	Cortisol and endocrine labs 2, 4, and 6 weeks after surgery MRI 2 months after surgery	Cortisol every 6 hours until less than 2 for 2–3 days after surgery MRI 3 months after surgery
Follow-up visits	1 week after surgery for neuroendocrinology 2 weeks after surgery for ENT 6 weeks after surgery for neurosurgery	3 months after surgery for neurosurgery Continual follow-up with ENT 3 months after surgery for endocrinology	2 months after surgery with neurosurgery 2 weeks after surgery with endocrinology	10 days, 6 weeks, 3 months, and annually after surgery
Adjuvant treatment for lack of biochemical cure	Little or no biochemical response: possible resection or partial/total hypophysectomy Partial biochemical response: observation for 3 months, then SRS, and then bilateral adrenalectomy	No cure: repeat surgery if visible tumor seen and accessible; medical or radiation if no visible tumor seen or residual tumor is inaccessible	No cure: repeat surgery if lesion evident on scans or radiation if no lesion apparent	SRS or medical management

ACOM, anterior communicating artery; *BMP*, basic metabolic panel; *CSF*, cerebrospinal fluid; *CT*, computed tomography; *ENT*, ear, nose, and throat; *HPA*, hypothalamic-pituitary axis; *ICA*, internal carotid artery; *ICU*, intensive care unit; *LD*, lumbar drain; *MRI*, magnetic resonance imaging; *OCT*, optical coherence tomography; *SIADH*, syndrome of inappropriate antidiuretic hormone; *SRS*, stereotactic radiosurgery.

Differential diagnosis and actual diagnosis

- Pituitary adenoma
- Rathke cleft cyst

Important anatomic and preoperative considerations

The sellar anatomy is discussed in Chapters 56 and 57, whereas the cavernous sinus anatomy is discussed in Chapter 50. The most common cause of Cushing syndrome is administration of exogenous steroids.[1,2] The causes of endogenous hypercortisolism are either ACTH-dependent (pituitary adenoma, ectopic tumor) or ACTH-independent (adrenal tumor).[1,2] ACTH levels greater than 10 pg/mL signify an ACTH-dependent cause, in which ACTH-dependent causes can be distinguished by either corticotropin-releasing hormone stimulation (pituitary adenoma has >50% increase in ACTH and 20% increase in cortisol) or high-dose (8 mg) dexamethasone suppression test (cortisol suppression by >50%).[1,2] The diagnosis of Cushing disease prompts a magnetic resonance imaging (MRI) scan, which detects a pituitary adenoma in 60% to 70% of the time, in which the lack of sensitivity is because of the reduced signal-to-noise imaging ratio at the sellar-sphenoid bone-air interface, but modalities, such as high-resolution MRI, spoiled gradient

recalled acquisition, and injecting the sphenoid sinus to eliminate the air-bone interface, can increase the sensitivity in diagnosing these lesions as they are typically microadenomas.[1,2] Alternatively, inferior petrosal sampling with corticotropin-releasing hormone stimulation can aid in diagnosis in MRI-negative Cushing disease.[1,2]

Once an adenoma is diagnosed on MRI, surgery is typically pursued.[1,2] The factors associated with surgical outcomes are preoperative MRI, dural invasion, and adenoma size.[1,2] The MRI features associated with improved surgical outcomes are presence of lesion and absence of cavernous sinus invasion.[1,2] When these tumors invade the cavernous sinus, they can also invade the dural wall, which can make curative resection unlikely.[1,2] Exceedingly small adenomas less than 5 mm that are difficult to target and large macroadenomas greater than 2.5 cm are associated with poor surgical outcomes.[1,2] Typically within 48 hours after surgery, most patients who achieve Cushing disease remission develop glucocorticoid withdrawal syndrome associated with cortisol levels of 2 ug/dL or less. Unsuccessful surgery is associated with incidental adenomas, lack of lesion targeting, and/or incomplete removal.[1,2] Despite successful surgery, recurrence can occur with growth of residual tumor.[1,2] Biochemical remission is defined as less than 2 ug/dL morning cortisol, less than 20 ug/24-hour urine free cortisol, and/or low midnight salivary cortisol, whereas the morning serum cortisol less than 1 ug/dL is associated with a 96% positive predictive value of lasting biochemical remission.[1,2] It should be noted that higher subnormal values do not exclude biochemical remission.[1,2] For failed surgery or patients who cannot tolerate surgery, options include radiation therapy (radiosurgery or fractionated therapy, 46%–84% incidence of remission, with 20%–40% of loss of pituitary function at 10 years after radiation therapy); adrenalectomy (95% incidence of remission, 18% morbidity rate, 28% of adrenal crisis, 9% mortality from stroke or myocardial infarction, 21% rate of Nelson syndrome); and medical therapy (with steroidogenesis inhibitors, where 30%–50% have cortisol normalization).[1,2]

The Hardy and Knosp classification schemes are used to describe sellar changes and tumor extension and cavernous sinus involvement, respectively (Chapter 56, Figs. 56.3 and 56.4).[3,4] The tumor presented in this case is a Hardy grade 2B with expansion of the sella with size greater than 10 mm, and the tumor reaches floor of the third ventricle, and a Knosp grade 1 in which the tumor does extends past the medial line.

Approaches to this lesion

The approaches for sellar pathology are discussed in detail in Chapter 56, Fig. 56.2. These approaches can be divided into transsphenoidal and transcranial approaches.[3–7] For pituitary adenomas, the most commonly used approach is an endoscopic endonasal transsphenoidal approach with or without the assistance of otolaryngology.[3–7] In this approach, one or both nares are used to access the sphenoid sinus to enter the lesion through the sella.[3–7]

What was actually done

The patient was taken to surgery for an endoscopic expanded endonasal resection of a Cushing macroadenoma with otolaryngology with general anesthesia and no intraoperative monitoring. The patient was induced and intubated per routine. An electromagnetic navigation system with preoperative MRI and computed tomography was used to avoid the need for head pinning. The left lower abdominal quadrant was prepped in case a fat graft was needed. The patient was draped in the usual standard fashion and given cefazolin, and steroids were withheld. With the assistance of a rhinologist, the right middle turbinate was removed, and the right inferior turbinate was displaced laterally. A right maxillary antrostomy and right anterior and posterior ethmoidectomies were done. A right nasal septal flap was raised and placed into the nasopharynx. A posterior septectomy was done to allow bilateral nasal access. The sphenoid ostia were opened bilaterally, and the intersinus septation was drilled flush with the sellar face. The bone overlying the sella was thinned with a diamond drill until the dura was identified. A nerve hook was used to dissect the dura in the epidural plane, and up- and down-going Kerrison punches were used to remove the bone until both cavernous sinuses were identified, as well as the floor of the sella and the planum sphenoidale. The tuberculum was then removed. The dura was opened in a cruciate fashion with an arachnoid knife, and the dura was removed with a side-cutting tissue-biting device (Myriad, NICO Corporation, Indianapolis, IN). The tumor was debulked first at the inferior aspect by identifying the floor, followed by the bilateral cavernous sinuses, and moving upward until the diaphragma sellae fell into the sellar cavity. The tumor was debulked until no more tumor was visible. Preliminary pathology was pituitary adenoma. A couple rounds of Valsalva were used to see if more tumor would fall into the cavity. A small cerebrospinal fluid leak was encountered, and the sella was packed with gelfoam, followed by a dural substitute in the epidural plane, and tucked into the bone edges of the sella. The nasoseptal flap was used to reinforce the opening. Nasal packings were placed bilaterally. No lumbar drain or fat graft was used.

The patient awoke at their neurologic baseline and was taken to the intensive care unit for recovery. An MRI scan was done within 24 hours after surgery and showed gross total resection (Fig. 59.2). The sodium, urine specific gravity, and cortisol were checked every 6 hours. The cortisol nadir was less than 0.1 ug/dL, and she had one episode of diabetes insipidus requiring desmopressin. The patient was started on hydrocortisone after the nadir was confirmed (20 mg in the morning and 10 mg in the afternoon). The nasal packings were removed 24 hours after surgery. The patient participated with physical therapy and was discharged to home on postoperative day 3 with 7 days of cefdinir. The

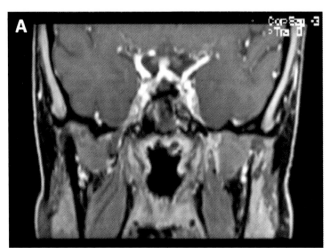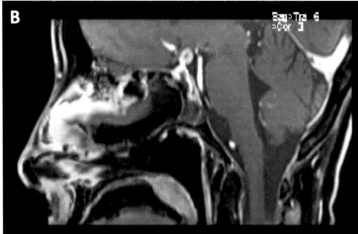

Fig. 59.2 Postoperative magnetic resonance imaging. (A) T1 coronal image with gadolinium contrast; **(B)** T1 sagittal image with gadolinium contrast magnetic resonance imaging scan demonstrating gross total resection of the lesion.

patient was seen in the ear, nose, and throat clinic for endoscopic examination and cleaning on postoperative day 7. The patient was seen at 2 weeks postoperatively and remained neurologically intact. Pathology was pituitary adenoma and hormonal stains were positive for ACTH. The patient remains in biochemical remission for 24 months.

Commonalities among the experts

The majority of surgeons opted for the patient to undergo ophthalmology evaluation for baseline visual functioning assessment, endocrinology evaluation for pituitary hormonal functioning, and high-resolution MRI for better delineation of the tumor and pituitary gland prior to surgery. All surgeons pursued an endoscopic endonasal transsphenoidal approach (half would supplement with a transtubercular approach), and all surgeons aimed for maximal resection with most aiming for biochemical cure. Most surgeons would perform the surgery in combination with otolaryngology. Most surgeons were cognizant of the parasellar carotid arteries, optic nerves, and infundibulum. The most feared complications were internal carotid artery injury, cerebrospinal fluid leak, and pituitary damage. Surgery was generally pursued with surgical navigation, endoscopic equipment, and cranial Doppler, with most surgeons not requesting perioperative steroids. The majority of surgeons advocated for use of nasal septal flaps, wide sellar opening, and extracapsular dissection. Following surgery, most surgeons admitted their patients to the intensive care unit or intermediate care, half performed cortisol evaluations while the patient was in the hospital, and most requested imaging 3 months after surgery to assess for extent of resection.

SUMMARY OF QUALITY OF EVIDENCE TO GUIDE SPECIFIC INTERVENTIONS FOR THIS CASE

- Surgery for Cushing disease—Class III.
- Endoscopic endonasal versus microscopic approach—Class II-2.
- One nostril versus two nostrils for endoscopic endonasal approaches—Class III.

REFERENCES

1. Bansal V, El Asmar N, Selman WR, Arafah BM. Pitfalls in the diagnosis and management of Cushing's syndrome. *Neurosurg Focus*. 2015;38:E4.
2. Lonser RR, Nieman L, Oldfield EH. Cushing's disease: pathobiology, diagnosis, and management. *J Neurosurg*. 2017;126:404–417.
3. Eseonu CI, ReFaey K, Pamias-Portalatin E, et al. Three-hand endoscopic endonasal transsphenoidal surgery: experience with an anatomy-preserving mononostril approach technique. *Oper Neurosurg (Hagerstown)*. 2018;14:158–165.
4. Eseonu CI, ReFaey K, Rincon-Torroella J, et al. Endoscopic versus microscopic transsphenoidal approach for pituitary adenomas: comparison of outcomes during the transition of methods of a single surgeon. *World Neurosurg*. 2017;97:317–325.
5. Liu JK, Weiss MH, Couldwell WT. Surgical approaches to pituitary tumors. *Neurosurg Clin N Am*. 2003;14:93–107.
6. Couldwell WT. Transsphenoidal and transcranial surgery for pituitary adenomas. *J Neurooncol*. 2004;69:237–256.
7. Eseonu CI, ReFaey K, Garcia O, Salvatori R, Quinones-Hinojosa A. Comparative cost analysis of endoscopic versus microscopic endonasal transsphenoidal surgery for pituitary adenomas. *J Neurol Surg B Skull Base*. 2018;79:131–138.

60

Growth hormone pituitary adenoma

Case reviewed by Luigi Maria Cavallo, Edward R. Laws, Daniel Donoho,
Eslam Mohsen Mahmoud Hussein, Daniel M. Prevedello

Introduction

Growth hormone (GH)-secreting pituitary adenomas result in symptoms of acromegaly in adults and gigantism in children.[1] It is caused by elevated levels of GHs and insulin-like growth factor-1 (IGF-1).[1] Acromegaly is diagnosed with elevated IGF-1 and a failed oral glucose suppression test in which GH levels do not decrease to lower than 1 ng/mL with oral glucose adminsitration.[1] Acromegaly is typically caused by a pituitary adenoma that secretes GH, which stimulates secretion of IGF-1 by the liver and leads to cardiovascular disease, musculoskeletal changes, diabetes, and risk of several malignancies, in which the risk of death is twofold compared with the general population.[1] Surgery is the first-line treatment for acromegaly.[2–5] Biochemical control is achieved in 75% to 95% of patients with microadenomas but only 40% to 68% of patients with macroadenomas.[2–5] The cure rates have decreased because of more stringent criteria of biochemical remission in recent years, and the median biochemical remission rate following surgery is approximately 50%.[5] In this chapter, we present a case of a patient with a GH-secreting pituitary macroadenoma.

Example case

Chief complaint: facial and hand changes
History of present illness
A 36-year-old, right-handed man with no significant past medical history presented with facial and hand changes. His family noticed that his face had changed over the years. On questioning, his ring size had increased, as well as his shoe size from 10 to 12 over the past 2 years. He also complained of headaches and joint pain. He was seen by an endocrinologist who performed laboratory assessments and ordered magnetic resonance imaging (MRI) (Fig. 60.1).

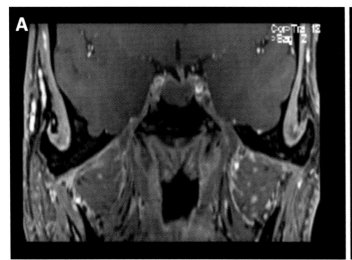
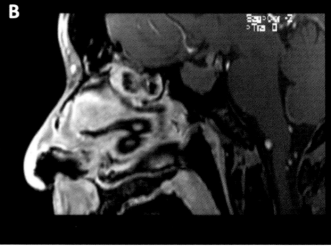

Fig. 60.1 Preoperative magnetic resonance imaging. (A) T1 coronal image with gadolinium contrast; **(B)** T1 sagittal image with gadolinium contrast magnetic resonance imaging scan demonstrating a hypoenhancing lesion involving the sella with displacement of the gland superiorly.

Medications: None.
Allergies: No known drug allergies.
Past medical and surgical history: None.
Family history: No history of intracranial malignancies.
Social history: Firefighter, no smoking or alcohol.

Physical examination: Awake, alert, oriented to person, place, and time; Cranial nerves II to XII intact, visual fields full to confrontation; No drift, moves all extremities with full strength.
Pituitary labs: IGF-1elevated, failed glucose suppression test; cortisol, prolactin, thyroid stimulating hormone/T4 all within normal limits.

	Luigi Maria Cavallo, MD, PhD, University of Naples Federico II, Naples, Italy	Edward R. Laws, MD, Daniel Donoho, MD, Brigham and Women's Hospital, Boston, MA, United States	Eslam Mohsen Mahmoud Hussein, MBBS, MSc, Ain Shams University, Cairo, Egypt	Daniel M. Prevedello, MD, Ohio State University, Columbus, OH, United States
Preoperative				
Additional tests requested	Sinus CT Laryngoscopy Colonoscopy Echocardiogram	Total testosterone, HgbA1c, serum Ca Sleep study if needed Hypertension, cardiac function evaluation	Ophthalmology evaluation (visual fields, fundus) Endocrinology evaluation ENT evaluation CT maxillofacial	Endocrinology evaluation CT maxillofacial
Surgical approach selected	Endoscopic endonasal transsphenoidal	Endoscopic endonasal transsphenoidal	Endoscopic endonasal transsphenoidal	Endoscopic endonasal transsellar
Other teams involved during surgery	ENT	ENT	ENT	ENT
Anatomic corridor	Transnasal transsphenoidal	Transnasal transsphenoidal	Transnasal transsphenoidal	Transnasal transsphenoidal
Goal of surgery	Gross total resection, preservation of normal pituitary gland	Gross total resection, biochemical cure, preservation of normal pituitary gland	Radical excision	Gross total resection
Perioperative				
Positioning	Supine without pins	Supine with pins	Supine with left head tilt without pins	Supine without pins
Surgical equipment	Endoscope Microdoppler	Endoscope Microdoppler Microdebrider Ring curettes	Surgical navigation Endoscope Microdoppler	Surgical navigation Endoscope Microdebrider
Medications	Steroids	None	Steroids	None
Anatomic considerations	ICAs, clival recess	ICA, midline structures, tuberculum, clival recess, opticocarotid recess, Onodi cells if present	ICA, cavernous sinus, arachnoid of suprasellar cistern, optic nerves, pituitary stalk and gland	ICA, optic nerves, pituitary gland (including posterior pituitary), cavernous sinuses
Complications feared with approach chosen	ICA injury, CSF leak	Visual loss, hypopituitarism, carotid/cavernous sinus injury	ICA injury, vision loss, CSF leak	CSF leak, residual tumor, ICA injury, vision loss, diabetes insipidus
Intraoperative				
Anesthesia	General	General	General	General
Skin incision	None	None	None	None
Bone opening	Sphenoid osteotomy, removal of sellar bone	Wide sphenoid osteotomy, removal of sellar bone	Wide sphenoid osteotomy, removal of sellar bone	Wide sphenoid osteotomy, removal of sellar bone
Brain exposure	Sella	Sella	Sella	Sella

(continued on next page)

	Luigi Maria Cavallo, MD, PhD, University of Naples Federico II, Naples, Italy	Edward R. Laws, MD, Daniel Donoho, MD, Brigham and Women's Hospital, Boston, MA, United States	Eslam Mohsen Mahmoud Hussein, MBBS, MSc, Ain Shams University, Cairo, Egypt	Daniel M. Prevedello, MD, Ohio State University, Columbus, OH, United States
Method of resection	Decongestion of nasal mucosa, lateralization of both middle turbinates, anterior sphenoidotomy, flattening of sphenoid septa, open sellar floor, dural incision, remove tumor	Lateralize bilateral middle turbinates, posterior septectomy with preservation of rescue flaps, exposure of sphenoid ostia, removal of sphenoid face out to lateral recesses and rostral aspect of sphenoid, removal of sphenoid sinus septations and mucosa, remove sellar face, open dura, resect tumor extracapsularly if possible, evaluate for CSF leak, abdominal fat if leak present, reconstruct sellar face with medpore/septal cartilage or bone, medialize middle turbinates	Mucosa incised in midline, vomer removed, insertion of nasal speculum with keel used as landmark, bone removed between sphenoid ostia, mucosa removed, sphenoid floor is drilled if thick, dura opened in cruciate fashion, tumor removed with ring curettes, Valsalva to facilitate tumor descent, if CSF leak, the sella is packed with abdominal fat and lumbar drain is inserted, nasal packs for 24–48 hours	Midline turbinates lateralized, bilateral rescue flaps raised, sphenoid rostrum exposed and drilled, anterior sphenoidotomy, septations are drilled, face of sella is drilled, dural opening with feather blade, plane between tumor and gland identified, extracapsular dissection, inspect cavity with 45-degree endoscope for residual, hydrogen peroxide to cavity, synthetic dural for replacement, splints placed bilaterally
Complication avoidance	Leave middle turbinates, wide sellar opening, cognizant of spheno-palatine branches	Leave middle turbinates, wide sellar opening, extracapsular dissection, inspection for residual and CSF leaks	Use keel as midline landmark, Valsalva to facilitate tumor descent, CSF leak repaired with abdominal fat and lumbar drain	Extracapsular dissection, hydrogen peroxide
Postoperative				
Admission	Floor	Floor	Intermediate care	Intermediate care
Postoperative complications feared	Nasal bleeding, CSF leak	Hypopituitarism, hyponatremia, visual loss, arterial injury, airway issues	Diabetes insipidus, CSF leak, vascular injury, visual deficit	Diabetes insipidus, CSF leak
Follow-up testing	Growth hormones 1 and 3 days after surgery with goal <1 Sodium and electrolytes 10 days after surgery MRI 3 months after surgery	Growth hormone levels until <1 while admitted Sodium and cortisol 1 week after surgery Full endocrine labs at 6 weeks after surgery MRI 3 months after surgery	Growth hormone levels for 3 days Full hormonal panel and electrolytes Visual acuity and field testing MRI within 36 hours after surgery	Growth hormone level before, during, end of resection and postoperative day 1 CT after surgery Sodium and specific gravity every 6 hours MRI 3 months after surgery
Follow-up visits	10 days after surgery	1 week after surgery for neuroendocrinology 3 months after surgery for neurosurgery	Daily after surgery for 1 week for ENT 7 days after surgery for neurosurgery	6 weeks with neurosurgery 7 days with ENT and endocrinology
Adjuvant therapies recommended	Medical treatment if disease not controlled, consider radiation or repeat surgery upon failure	Somatostatin analogues at 6–12 months	Somatostatins or SRS	Second surgery if residual, somatostatin if nonsurgical

Ca, calcium; *CSF*, cerebrospinal fluid; *CT*, computed tomography; *ENT*, ear, nose, and throat; *HgbA1c*, hemoglobin A1c; *ICA*, internal carotid artery; *MRI*, magnetic resonance imaging; *SRS*, stereotactic radiosurgery.

Differential diagnosis and actual diagnosis

- Pituitary adenoma
- Rathke cleft cyst

Important anatomic and preoperative considerations

Sellar anatomy is discussed in Chapters 56 and 57, whereas the cavernous sinus anatomy is discussed in Chapter 50. Once acromegaly is suspected, diagnosing acromegaly involves testing IGF-1 and, when elevated, an oral glucose tolerance test in which 75 g of sugar are given and GH levels are checked at 30, 60, 90, and 120 minutes, in which GH levels greater than 1 ng/mL are standards for diagnosing acromegaly.[1] Some 95% of acromegaly cases are caused by a pituitary tumor, and biochemical evidence of acromegaly leads to an MRI.[1] Surgery is the first-line treatment for acromegaly.[2–5] The factors associated with biochemical remission for acromegaly are tumor size and cavernous sinus involvement, in which larger tumor sizes and cavernous sinus involvement are associated with lack of biochemical remission.[2–5] Following surgery, the most recent consensus statement in 2010 for biochemical remission was defined as IGF-1 levels within the age- and sex-adjusted normal range, and a random GH of less than 1 ug/L or GH levels less than 0.4 ug/L after oral glucose suppression tests.[5] This is different from prior consensus statements, as there are more sensitive immunoassays for detecting GH levels less than 1 ug/L.[5] In the immediate postoperative period, random GH less than 2.5 ug/L are associated were significant predictors of remission.[4,5] At 3 months follow-up, however, in some series, patients with GH levels of 0.4 to 1 µg/L on glucose challenge and MRI sequences showing no tumor can still result in remission at 1-year follow-up.[4,5] For patients who fail surgical therapy, options include radiation therapy and medical therapy.[4,5]

The Hardy and Knosp classification schemes are used to describe sellar changes and tumor extension and cavernous sinus involvement, respectively (Chapter 56, Figs. 56.3 and 56.4).[6,7] The tumor presented in this case is a Hardy grade 2A with expansion of the sella with a size greater than 10 mm, and the tumor bulges into the chiasmatic cistern and a Knosp grade 1 in which the tumor does not extend past the medial line.

Approaches to this lesion

The approaches for sellar pathology are discussed in detail in Chapter 56, Fig. 56.2. These approaches can be divided into transsphenoidal and transcranial approaches.[8–12] For pituitary adenomas, the most commonly used approach is an endoscopic endonasal transsphenoidal approach with or without the use assistance of otolaryngology.[8–12] In this approach, one or both nares are used to access the sphenoid sinus to enter the lesion through the sella.[8–12]

What was actually done

The patient was taken to surgery for an endoscopic expanded endonasal resection of a GH-producing macroadenoma with otolaryngology with general anesthesia and no intraoperative monitoring. The patient was induced and intubated per routine. An electromagnetic navigation system with preoperative MRI and computed tomography was used to avoid the need for head pinning. The patient was draped in the usual standard fashion and given cefazolin and steroids. With the assistance of a rhinologist, the right middle turbinate was removed, and the right inferior turbinate was displaced laterally. A right maxillary antrostomy and right anterior and posterior ethmoidectomies were done. A right nasal septal flap was raised and placed into the nasopharynx. A posterior septectomy was done to allow bilateral nasal access. The sphenoid ostia were opened bilaterally, and the intersinus septation was drilled flush with the sellar face. The bone overlying the sella was thinned with a diamond drill until the dura was identified. A nerve hook was used to dissect the dura in the epidural plane, and up- and down-going Kerrison punches were used to remove the bone until both cavernous sinuses were identified, as were the floor of the sella and tuberculum. The dura was opened in a cruciate fashion with an arachnoid knife and removed with a side-cutting tissue biting device (Myriad, NICO Corporation, Indianapolis, IN). The tumor was debulked first at the inferior aspect by identifying the floor, followed by the bilateral cavernous sinuses, and moving upward until the diaphragma sellae fell into the sellar cavity. The tumor was debulked until no more tumor was visible, and the gland was identified at the superior resection cavity margin. Preliminary pathology was pituitary adenoma. A couple of rounds of Valsalva were used to see if more tumor would fall into the cavity, and the cavity was examined with a 30-degree endoscope. No cerebrospinal fluid (CSF) leak was encountered, and the sella was packed with gelfoam, followed by a dural substitute in the epidural plane, and tucked into the bone edges of the sella. The nasoseptal flap was replaced as no CSF leak was encountered. Nasal packings were placed bilaterally. No lumbar drain or fat graft was used.

The patient awoke at their neurologic baseline and was taken to the intensive care unit for recovery. An MRI was done within 24 hours after surgery that showed gross total resection (Fig. 60.2). The sodium, urine specific gravity, and GHs levels were checked every 6 hours. The GH nadir was less than 0.1 ug/dL, and he had no episodes of diabetes insipidus. The patient was started on hydrocortisone (20 mg in the morning and 10 mg in the afternoon). The nasal packings were removed 24 hours after surgery. The patient participated with physical therapy and was discharged to home on postoperative day 3 with 7 days of cefdinir. The patient was seen in the ear, nose, and throat clinic for endoscopic examination and cleaning on postoperative day 7. The patient was seen at 2 weeks postoperatively and remained neurologically intact. Pathology was pituitary adenoma, and hormonal stains were positive for GH. The patient underwent 3-month postoperative IGF-1 and oral glucose suppression test, and levels were consistent with biochemical remission. He remains in biochemical remission at 36 months following surgery.

Commonalities among the experts

The majority of surgeons opted for the patient to undergo computed tomography to better define bony anatomy, half requested endocrinology evaluation for pituitary hormonal functioning, and half requested additional testing for conditions associated with acromegaly (sleep study, colonoscopy,

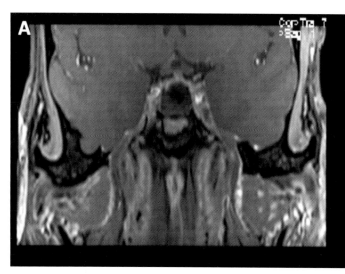 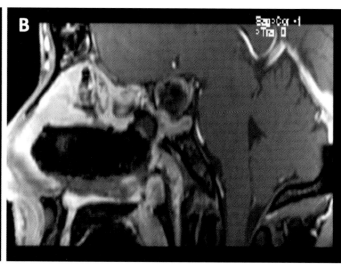

Fig. 60.2 Postoperative magnetic resonance imaging. (A) T1 coronal image with gadolinium contrast; **(B)** T1 sagittal image with gadolinium contrast magnetic resonance imaging scan demonstrating gross total resection of the lesion.

etc.) prior to surgery. All surgeons pursued an endoscopic endonasal transsphenoidal approach, and most aimed for gross total resection. All surgeons would perform the surgery in combination with ear, nose, and throat. Most surgeons were cognizant of the parasellar carotid arteries, optic nerves, and pituitary gland. The most feared complications were internal carotid artery injury, vision loss, and CSF leak. Surgery was generally pursued with surgical navigation, endoscopic equipment, and cranial Doppler, with half administering perioperative steroids. The majority of surgeons advocated for preservation of turbinates and extracapsular dissection. Following surgery, half of the surgeons admitted their patients to intermediate care and the other half to the floor, all surgeons performed GH evaluations while the patient was in the hospital, and most requested imaging 3 months after surgery to assess for extent of resection.

SUMMARY OF QUALITY OF EVIDENCE TO GUIDE SPECIFIC INTERVENTIONS FOR THIS CASE

- Surgery for acromegaly—Class III.
- Endoscopic endonasal versus microscopic approach—Class II-2.
- One nostril versus two nostrils for endoscopic endonasal approaches—Class III.

REFERENCES

1. Buchfelder M, Schlaffer SM. The surgical treatment of acromegaly. *Pituitary*. 2017;20:76–83.
2. Babu H, Ortega A, Nuno M, et al. Long-term endocrine outcomes following endoscopic endonasal transsphenoidal surgery for acromegaly and associated prognostic factors. *Neurosurgery*. 2017;81:357–366.
3. Chen CJ, Ironside N, Pomeraniec IJ, et al. Microsurgical versus endoscopic transsphenoidal resection for acromegaly: a systematic review of outcomes and complications. *Acta Neurochir (Wien)*. 2017;159:2193–2207.
4. Kim JH, Hur KY, Lee JH, et al. Outcome of endoscopic transsphenoidal surgery for acromegaly. *World Neurosurg*. 2017;104:272–278.
5. Hazer DB, Isik S, Berker D, et al. Treatment of acromegaly by endoscopic transsphenoidal surgery: surgical experience in 214 cases and cure rates according to current consensus criteria. *J Neurosurg*. 2013;119:1467–1477.
6. Knosp E, Steiner E, Kitz K, Matula C. Pituitary adenomas with invasion of the cavernous sinus space: a magnetic resonance imaging classification compared with surgical findings. *Neurosurgery*. 1993;33:610–617; discussion 617–618.
7. Mooney MA, Hardesty DA, Sheehy JP, et al. Rater reliability of the hardy classification for pituitary adenomas in the magnetic resonance imaging era. *J Neurol Surg B Skull Base*. 2017;78:413–418.
8. Liu JK, Weiss MH, Couldwell WT. Surgical approaches to pituitary tumors. *Neurosurg Clin N Am*. 2003;14:93–107.
9. Couldwell WT. Transsphenoidal and transcranial surgery for pituitary adenomas. *J Neurooncol*. 2004;69:237–256.
10. Eseonu CI, ReFaey K, Garcia O, Salvatori R, Quinones-Hinojosa A. Comparative cost analysis of endoscopic versus microscopic endonasal transsphenoidal surgery for pituitary adenomas. *J Neurol Surg B Skull Base*. 2018;79:131–138.
11. Eseonu CI, ReFaey K, Pamias-Portalatin E, et al. Three-hand endoscopic endonasal transsphenoidal surgery: experience with an anatomy-preserving mononostril approach technique. *Oper Neurosurg (Hagerstown)*. 2018;14:158–165.
12. Eseonu CI, ReFaey K, Rincon-Torroella J, et al. Endoscopic versus microscopic transsphenoidal approach for pituitary adenomas: comparison of outcomes during the transition of methods of a single surgeon. *World Neurosurg*. 2017;97:317–325.

61

Prolactinomas

Case reviewed by Carlos E. Briceno, William T. Curry, Nasser M. F. El-Ghandour, Theodore H. Schwartz

Introduction

Pituitary tumors account for approximately 14% of primary intracranial tumors, and their overall prevalence in the general population is estimated at 17%.[1-3] Among pituitary tumors, the range of functional pituitary adenomas is 46% to 64% in several series, in which prolactinomas account for 32% to 51% of pituitary adenomas, or 69% to 80% of clinically functional pituitary adenomas.[1-3] Female patients typically present earlier with smaller tumors, in which their symptoms include amenorrhea, galactorrhea, headache, infertility, and/or mass effect, whereas male patients present later with larger tumor sizes and have symptoms of visual loss (~40%), premature ejaculation, erective dysfunction, hypogonadism, and symptoms of mass effect.[1-3] The conventional management is the use of dopamine agonists (bromocriptine, cabergoline); however, this is not always feasible because of patient's symptoms, social situations, and economic status.[4,5] In this chapter, we present a case of a patient with a prolactin-secreting pituitary macroadenoma.

Chief complaint: visual loss
History of present illness
A 24-year-old, right-handed man with severe mental retardation and Down syndrome and lymphoma presented with acute vision loss. He is nonverbal at baseline, but family noted that he was walking into walls and did not appear to be able to see anything. He was seen in the emergency room, and imaging revealed a sellar mass (Fig. 61.1).
Medications: None.

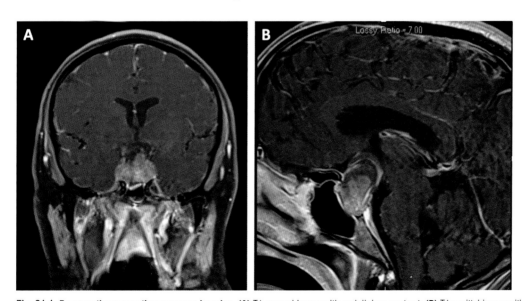

Fig. 61.1 Preoperative magnetic resonance imaging. (A) T1 coronal image with gadolinium contrast; **(B)** T1 sagittal image with gadolinium contrast magnetic resonance imaging scan demonstrating a hypoenhancing lesion involving the sella with displacement of the optic chiasm.

Allergies: No known drug allergies.
Past medical and surgical history: Down syndrome, lymphoma (controlled).
Family history: No history of intracranial malignancies.
Social history: Not independent with activities of daily living, no smoking or alcohol.

Physical examination: Awake, alert, nonverbal; Cranial nerves III to XII intact but unable to detect threat in either eye; Moves all extremities with good strength.
Pituitary labs: Prolactin 560 (with dilution), insulin-like growth factor-1, cortisol, thyroid stimulating hormone/T4 all within normal limits.

	Carlos E. Briceno, MD, Paitilla Medical Center, Panama City, Panama	William T. Curry, MD, Massachusetts General Hospital, Boston, MA, United States	Nasser M. F. El-Ghandour, MD, Cairo University, Cairo, Egypt	Theodore H. Schwartz, MD, Cornell University, New York, NY, United States
Preoperative				
Additional tests requested	CT head to evaluate paranasal sinus MRA Endocrinology evaluation Ophthalmology evaluation	CT and CT angiogram	CT head to evaluate paranasal sinus	CT head Macroprolactin test
Surgical approach selected	Endoscopic transnasal transsphenoidal	Endoscopic transnasal transsphenoidal	Endoscopic transnasal transsphenoidal	Endoscopic transnasal transsphenoidal
Other teams involved during surgery	ENT	ENT	ENT	ENT
Anatomic corridor	Transnasal transsphenoidal	Transnasal transsphenoidal	Transnasal transsphenoidal	Transnasal transsphenoidal
Goal of surgery	Decompress optic apparatus, maintain normal endocrine function	Decompress optic apparatus	Decompress optic apparatus	Decompress optic apparatus, remove as much tumor as possible with preservation of gland
Offer surgery if no vision deficit	No	Yes	No	No
Perioperative				
Positioning	Supine neutral with pins and 20 degree head elevation	Supine with pins	Supine neutral with pins	Supine neutral with pins
Surgical equipment	Surgical navigation Endoscopes Doppler	Surgical navigation Endoscopes	Surgical navigation Fluoroscopy Endoscopes	Endoscopes Doppler
Medications	Steroids	Steroids	Steroids	Steroids
Anatomic considerations	Sphenopalatine artery, ICA, optic nerves and chiasm, pituitary stalk, pituitary gland, cavernous sinuses	ICA, pituitary stalk, optic nerves and chiasm	Sphenoid sinus, sella, optic apparatus, ICA, cavernous sinus, cranial nerves III–VI, diaphragma sellae, pituitary gland, infundibulum	ICA, sphenoid septations
Complications feared with approach chosen	Brain retraction injury, CSF leak, meningitis, worsening visual deficit, panhypopituitarism, ICA or cavernous sinus injury, diabetes insipidus, electrolyte abnormalities, cranial neuropathy, hydrocephalus	Injury of pituitary gland, CSF leak	Injury of pituitary gland, CSF leak	Injury of pituitary gland
Intraoperative				
Anesthesia	General	General	General	General
Skin incision	None	None	None	None

	Carlos E. Briceno, MD, Paitilla Medical Center, Panama City, Panama	William T. Curry, MD, Massachusetts General Hospital, Boston, MA, United States	Nasser M. F. El-Ghandour, MD, Cairo University, Cairo, Egypt	Theodore H. Schwartz, MD, Cornell University, New York, NY, United States
Bone opening	Sphenoid ostia, sphenoid rostrum, anterior sphenoid sinus wall, sellar face	+/– right middle turbinate, anterior sphenoid sinus wall, sellar face	Sphenoid rostrum, anterior sphenoid sinus wall, sellar face	Sphenoid rostrum, anterior sphenoid sinus wall, posterior ethmoids, sellar face
Brain exposure	Sella	Sella	Sella	Sella
Method of resection	Pack both nostrils with oxymetazoline, prep with antibiotics and antiseptic solutions, compress inferior/middle/superior turbinates laterally in right nostril, coagulate mucosa over rostrum of sphenoid sinus, nasal septum out fractured, submucosal dissection along contralateral rostrum to visualize contralateral sphenoid ostia for binostril approach, harvest nasoseptal mucosa and hide in nasopharynx, open both sphenoid ostia with Kerrison rongeurs first inferiorly, remove rostrum and anterior wall of sphenoid sinus, skeletonize walls of sphenoid sinus, identify landmarks (clivus, sellar floor, carotid prominences, optic prominences), use microdoppler to confirm ICA, open dura, piecemeal resection in the midline, debulk inferior part and remove until encounter posterior sella, resect tumor laterally off cavernous sinus walls, remove superior portion extracapsular if possible, inspection with 30-degree scope for residual, use abdominal fat and fascia for dural reconstruction, bone from vomer and nasoseptal flap to reconstruct sella, dural sealant, avoid packing nostrils	+/– removal of right middle turbinate, identify and expand sphenoid ostia to enter sphenoid sinus, remove sphenoid face, posterior nasal septectomy preserving sphenopalatine artery, remove intersinus septations, identify sellar anatomy, remove sellar face from carotid to carotid up to tuberculum, open dura, observe for diaphragm, no need to be aggressive in cavernous sinuses because expect medical therapy to be effective, seal dural defect with free mucosa, +/– abdominal fat graft	Antiseptic nasal wash, lateralization of bilateral middle turbinates, C-shaped incisions in bilateral septal mucosa, elevation of nasoseptal flaps, removal of sphenoid rostrum, enlargement of sphenoid ostia and removal of anterior sphenoid sinus wall, removal of sellar face after confirmation with lateral fluoroscopy, needle to confirm not carotid before dural opening, tumor debulking in piecemeal with ring curettes, Valsalva to cause descent of tumor, inspection with angled endoscopes. If CSF leak, then harvest fat, fascia lata or dural substitute, and fibrin glue, with lumbar drain for 3 days.	ENT opening, removal of anterior sphenoid wall/rostrum/posterior ethmoids, compare sphenoid septations to preoperative imaging to understand location of ICA and location of normal gland, sella opened from medial cavernous to cavernous sinus and from superior intercavernous sinus to floor, Doppler to identify ICAs, dura opened cruciate fashion, debulking at center and inferior of tumor and then laterally until medial wall of cavernous sinus identified, roof of the tumor attempted at en bloc, harvest fat for CSF leak, gelfoam for cavernous sinus bleeding

(continued on next page)

	Carlos E. Briceno, MD, Paitilla Medical Center, Panama City, Panama	William T. Curry, MD, Massachusetts General Hospital, Boston, MA, United States	Nasser M. F. El-Ghandour, MD, Cairo University, Cairo, Egypt	Theodore H. Schwartz, MD, Cornell University, New York, NY, United States
Complication avoidance	Preserve sphenopalatine artery and nasoseptal flap, identify key anatomic landmarks, microdoppler to confirm ICA, remove superior portion extracapsular, abdominal fat and fascia for dural reconstruction, use bone to reconstruct sella	Preserve sphenopalatine artery and nasoseptal flap, large sellar face opening, observe for diaphragm, conservative approach in cavernous sinus	Avoid removal of middle turbinates, large sphenoid opening, fluoroscopy to identify sellar anatomy, needle to confirm absence of vascular structures, harvesting of nasoseptal flaps	Study sphenoid septations to identify ICA location, study gland location, debulk center and inferior portion of tumor first, en bloc resection of superior component, abdominal fat for CSF leaks
Postoperative				
Admission	ICU	Floor	ICU	Intermediate care
Postoperative complications feared	CSF leak, worsening visual deficit, panhypopituitarism, carotid or cavernous sinus injury, diabetes insipidus, electrolyte abnormality, cranial neuropathy, hydrocephalus	Recurrent hemorrhage, diabetes insipidus, CSF leak	Diabetes insipidus, panhypopituitarism, CSF leak	Diabetes insipidus, panhypopituitarism
Follow-up testing	Prolactin levels until <20, serum sodium/urea/creatinine postoperative and daily, a.m. cortisol MRI within 48 hours after surgery	Serum sodium, urine output and osmolarity (serum sodium every 3 days for several weeks), a.m. cortisol MRI prior to discharge	Prolactin at 2 and 6 weeks, then every 3 months after surgery Pituitary hormonal analysis 1 day after surgery Lumbar drain for 3 days if CSF leak MRI within 24 hours after surgery	Prolactin daily until discharge MRI within 48 hours after surgery Serum sodium and urine output every 6 hours initially
Follow-up visits	2 weeks after surgery	ENT 1 week after surgery Endocrinology 30 days after surgery Neurosurgery 6 weeks after surgery 7 days after surgery with ENT and endocrinology	2 weeks, 6 weeks, 3 months after surgery	Endocrinology 1 week after surgery ENT 1 week after surgery Neurosurgery 3 months after surgery
Adjuvant therapies recommended	Reoperation or radiation therapy if treatment failure	Defer to endocrinology	Craniotomy for residual	Defer to endocrinology

CSF, cerebrospinal fluid; *CT*, computed tomography; *ICA*, internal carotid artery; *ICU*, intensive care unit; *ENT*, ear, nose, and throat; *MRA*, magnetic resonance angiography; *MRI*, magnetic resonance imaging.

Differential diagnosis and actual diagnosis

- Pituitary adenoma
- Craniopharyngioma
- Metastatic brain tumor

Important anatomic and preoperative considerations

Sellar anatomy is discussed in Chapters 56 and 57, whereas the cavernous sinus anatomy is discussed in Chapter 50. Prolactin is normally inhibited by dopamine from the hypothalamus, and therefore prolactinomas, hypothalamic or pituitary stalk dysfunction, medications that block dopamine receptors (i.e., haloperidol, phenothiazines, tricyclic antidepressants, monoamine-oxidase inhibitors), and several medical conditions (i.e., pregnancy, hypothyroidism, renal insufficiency) can all cause prolactin elevation.[1-3] Once a prolactinoma is considered, it is important to rule out other causes of elevated prolactin and to assess serum thyrotropin and creatinine.[1-3] Once these other conditions are ruled out, magnetic resonance imaging (MRI) will help determine the presence of a pituitary adenoma, in which 90% of prolactinomas are microadenomas.[1-3] Nonprolactin-producing macroadenomas can also cause elevated prolactin by mass effect on the stalk or hypothalamus, in which prolactin levels more than 200 μg/L are typically considered to be caused by prolactinomas.[1–3] If the tumor is large with high prolactin levels (usually >10,000 μg/L), elevated prolactins can saturate the antibodies in some assays leading to artifactually low results, and therefore should undergo dilutional assessments.[1–3] The goals of medical treatment are to restore normal gonadal function and fertility and to reduce tumor size for macroadenomas.[1–3] For patients with minimal symptoms with normal gonadal function, these prolactinomas can be monitored conservatively with serial MRI scans and prolactin levels.[1–3] The most common treatment for patients with prolactinomas is the use of dopamine agonists, in which cabergoline has been shown to be more effective in normalizing prolactin values, reducing tumor size, and has fewer side effects than bromocriptine, in which patients should be followed with serial echocardiograms for patients exceeding 2 mg per week.[1–3] Other potential side effects are compulsive behavior, chest pain, shortness of breath, persistent cough, swelling of extremities, nausea/vomiting, headaches, depressed mood, and dizziness.[1–3] Surgery is typically considered for medically refractory tumors (3%–12%), patients with significant side effects (3%–11%), and younger patients of childbearing age, in which surgery can normalize prolactin in 65% to 85% of patients with microadenomas and 30% to 40% of macroadenomas with recurrence rates of 20% over 10 years.[1–3,6] The factors associated with biochemical remission following surgery are microprolactinomas and lower preoperative prolactin levels (<200 ug/L).[1–3,6] Postoperative prolactin levels less than 10 μg/L are associated with long-term surgical remission.[1–3,6] Other therapies include radiation therapy for patients who cannot be controlled with dopamine agonists and/or surgery, and more recently temozolomide has been used with limited success.[1–3]

The Hardy and Knosp classification schemes are used to describe sellar changes and tumor extension and cavernous sinus involvement, respectively (Chapter 56, Figs. 56.3 and 56.4).[7,8] The tumor presented in this case is a Hardy grade 2B with expansion of the sella with a size greater than 10 mm, and the tumor reaches the floor of the third ventricle, and a Knosp grade 3 in which the tumor extends past the internal carotid artery lateral line but does not circumferentially involve the internal carotid artery.

Approaches to this lesion

The approaches for sellar pathology are discussed in detail in Chapter 56, Fig. 56.2. These approaches can be divided into transsphenoidal and transcranial approaches.[9–13] For pituitary adenomas, the most commonly used approach is an endoscopic endonasal transsphenoidal approach with or without the use assistance of otolaryngology.[9–13] In this approach, one or both nares are used to access the sphenoid sinus to enter the lesion through the sella.[9–13] This approach allows for minimal nasal dissection, no brain retraction, and panoramic view within the sella, which facilitates resection within the cavernous sinus; however, it is associated with a loss of stereoscopic visualization, small working corridor, and risk of cerebrospinal fluid (CSF) leak.[9–13]

What was actually done

The patient was taken to surgery for an endoscopic expanded endonasal resection of a prolactin-producing macroadenoma with otolaryngology with general anesthesia and no intraoperative monitoring. It was decided to proceed with surgery because of the vision loss, poor compliance with medication, and young age of the patient, in which the goal was optic chiasm decompression rather than biochemical remission because of the large size of the tumor and elevated prolactin levels. The patient was induced and intubated per routine. An electromagnetic navigation system with preoperative MRI and computed tomography was used to avoid the need for head pinning. The patient was draped in the usual standard fashion and given cefazolin and steroids. With the assistance of a rhinologist, the right middle turbinate was removed, and the right inferior turbinate was displaced laterally. A right maxillary antrostomy and right anterior and posterior ethmoidectomies were done. A right nasal septal flap was raised and placed into the nasopharynx. A posterior septectomy was done to allow bilateral nasal access. The sphenoid ostia were opened bilaterally, and the intersinus septation was drilled flush with the sellar face. The bone overlying the sella was thinned with a diamond drill until the dura was identified. A nerve hook was used to dissect the dura in the epidural plane, and up- and down-going Kerrison punches were used to remove the bone until both cavernous sinuses were identified, as were the floor of the sella and tuberculum. The tuberculum was removed to facilitate suprasellar access. The dura was opened in a cruciate fashion with an arachnoid knife, and the dura was removed with a side-cutting tissue biting device (Myriad, NICO Corporation, Indianapolis, IN). The tumor was debulked first at the inferior aspect by identifying the floor, followed by the bilateral cavernous sinuses, and moving upward until the diaphragma sellae fell into the sellar cavity. The tumor was debulked until no more tumor was visible. Preliminary pathology was pituitary adenoma. A couple of rounds of Valsalva were used to see if more tumor would fall into the cavity, and the cavity was examined with a 30-degree endoscope. A CSF leak was encountered, and the sella was packed with gelfoam, followed by a dural substitute in the epidural plane, and tucked into the bone edges of the sella. The nasoseptal flap was mobilized to cover the sella. Nasal packings were placed bilaterally. A lumbar drain was placed and drained for 72 hours (5–10 cc/hr) and removed. The lumbar drain was placed because of anticipated poor patient compliance.

The patient awoke at their neurologic baseline and was taken to the intensive care unit for recovery. An MRI was done within 24 hours after surgery that showed gross total resection (Fig. 61.2). The sodium, urine specific gravity, and prolactin levels were checked every 6 hours. The prolactin nadir was 7 ug/dL, and he had two episodes of diabetes insipidus requiring vasopressin. The patient was started on hydrocortisone (20 mg in the morning and 10 mg in the afternoon). The nasal packings were removed 24 hours after surgery. The patient participated with physical therapy and was discharged to home on postoperative day 6 with 7 days of cefdinir. The patient was seen at 2 weeks postoperatively and remained at their neurologic baseline with vision present. Pathology was pituitary adenoma, and hormonal stains

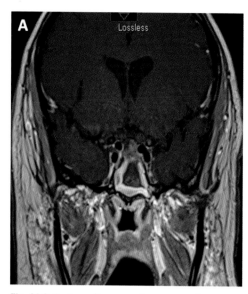 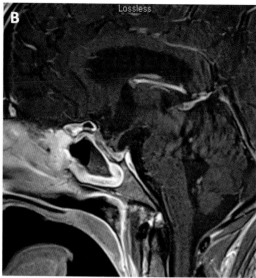

Fig. 61.2 Postoperative magnetic resonance imaging. (A) T1 coronal image with gadolinium contrast; **(B)** T1 sagittal image with gadolinium contrast magnetic resonance imaging scan demonstrating gross total resection of the lesion.

were positive for prolactin. The patient underwent 3-month postoperative serum prolactin evaluations, and levels were consistent with biochemical remission. He remains in biochemical remission at 36 months following surgery.

Commonalities among the experts

All surgeons opted for the patient to undergo computed tomography to better define bony and sinus anatomy prior to surgery. All surgeons pursued an endoscopic endonasal transsphenoidal approach, and all aimed to decompress the optic apparatus. If the patient did not have visual deficits, then all surgeons advocated for medical therapy. All surgeons would perform the surgery in combination with otolaryngology. Most surgeons were cognizant of the parasellar carotid arteries, optic nerves, pituitary gland, and infundibulum. Surgery was generally pursued with surgical navigation, endoscopic equipment, and cranial Doppler, with all surgeons administering perioperative steroids. The majority of surgeons advocated for preservation of the sphenopalatine artery, harvesting of a nasal septal flap, conservative resection in cavernous sinus, and abdominal fat if CSF leak occurs. Following surgery, most of the surgeons admitted their patients to intermediate care or the intensive care unit, half performed prolactin hormone evaluations while the patient was in the hospital, and most requested imaging within 48 hours after surgery to assess for extent of resection and/or possible complications.

SUMMARY OF QUALITY OF EVIDENCE TO GUIDE SPECIFIC INTERVENTIONS FOR THIS CASE

- Surgery as opposed to medical therapies for prolactinomas—Class III.
- Endoscopic endonasal versus microscopic approach—Class II-2.
- One nostril versus two nostrils for endoscopic endonasal approaches—Class III.

REFERENCES

1. Maiter D. Management of dopamine agonist-resistant prolactinoma. *Neuroendocrinology.* 2019;109:42–50.
2. Mehta GU, Lonser RR. Management of hormone-secreting pituitary adenomas. *Neuro Oncol.* 2017;19:762–773.
3. Molitch ME. Diagnosis and treatment of pituitary adenomas: a review. *JAMA.* 2017;317:516–524.
4. Duan L, Yan H, Huang M, Zhang Y, Gu F. An economic analysis of bromocriptine versus trans-sphenoidal surgery for the treatment of prolactinoma. *J Craniofac Surg.* 2017;28:1046–1051.
5. Jethwa PR, Patel TD, Hajart AF, Eloy JA, Couldwell WT, Liu JK. Cost-effectiveness analysis of microscopic and endoscopic transsphenoidal surgery versus medical therapy in the management of microprolactinoma in the United States. *World Neurosurg.* 2016;87:65–76.
6. Babey M, Sahli R, Vajtai I, Andres RH, Seiler RW. Pituitary surgery for small prolactinomas as an alternative to treatment with dopamine agonists. *Pituitary.* 2011;14:222–230.
7. Knosp E, Steiner E, Kitz K, Matula C. Pituitary adenomas with invasion of the cavernous sinus space: a magnetic resonance imaging classification compared with surgical findings. *Neurosurgery.* 1993;33:610–617; discussion 617–618.
8. Mooney MA, Hardesty DA, Sheehy JP, et al. Rater reliability of the hardy classification for pituitary adenomas in the magnetic resonance imaging era. *J Neurol Surg B Skull Base.* 2017;78:413–418.
9. Liu JK, Weiss MH, Couldwell WT. Surgical approaches to pituitary tumors. *Neurosurg Clin N Am.* 2003;14:93–107.
10. Couldwell WT. Transsphenoidal and transcranial surgery for pituitary adenomas. *J Neurooncol.* 2004;69:237–256.
11. Eseonu CI, ReFaey K, Garcia O, Salvatori R, Quinones-Hinojosa A. Comparative cost analysis of endoscopic versus microscopic endonasal transsphenoidal surgery for pituitary adenomas. *J Neurol Surg B Skull Base.* 2018;79:131–138.
12. Eseonu CI, ReFaey K, Pamias-Portalatin E, et al. Three-hand endoscopic endonasal transsphenoidal surgery: experience with an anatomy-preserving mononostril approach technique. *Oper Neurosurg (Hagerstown).* 2018;14:158–165.
13. Eseonu CI, ReFaey K, Rincon-Torroella J, et al. Endoscopic versus microscopic transsphenoidal approach for pituitary adenomas: comparison of outcomes during the transition of methods of a single surgeon. *World Neurosurg.* 2017;97:317–325.

62

Craniopharyngiomas

Case reviewed by Peter Bullock, Edward R. Laws, Daniel Donoho, James Rutka, Theodore H. Schwartz

Introduction

Craniopharyngiomas are rare intracranial tumors with an incidence of 1 to 2 cases per million persons per year that are derived from pituitary gland embryonic tissue, and have a bimodal clinical presentation in which it most commonly occurs in children between the ages of 5 to 14 years (30%–50%), but can also occur in adults 50 to 74 years.[1,2] Childhood-onset craniopharyngiomas are typically adamantinomatous in histology and have an 87% to 95% 20-year overall survival rate, but are associated with a poor quality of life owing to injury of the optic apparatus and hypothalamic-pituitary axis, whereas adult-onset craniopharyngiomas are typically papillary in histology and have a 19-fold higher cerebrovascular mortality than the general population.[2] Childhood craniopharyngiomas usually present late with prolonged symptoms of mass effect (headaches, nausea, vomiting), visual impairment, and endocrine deficits, whereas adults typically present with hormonal deficits (growth hormone, gonadotropins, adrenocorticotropic hormone, thyroid stimulating hormone).[2] Surgery is typically first-line therapy in most patients; however, there is controversy over the best treatment strategy (gross total resection vs. partial resection and radiation therapy, as well as endoscopic vs. transcranial approaches).[3–8] In this chapter, we present a case of a patient with a craniopharyngioma.

Example case

Chief complaint: headaches

History of present illness

A 14-year-old, right-handed boy with no significant past medical history presented with worsening headaches. For the past 2 to 3 months, he complained of worsening headaches that were exacerbated by activity and associated with nausea and vomiting. Primary care ordered imaging that showed a large brain lesion (Fig. 62.1).

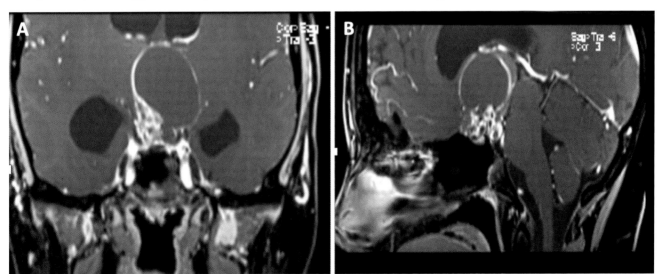

Fig. 62.1 Preoperative magnetic resonance imaging. (A) T1 coronal image with gadolinium contrast; **(B)** T1 sagittal image with gadolinium contrast magnetic resonance imaging scan demonstrating a heterogeneously enhancing lesion involving the sellar, suprasellar space, and third ventricle with obstructive hydrocephalus.

Medications: None.
Allergies: No known drug allergies.
Past medical and surgical history: Tonsillectomy.
Family history: No history of intracranial malignancies.
Social history: Eighth grade honors student, no smoking or alcohol.

Physical examination: Awake, alert, oriented to person, place, time; Cranial nerves II to XII intact, except bitemporal hemianopsia; Moves all extremities with good strength.
Pituitary labs: Prolactin, insulin-like growth factor-1, cortisol, thyroid-stimulating hormone/T4 all within normal limits.

	Peter Bullock, FRCS, MRCP, London Clinic, London, England	Edward R. Laws, MD, Daniel Donoho, MD, Brigham and Women's Hospital, Boston, MA, United States	James Rutka, MD, PhD, University of Toronto Sick Kids, Toronto, Canada	Theodore H. Schwartz, MD, Cornell University, New York, NY, United States
Preoperative				
Additional tests requested	CT Neuroophthalmology evaluation Neuroendocrinology evaluation Neuropsychological assessment	CT and CTA Neuroophthalmology evaluation (papilledema, OCT) Neuropsychological assessment BMI and diabetes insipidus evaluation	CT Neuroophthalmology evaluation Neuroendocrinology evaluation Neuropsychological Neurology evaluation	CT Neuroophthalmology evaluation (visual fields) Neuroendocrinology evaluation Neuropsychological assessment
Surgical approach selected	Expanded endoscopic endonasal	Right frontotemporal craniotomy with IOM (MEP/SSEP)	Endoscopic endonasal	EVD and endoscopic endonasal
Other teams involved during surgery	ENT	None	ENT	ENT
Anatomic corridor	Transsphenoidal, transplanum, transtuberculum	Right frontotemporal, trans-Sylvian	Transsphenoidal	Transsphenoidal, transplanum, transtubercular
Goal of surgery	Gross total resection, maintain or improve vision, preserve endocrine function	Diagnosis, optic compression, maximal safe resection, cyst decompression	Gross total resection	EVD to relieve hydrocephalus, decompression of optic chiasm, gross total resection without injuring hypothalamus
Perioperative				
Positioning	Supine with pins with left rotation	Supine with left rotation	Supine neutral in pins	Supine neutral in pins
Surgical equipment	Surgical navigation Endoscopes Ring curettes	Surgical navigation IOM (MEP/SSEP) Surgical microscope Ultrasonic aspirator Ring curettes	Surgical navigation Endoscopes	Surgical navigation Endoscopes with scope holder Tissue biting device
Medications	Steroids	Antiepileptics Mannitol if necessary	None	Steroids
Anatomic considerations	Sella, clivus, carotid prominences, optic canals, medial and lateral optico-carotid recesses	ICA	Optic nerves and chiasm, pituitary gland and stalk, ICA/ACA, hypothalamus	Tuberculum, sella, ICAs, optic chiasm and nerves
Complications feared with approach chosen	Diabetes insipidus, vision loss, CSF leak, ICA injury, meningitis	Visual deficit	Injury to hypothalamus, optic apparatus, cerebrovasculature, CSF leak	Injury to optic nerves, hypothalamic injury, CSF leak, anosmia, panhypopituitarism
Intraoperative				
Anesthesia	General	General	General	General
Skin incision	None	Pterional	None	None

	Peter Bullock, FRCS, MRCP, London Clinic, London, England	Edward R. Laws, MD, Daniel Donoho, MD, Brigham and Women's Hospital, Boston, MA, United States	James Rutka, MD, PhD, University of Toronto Sick Kids, Toronto, Canada	Theodore H. Schwartz, MD, Cornell University, New York, NY, United States
Bone opening	Anterior wall of sphenoid sinus, posterior ethmoidectomy, sella, planum tuberculum	Frontotemporal	Anterior wall of sphenoid sinus, sella	Sphenoid rostrum, anterior sphenoid sinus wall, posterior ethmoids, sellar face, tuberculum, planum
Brain exposure	Sella, tuberculum, planum	Frontotemporal	Sella	Sella, tuberculum, planum
Method of resection	ENT starts the approach, sphenoid sinus opened widely, nasoseptal flap raised and tucked into nasopharynx, identification of ICA/ optic canals, removal of tuberculum and sellar bone, neurosurgeon exposes medial edge of cavernous sinuses and thins bone over planum and tuberculum with drill, remove medial aspects of borth optic canals, carotid and ophthalmic arteries identified with Doppler, dura opened with diamond knife and coagulating and dividing intercavernous sinus, suprasellar space entered and diaphragm opened, chiasm and supraclinoid ICA identified, cyst decompressed on left, chiasm dissected from tumor making sure to prescrvc perforators to the chiasm and pituitary, extra capsular dissection of solid elements with internal tumor debulking, stalk may need to be sacrificed to compelte resection, peel superior cyst wall from inside ventricle, close with a multi-layer reconstruction using nasoseptal flap rotated into position and held in position with surgicell / tissue glue / nasopore	Pterional craniotomy, dural opening, Sylvian fissure opening, mannitol if necessary, tumor resection of solid and cystic component with sparing hypothalamus	Nasal septal flap, exposure of sphenoid sinus, remove sellar face, puncture and drain cyst, mobilize capsule, dissect capsule from surrounding neurovasculature structures, preserve pituitary stalk, angled endoscope to observe for residual, closure of sella with bone, fat, and nasoseptal flap nasal packing	EVD placement, ENT approach with harvesting of nasoseptal flap and opening of sphenoid sinus posterior ethmoids, partial removal of left middle turbinate, removal of the keel and then entry into sphenoid sinus, remove all mucosa within the sphenoid sinus, open bone from the top of the sella just below the superior intercavernous sinus to the planum from medial OCR to medial OCR, opening of dura starting below intercavernous sinus with dural removal, identification of SHA and dissected away from tumor, tumor entered and debulked, capsule dissected free from arachnoid, stalk identified and attempted at preservation unless it compromises complete resection, tumor removed from optic chiasm and hypothalamus with caution, dura reconstructed with alloderm of fascia lata and countersunk with medpore implant and nasoseptal flap

(continued on next page)

	Peter Bullock, FRCS, MRCP, London Clinic, London, England	Edward R. Laws, MD, Daniel Donoho, MD, Brigham and Women's Hospital, Boston, MA, United States	James Rutka, MD, PhD, University of Toronto Sick Kids, Toronto, Canada	Theodore H. Schwartz, MD, Cornell University, New York, NY, United States
Complication avoidance	Wide bony opening, drain cyst early, extracapsular dissection, nasal septal flap and multi-layered closure	Sylvian fissure opening, leave tumor adherent to hypothalamus	Drain cyst first, dissect capsule from surrounding structures but care to hypothalamus and pituitary stalk, nasoseptal flap	EVD, nasoseptal flap, remove all sphenoid sinus mucosa, identify SHA, leave piece along hypothalamus if cannot be dissected, countersinking layered closure, leave EVD at opening pressure of 0 to reduce intracranial pressure for 48 hours
Postoperative				
Admission	High dependency unit	ICU	ICU	ICU
Postoperative complications feared	CSF leak, hypopituitarism, diabetes insipidus, visual decline	Hypopituitarism, hyponatremia, visual loss, injury to arteries and hypothalamus, obesity, memory loss	CSF leak, panhypopituitarism, visual impairment	Diabetes insipidus, adrenal insufficiency, CSF leak, vision loss
Follow-up testing	Maintain strict fluid balance Vision checked every 4 hours MRI within 24 hours after surgery	Sodium and cortisol 1 week after surgery Full endocrine panel 6 weeks after surgery MRI 3 months after surgery	MRI within 24 hours after surgery Neuroophthalmology evaluation	EVD MRI within 48 hours after surgery after EVD removal
Follow-up visits	2 weeks and 3 months after surgery with neurosurgery 1 week after surgery with ENT	3 months after surgery	4–6 weeks after surgery	7 days after surgery with ENT and endocrine 3 months after surgery with neurosurgery
Adjuvant therapies recommended for residual	Radiation	Radiation, BRAF inhibitor, or repeat surgery if necessary	Radiation therapy or radiosurgery, repeat surgery if necessary	Observation for gross total resection, early radiation for subtotal resection

ACA, anterior cerebral artery; *BMI*, body mass index; *CSF*, cerebrospinal fluid; *CT*, computed tomography; *CTA*, computed tomography angiography; *ENT*, ear, nose, and throat; *EVD*, external ventricular drain; *ICA*, internal carotid artery; *ICU*, intensive care unit; *IOM*, intraoperative monitoring; *MEP*, motor evoked potential; *MRI*, magnetic resonance imaging; *OCR*, opticocarotid recess; *OCT*, optical coherence tomography; *SHA*, superior hypophyseal artery; *SSEP*, somatosensory evoked potential.

Differential diagnosis and actual diagnosis

- Craniopharyngioma
- Pituitary adenoma
- Metastatic brain tumor

Important anatomic and preoperative considerations

Sellar anatomy is discussed in Chapters 56 and 57, whereas the cavernous sinus anatomy is discussed in Chapter 50. Craniopharyngiomas can be classified by pathology and location.[9] Pathologically, craniopharyngiomas can be divided into adamantinomatous (90% of craniopharyngiomas, more common in children, cystic and solid components with frequent calcifications, contain nodules of wet keratin/

palisading basal layer of cells/Rosenthal fibers) and papillary (10% of craniopharyngiomas, more common in adults, mostly solid, mature squamous epithelium and pseudopapillae).[9] By location, craniopharyngiomas can occur anywhere along the craniopharyngeal canal, but most rise in the sellar and parasellar regions, although there are reports of ectopic locations.[9] As a result of these diverse craniopharyngeal locations, there are a variety of classification schemes (Table 62.1).[7–10] The Yasargil et al.[8] classification scheme is based on the tumor location in relation to the diaphragma sella, in which the tumors can be classified as infradiaphragmatic (purely intrasellar), infra- and supradiaphragmatic (both intra- and suprasellar), supradiaphragmatic parachiasmatic (suprasellar but extraventricular), paraventricular (intra- and extraventricular), and intraventricular. This was primarily used to help guide transcranial surgical approaches.[8] Similarly, Samii and Tatagiba[7] categorized

Table 62.1 Common craniopharyngioma classification schemes		
Classification Schemes	**Reference Structure**	**Categories**
Yasargil et al.[8]	Diaphragma sella	Infradiaphragmatic–intrasellar Infra- and supradiaphragmatic–intra/suprasellar Supradiaphragmatic parachiasmatic–extraventricular Intra- and extraventricular Paraventricular Intraventricular
Samii and Tatagiba[7]	Tumor extension	I: Intrasellar II: Suprasellar cistern with/without intrasellar involvement III: Lower half of the third ventricle IV: Upper half of the third ventricle V: Reaching lateral ventricle
Hoffman[11]	Optic chiasm	Sellar Prechiasmatic Retrochiasmatic
Kassam et al.[10]	Infundibulum	Preinfundibular Transinfundibular Retroinfundibular Isolated intraventricular

craniopharyngiomas from I to V, in which I were intrasellar, II were suprasellar with or without intrasellar involvement, III involved the lower half of the third ventricle, IV reached the upper half of the third ventricle, and V reached the

lateral ventricle, and was used to define skull base versus transcranial approaches. Hoffman[11] described the location of the tumor in relation to the optic chiasm, in which they are divided into sellar, prechiasmatic, and retrochiasmatic, which can dictate a subfrontal or anterolateral transcranial approach. With the advances in endoscopic surgery, Kassam et al.[10] categorized craniopharyngiomas based on the location of the infundibulum, in which tumors were either preinfundibular, transinfundibular, retroinfundibular, and intraventricular.[7]

Approaches to this lesion

The approaches for craniopharyngiomas are varied, which is the reason why several classification schemes exist to try and identify the best surgical routes with the lowest morbidity.[7,8,10,11] As with pituitary tumors, the approaches can be divided into endonasal transsphenoidal and transcranial approaches (Fig. 62.2).[12–16] The endonasal transsphenoidal approach can be expanded by opening the tuberculum (transtuberculum) and/or planum sphenoidale (transplanum) to allow more superior and anterior access.[10] However, other than cases of purely intrasellar involvement, the transsphenoidal approach must traverse "normal tissue," including the pituitary gland and stalk, which can lead to pituitary dysfunction.[6] The advantages of the endonasal transsphenoidal with or without transtubercular and/or transplanar approaches include minimal nasal dissection, no brain retraction, and the approach is not dictated by the position of the optic chiasm, whereas the disadvantages include difficult vascular control for tumors involving intracranial vessels, need for skull base reconstruction, risk of cerebrospinal fluid leak, potential pituitary dysfunction, and difficulty

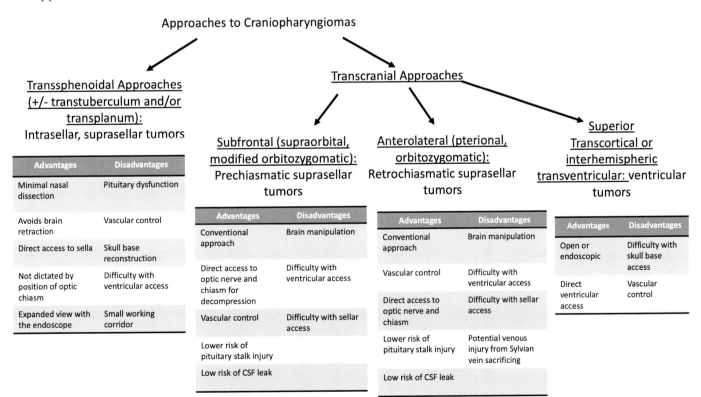

Fig. 62.2 Diagram of approaches to craniopharyngiomas. *CSF,* cerebrospinal fluid.

with ventricular access.[10] For transcranial approaches, the options are varied and include anterolateral approaches, such as a pterional and orbitozygomatic via trans-Sylvian, opticocarotid, interoptic, and carotid-oculomotor triangles, as well as lamina terminalis; subfrontal approaches, such as transpalpebral/transciliary, orbitozygomatic, and pterional, through the same skull base triangles and/or lamina terminalis; and superior approaches, such as transcortical or interhemispheric transventricular.[7,8,11] These approaches are typically dictated by the position of the optic chiasm for skull base approaches, and tumor extension for superior approaches.[7,8,11] In general, intrasellar tumors (whether they are purely intrasellar or sellar/suprasellar) are typically operated on with an endonasal approach; prechiasmatic tumors are done through an endonasal or subfrontal transcranial approach; retrochiasmatic tumors are done through an endonasal or anterolateral transcranial approach; and tumors in the ventricle are done through a superior transcranial approach unless there is sellar or suprasellar involvement that allows access through an endonasal approach.[7,8,11]

What was actually done

The patient was taken to surgery for an endoscopic expanded endonasal resection of a craniopharyngioma and lumbar drain placement with otolaryngology with general anesthesia and no intraoperative monitoring. The goal was to do an endonasal approach, as most of the lesion was in the intrasellar/suprasellar space, and it was believed the cyst could be accessed from below. The patient was induced and intubated per routine. A lumbar drain was placed in the lateral decubitus position. The patient was turned supine, and an electromagnetic navigation system with preoperative magnetic resonance imaging (MRI) and computed tomography was used to avoid the need for head pinning. The patient was draped in the usual standard fashion and given cefazolin and steroids. With the assistance of a rhinologist, the right middle turbinate was removed, and the right inferior turbinate was displaced laterally. A right maxillary antrostomy and bilateral anterior and posterior

ethmoidectomies were done. A right nasal septal flap was raised and placed into the nasopharynx. A posterior septectomy was done to allow bilateral nasal access. The sphenoid ostia were opened bilaterally, and the intersinus septation was drilled flush with the sellar face. The bone overlying the sella was thinned with a diamond drill until the dura was identified. A nerve hook was used to dissect the dura in the epidural plane, and up- and down-going Kerrison punches were used to remove the bone until both cavernous sinuses were identified, as were the floor of the sella and tuberculum. The tuberculum and posterior portion of the planum sphenoidale were removed to facilitate suprasellar access and to identify the optic nerves. The floor of the sella was also removed to allow downward displacement of the pituitary gland to facilitate superior access. The dura was opened in a cruciate fashion with an arachnoid knife, and the dura was removed with a side-cutting tissue-biting device (Myriad, NICO Corporation, Indianapolis, IN). The pituitary gland was dissected from the tumor and retracted downward with a cottonoid. The tumor was debulked first at the inferior aspect and then dissecting the lesion from the cavernous walls laterally, optic chiasm anteriorly and superiorly. The cyst was then encountered and drained, which facilitated dissection from the third ventricle. Preliminary pathology was a craniopharyngioma. The cavity was examined with a 30-degree endoscope, and no residual tumor was seen. The bilateral foramen of Monro, pituitary stalk, and optic nerves and chiasm were identified. The gland was displaced superiorly from the floor, and gelfoam was placed underneath to bolster the gland to act as a vascularized graft. A dural substitute was placed both in the subdural and epidural planes, and tucked into the bone edges of the sella. The nasoseptal flap was mobilized to cover the bony opening. Nasal packings were placed bilaterally.

The patient awoke at their neurologic baseline with intact vision and was taken to the intensive care unit for recovery. An MRI was done within 24 hours after surgery that showed gross total resection (Fig. 62.3). The sodium and urine specific gravity were checked every 6 hours. The patient was started on hydrocortisone (20 mg in the morning and 10 mg

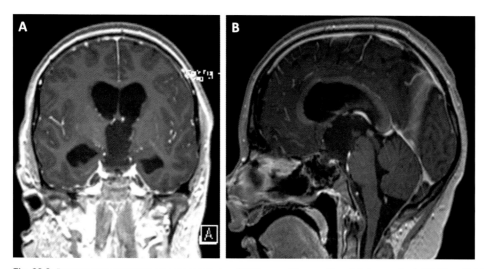

Fig. 62.3 Postoperative magnetic resonance imaging. (A) T1 coronal image with gadolinium contrast; **(B)** T1 sagittal image with gadolinium contrast magnetic resonance imaging scan demonstrating gross total resection of the lesion.

in the afternoon) and required several doses of vasopressin for diabetes insipidus. The lumbar drain was drained for 72 hours (5–10 cc/hr) and removed. The nasal packings were removed 24 hours after surgery. The patient participated with physical therapy and was discharged to home on postoperative day 5 with 7 days of cefdinir, hydrocortisone, and vasopressin. The patient was seen at 2 weeks postoperatively and remained at their neurologic baseline with intact vision. Pathology was an adamantinomatous craniopharyngioma. The patient underwent hormonal analysis and was placed on pituitary replacements for panhypopituitarism (levothyroxine, hydrocortisone, and vasopressin). The patient underwent formal visual field examination at 3 months postoperatively and had full visual fields. The lesion was observed with serial MRI examinations at 3- to 6-month intervals, and no recurrence has been noted for 36 months.

Commonalities among the experts

All of the surgeons opted for the patient to undergo computed tomography to better define bony anatomy, ophthalmology evaluation to asses preoperative vision status, and endocrinology to assess baseline pituitary hormone functioning, as well as the majority of surgeons requesting neuropsychological evaluation for baseline neurocognitive functioning. The majority of surgeons would pursue surgery through an endoscopic endonasal approach with ear, nose, and throat, whereas one would perform a frontotemporal craniotomy. Only one surgeon would place an external ventricular drain prior to surgery. The goal was extensive or gross total resection with decompression of the optic apparatus. Most surgeons were cognizant of the parasellar and intracranial carotid arteries and optic apparatus. The most feared complications were vision loss and internal carotid artery injury. Surgery was generally pursued with surgical navigation and endoscopic equipment, with half of the surgeons administering perioperative steroids. The majority of surgeons advocated for wide bony opening of the sella and parasellar region, early cyst drainage, sharp dissection and preservation of hypothalamus, and nasoseptal flap for reconstruction. Following surgery, the majority of the surgeons admitted their patients to the intensive care unit, and most surgeons requested imaging within 48 hours to assess for extent of resection and/or evaluate for complications. All surgeons advocated for radiation for regrowth or residual lesion.

SUMMARY OF QUALITY OF EVIDENCE TO GUIDE SPECIFIC INTERVENTIONS FOR THIS CASE

- Endoscopic endonasal surgery for sellar/suprasellar/ventricular craniopharyngiomas–Class III.
- Gross total resection versus subtotal resection and radiation therapy—Class III.

REFERENCES

1. Fujio S, Juratli TA, Arita K, et al. A clinical rule for preoperative prediction of BRAF mutation status in craniopharyngiomas. *Neurosurgery*. 2019;85:204–210.
2. Muller HL. Craniopharyngioma. *Endocr Rev*. 2014;35:513–543.
3. Feng SY, Zhang YY, Yu XG, et al. Microsurgical treatment of craniopharyngioma: experiences on 183 consecutive patients. *Medicine (Baltimore)*. 2018;97:e11746.
4. Forbes JA, Ordonez-Rubiano EG, Tomasiewicz HC, et al. Endonasal endoscopic transsphenoidal resection of intrinsic third ventricular craniopharyngioma: surgical results. *J Neurosurg*. 2019;131:1152–1162.
5. Losa M, Pieri V, Bailo M, et al. Single fraction and multisession Gamma Knife radiosurgery for craniopharyngioma. *Pituitary*. 2018;21:499–506.
6. Ordonez-Rubiano EG, Forbes JA, Morgenstern PF, et al. Preserve or sacrifice the stalk? Endocrinological outcomes, extent of resection, and recurrence rates following endoscopic endonasal resection of craniopharyngiomas. *J Neurosurg*. 2019;131:1163–1171.
7. Samii M, Tatagiba M. Surgical management of craniopharyngiomas: a review. *Neurol Med Chir (Tokyo)*. 1997;37:141–149.
8. Yasargil MG, Curcic M, Kis M, Siegenthaler G, Teddy PJ, Roth P. Total removal of craniopharyngiomas. Approaches and long-term results in 144 patients. *J Neurosurg*. 1990;73:3–11.
9. Lubuulwa J, Lei T. Pathological and topographical classification of craniopharyngiomas: a literature review. *J Neurol Surg Rep*. 2016;77:e121–e127.
10. Kassam AB, Gardner PA, Snyderman CH, Carrau RL, Mintz AH, Prevedello DM. Expanded endonasal approach, a fully endoscopic transnasal approach for the resection of midline suprasellar craniopharyngiomas: a new classification based on the infundibulum. *J Neurosurg*. 2008;108:715–728.
11. Hoffman HJ. Surgical management of craniopharyngioma. *Pediatr Neurosurg*. 1994;21(Suppl 1):44–49.
12. Liu JK, Weiss MH, Couldwell WT. Surgical approaches to pituitary tumors. *Neurosurg Clin N Am*. 2003;14:93–107.
13. Couldwell WT. Transsphenoidal and transcranial surgery for pituitary adenomas. *J Neurooncol*. 2004;69:237–256.
14. Eseonu CI, ReFaey K, Garcia O, Salvatori R, Quinones-Hinojosa A. cost analysis of endoscopic versus microscopic endonasal transsphenoidal surgery for pituitary adenomas. *J Neurol Surg B Skull Base*. 2018;79:131–138.
15. Eseonu CI, ReFaey K, Pamias-Portalatin E, et al. Three-hand endoscopic endonasal transsphenoidal surgery: experience with an anatomy-preserving mononostril approach technique. *Oper Neurosurg (Hagerstown)*. 2018;14:158–165.
16. Eseonu CI, ReFaey K, Rincon-Torroella J, et al. Endoscopic versus microscopic transsphenoidal approach for pituitary adenomas: comparison of outcomes during the transition of methods of a single surgeon. *World Neurosurg*. 2017;97:317–325.

63

Pituicytomas

Case reviewed by Luigi Maria Cavallo, William T. Curry, James J. Evans, Tomas Garzon-Muvdi, Tetsuro Sameshima

Introduction

Pituicytomas are rare low-grade tumors (World Health Organization grade I) that are derived from pituicytes that are specialized glial cells of the neurohypophysis and infundibulum.[1–5] Pituicytes are glial cells that function to support the hypothalamic-axons that secrete vasopressin and oxytocin and are comprised of oncocytic, ependymal, and granular cell types.[1–5] Their description is primarily limited to case reports, with approximately 80 reported in the literature.[1–5] However, they closely resemble meningiomas and pituitary adenomas both clinically and radiologically, and therefore their surgical management is similar to these lesions.[1–5] Surgical treatment, however, is challenging because of the hypervascularity of these lesions.[1–5] In this chapter, we present a case of a patient with a suprasellar third ventricular pituicytoma.

Example case

Chief complaint: seizures
History of present illness
A 49-year-old, right-handed woman with a history of hypertension, anxiety, and depression presented after a seizure. She was working when she had an acute loss of consciousness with generalized tonic-clonic activity. She was taken to the emergency room where imaging was obtained (Fig. 63.1). On further questioning, she complained of progressive confusion and diminished peripheral vision over several months.
Medications: Lithium, hydrochlorothiazide.
Allergies: No known drug allergies.
Past medical and surgical history: Tonsillectomy, hysterectomy.
Family history: No history of intracranial malignancies.
Social history: Accountant, 30 pack per year smoking history, occasional alcohol.

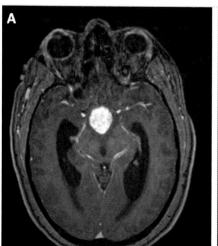 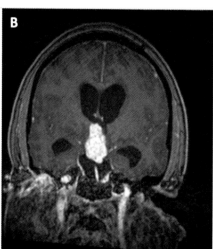 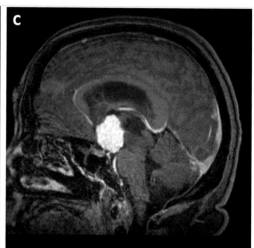

Fig. 63.1 Preoperative magnetic resonance imaging. (A) T1 axial image with gadolinium contrast; **(B)** T1 coronal image with gadolinium contrast; **(C)** T1 sagittal image with gadolinium contrast magnetic resonance imaging scan demonstrating a homogenously enhancing lesion involving the third ventricle, with extension near the right foramen of Monro and hydrocephalus.

Physical examination: Awake, alert, oriented to person, place, time; Cranial nerves II to XII intact, except mild bitemporal hemianopsia; Moves all extremities with good strength.

Pituitary labs: Prolactin, insulin-like growth factor-1, cortisol, thyroid stimulating hormone/T4 all within normal limits.

	Luigi Maria Cavallo, MD, PhD, University of Naples Federico II, Naples, Italy	William T. Curry, MD, Massachusetts General Hospital, Boston, MA, United States	James J. Evans, MD, Tomas Garzon-Muvdi, MD, Thomas Jefferson University, Philadelphia, PA, United States	Tetsuro Sameshima, MD, PhD, Hamamatsu University, Hamamatsu, Shizuoka, Japan
Preoperative				
Additional tests requested	MRI FIESTA and DTI Neuropsychological assessment Neuroophthalmology (OCT, visual field)	CT/CT angiography Endocrine evaluation	CT/CT angiography EVD Endocrine evaluation	MRI FIESTA ASL MRI Pituitary hormonal evaluation Neuroophthalmology evaluation
Surgical approach selected	Right frontal endoscopic transventricular	Right frontal orbital craniotomy with left EVD	Endoscopic endonasal transtubercular, transplanum	Bifrontal basal interhemispheric
Other teams involved during surgery	None	None	ENT	None
Anatomic corridor	Right frontal transventricular	Translamina terminalis	Endonasal transtubercular, transplanum	Interhemispheric trans-lamina terminalis
Goal of surgery	Maximal resection	Maximal resection, resolution of hydrocephalus	Diagnosis, decompression, maximal resection	Total resection
Perioperative				
Positioning	Supine neutral	Right supine with left 15-degree rotation	Supine without pins	Supine neutral
Surgical equipment	Surgical navigation Endoscopes Neuroport	Surgical navigation Surgical microscope	Surgical navigation Endoscope Ultrasonic aspirator	Surgical navigation Surgical microscope Ultrasonic aspirator
Medications	Steroids	Antiepileptics	Steroids	Steroids
Anatomic considerations	Foramen of Monro, aqueduct, third ventricular floor, infundibular recess, anterior commissure	Optic chiasm, ACA and branches, hypothalamus, pituitary stalk, mammillary bodies, walls of the third ventricle	Pituitary stalk, optic nerves, ICA, ACA, superior hypophyseal arteries	Optic nerves, hypothalamus, infundibulum
Complications feared with approach chosen	Pituitary dysfunction, hypothalamic disorder fornix injury, CSF leak	Injury to hypothalamus, optic apparatus	Brain retraction	Visual decline, diabetes insipidus, panhypopituitarism
Intraoperative				
Anesthesia	General	General	General	General
Skin incision	Linear	Frontotemporal linear	Fascia lata	Bicoronal
Bone opening	Right frontal mini-craniotomy	Left frontal burr hole, right frontotemporal/orbital roof	Sphenoid bone, sella, tuberculum sellae, planum sphenoidale	Bifrontal
Brain exposure	Right frontal lobe	Right frontotemporal	Anterior skull base	Bifrontal eccentric to the right

(continued on next page)

	Luigi Maria Cavallo, MD, PhD, University of Naples Federico II, Naples, Italy	William T. Curry, MD, Massachusetts General Hospital, Boston, MA, United States	James J. Evans, MD, Tomas Garzon-Muvdi, MD, Thomas Jefferson University, Philadelphia, PA, United States	Tetsuro Sameshima, MD, PhD, Hamamatsu University, Hamamatsu, Shizuoka, Japan
Method of resection	Right frontal mini-craniotomy based on navigation, small corticectomy, placement of neuroport in right lateral ventricle, bimanual debulking of tumor through foramen of Monro, dissection of tumor from third ventricular walls, third ventriculostomy	Left frontal burr hole, right frontotemporal craniotomy, removal of superior and lateral orbital rims and orbital roof, open dura, subfrontal dissection with identification of olfactory nerve and optic nerves, sharply open cisterns and proximal Sylvian fissure, identify chiasm/ACA/ACOM, dynamic retraction, debulk tumor and follow into third ventricle and dissect from lateral walls, aim for maximal resection	ENT to assist, nasoseptal flap harvest and placed in choanae, lateralization of bilateral middle turbinates, wide right sphenoidotomy, anterior skull base osteotomy of sella/tuberculum/planum using drills and punches, decompress optic nerves proximally, dura opened along midline, sharp dissection to expose anterior tumor, preserve blood vessels supplying optic chiasm and infundibulum, tumor cauterized and opened sharply and debulked followed by extracapsular microdissection, resect as much as possible, fascia lata harvested and button repair of dura is done and reinforced with nasoseptal flap and dural sealant	Bifrontal craniotomy, open dura, sagittal sinus ligation, interhemispheric opening, expose tumor identify key anatomic landmarks (optic nerve, pituitary stalk, hypothalamus), removal of tumor
Complication avoidance	Use port, avoid forniceal injury, avoid vascular injury inside the ventricle, mindful of floor of third ventricle, third ventriculostomy	EVD, cistern opening, dynamic retraction, follow tumor into third ventricle	Nasoseptal flap and fascia lata, large anterior skull base opening, internal debulking before extracapsular dissection, EVD placement	Bifrontal interhemispheric approach, identify and protect key anatomic landmarks
Postoperative				
Admission	ICU	ICU	ICU	ICU
Postoperative complications feared	Hypothalamic dysfunction, diabetes insipidus, hypopituitarism, visual decline	Cognitive decline, endocrine dysfunction, visual decline	CSF leak, hypopituitarism	Visual decline, hormonal dysfunction
Follow-up testing	Head CT immediately after surgery MRI within 48 hours after surgery Pituitary hormone analysis Visual field assessment	MRI 6 weeks after surgery if GTR, or MRI prior to discharge if STR	MRI 3 months after surgery Pituitary panel after surgery Sodium/SG if UOP >250 cc/hr for 2 hours	Hormonal evaluation CT immediately after and 1 day after surgery MRI 7 days after surgery
Follow-up visits	1 month after surgery with neuropsychology, endocrinology, and visual field testing	6 weeks after surgery with neurosurgery 1 month after surgery with endocrinology	1 week after surgery with ENT and neurosurgery	3 months after surgery
Adjuvant therapies recommended	Observation, repeat surgery or radiation therapy with recurrence	Observation, repeat surgery or radiation therapy with recurrence	Observation and possible radiotherapy with growth	Observation and repeat surgery with recurrence

ACA, anterior cerebral artery; *ACOM*, anterior communicating artery; *ASL*, arterial spin labeling; *CSF*, cerebrospinal fluid; *CT*, computed tomography; *DTI*, diffusion tensor imaging; *ENT*, ear, nose, and throat; *EVD*, external ventricular drain; *FIESTA*, fast imaging employing steady-state acquisition; *GTR*, gross total resection; *ICA*, internal carotid artery; *ICU*, intensive care unit; *MRI*, magnetic resonance imaging; *OCT*, optical coherence tomography; *SG*, specific gravity; *STR*, subtotal resection; *UOP*, urine output.

Differential diagnosis and actual diagnosis

- Meningioma
- Pituitary adenoma
- Craniopharyngioma
- Pilocytic astrocytoma
- Metastatic brain tumor
- Pituicytoma

Important anatomic and preoperative considerations

Sellar anatomy is discussed in Chapters 56 and 57, and lateral ventricular anatomy in Chapter 37. The third ventricle is a midline cavity that communicates with the lateral ventricles through the foramen of Monro, and with the fourth ventricle through the aqueduct of Sylvius.[6] The anterior wall of the third ventricle is the lamina terminalis; the superior wall consists of the fornices and hippocampal commissure, superior membrane of the tela choroidea, internal cerebral veins and branches of the medial posterior choroidal arteries, and the inferior membrane of the tela choroidea; the lateral wall consists of the hypothalamic sulcus that runs from the foramen of Monro to the aqueduct that divides the thalamus above from the hypothalamus below; the posterior wall is formed by the superior pineal recess, habenular commissure, pineal recess, and posterior commissure; and the inferior wall is formed by the optic recess, infundibular recess, tuber cinereum, mammillary bodies, and posterior perforated substance.[6] The superior membrane of the tela choroidea extends laterally to the choroid plexus on the lateral ventricles, and the inferior membrane attaches to the lateral side of the thalamus via the stria medullaris thalami, and is where choroid plexus along the roof of the third ventricle is attached.[6] The space between the superior and inferior layer of tela choroidea is the velum interpositum.[6]

Approaches to this lesion

The approaches to the third ventricle can be divided into anterior, superior, lateral, and posterior approaches based on the wall of the third ventricle that is targeted.[6] Anterior approaches involve opening the lamina terminalis, which can be done through pterional, subfrontal, and orbitozygomatic craniotomies, among others.[7–9] In these approaches, the olfactory nerve is followed to the optic nerve, and the lamina terminalis is identified and opened. Inferior approaches involve accessing the third ventricle through the floor of the third ventricle, typically through endoscopic approaches.[10] This typically requires tumors in the interpeduncular cistern that extend to the third ventricle.[10] In these approaches, the sphenoid sinus is accessed through the nose, and the sella, tuberculum, and/or planum are opened to allow superior access through the floor of the third ventricle.[10] Posterior approaches primarily involve a supracerebellar infratentorial approach, and is typically used for pineal region tumors that extend through the suprapineal recess.[11] This is typically done in a sitting or Concorde position, whereby the space between the cerebellum and the tentorium are used to access the pineal region.[11] Superior approaches primarily involve the foramen of Monro with or without a transchoroidal approach that allows expansion of the foramen of Monro to minimize manipulation of the fornix.[12] In

this approach, the lateral ventricles can be reached through a transcallosal or transcortical approach, and then the choroidal fissure is typically opened on the forniceal side of the fissure, thereby avoiding the veins of the thalamic side and proceeding medially between the internal cerebral veins.[12] The superior approach is typically used for tumors located near the foramen of Monro and/or body of the third ventricle.[12]

What was actually done

The patient was taken to surgery for a right frontal transcortical, transchoroidal approach for resection of a third ventricular tumor, with a tubular retractor along with general anesthesia and intraoperative monitoring (motor evoked potential, somatosensory evoked potentials, and electroencephalography). The goal was to decompress the ventricles and open the foramen of Monro to obviate the need for a shunt. The patient was induced and intubated per routine. The head was fixed in neutral position, with two pins centered over the left external auditory meatus and one pin over the right external auditory meatus. The patient's head was flexed and kept neutral. A linear incision was planned in the coronal plane over the right frontal region over the Kocher point with the use of surgical navigation. The patient was draped in the usual standard fashion and given dexamethasone, levetiracetam, and cefazolin. The incision was made, and the skin was retracted with a Weitlaner retractor. A keyhole craniotomy was made over the right frontal lobe. The dura was opened in a cruciate fashion and tacked up. The sulcus underlying the dural opening was identified and opened under exoscopic visualization. The 65-mm tubular retractor was passed under navigation into the superficial aspect of the ventricle. The roof of the third ventricle was identified, and the choroidal fissure was opened posteriorly from the right foramen of Monro. The lesion was identified and was coagulated and removed piecemeal with a suction/cutting device (Nico Myriad, NICO Corporation, Indianapolis, IN). The lesion was quite hypervascular and required extensive bipolar cautery before removing piecemeal. Preliminary pathology was a fibrous tumor. After several rounds of cautery and resection, the foramen of Monro was decompressed, and the ventricle was collapsed. It was determined to stop the surgery at this point because of relief of hydrocephalus and the hypervascularity of the lesion. An external ventricular drain was placed through the retractor, and the retractor was withdrawn. The dura, bone, and skin were closed in standard fashion.

The patient awoke at their neurologic baseline with mild bitemporal hemianopsia and was taken to the intensive care unit for recovery. Magnetic resonance imaging (MRI) was done within 48 hours after surgery and showed subtotal resection with residual in the third ventricle along the thalamic walls (Fig. 63.2). The patient participated with physical and occupational therapy. The external ventricular drain was allowed to drain for 48 hours and then clamped and removed on postoperative day 3. The patient was discharged to inpatient rehabilitation on postoperative day 5. The patient was prescribed levetiracetam for 3 months, and dexamethasone that was tapered to off over 14 days. The patient was seen at 2 weeks postoperatively for staple removal and remained neurologically stable with improved but still present mild bitemporal hemianopsia. Pathology was a pituicytoma. The lesion was observed with serial MRI examinations at 3- to

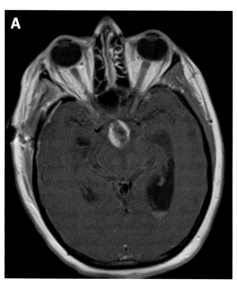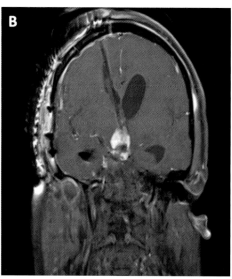

Fig. 63.2 Postoperative magnetic resonance imaging. (A) T1 axial image with gadolinium contrast; **(B)** T1 coronal image with gadolinium contrast magnetic resonance imaging scan demonstrating subtotal resection of the lesion, with improvement in the caliber of the ventricles.

6-month intervals and had recurrence at 8 months and underwent fractionated radiotherapy. The patient developed memory difficulties and vision changes 18 months after surgery and 6 months after radiation therapy.

Commonalities among the experts

Half of the surgeons opted for the patient to undergo MRI fast imaging employing steady-state acquisition for better resolution of the sellar anatomy, ophthalmology evaluation to assess preoperative vision status, and endocrinology to assess baseline pituitary hormone functioning. The approach differed, in which the majority of surgeons favored a cranial-based approach that varied from subfrontal translamina terminalis to endoscopic transventricular. The goal in most was maximal extensive resection. Most surgeons were cognizant of the optic apparatus, internal carotid artery and anterior cerebral artery vessels, hypothalamus, pituitary gland, and infundibulum. The most feared complication was vision loss. Surgery was generally pursued with surgical navigation, endoscope or microscope, and ultrasonic aspirator, with perioperative steroids. Because the approach greatly varied, surgical nuances were distinct, but most surgeons shared the concept of identifying and preserving critical neurovascular anatomy. Following surgery, all surgeons admitted their patients to the intensive care unit, and half requested imaging within 48 hours to assess for extent of resection and/or evaluate for complications. Most surgeons advocated for observation of residual and re-resection with recurrence.

SUMMARY OF QUALITY OF EVIDENCE TO GUIDE SPECIFIC INTERVENTIONS FOR THIS CASE

- Transcortical transchoroidal approach for third ventricular tumors—Class III.
- Radiation therapy for residual/recurrent pituicytomas—Class III.

REFERENCES

1. Chakraborti S, Mahadevan A, Govindan A, et al. Pituicytoma: report of three cases with review of literature. *Pathol Res Pract.* 2013;209:52–58.
2. Yang X, Liu X, Li W, Chen D. Pituicytoma: a report of three cases and literature review. *Oncol Lett.* 2016;12:3417–3422.
3. Zygourakis CC, Rolston JD, Lee HS, Partow C, Kunwar S, Aghi MK. Pituicytomas and spindle cell oncocytomas: modern case series from the University of California, San Francisco. *Pituitary.* 2015;18:150–158.
4. El Hussein S, Vincentelli C. Pituicytoma: review of commonalities and distinguishing features among TTF-1 positive tumors of the central nervous system. *Ann Diagn Pathol.* 2017;29:57–61.
5. Lefevre E, Bouazza S, Bielle F, Boch AL. Management of pituicytomas: a multicenter series of eight cases. *Pituitary.* 2018;21:507–514.
6. Rhoton Jr AL. The lateral and third ventricles. *Neurosurgery.* 2002;51:S207–S271.
7. Ruzevick J, Raza SM, Recinos PF, et al. Technical note: orbitozygomatic craniotomy using an ultrasonic osteotome for precise osteotomies. *Clin Neurol Neurosurg.* 2015;134:24–27.
8. Raza SM, Garzon-Muvdi T, Boaehene K, et al. The supraorbital craniotomy for access to the skull base and intraaxial lesions: a technique in evolution. *Minim Invasive Neurosurg.* 2010;53:1–8.
9. Raza SM, Quinones-Hinojosa A, Lim M, Boahene KD. The transconjunctival transorbital approach: a keyhole approach to the midline anterior skull base. *World Neurosurg.* 2013;80:864–871.
10. Kassam AB, Gardner PA, Snyderman CH, Carrau RL, Mintz AH, Prevedello DM. Expanded endonasal approach, a fully endoscopic transnasal approach for the resection of midline suprasellar craniopharyngiomas: a new classification based on the infundibulum. *J Neurosurg.* 2008;108:715–728.
11. Mottolese C, Szathmari A, Ricci-Franchi AC, Gallo P, Beuriat PA, Capone G. Supracerebellar infratentorial approach for pineal region tumors: our surgical and technical considerations. *Neurochirurgie.* 2015;61:176–183.
12. Bozkurt B, Yagmurlu K, Belykh E, et al. Quantitative anatomic analysis of the transcallosal-transchoroidal approach and the transcallosal-subchoroidal approach to the floor of the third ventricle: an anatomic study. *World Neurosurg.* 2018;118:219–229.

64

Sinonasal malignancies

Case reviewed by Luigi Maria Cavallo, Kenji Ohata, Gustavo Pradilla, Shaan M. Raza

Introduction

The sinonasal cavities, which include the nasal cavity and paranasal sinuses (maxillary, sphenoid, frontal, and ethmoid), occupy a relatively small anatomic space, but can be afflicted by a variety of distinct benign and malignant tumors.[1-6] Sinonasal tumors occur in 1 per 100,000 people per year, and the most common are squamous cell and adenocarcinoma, which account for 80% of these tumors.[1-6] In terms of malignant tumors, the primary tumors that involve the sinonasal cavities include sinonasal squamous cell carcinoma (50%), intestinal type adenocarcinoma (13%), mucosal melanoma (7%), esthesioneuroblastoma (7%), adenoid cystic carcinoma (7%), and sinonasal undifferentiated carcinoma (SNUC) (3%).[6] The region where these tumors occur is a complex anatomic area in close proximity to the eye and brain.[1-6] Although this region is more pertinent to otolaryngologists, tumors in this region can invade the anterior skull base, and therefore can also be relevant to neurosurgeons.[1-6] In this chapter, we present a case of a patient with a sinonasal malignancy that involves the anterior skull base.

Example case

Chief complaint: epistaxis
History of present illness
A 64-year-old, right-handed man with a history of sleep apnea on continuous positive airway pressure, hypertension, and hypercholesterolemia presented with persistent right naris epistaxis. He complained of unprovoked nosebleeds for several months, and saw an ear, nose, and throat doctor who did a biopsy of a sinonasal mass consistent with SNUC. This led to magnetic resonance imaging (MRI) (Fig. 64.1), and he was referred for evaluation and management.

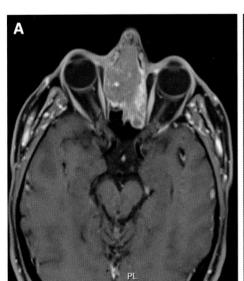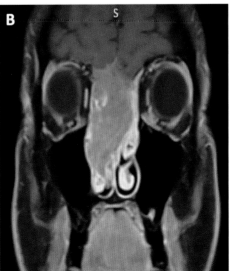

Fig. 64.1 Preoperative magnetic resonance imaging. (A) T1 axial image with gadolinium contrast; **(B)** T1 coronal image with gadolinium contrast magnetic resonance imaging scan demonstrating a heterogeneously enhancing lesion involving the right nasal cavity.

Medications: Lisinopril, atorvastatin.
Allergies: No known drug allergies.
Past medical and surgical history: None.
Family history: No history of intracranial malignancies.
Social history: Business owner, no smoking or alcohol.

Physical examination: Awake, alert, oriented to person, place, time; Cranial nerves II to XI; Moves all extremities with good strength.
Positron emission tomography scan: Hypermetabolic lesion in the right nasal cavity without any evidence of systemic disease.

	Luigi Maria Cavallo, MD, PhD, University of Naples Federico II, Naples, Italy	Kenji Ohata, MD, PhD, Osaka City University, Osaka, Japan	Gustavo Pradilla, MD, Emory University, Atlanta, GA, United States	Shaan M. Raza, MD, MD Anderson Cancer Center, Houston, TX, United States
Preoperative				
Additional tests requested	High-resolution CT Neck ultrasound	High-resolution CT CTA Neuroophthalmology evaluation (OCT, visual fields)	Staging scans including PET CTA head and neck CT sinus ENT evaluation Neuroophthalmology evaluation	Pathology consultation Head and neck medical and radiation oncology evaluation Ophthalmology evaluation
Neoadjuvant therapy	Yes	No	Yes	Yes Induction chemotherapy with platinum-based therapy
Surgical approach selected	Endoscopic nasoethmoidal	Endoscopic endonasal combined transcranial frontobasal	Endoscopic endonasal transcribriform, transplanum	Endoscopic endonasal approach with pericranial flap reconstruction
Other teams involved during surgery	ENT	ENT	ENT	ENT
Anatomic corridor	Transnasal trancribriform	Transnasal and transcranial	Transnasal transcribriform, transplanum	Transnasal transcribriform, transplanum
Goal of surgery	Radical resection after neoadjuvant radiation	Radical resection	Radical resection	Oncologic resection with negative margins, protection of critical neurovascular structures, optimal aesthetic outcome
Perioperative				
Positioning	Supine neutral	Supine neutral	Supine neutral, no pins	Supine neutral with head of bed at 30 degrees and neck extension
Surgical equipment	Surgical navigation Endoscopes Ultrasonic aspirator	Surgical navigation Endoscopes	Surgical navigation IOM (SSEP) Endoscopes	Endoscopes Tissue implants
Medications	None	Mannitol	None	None
Anatomic considerations	Posterior wall of frontal sinus, ethmoidal arteries, medial orbital walls, lacrimal ducts	Crista galli, cribriform plate, planum sphenoidale, orbital roofs	Orbits, orbital nerve, medial rectus, frontal lobes, olfactory nerves, orbito-frontal / fronto-polar / anterior and posterior ethmoidal arteries	Nasal septum, nasal floor, posterior nasopharynx, lamina papyracea, frontal sinuses, sphenoid sinus, anterior skull base dura, orbital contents, frontal lobes
Complications feared with approach chosen	Ethmoidal artery injury, orbital hematoma, epistaxis, frontal lobe hematoma, CSF leak	Brain contusion, visual decline	Frontal lobe retraction, orbital hematoma, CSF leak	Positive margins, orbital injury, frontal lobe injury, reconstruction failure
Intraoperative				
Anesthesia	General	General	General	General
Skin incision	None	Bicoronal	None	Bicoronal incision for pericranial graft harvest

	Luigi Maria Cavallo, MD, PhD, University of Naples Federico II, Naples, Italy	Kenji Ohata, MD, PhD, Osaka City University, Osaka, Japan	Gustavo Pradilla, MD, Emory University, Atlanta, GA, United States	Shaan M. Raza, MD, MD Anderson Cancer Center, Houston, TX, United States
Bone opening	Nasoethmoidal	Bifrontal	Posterior nasal septum, bilateral sphenoidotomies, sphenoid septum, sphenoid rostrum, posterior frontal sinuses, medial maxillectomy, medial orbital walls, cribriform and planum	Nasal septectomy, right maxillary antrostomy, right MT/IT, left anterior and posterior ethmoids, right lamina papyracea, Draf III, frontal sinusotomy, anterior skull base from posterior frontal sinus wall to planum sphenoidale
Brain exposure	Frontal	Bifrontal	Bifrontal	Anterior cranial fossa
Method of resection	Draf III procedure, identify anterior border of tumor, bilateral ethmoidectomy with lamina papyracea removal, identification of ethmoidal arteries and lateral border of tumors, nasal septectomy and identification of inferior tumor border, opening of cribriform plate and removal of intradural component, biopsy of dural borders, multilayer reconstruction	Transcranial approach first with bicoronal incision, harvesting pericranial flap, low bifrontal craniotomy, curetting of frontal sinuses, separate subfrontal dura from anterior skull base, remove tumor from orbit and anterior cranial fossa bone with negative margins, reconstruction with pericranium, endonasal resection by ENT.	Nares packed with epinephrine solution, ENT and neurosurgeon work together with four handed technique, mass debulked once encountered, posterior two-thirds of nasal septum, bilateral sphenoidotomies, removal of sphenoid septum and sphenoid rostrum, Draf III approach to frontal sinus, opening of the entire frontal sinus, define anterior and superior boundary of resection, identify lamina papyracea to define lateral extent of resection, identify posterior and ethmoid arteries identified and ligated, osteotomies made posterior to front sinus at lamina papyracea, expose frontal lobes, widen osteotomies to medial wall of orbit, medial maxillectomy on right to confirm negative margin, continue centripetal piecemeal resection with care to preserve normal anatomy, exposed frontal lobe dura exposed and incised, biopsy of olfactory bulbs and periorbital fat to confirm negative margins, closure of anterior skull base in layers with collagen inlay in subdural space and allograft in epidural space, dural sealant, nasal tampons, lumbar drain	Nasal approach first, septectomy from inferior to tumor to maxillary crest and posterior to sphenoid rostrum to clear inferior portion of tumor and allow binasal access, wide right maxillary antrostomy, removal of right IT and MT, open right anterior and posterior ethmoid sinus, mucosal margins of maxillary sinus taken, identification and ligation of SPA, opening of left maxillary sinus and margin taken, preservation of left IT if no tumor involvement, open sphenoid sinus and removal of septations with mucosa taken as margin, open left anterior and posterior ethmoids to identify fovea ethmoidalis with sacrifice of the left anterior and posterior ethmoidal arteries, resection of lamina papyracea on right side with periorbita taken as margin, identify right fovea ethmoidalis after sacrificing right anterior and posterior ethmoidal arteries, Draf III frontal sinusotomy to identify crista galli and posterior frontal sinus wall, anterior skull base removal from posterior frontal sinus wall to planum sphenoidale and extending from orbital roof to orbital roof, dura circumferentially incised along with falx with transection of the olfactory bulbs from the frontal lobes with margins along dura and olfactory bulbs, reconstruction with button graft (fascia lata) in subdural and epidural space, observe for CSF leak, harvest pericranial flap and rotate into nasal cavity via opening at nasofrontal suture

(continued on next page)

	Luigi Maria Cavallo, MD, PhD, University of Naples Federico II, Naples, Italy	Kenji Ohata, MD, PhD, Osaka City University, Osaka, Japan	Gustavo Pradilla, MD, Emory University, Atlanta, GA, United States	Shaan M. Raza, MD, MD Anderson Cancer Center, Houston, TX, United States
Complication avoidance	Identification of ethmoidal arteries, delineate tumor borders	Pericranial harvest and reconstruction, two stage approach, use of ENT for endonasal component	Wide bony exposure, centripetal resection, biopsy of margins to confirm tumor-free margins, lumbar drain	Wide bony exposure, circumferential and anatomic margins, removal of anterior skull base dura in one piece
Postoperative				
Admission	ICU	ICU	ICU	Intermediate care
Postoperative complications feared	Orbital hematoma, epistaxis, frontal lobe hematoma, CSF leak	CSF leak	CSF leak	CSF leak, orbital dysfunction (diplopia secondary to medial rectus injury), epiphora
Follow-up testing	CT within 24 hours after surgery MRI 1 month after surgery	CT immediately after surgery MRI 1 week after surgery Neuroophthalmology evaluation	Lumbar drain for 3 days MRI within 24 hours after surgery Physical and occupational therapy	Confirmation of margins by pathology MRI within 48 hours after surgery
Follow-up visits	1 week after surgery	Follow-up with ENT	2 weeks after surgery with ENT	2 weeks after surgery
Adjuvant therapies recommended	PET/neck ultrasound, second attempt, palliative measures with diffuse disease	Radiation/ chemotherapy	Radiation/chemotherapy	Radiation/chemotherapy

BMI, body mass index; *CSF*, cerebrospinal fluid; *CT*, computed tomography; *CTA*, computed tomography angiography; *ENT*, ear, nose, and throat; *ICA*, internal carotid artery; *ICU*, intensive care unit; *IOM*, intraoperative monitoring; *IT*, inferior turbinate; *MRI*, magnetic resonance imaging; *MT*, middle turbinate; *OCT*, optical coherence tomography; *PET*, positron emission tomography; *SPA*, sphenopalatine artery; *SSEP*, somatosensory evoked potential.

Differential diagnosis and actual diagnosis

- Squamous cell carcinoma
- Adenocarcinoma
- Mucosal melanoma
- Adenoid cystic carcinoma
- Esthesioneuroblastoma
- SNUC

Important anatomic and preoperative considerations

The nasal cavity extends from the nasal vestibule to the nasopharynx and is separated in the middle by the nasal septum into nostrils that can be further divided into the roof, floor, medial, and lateral walls.[7] The lateral wall of each nasal cavity is mainly comprised of the maxilla, as well as the perpendicular plate of the palatine bone, medial pterygoid plate, labyrinth of the ethmoid bone, and the inferior turbinate.[7] The majority of the paranasal sinuses communicate with the nasal cavity through the lateral nasal wall via the infundibulum, which is bound by the uncinate process.[7] The roof of the nasal cavity is formed by the nasal bone superiorly and the junction of the upper lateral cartilage and nasal septum inferiorly, and the floor is made up of the palatine process of the maxilla anteriorly and the horizontal plate of the palatine bone posteriorly.[7] On the lateral sides of the nasal cavity are the turbinates, and under each turbinate are meatuses.[7] The major blood supply to the nasal cavity comes from branches of the internal maxillary (sphenopalatine artery and greater palatine artery), ophthalmic (anterior and posterior ethmoidal arteries), and facial arteries (septal branches of the superior labial artery).[7] The olfactory nerve sends microscopic fibers from the olfactory bulb through the cribriform plate to reach the nasal cavity, and sensation primarily comes from branches of the ophthalmic (nasociliary) and maxillary divisions (nasopalatine, posterior nasal branches) of the trigeminal nerve. The paranasal sinuses consist of the paired maxillary, frontal, ethmoidal, and sphenoidal sinuses.[7] The maxillary sinuses are connected to the nasal cavity by the semilunar hiatus and reside under the eyes; the frontal sinuses open into the anterior part of the middle nasal meatus through the frontonasal duct that traverses the anterior part of the ethmoid labyrinth and open into the semilunar hiatus and reside superior to the eyes; the ethmoidal sinuses are divided into anterior and posterior groups by the basal lamella in which the posterior ethmoid sinuses drain into the superior meatus above the middle turbinate, and the anterior ethmoid sinus drains into the middle meatus via the infundibulum into the semilunar hiatus, and both anterior and posterior ethmoid sinuses reside between the eyes; and the sphenoid sinus opens into the roof of the nasal cavity into the sphenoethmoidal recess and resides behind the eyes.[7] The semilunar hiatus is a crescent-shaped groove within the lateral wall of the nasal cavity just inferior to the ethmoid bulla that is limited inferiorly by the uncinate process of the ethmoid, and superiorly by the anterior ethmoid cells within the ethmoid bulla.[7]

Paranasal tumors can also be classified according to the tumor, node, metastasis (TNM) staging system (Table 64.1), which can be subclassified into maxillary, as well as nasal cavity and ethmoid sinus criteria, whereas tumors that originate from the frontal or sphenoid sinus do not apply and are nonetheless rarer.[1] However, regardless of the histology, sinonasal malignancies are associated with poor outcomes in which the overall 5-year survival rates ranges from 30% to 50%, in which the factors associated with survival include tumor histology and disease stage.[1] For sinonasal squamous cell carcinoma the 5-year overall survival rate is 50%, intestinal type adenocarcinoma is 60%, mucosal melanoma is 35%, esthesioneuroblastoma is 70%, adenoid cystic adenocarcinoma is 70%, and SNUC is 35%.[1]

Table 64.1 **TNM staging system**

TNM Staging of Paranasal Sinus Tumors	
	Maxillary sinus
T1	Limited to maxillary sinus mucosa with no bone erosion
T2	Bone erosion including hard palate and/or middle meatus extension
T3	Invasion of posterior wall maxillary sinus, subcutaneous tissues, floor or medial wall of orbit, pterygoid fossa, or ethmoid sinuses
T4a	Invasion of anterior orbital contents, skin of cheek, pterygoid plates, infratemporal fossa, cribriform plate, sphenoid or frontal sinuses
T4b	Invasion of orbital apex, dura, brain, middle cranial fossa, cranial nerves other than V2, nasopharynx, or clivus
	Nasal cavity and ethmoid sinus
T1	Limited to any one site, with or without bony invasions
T2	Invasion into two subsites or tension into adjacent nasoethmoidal complex, with or without bony invasion
T3	Invasion of medial wall or floor of orbit, maxillary sinus, palate, or cribriform plate
T4a	Invasion of anterior orbital contents, skin of nose or cheek, minimal extension to anterior cranial fossa, pterygoid plates, sphenoid or frontal sinuses
T4b	Invasion or orbital apex, dura, brain, middle cranial fossa, cranial nerves other than V2, nasopharynx, or clivus
N0	No LN involvement
N1	Spread to a single LN on the same side of the neck as the tumor and <3 cm in diameter
N2	Spread to a single LN on the same size of the neck as the tumor and >3 but <6 cm in diameter, spread to >1 LN on the same side of the neck as the tumor and none are >6 cm, or has spread to at least one LN on the other side of the neck and none are >6 cm
N3	Spread to at least one LN that is >6 cm or spread to an LN and then grown outside the LN
M0	Has not spread to other parts of the body
M1	Has spread to other parts of the body

LN, lymph node; *TNM*, tumor, node, metastasis.

In addition, independent of the treatment type and the histology of sinonasal malignancies, the 5-year survival rate is 80% for patients with T1 disease, and 30% for T4 tumors.[1] The patient in this case had a TNM staging of T4bN0M0 because of dural invasion.

Approaches to this lesion

Sinonasal malignancies typically have skull base involvement.[1–6] Involvement of the orbital contents and skull base are typically the challenging component of surgery, as these are the areas in which it is difficult to obtain negative margins without significant morbidity.[1–6] Because of the rarity of these lesions, there is no standard treatment protocol, and therefore treatment paradigms range from surgery followed by postoperative radiation therapy, to chemotherapy and/or radiation without surgery, to induction chemoradiation followed by surgery.[1–6] Treatment of sinonasal malignancies vary and include some combination of surgical resection, radiation therapy, and chemotherapy, depending on several factors including the patient age, medical comorbidities, tumor staging, and histology.[1–6] Biopsies are usually done first to determine tumor type, and the patients typically undergo systemic imaging to stage the tumor.[1–6] In a retrospective study on SNUC, Amit et al.[8] found that patients who achieve a favorable response to induction chemotherapy followed by definitive chemoradiation therapy had improved survival as compared with those who underwent surgery, whereas for patients who did not have a favorable response to induction chemotherapy, surgery appeared to provide better outcomes as salvage therapy. Surgery can include some combination of open craniofacial resection, endoscopic endonasal resection, or endoscopically assisted craniofacial resection depending on the extent and location of the disease, and may include neck dissections in patients with lymph node metastases.[8] For sinonasal squamous cell carcinoma, most studies have shown improved outcomes for patients who undergo induction chemoradiation therapy followed by wide surgical resection, whereas others have shown increased efficacy with definitive radiotherapy.[9] For sinonasal adenocarcinoma, for localized disease in a patient who is amenable to surgical therapy, treatment usually involves surgical resection with negative margins followed by radiation therapy.[10] For sinonasal melanoma, outcomes are poor, and a recent meta-analysis found that multimodal therapy improved outcomes, in which there was a nonsignificant increase in survival for patients treated with surgery and radiation versus surgery alone, statistically significant increase in survival for surgery and chemotherapy versus chemotherapy or surgery alone, but patients who had surgery, radiation, and chemotherapy had worsened outcomes likely as a result of having more advanced disease.[11] For adenoid cystic carcinoma, most studies show that wide surgical excision followed by postoperative radiation therapy has the best outcomes.[12,13] Esthesioneuroblastoma will be discussed in Chapter 65. Regardless, the management of sinonasal malignancies is controversial, as the studies are all retrospective in design and subject to treatment bias and have disparate TNM stages tumors, which makes outcome analyses challenging to interpret.

What was actually done

The patient was discussed at a multidisciplinary tumor board, and the plan was to proceed with induction chemotherapy with cisplatin and fractionated radiotherapy. The patient had an intermediate response to induction chemoradiotherapy, and the plan was to proceed with salvage surgical therapy. The patient underwent surgery for endoscopic endonasal resection of the lesion, with the goal of negative microscopic margins under general anesthesia without intraoperative monitoring with otolaryngology and neurosurgery. The patient was induced and intubated per routine. The patient was placed in a Mayfield horseshoe headrest, and electromagnetic computed tomography and MRI navigation were used to avoid the need for pinning. The patient was draped in the usual standard fashion and given cefazolin. The lesion was identified and dissected from the nasal septum, followed by removal of the right middle turbinate, and then dissected from the skull base. The tumor was dissected with a combination of suction cautery and sharp dissection. After the lesion was removed, biopsies were taken from the nasal septum, maxillary sinus, nasal floor, and ethmoid sinuses. The dura at the right cribriform plate was positive, and therefore bone on the right anterior cranial fossa was removed with a drill and Kerrison punches to identify the dura over the right olfactory bulb. The dura was then removed circumferentially until margins were negative. A right fascia lata graft was obtained, and the dura was reconstructed with a dural substitute placed in the subdural space and fascia lata placed in the epidural space. Dural sealant was used to reinforce the opening. No nasal septal flap was available because of the tumor involvement. All margins were negative. Nasal stents were placed bilaterally.

The patient awoke at their neurologic baseline with an intact examination and was taken to the intensive care unit for recovery. An MRI was done within 48 hours after surgery and showed gross total resection of the mass (Fig. 64.2).

The nasal stents were removed on postoperative day 2. The patient participated with physical and occupational therapy and was discharged to home on postoperative day 3. The patient was prescribed cefdinir for 7 days. The patient was seen at 2 weeks postoperatively and remained neurologically intact. Microscopic margins were negative. The surgical site was observed with serial MRI examinations at 3- to 6-month intervals, and systemic disease was evaluated with serial positron emission tomography scans. The patient is without local or distal recurrence for 12 months.

Commonalities among the experts

Most of the surgeons opted for the patient to undergo high-resolution computed tomography to better evaluate bony anatomy, and ophthalmology evaluation to asses preoperative vision status. The majority of surgeons would pursue neoadjuvant therapy before attempted surgical resection. All surgeons would pursue surgery primarily through an endonasal transcribriform approach with otolaryngology, and half would combine potentially with a craniotomy to establish negative margins. All surgeons aimed for radical resection with negative margins. Most surgeons were cognizant of the medial orbital walls, anterior cranial fossa, and posterior wall of the frontal sinus. The most feared complications were frontal lobe injury, vision loss, and cerebrospinal fluid leak. Surgery was generally pursued with surgical navigation and endoscopes, with no special perioperative medications. Because the approach greatly varied, surgical nuances were distinct, but most surgeons shared the concept of identifying and preserving critical neurovascular anatomy. Following surgery, most surgeons admitted their patients to the intensive care unit, and all requested imaging within 48 hours to assess for extent of resection and/or evaluate for complications. Most surgeons advocated for chemotherapy and radiation therapy for residual disease.

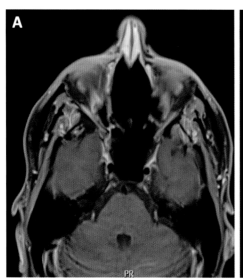 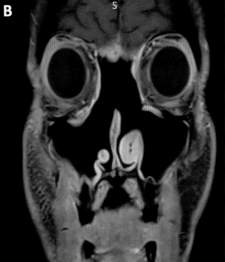

Fig. 64.2 Postoperative magnetic resonance imaging. (A) T1 axial image with gadolinium contrast; **(B)** T1 coronal image with gadolinium contrast magnetic resonance imaging scan demonstrating gross total resection of the lesion.

SUMMARY OF QUALITY OF EVIDENCE TO GUIDE SPECIFIC INTERVENTIONS FOR THIS CASE

- Induction chemotherapy prior to resection of sinonasal malignancy—Class III.
- Salvage surgical resection for residual disease after induction chemoradiotherapy—Class III.

REFERENCES

1. Eloy JA, Marchiano E, Vazquez A, et al. Management of skull base defects after surgical resection of sinonasal and ventral skull base malignancies. *Otolaryngol Clin North Am*. 2017;50:397–417.
2. Govindaraj S, Iloreta AM, Tong CC, Hernandez-Prera JC. Evaluation of patients with sinonasal and ventral skull base malignancies. *Otolaryngol Clin North Am*. 2017;50:221–244.
3. Kashat L, Le CH, Chiu AG. The role of targeted therapy in the management of sinonasal malignancies. *Otolaryngol Clin North Am*. 2017;50:443–455.
4. Kawaguchi M, Kato H, Tomita H, et al. Imaging characteristics of malignant sinonasal tumors. *J Clin Med*. 2017;6:116.
5. Khoury T, Jang D, Carrau R, Ready N, Barak I, Hachem RA. Role of induction chemotherapy in sinonasal malignancies: a systematic review. *Int Forum Allergy Rhinol*. 2019;9:212–219.
6. Mahalingappa YB, Khalil HS. Sinonasal malignancy: presentation and outcomes. *J Laryngol Otol*. 2014;128:654–657.
7. Cappello ZJ, Dublin AB. *Anatomy, Head and Neck, Nose Paranasal Sinuses*. StatPearls [Internet]. Treasure Island, FL: StatPearls Publishing; 2020.
8. Amit M, Abdelmeguid AS, Watcherporn T, et al. Induction chemotherapy response as a guide for treatment optimization in sinonasal undifferentiated carcinoma. *J Clin Oncol*. 2019;37:504–512.
9. Pare A, Blanchard P, Rosellini S, et al. Outcomes of multimodal management for sinonasal squamous cell carcinoma. *J Craniomaxillofac Surg*. 2017;45:1124–1132.
10. Lund VJ, Chisholm EJ, Takes RP, et al. Evidence for treatment strategies in sinonasal adenocarcinoma. *Head Neck*. 2012;34:1168–1178.
11. Gore MR, Zanation AM. Survival in sinonasal melanoma: a meta-analysis. *J Neurol Surg B Skull Base*. 2012;73:157–162.
12. Lupinetti AD, Roberts DB, Williams MD, et al. Sinonasal adenoid cystic carcinoma: the M.D. Anderson Cancer Center experience. *Cancer*. 2007;110:2726–2731.
13. Rhee CS, Won TB, Lee CH, et al. Adenoid cystic carcinoma of the sinonasal tract: treatment results. *Laryngoscope*. 2006;116:982–986.

65

Esthesioneuroblastoma

Case reviewed by William T. Curry, José Hinojosa Mena-Bernal, Shaan M. Raza, Henry W. S. Schroeder

Introduction

Esthesioneuroblastoma (ENB), which is also known as an olfactory neuroblastoma, is an uncommon sinonasal malignancy that has a propensity for local invasion into surrounding paranasal structures, including the eye and brain, as well as systemic metastases.[1–3] These tumors are thought to arise from neuroendocrine cells in the olfactory epithelium, and account for approximately 3% to 6% of all sinonasal cancers.[1–3] They usually present with symptoms of nasal obstruction and epistaxis, but can also result in symptoms of cerebral mass effect (headaches, nausea, vomiting) and vision loss.[1–3] The outcomes for patients with ENB are dictated by the extent of disease and tumor grade at presentation, in which the overall 5- and 10-year survival rates were 62.1% and 45.6%, respectively.[1] The typical goal of treatment for ENB is complete surgical resection with negative margins,

and in cases in which negative margins are not obtained or in patients with distant metastases, adjuvant radiation and chemotherapy are often offered.[1–3] However, treatment plans should be administered on an individual basis.[1–3] In this chapter, we present a case of a patient with an ENB.

Example case

Chief complaint: acute vision loss

History of present illness

A 73-year-old, right-handed woman with a history of hypertension and hypercholesterolemia presented with acute vision loss. She noticed visual decline over several months; however, over the past 24 hours her vision deteriorated to the point in which she only had light perception in both eyes. She was taken to the emergency room, and imaging revealed a large skull base lesion (Fig. 65.1).

Medications: Hydrochlorothiazide, simvastatin.

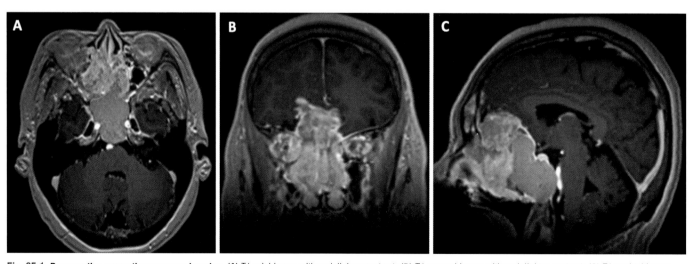

Fig. 65.1 Preoperative magnetic resonance imaging. (A) T1 axial image with gadolinium contrast; **(B)** T1 coronal image with gadolinium contrast; **(C)** T1 sagittal image with gadolinium contrast magnetic resonance imaging scan demonstrating a heterogeneously enhancing lesion involving the nasal cavity, paranasal sinuses, anterior cranial fossa, and right periorbita with an obstructive mucocele.

Allergies: No known drug allergies.
Past medical and surgical history: Hypertension, hypercholesterolemia.
Family history: No history of intracranial malignancies.
Social history: Retired school teacher, no smoking or alcohol.

Physical examination: Awake, alert, oriented to person, place, time; Cranial nerves II to XI; Moves all extremities with good strength.
Chest/abdomen/pelvis computed tomography (CT): No evidence of systemic disease.

	William T. Curry, MD, Massachusetts General Hospital, Boston, MA, United States	José Hinojosa Mena-Bernal, MD, PhD, Sant Joan de Deu, Barcelona, Spain	Shaan M. Raza, MD, MD Anderson Cancer Center, Houston, TX, United States	Henry W. S. Schroeder, MD, PhD, University of Greifswald, Greifswald, M-V, Germany
Preoperative				
Additional tests requested	CT maxillofacial	Ophthalmology evaluation (visual fields, OCT) Endocrinology evaluation CT chest, abdomen, pelvis Anosmia evaluation	Medical oncology evaluation Radiation oncology evaluation Ophthalmology evaluation MRI face/neck/orbits with fat saturation Biopsy of mass, drainage of sphenoid Based on esthesioneuroblastoma pathology, potential urgent platinum based chemotherapy for Hyams III/IV or urgent curative surgery for Hyams I/II	Ophthalmology evaluation (visual fields) Endocrinology evaluation Anesthesia evaluation CT maxillofacial
Surgical approach selected	Bifrontal craniotomy and endoscopic endonasal	Endoscopic endonasal +/− bifrontal craniotomy	Craniotomy and endoscopic endonasal	Bifrontal craniotomy and endoscopic endonasal
Other teams involved during surgery	ENT	ENT	ENT	ENT
Anatomic corridor	Bifrontal and craniofacial	Transcribriform/ transplanum, bifrontal if needed	Bifrontal and endonasal	Bifrontal and endonasal
Goal of surgery	Restoration of vision, total resection, skull base reconstruction	Radical tumor resection with negative margins	For Hyams I/II, gross total resection without orbitectomy. For Hyams III/IV, induction chemotherapy	Radical tumor resection
Perioperative				
Positioning	Supine neutral	Supine neutral	Supine neutral with slight extension	Supine with right rotation, left tilt
Surgical equipment	Surgical microscope Endoscope	Surgical navigation Endoscopes Ultrasonic aspirator Ultrasonic bone cutter Surgical microscope Microdoppler	Surgical microscope Ultrasonic aspirator Endoscope	Surgical navigation Surgical microscope Endoscopes Ultrasonic aspirator
Medications	Mannitol Diuretics Steroids Antiepileptics	Steroids	Mannitol Steroids	Steroids
Anatomic considerations	Optic nerves, ICA, ACA	Optic nerves and chiasm, ICA, ACA, ACOM	Olfactory bulbs, orbital roofs, planum sphenoidale, frontal/sphenoid/ethmoid/maxillary sinuses, nasal septum, right orbital apex, anterior/posterior ethmoidal arteries, sphenopalatine arteries, right orbital apex (periorbita, medial/superior rectus, superior division of CN III)	ICA, optic nerves
Complications feared with approach chosen	Visual decline, lack of negative margins	CSF leak, epiphora, facial scarring, venous thrombosis, vascular injury	Brain and orbital manipulation, positive margins	Injury to critical neurovascular structures

(continued on next page)

	William T. Curry, MD, Massachusetts General Hospital, Boston, MA, United States	José Hinojosa Mena-Bernal, MD, PhD, Sant Joan de Deu, Barcelona, Spain	Shaan M. Raza, MD, MD Anderson Cancer Center, Houston, TX, United States	Henry W. S. Schroeder, MD, PhD, University of Greifswald, Greifswald, M-V, Germany
Intraoperative				
Anesthesia	General	General	General	General
Skin incision	Bicoronal	Bicoronal if needed	Bicoronal	Bicoronal
Bone opening	Bifrontal, anterior skull base	Cribriform plate, planum, bifrontal if needed	Bifrontal, anterior skull base	Bifrontal, anterior skull base
Brain exposure	Bilateral frontal lobes, anterior skull base	Anterior skull base and bilateral frontal lobes if needed	Bilateral frontal lobes	Bilateral frontal lobes
Method of resection	Harvest pericranial flap, bifrontal craniotomy, open dura bilaterally with ligation of superior sagittal sinus, divide falx posterior to tumor, dissect tumor off of frontal lobes and mobilize ACA, remove tumor down to skull base, amputate cribriform, dissect tumor off of optic nerves, watertight dura closure with synthetic material or pericranium, ENT to resect sinonasal component, drainage of mucocele, dissect tumor from lamina papyracea/sphenoid sinus/maxillary sinus, palate, drill through craniotomy site to define posterior margin and remove from orbit, remove from frontal sinus, sectioning of anterior and posterior nasal septum, check margins, tack down pericranial flap	Endonasal first, middle and superior turbinates removed, middle meatal antrostomy, tumor debulking with suction and ultrasonic aspiration, sphenoidotomy, sphenoethmoidectomy, expose periorbita on both sides, coagulate anterior and posterior ethmoidal arteries, remove cribriform plate and roof of ethmoidal sinuses and posterior nasal septum, identify olfactory nerves and spare if not invaded, Draf III frontal sinusotomy approach, open dura, transect falx, deliver tumor along with underlying dura paying attention to separation ACA and ACOM, multilayer reconstruction with fascia lata and abdominal fat graft with nasoseptal flap, if any of the tumor cannot be reached, then an anterior bifrontal craniotomy is done with pericranial graft, dura is opened and SSS is ligated, retraction of frontal lobe, remove any intracranial extension, ultrasonic bone scalpel into ethmoid to establish negative margins, en bloc removal of cribriform plate, reconstruction with vascularized pericranium, watertight dural closure	Bicoronal incision with two-layer scalp dissection (scalp/pericranium), subfascial dissection laterally, low bifrontal craniotomy to level of nasofrontal suture in midline after bilateral McCarty burr holes, unify frontal sinuses with removal of posterior table and opening of nasofrontal ostia widely and mucosal margins taken, resect crista galli along the medial aspect of orbital roofs, coagulate and cut anterior/posterior ethmoidal arteries in orbit, open dura over both frontal lobes and ligate and cut SSS and falx above foramen cecum, intracranial portion of tumor debulked internally and capsule dissected from basal surface of both frontal lobes, cuff of brain is resected as margin, dissect olfactory bulbs posteriorly beyond gross disease and obtain margin, anterior skull base dura is incised circumferentially around gross disease where posterior limit of dural incision is just anterior to optic canals, resect lamina papyracea bilaterally and drilling planum sphenoidale to access sphenoid sinus with margins obtained, endoscopic approach next, septectomy with septal margins, bilateral maxillary antrostomies with mucosal margins and resection of superior/middle/inferior turbinates, SPA identified and sacrificed, inspect right nasolacrimal duct and extend medial maxillectomy and transect duct if necessary, resect remnants of medial orbital walls and biopsy left medial periorbita if necessary for margin, right periorbita incised anteriorly/superiorly/inferiorly, resect all gross disease from orbital apex after identifying superior rectus, dura reconstruction with pericranial flap that is rotated and sutured to planum sphenoidale	Harvest pericranial flap, bifrontal craniotomy, resection of intradural portion until skull base is reached, decompress bilateral optic nerves, resection of infiltrated dura, continue resection into paranasal sinuses with removal of tumor in ethmoid air cells and sphenoid sinus, parallel ENT access from below, resection of intraorbital portion of tumor on right, repair defect with pericranial flap and augmented with free pericranium fixed with sutures and fibrin glue, nasal pledgets, lumbar drain if CSF leak occurs

	William T. Curry, MD, Massachusetts General Hospital, Boston, MA, United States	José Hinojosa Mena-Bernal, MD, PhD, Sant Joan de Deu, Barcelona, Spain	Shaan M. Raza, MD, MD Anderson Cancer Center, Houston, TX, United States	Henry W. S. Schroeder, MD, PhD, University of Greifswald, Greifswald, M-V, Germany
Complication avoidance	Harvest pericranium, large craniotomy, intradural portion first and then closure, communicate endonasal with transcranial component, check margins, reconstruction	Endonasal first, wide bony opening of anterior skull base, careful dissection of ACA and ACOM, multilayer closure, bifrontal craniotomy with wide bony opening if necessary, pericranial flap	Harvest pericranium, craniotomy first with sequential margins, devascularize skull base with ethmoidal arteries, devascularize nasal cavity with SPA, leave right periorbita for last, vascularized pericranium for dura closure	Harvest pericranium for reconstruction, multilayered closure, concomitant surgery with ENT, lumbar drain if CSF leak
Postoperative				
Admission	ICU	ICU	Intermediate care	Intermediate care
Postoperative complications feared	CSF leak	CSF leak, visual deterioration, endocrine dysfunction, cognitive decline, anosmia	CSF leak, pericranial flap breakdown, frontal lobe injury, orbital injury (muscular or cranial nerve)	CSF leak, visual deterioration
Follow-up testing	MRI within 72 hours after surgery	MRI within 24 hours after surgery PET for systemic disease	MRI within 48 hours after surgery Adjuvant therapy 4 weeks after surgery	MRI within 24 hours after surgery Lumbar drain for 5 days if CSF leak
Follow-up visits	14 days after surgery with neurosurgery 14 days after surgery with oncology and radiation oncology	10–15 days after surgery	10 days after surgery	Continual follow-up with ENT 3 months after surgery with neurosurgery
Adjuvant therapies recommended	Surgery or radiation therapy depending on resectability	Second look surgery if possible, radiation for modified Kadish stage 3 without prophylactic neck radiation	Hyams I/II: adjuvant radiation therapy Hyams III/IV: adjuvant chemoradiation therapy	Surgery for remnant, radiation therapy after surgery

ACA, anterior cerebral artery; *ACOM*, anterior communicating artery; *CN*, cranial nerve; *CSF*, cerebrospinal fluid; *CT*, computed tomography; *ENT*, ear, nose and throat; *ICA*, internal carotid artery; *ICU*, intensive care unit; *MRI*, magnetic resonance imaging; *OCT*, optical coherence tomography; *PET*, positron emission tomography; *SPA*, sphenopalatine arteries; *SSS*, superior sagittal sinus.

Differential diagnosis and actual diagnosis

- Squamous cell carcinoma
- Adenocarcinoma
- Mucosal melanoma
- Adenoid cystic carcinoma
- ENB
- Sinonasal undifferentiated carcinoma

Important anatomic and preoperative considerations

A complete discussion of the nasal cavity and paranasal sinus is presented in Chapter 64. ENB have a propensity to invade into surrounding structures from the nasal cavity, and the most commonly used staging system is the Kadish staging system that was originally devised in 1976, in which Kadish A are tumors confined to the nasal cavity, Kadish B are tumors that extend from the nasal cavity to paranasal sinuses, Kadish C are tumors that extend beyond the nasal cavity and paranasal sinuses, and Kadish D are metastatic tumors (Table 65.1).[1,4] Based on a population study, the overall survival at 10 years was 83.4% for patients with stage A, 49% for stage B, 39% for stage C, and 13% for stage D.[1] The tumor in this case is a Kadish stage C tumor because of involvement of the anterior skull base. In addition to staging by tumor location, ENB can also be graded by histology.[5] The most commonly used grading system was originally described by Hyams, which is based on mitotic activity, nuclear polymorphism, amount of fibrillary matrix, rosette formation, and necrosis (Table 65.2).[5] The prognostic role of the Hyams grading system has been questioned, but in one study showed that Hyams grade I or II had a median survival of 9.8 years as compared with 6.9 years for Hyams grade III or IV tumors.[5]

Table 65.1	Modified Kadish staging system
A	Tumor limited to nasal cavity
B	Extension to paranasal sinuses
C	Extension beyond nasal cavity/paranasal sinuses
D	Metastatic disease

Table 65.2 Hyams histological grading system

	Architecture	Pleomorphism	Neurofibrillary matrix	Rosettes	Mitoses	Necrosis	Calcification
Grade I	Lobular	Absent or Minimal	Prominent	Homer-Wright	Absent	Absent	Variable
Grade II	Lobular	Present	Present	Homer-Wright	Present	Absent	Variable
Grade III	+/– Lobular	Prominent	May be present	Flexner-Wintersteiner	Prominent	Present	Absent
Grade IV	+/– Lobular	Marked	Present	Flexner-Wintersteiner	Marked	Prominent	Absent

ENB typically involve the anterior skull base.[6] The anterior skull base can be divided into medial and lateral compartments.[6] The medial compartment is comprised of the ethmoid, sphenoid, and frontal bones, in which the anterior portion is comprised of the frontal bones containing the frontal sinuses, and below this area is the nasal cavity anteriorly and the sphenoid sinus within the sphenoid body posteriorly.[6] Intracranially, the gyrus rectus of the frontal lobes and olfactory bulbs rest on the anteromedial skull base, and the roof of the ethmoid bone forms the cribriform plate anteriorly, and the olfactory rootlets from the olfactory bulb penetrate the cribriform plate to enter the nasal cavity.[6] Within the nasal cavity, the perpendicular plate of the ethmoid bone joins the vomer to form the posterior nasal septum, whereas the lateral ethmoid plates contribute to the medial orbital walls.[6] The superior turbinates emanate from the roof of the ethmoid into the nasal cavity and reside lateral to the cribriform plate.[6] The sphenoethmoidal recesses and sphenoid ostia are posterior and superior to the superior turbinates.[6] The lateral portion of the anterior skull base is mainly in the orbital region, in which the roof of the orbit is formed by the lesser sphenoid wing and the zygomatic bone; the inferior orbit by the zygomatic, maxillary, and palatine bones; and the medial wall by the maxilla, lacrimal bone, and ethmoid bones.[6] On the intracranial side of the lateral skull base it the orbital gyri.[6] The anterior and posterior ethmoidal foramina transmit the anterior and posterior ethmoidal arteries that are branches of the ophthalmic artery, and traverse the superomedial orbital walls from the orbit to the nasal cavity.[6] Also within the orbit is the supratrochlear foramen medially and the supraorbital foramen laterally.[6] In the posterior orbit, the optic canal is formed by the frontal bone and lesser sphenoid wing and transmits the optic nerve and ophthalmic arteries.[6] The superior orbital fissure is between the lesser and greater sphenoid wings and transmits the oculomotor, trochlear, branches of the ophthalmic division of the trigeminal nerve (frontal, lacrimal, nasociliary), abducens, ophthalmic vein, and sympathetic fibers.[6] The inferior orbital fissure is between the greater sphenoid wing and the anterior orbital floor formed by the maxillary and palatine bones, and transmits the maxillary nerve and its zygomatic branch, as well as the ascending branches of the pterygopalatine ganglion.[6] The infraorbital canal transmits the infraorbital artery and vein.[6]

Approaches to this lesion

The goal of surgery for ENB is to achieve complete removal of the tumor with negative margins, but it is important that the treatment plan be individualized for each patient. When negative margins cannot be achieved either because of tumor invasion, patient condition, or presence of systemic disease, adjuvant therapy consisting of radiation and/or chemotherapy are often used. Because ENB typically involves the anterior skull base, access can be achieved by several approaches, including a bifrontal, subfrontal-transglabellar, transnasal, and transmaxillary-transnasal approaches, through open-end endoscopic routes.[6] The traditional approach for ENB have typically been craniofacial resections that usually involve a bifrontal craniotomy combined with a transfacial approach, which is typically achieved with a lateral rhinotomy or Weber-Ferguson incision.[1–3] All tumors that reach the anterior skull base are by definition at least Kadish B or C and require resection of the dura and olfactory tracts, and therefore require dural closure with a vascularized pericranial graft.[1–3] For tumors limited to the midline nasal cavity, a lateral rhinotomy incision with transnasal approach can be used but may require a lip-split with a gingivobuccal incision or even a Weber-Ferguson facial flap to increase lateral exposure.[1–3] Another approach that has been used in the past is a facial degloving procedure but can be associated with cosmetic deformity to the lower nasal cartilages and nose.[1–3] For orbital involvement, the orbit can be spared if the periorbita is not invaded, but once the tumor has involved orbital fat, extraocular muscles, or other intraorbital contents, the eye cannot be saved.[1–3] In addition to these conventional approaches, there are other approaches that have become more commonplace for ENB.[1–3] The transglabellar-subcranial approach involves the use of a bicoronal skin incision, preservation of the pericranium, and frontal craniotomy in which the inferior cuts across the nasal bridge and superior orbital rims and fractures along the crista galli and nasal septum.[1–3] In addition, endoscopic surgery can also be done in combination with craniofacial resections, as with a gingival-buccal, transmaxillary (Caldwell-Luc), or purely transnasal approaches.[1–3] For ENB that involve the cervical lymph nodes, management has been varied.[1–3] The incidence of cervical lymph node involvement at the time of presentation has ranged from 5% to 10%, but increased to 20% to 25% with disease progression.[1–3] Neck dissection is usually done for patients who present with clinical or radiographic evidence of lymph node involvement, or for those who develop lymph node involvement after treatment of the primary site if it allows complete resection of known disease.[1–3]

Radiation can be delivered as the primary modality of treatment, preoperatively, or most commonly following surgery.[1–3] Radiation is typically delivered using intensity-modulated radiation therapy, in which the gross tumor is treated with 1.8 to 2 Gy fractions up to a total dose of 65 to 70 Gy; however, there are recent studies demonstrating the efficacy of proton beam therapy.[1–3] The majority of studies have shown that surgery with radiation is superior to radiation alone.[1–3] The goal of radiation after surgery is to treat microscopic residual disease to minimize local-regional recurrence.[1–3] The majority of studies show a trend in benefit toward surgery followed by radiation versus complete resection alone.[1–3] Radiation can also be administered preoperatively in which the advantages are improved accuracy in delineating the target volume and sparing noninvolved structures, and may reduce tumor volume to improve resectability, but studies have failed to show that it is advantageous over postoperative radiation therapy.[1–3] In regard to neck radiation, it remains controversial whether neck radiation leads to improved local-regional control when the neck is not involved when treating the primary site.[1–3] Chemotherapy can be used in combination with radiation therapy in the preoperative induction setting when there is involvement of intracranial space or the orbits, or postoperatively when there is a high risk of local-regional recurrence, as well as a single modality typically for palliation.[1–3] The most commonly used chemotherapeutic drugs are cisplatin and etoposide or cyclophosphamide and vincristine for induction therapy when there is significant intracranial or orbital invasion.[1–3]

In general, for Kadish A tumors, many advocate that surgery alone with clear margins is sufficient, in which adjuvant radiation therapy is indicated for positive margins or when there is residual disease, but there is no role for adjuvant chemotherapy.[1–3] For Kadish B, surgery followed by adjuvant radiation therapy regardless of resection margins, in which the role of adjuvant chemotherapy is controversial, and induction chemoradiation therapy has been used in inoperable cases.[1–3] For Kadish C, surgery, radiation, and chemotherapy are typically all used, in which induction chemoradiation therapy is typically preferred, as well as the definitive role of chemotherapy.[1–3] For Kadish D, most advocate for systemic chemotherapy and palliative radiation to the local and metastatic sites.[1–3] In cases of local recurrence and/or distal metastases, salvage treatment involves some combination of surgery, surgery and postoperative radiation

therapy, radiation therapy alone, palliative chemotherapy, or supportive/palliative care.[1–3] Local recurrence rates ranges around 30%, regional recurrence 15% to 20%, and distal recurrence 15% to 20%.[1–3]

What was actually done

The patient underwent emergent surgery for endoscopic endonasal resection of the lesion, with the goal of debulking the extracranial or sinonasal component of the tumor to relieve pressure on the optic apparatus because of the acute vision decline. The plan was for possible staged procedure for the intracranial tumor component at a later date. The patient underwent endoscopic endonasal debulking of tumor under general anesthesia without intraoperative monitoring with otolaryngology and neurosurgery. The patient was induced and intubated per routine. The patient was placed in a Mayfield horseshoe headrest, and electromagnetic CT and magnetic resonance imaging (MRI) navigation was used to avoid the need for pinning. The patient was draped in the usual standard fashion and given cefazolin and dexamethasone. The lesion was debulked internally and continued into the sphenoid sinus to relieve the pressure of the mucocele, removal of the right middle turbinate and a right maxillary antrostomy, and continued until the anterior skull base was reached. The tumor was not pursued into the anterior cranial fossa. The tumor was dissected with a combination of suction cautery and sharp dissection. After the lesion was removed, biopsies were taken from the nasal septum, maxillary sinus, nasal floor, ethmoid sinuses, and right periorbita. Positive margins were obtained at the right periorbita. Nasal stents were placed bilaterally.

The patient awoke at their neurologic baseline with improved vision and was taken to the intensive care unit for recovery. An MRI was done within 48 hours after surgery and showed expected subtotal resection with residual in the anterior cranial fossa (Fig. 65.2). A positron emission tomography scan was done and only showed disease at the anterior

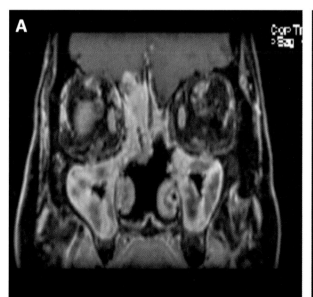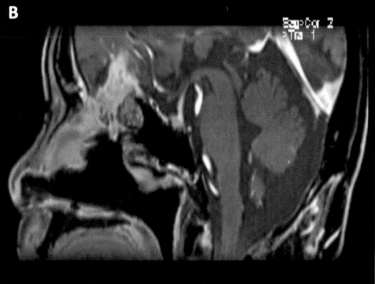

Fig. 65.2 Postoperative magnetic resonance imaging. (A) T1 axial image with gadolinium contrast; **(B)** T1 coronal image with gadolinium contrast magnetic resonance imaging scan demonstrating subtotal resection of the lesion with residual lesion along the anterior skull base.

skull base and no lymph node or systemic involvement. The nasal stents were removed on postoperative day 2. The patient participated with physical and occupational therapy and was discharged to home on postoperative day 3. The patient was prescribed cefdinir for 7 days. The patient was seen at 2 weeks postoperatively and had intact vision with full visual fields. Final pathology was consistent with Hyams grade IV ENB. The patient refused to pursue further surgery and instead underwent postoperative radiation and chemotherapy (cisplatin). The surgical site was observed with serial MRI examinations at 3- to 6-month intervals, and systemic disease was evaluated with serial positron emission tomography scans. The patient is without local or distal recurrence for 12 months.

Commonalities among the experts

Most of the surgeons opted for the patient to undergo ophthalmology evaluation to assess preoperative vision status, and half requested high-resolution CT to better evaluate bony anatomy. The majority of surgeons would pursue a combination of bifrontal craniotomy combined with endoscopic endonasal, and one pursued primarily an endonasal with possible bifrontal craniotomy, in which otolaryngology would assist with the endonasal component of the surgery. Most surgeons aimed for radical resection with negative margins. Most surgeons were cognizant of the optic nerves, internal carotid artery, and anterior cerebral artery. The most common feared complication was vision loss. Surgery was generally pursued with surgical navigation, surgical microscope, endoscope, and ultrasonic aspirator, with perioperative steroids and mannitol. Most surgeons advocated for harvesting pericranium, wide boney opening,

communicating the cranial with the endonasal areas, and multilayer closure. Following surgery, all surgeons admitted their patients to the intensive care unit or intermediate care, and all requested imaging within 72 hours to assess for extent of resection and/or evaluate for complications. Most surgeons advocated for repeat surgery for residual disease.

SUMMARY OF QUALITY OF EVIDENCE TO GUIDE SPECIFIC INTERVENTIONS FOR THIS CASE

- Postoperative radiation and chemotherapy for residual ENB—Class III.

REFERENCES

1. Konuthula N, Iloreta AM, Miles B, et al. Prognostic significance of Kadish staging in esthesioneuroblastoma: an analysis of the National Cancer Database. *Head Neck.* 2017;39:1962–1968.
2. Ow TJ, Bell D, Kupferman ME, Demonte F, Hanna EY. Esthesioneuroblastoma. *Neurosurg Clin N Am.* 2013;24:51–65.
3. Roxbury CR, Ishii M, Gallia GL, Reh DD. Endoscopic management of esthesioneuroblastoma. *Otolaryngol Clin North Am.* 2016;49:153–165.
4. Kadish S, Goodman M, Wang CC. Olfactory neuroblastoma. A clinical analysis of 17 cases. *Cancer.* 1976;37:1571–1576.
5. Gallagher KK, Spector ME, Pepper JP, McKean EL, Marentette LJ, McHugh JB. Esthesioneuroblastoma: updating histologic grading as it relates to prognosis. *Ann Otol Rhinol Laryngol.* 2014;123:353–358.
6. Cappello ZJ, Dublin AB. *Anatomy, Head and Neck, Nose Paranasal Sinuses.* In StatPearls [Internet]. Treasure Island, FL: StatPearls Publishing; 2020.

66

Chordoma

Case reviewed by William T. Couldwell, Paul A. Gardner, Carl H. Snyderman, Gerardo D. Legaspi, Henry W. S. Schroeder

Introduction

Chordomas are rare World Health Organization grade I slow-growing neoplasms that are thought to arise from remnants of the notochord.[1–6] As a result, these tumors can occur anywhere along the spinal axis, in which the majority occur in the sacral region followed by the spheno-occipital or clival region, in which approximately 25% arise in the clivus and account for 0.1% of primary intracranial neoplasms.[1–6] Chordomas typically involve the spheno-occipital synchondrosis, and those that involve the upper clivus (basisphenoid) can affect the upper cranial nerves, pituitary gland, and hypothalamus, whereas those involving the lower clivus (basiocciput) typically affect the lower cranial nerves.[1–6] They can also involve the petrous apex, sellar region, sphenoid sinus, nasopharynx, maxilla, and paranasal sinuses, among others.[1–6] Although these lesions are considered to

be low-grade, they are highly invasive, radioresistant, and recurrent.[1–6] They come in three histologic variants: classical, chondroid, and dedifferentiated.[1–6] In this chapter, we present a case of a patient with clival chordoma.

Example case

Chief complaint: deviated tongue and neck stiffness
History of present illness
A 21-year-old, right-handed woman with no significant past medical history presented with deviated tongue and neck stiffness. Three months prior, she was involved in a motor vehicle collision, and since then has complained of neck stiffness. However, 7 days prior to evaluation, she noticed that her tongue deviated to her left. She was seen at a local emergency room for stroke evaluation, and imaging revealed a skull base lesion (Fig. 66.1). She underwent endonasal biopsy consistent with chordoma.

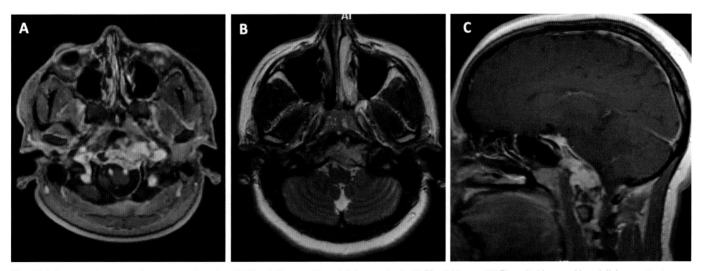

Fig. 66.1 Preoperative magnetic resonance imaging. (A) T1 axial image with gadolinium contrast; **(B)** T2 axial image; **(C)** T1 sagittal image with gadolinium contrast magnetic resonance imaging scan demonstrating a heterogeneously enhancing lesion involving the clivus, odontoid, left hypoglossal canal, and left vertebral artery, with mass effect on the cervicomedullary junction.

Medications: Diazepam.
Allergies: No known drug allergies.
Past medical and surgical history: None.
Family history: No history of intracranial malignancies.

Social history: Military, no smoking or alcohol.
Physical examination: Awake, alert, oriented to person, place, time; Cranial nerves II to XI, except left tongue deviation; Moves all extremities with good strength.

	William T. Couldwell, MD, PhD, University of Utah, Salt Lake City, UT, United States	Paul A. Gardner, MD, Carl H. Snyderman, MD, MBA, University of Pittsburgh, Pittsburgh, PA, United States	Gerardo D. Legaspi, MD, Philippine General Hospital, Manila, Philippines	Henry W. S. Schroeder, MD, PhD, University of Greifswald, Greifswald, M-V, Germany
Preoperative				
Additional tests requested	High-resolution CT Swallowing evaluation	High-resolution CT CT angiogram ENT evaluation Spine MRI	High-resolution CT	CT scan to assess stability of craniocervical junction
Surgical approach selected	Extreme lateral transodontoid resection, occipital-cervical fusion	Endoscopic endonasal transclival, left transpterygoid, possible partial transodontoid	Left suboccipital craniotomy with far lateral extension	Endoscopic endonasal transclival, occipital-C2 fusion
Other teams involved during surgery	ENT	ENT	None	ENT
Anatomic corridor	Extreme lateral transodontoid	Transnasal, transclival, left transpterygoid	Left far lateral transcondylar	Transnasal, transclival
Goal of surgery	Radical resection	Radical resection	Maximal safe resection	Radical resection
Perioperative				
Positioning	Left lateral	Supine with right rotation	Left lateral	Supine for endonasal; prone for fusion
Surgical equipment	IOM (MEP, SSEP, cranial nerves IX–XII) Surgical navigation Ultrasonic aspirator	IOM (SSEP) Surgical navigation Endoscope Microdoppler	Surgical microscope Ultrasonic aspirator	Surgical navigation Endoscope Microdoppler
Medications	Steroids	Steroids	None	None
Anatomic considerations	Hypoglossal nerve, brainstem, odontoid, anterior arch C1, vertebral artery	Parapharyngeal ICAs, Eustachian tubes, hypoglossal canals, inferior petrosal sinus, foramen lacerum, vertebrobasilar junction	Hypoglossal nerve, lower cranial nerves, vertebral artery	Cranial nerves IX–XII, vertebral artery
Complications feared with approach chosen	Lower cranial nerve injury	Lower cranial nerves and vertebrobasilar injury	Brainstem injury, vertebral artery injury	Injury to petrosal carotid artery and lower cranial nerves
Intraoperative				
Anesthesia	General	General	General	General
Skin incision	L-shaped inverted hockey stick	None	Linear 3 cm medial to mastoid from transverse sinus to C2	Midline posterior for fusion
Bone opening	Left retrosigmoid suboccipital, posterior arch/lateral mass/ condylar joint of C1, C2 lamina/superior articular process/ odontoid	Sphenoidotomy, bilateral maxillary antrostomy, left pterygoid wedge, left vidian canal, middle/lower clivus, left hypoglossal canal	Left retrosigmoid incorporating foramen magnum, left occipital condyle, partial anterior petrosectomy	Sphenoidotomy, clivus, anterior arch of C1 and infiltrated dens

	William T. Couldwell, MD, PhD, University of Utah, Salt Lake City, UT, United States	Paul A. Gardner, MD, Carl H. Snyderman, MD, MBA, University of Pittsburgh, Pittsburgh, PA, United States	Gerardo D. Legaspi, MD, Philippine General Hospital, Manila, Philippines	Henry W. S. Schroeder, MD, PhD, University of Greifswald, Greifswald, M-V, Germany
Brain exposure	Extreme lateral	Transclival	Far lateral transcondylar	Transclival
Method of resection	L-shaped incision, identify suboccipital triangle, release muscle attachments to C1 transverse process to identify vertebral artery and C1 root, division of the C2 root and transpose vertebral artery, small retrosigmoid suboccipital craniectomy, inferior foramen magnum removed to identify dural entry of vertebral artery, posterior arch/lateral mass/condylar joint of C1 drilled, remove anterior C1 ring, drill C2 lamina and superior articular process, remove odontoid, debulk tumor, leave dura intact, identify and preserve hypoglossal nerve, occipital-cervical fusion	Lateralize inferior turbinates, harvest right extended nasoseptal flap, wide sphenoidotomy, left maxillary antrostomy, open left pterygopalatine space, right maxillary antrostomy, nasal sleeves, inverted U nasopharyngeal/retropharyngeal flap down to anterior arch of C1, displace left pterygopalatine contents laterally to locate vidian canal, drill base of pterygoid/medial pterygoid wedge until flush with paraclival ICA, drill sphenoid rostrum and middle/lower clivus above pole of tumor, dissect until lateral margins identified, biopsy to confirm chordoma, localize left parapharyngeal ICA with Doppler, peel lateral prevertebral/preclival tumor from parapharyngeal space, resect bulk of tumor, inspect for residual, drill bony margins, dissect foramen lacerum, stimulate left hypoglossal nerve to clear tumor in canal and drill surrounding bone, drill tip of C2 as needed, resect inner layer of dura if involved, reconstruct dura with collagen inlay/fascia lata, fat graft to fill nasopharynx, nasoseptal and retropharyngeal flaps to protect lower borders, ICG endoscopic angiography to confirm vascularization, placement of lumbar drain	Linear incision carried down to periosteum, dissect and isolate left extracranial vertebral artery in areolar space, retract muscle flap laterally to sigmoid space and medially near midline, burr hole on the asterion, craniotomy flap, complete foramen magnum removal with drilling and bone punching, extend to the precondylar area with special extension to the hypoglossal nerve, partial anterior petrosectomy to expose more extradural tumor, debulk and excise tumor using combination of sharp and blunt dissection assisted by ultrasonic aspirator, attempt total excision and debulk maximally, close in layers	Harvest nasoseptal flap on right, reverse flap on left, enter sphenoid sinus, drill out clivus, resect tumor as far laterally and dorsally as possible, incise nasopharynx mucosa and create a flap, resection anterior arch of C1 and infiltrated dens, close defect with fat and nasoseptal flap/fibrin glue/nasal pledgets, reposition patient in prone position, midline skin incision and fusion with occipital plate-lateral mass of C1 and lamina of C2 after resection of dorsal part of condyle

(continued on next page)

	William T. Couldwell, MD, PhD, University of Utah, Salt Lake City, UT, United States	Paul A. Gardner, MD, Carl H. Snyderman, MD, MBA, University of Pittsburgh, Pittsburgh, PA, United States	Gerardo D. Legaspi, MD, Philippine General Hospital, Manila, Philippines	Henry W. S. Schroeder, MD, PhD, University of Greifswald, Greifswald, M-V, Germany
Complication avoidance	Large incision for fusion, early identification of vertebral artery, mobilization of vertebral artery, identification/ preservation of hypoglossal nerve, occipital-cervical fusion	Harvesting nasoseptal and retropharyngeal flaps, drill out for bony margins, inspect hypoglossal canal, multilayer dural reconstruction, ICG vascular flap assessment	Isolate vertebral artery, large craniotomy, far lateral transcondylar extension, anterior petrosectomy	Neuro-monitoring, navigation, harvest nasoseptal flap, drill out margins, multilayer closure
Postoperative				
Admission	ICU	Intermediate care or ICU	Floor	Intermediate care
Postoperative complications feared	Lower cranial nerve injury	CSF leak, worsened dysphagia, aspiration, craniocervical instability	Hypoglossal nerve injury, lower cranial neuropathy	CSF leak
Follow-up testing	MRI within 24 hours after surgery Swallow evaluation	Lumbar drain for 72 hours High-resolution CT within 1 day after surgery Swallow evaluation MRI within 48 hours after surgery	MRI within 48 hours after surgery	MRI within 24 hours after surgery CT within 24 hours after surgery
Follow-up visits	1 month after surgery	1 week after surgery with ENT 2 weeks after surgery with neurosurgery	1 week after surgery	3 months after surgery for neurosurgery Continual follow-up with ENT after surgery
Adjuvant therapies recommended	Reoperation to achieve gross total resection, proton beam radiation	Reoperation to achieve gross total resection, proton beam radiation	Proton beam radiation therapy	Reoperation to achieve gross total resection, radiation with proton beam or carbon ion radiation after 3 months

CSF, cerebrospinal fluid; *CT*, computed tomography; *ENT*, ear, nose, and throat; *ICA*, internal carotid artery; *ICG*, indocyanine green; *ICU*, intensive care unit; *IOM*, intraoperative monitoring; *MEP*, motor evoked potential; *MRI*, magnetic resonance imaging; *SSEP*, somatosensory evoked potential.

Differential diagnosis and actual diagnosis

- Chordoma
- Chondrosarcoma
- Metastatic brain tumor
- Giant cell tumor

Important anatomic and preoperative considerations

The clivus is located between the nasopharynx and the posterior cranial fossa, and in its upper half consists of the posterior sphenoid body (basisphenoid) and the lower half is the basilar part of the occipital bone (basioccipital).[7–9] The clivus is typically divided in upper, middle, and lower thirds.[7–9] The upper third is formed by the basisphenoid bone and usually faces the posterior component of the sphenoid sinus and contains the dorsum sellae, the middle third corresponds to the rostral part of the basioccipital bone and

is located by an imaginary line connecting the petroclival fissures, and the lower third is formed by the caudal portion of the basioccipital bone.[7–9] On the intracranial surface of the clivus is the pons and upper medulla, whereas on the extracranial surface of the upper clivus is the nasopharyngeal roof, the middle clivus is the pharyngeal tubercle to which the pharyngeal raphe is attached, and the lower third are the attachments of the longus capitis muscle on each side of midline that is covered by the prevertebral and pharyngobasilar fascia, as well as the superior pharyngeal constrictor muscle in the posterior nasopharyngeal wall.[7–9] The rectus capitis anterior lies posterolateral to the longus capitis and is attached to the lower clivus that is anterior to the occipital condyle.[7–9] Lateral to the rectus capitis anterior is the internal carotid artery (ICA) that is anteromedial to the internal jugular vein.[7–9] The lateral edge of the lower clivus contains the occipital condyles, jugular tubercles, and hypoglossal canal.[7–9] The hypoglossal canal is located in the middle one-third of the occipital condyle, and opens intracranially above the middle and posterior thirds of the condyle below the jugular tubercle, and opens extracranially above the middle thirds of the condyle and medial to the jugular foramen.[7–9] The abducens nerve ascends anterolaterally along the intracranial surface of the clivus and passes medial to the trigeminal nerve to enter the Dorello canal, which is bordered by the Gruber ligament (petrosphenoid ligament) superiorly and the petrous apex inferiorly.[7–9] The petrous portion of the temporal bone is connected to the upper and middle clivus bilaterally by the petroclival fissure, where on the intracranial side is the inferior petrosal sinus, and on the extracranial side is the inferior petroclival vein.[7–9]

The foramen magnum is the exit point of the brainstem from the cranial to the spinal compartments.[7–9] The anterior aspect of the foramen magnum is covered by the nasopharyngeal mucosa, pharyngobasilar fascia, superior pharyngeal constrictor muscle, longus capitis muscle, anterior longitudinal ligament (ALL), anterior atlantooccipital membrane, apical ligament, superior longitudinal band of the cruciform ligament, and tectorial membrane in order from anterior to posterior.[7–9] The ALL is attached to the inferior surface of the clivus and extends from the anterior tubercle of the atlas downward to the sacrum, and the tectorial membrane attaches to the middle and lower clivus and extends to the dorsal surface of the body of C2 and continues downward as the posterior longitudinal ligament.[7–9] Below the foramen magnum is the odontoid process that articulates anteriorly with the anterior arch of the atlas, and posteriorly with the cruciform ligament that is attached laterally to the medial surface of the lateral mass of the atlas.[7–9] The odontoid process is connected to the occipital bone by the apical and alar ligaments, in which the former arises at the tip of the odontoid and attaches to the anterior margin of the foramen magnum, and the latter arises from the posterolateral surface of the odontoid and attaches to the anteromedial surface of the occipital condyles.[7–9] The lateral mass of the atlas is the attachment of the rectus capitis lateralis, which reside anterior to the vertebral arteries that ascend through the transverse foramina and posterior to the ICA and internal jugular vein.[7–9] The dura facing the clivus is supplied by arteries from the dorsal meningeal branch of the meningohypophyseal trunk, anterior meningeal branch of the vertebral artery, and meningeal branches of the ascending pharyngeal artery.[7–9]

With advances in endoscopic surgery, a commonly used approach to the clivus and infratemporal fossa involves an endonasal transphenoidal transpterygoid approach.[7–9] Sphenoid sinus anatomy is discussed in detail in Chapter 56. After puberty, the sphenoid sinus pneumatizes, and as a result the intracavernous ICA produces the carotid prominence in the lateral wall of the sphenoid sinus.[7–9] The presellar segment of the carotid prominence corresponds to the anterior vertical segment and anterior bend, the infrasellar corresponds to the horizontal segment, and the retrosellar segment corresponds to the posterior bend and posterior vertical segment of the intracavernous ICA.[7–9] The optic canal is partially encircled by the sphenoid sinus and forms a prominence on the superoanterior portion of the lateral wall.[7–9] There is a bony depression between the optic canal medially and the presellar segment of the carotid prominence called the optico-carotid recess, which extends a variable distance into the optic strut that separates the optic canal from the superior orbital fissure.[7–9] The anterolateral

portion of the sphenoid sinus is in close juxtaposition to the posteromedial roof of the pterygopalatine fossa.[7–9] The maxillary sinus faces the lower nasal cavity medially, the orbit superiorly, the infratemporal fossa posterolaterally, and the pterygopalatine fossa postomedially.[7–9]

The goal of treatment for skull base chordomas is gross total resection, as complete resection improves overall survival (OS) and progression-free survival (PFS).[10] In a meta-analysis, the weighted average 5-year PFS and OS were 51% and 78%, respectively, in which gross total resection was associated with a higher 5-year PFS (87% vs. 50%) and OS (95% vs. 71%), as well as 10-year PFS (47% vs. 25%) and OS (95% vs. 53%) as compared with subtotal resections.[10] The use of postoperative radiation therapy is typically reserved for subtotal resections, whereas radiation is typically not used for complete resections.[1–6] The radiation that is typically required must be high dose and conformal because of the proximity to the brain and spinal cord, and therefore the most commonly used radiation therapies include proton beam therapy, radiosurgery, intensity modulated radiotherapy, and carbon ion.[1–6] In the same meta-analysis, there was no difference in 5-year PFS and OS between carbon ion, stereotactic radiosurgery, intensity modulated radiotherapy, and proton beam radiotherapy.[10]

Approaches to this lesion

There are a variety of skull base and/or endoscopic approaches for clival chordomas, which are dictated by tumor location, patient characteristics, and/or surgeon preference.[1–6] The typical goal of surgery is to achieve gross total resection; however, unlike in the sacrum, en bloc resection is not possible in this region.[1–6] The approaches to the clivus can be divided into anterior and lateral approaches.[1–6] There are a variety of anterior approaches including transcranial (bifrontal transbasal) transnasal (transsphenoidal, expanded endonasal), transfacial (lateral rhinotomy, Weber-Ferguson), transoral (transpalatal), and transcervical.[1–6] The lateral approaches include pterional, orbitozygomatic, infratemporal, transpetrosal, far lateral, and extreme far lateral, among others.[1–6] An approach that has been increasing in use for clival lesions is the expanded endoscopic transsphenoidal approach.[4,6,7] This approach allows access to midline structures from the frontal sinus to the odontoid based on patient anatomy.[4,6,7] In the expanded endonasal approach, the middle turbinate is typically removed, along with a maxillary antrostomy, anterior ethmoidectomy, and posterior ethmoidectomy to allow a wider corridor to the skull base, in which this is typically done on the right side because the endoscope is typically introduced through the right naris, but it can be done bilaterally as well.[4,6,7] In addition, a posterior septectomy is done to allow bilateral nasal access, removal of the sellar floor allows access to the upper clivus and dorsum sellae, and removal of the sphenoid floor allows visualization of the bilateral lateral recesses of the sphenoid sinus, as well as the middle and lower thirds of the clivus.[4,6,7] The lateral limit of the exposure are the clival carotid arteries, in which removal of the medial wall can increase exposure.[4,6,7]

Another commonly used approach for tumors that extend out of the reach of anterior approaches to the occipital condyle is the extreme lateral transcondylar approach.[11] In this approach, the suboccipital triangle is opened to expose the posterior arch and transverse processes of C1 and C2 and the dorsal root of C2.[11] The vertebral artery is identified at the sulcus arteriosus at the posterior arch of C1, removal of the C1 arch from the midline to the transverse foramen, and opening of the transverse foramen to allow transposition of the vertebral artery.[11] The vertebral artery can then be mobilized medially allowing access to the anterior rim of the foramen magnum and lateral mass of C1.[11] A suboccipital craniotomy is also done in the approach and includes the rim of the foramen magnum and is extended laterally to identify the posterior edge of the occipital condyle and sigmoid sinus, and the medial portion of the occipital condyle is removed after identification and transposition of the vertebral artery.[11]

What was actually done

The patient underwent a three-staged approach with an endoscopic endonasal transpterygoid transclival resection of the anterior portion of the tumor, followed by a left extreme far lateral transcondylar resection of the posterolateral component of the tumor, and occipital to C3 fusion for spinal instability. In the first stage, the patient underwent endoscopic endonasal transpterygoid transclival resection of the anterior portion of the tumor under general anesthesia, with intraoperative monitoring of cranial nerve XII, somatosensory evoked potentials, and motor evoked potentials with otolaryngology and neurosurgery. The patient was induced and intubated per routine. The patient was placed in pins, with two pins over the left external auditory meatus in the superior temporal line and one pin over the right external auditory meatus. Computed tomography and magnetic resonance imaging surgical navigation was used for surgical guidance. The patient was draped in the usual standard fashion and given cefazolin and dexamethasone. The base of the right middle turbinate was anesthetized with lidocaine and epinephrine and removed, followed by a right maxillary antrostomy and right anterior and posterior ethmoidectomies. The left middle turbinate had been displaced laterally and left anterior and posterior ethmoidectomies were done on the left. A right nasoseptal flap was raised and placed into the choanae. The sphenoid rostrum was identified, and the bilateral sphenoid ostia were opened to enter the sphenoid sinus, in which the intersinus septation was drilled flush with the sella. The bone overlying the clivus was thinned to enter the tumor, and the bone overlying the clival carotid arteries was thinned and removed to allow lateral mobilization. The floor of the sphenoid sinus was removed to identify the left vidian canal, which was traced to the petrous carotid artery. The tumor was removed piecemeal until the dura of the posterior fossa was identified. Preliminary pathology was consistent with chordoma. Once as much tumor could be removed as possible from this approach, the area was packed with fat, and nasal stents were placed bilaterally. The patient was placed in a halo because of removal of the ALL, tectorial membrane, and apical ligaments. Stage 2 of the approach was done 2 days later, and a left extreme lateral transcondylar approach was done under general anesthesia with intraoperative monitoring of the cranial nerves V and VII to XII, somatosensory evoked potentials, and motor

evoked potentials. The patient was induced and intubated per routine. The patient was positioned in the left modified park bench position after head pinning, and the halo was removed. A hockey stick incision was made in which the incision starts at the inion and extends down to around the C3 spinous process, and the upper end of the incision is extended laterally down toward the mastoid tip. The arch of C1 and spinous process of C2 and C3 were exposed, and the suboccipital muscles were reflected laterally. The dorsal ramus of C2 was identified between C1 and C2 and sectioned. The suboccipital muscles were dissected in layers in the following order: semispinalis, splenius, longus capitis, rectus major and minor, and superior and inferior obliques. A cuff was left at the superior nuchal line to allow for reapproximation. The vertebral artery was identified first at the sulcus arteriosus, followed into the suboccipital triangle underneath the superior oblique muscle, then between C1 and C2 in which it lay ventral to the C2 nerve root, and then followed into the transverse foramen of C1. The posterior aspect of the transverse foramen of C1 was removed using a high-speed drill and Kerrison rongeurs and was dissected to identify where it penetrated the dura from where it leaves the transverse foramen of C1, courses around the lateral mass of C1 to form the sulcus arteriosus at the upper C1 laminar surface before turning superiorly, anteriorly, and medially to penetrate the dura at the level of the foramen magnum. The occipital craniectomy was done that extended laterally passed the sigmoid sinus and incorporated the foramen magnum inferiorly and the mastoid tip laterally. The left C1 lamina was removed with a high-speed drill just lateral to the posterior tubercle and extended to the lateral mass, making sure to protect the vertebral artery. The occipital-C1 condyle was drilled lateral to the vertebral artery under microscopic visualization, and the bone was removed to the hypoglossal canal. The tumor was removed in piecemeal all the way up the hypoglossal canal. There was some microscopic disease present on the vertebral artery. The patient was temporarily closed and positioned prone with the halo. Stage 3 was completed on the same sitting and involved an occipital to C3 fusion. The halo was removed after prone positioning. The occipital bone was exposed, and subperiosteal dissection was carried laterally to expose the lateral mass of C1 bilaterally, the pedicles of C2, and the lateral mass of C3. An occipital plate was placed over the midline occipital bone, and a lateral mass screw was placed on the right C1, bilateral C2 pedicle screws, and bilateral C3 lateral mass screws followed by rods. The joints were decorticated, and bone mineral was placed in the lateral gutters. The muscle and skin were closed in the standard fashion. A cervical spine collar was placed.

The patient awoke at their neurologic baseline with baseline left tongue weakness and was taken to the intensive care unit for recovery and remained intubated overnight. Magnetic resonance imaging was done within 48 hours after surgery and showed gross total resection but with known microscopic disease. The patient participated with physical, occupational, and speech therapy and was discharged to rehabilitation on postoperative day 7 following the last procedure. The patient was seen at 2 weeks postoperatively and remained at their neurologic baseline. Final pathology was a chordoma. The patient underwent postoperative proton beam therapy 3 weeks after surgery.

Commonalities among the experts

All of the surgeons opted for the patient to undergo high-resolution computed tomography to better evaluate bony anatomy and spinal stability. Half of the surgeons would pursue surgery through an endoscopic endonasal transclival route, whereas the other half would pursue surgery through a posterolateral approach (far lateral in one and extreme lateral in another). Most surgeons would pursue surgery in combination with ear, nose, and throat. Most surgeons aimed for radical resection with negative margins. Most surgeons were cognizant of the hypoglossal nerve, vertebral artery, and stability of the occipital-C1 joint. The most common shared feared complications were lower cranial neuropathy and vertebral artery injury. Surgery was generally pursued with surgical navigation, intraoperative monitoring of lower cranial nerves, surgical microscope, endoscope, Doppler, and ultrasonic aspirator, with perioperative steroids. Most surgeons advocated for wide boney opening, identifying and preserving vertebral artery and hypoglossal nerve, and nasoseptal flap for the endonasal cases. Following surgery, most surgeons admitted their patients to the intensive care unit or intermediate care, and all surgeons requested imaging within 48 hours to assess for extent of resection and/or evaluate for complications. Most surgeons advocated for repeat surgery for residual disease, followed by proton beam therapy.

SUMMARY OF QUALITY OF EVIDENCE TO GUIDE SPECIFIC INTERVENTIONS FOR THIS CASE

- Staged procedure for clival chordomas—Class III.
- Endoscopic endonasal transsphenoidal transpterygoid and transclival resection of clival chordomas—Class III.
- Extreme lateral transcondylar resection of clival chordomas—Class III.
- Proton beam radiation therapy for microscopic residual—Class III.

REFERENCES

1. Erdem E, Angtuaco EC, Van Hemert R, Park JS, Al-Mefty O. Comprehensive review of intracranial chordoma. *Radiographics*. 2003;23:995–1009.
2. Higinbotham NL, Phillips RF, Farr HW, Hustu HO. Chordoma. Thirty-five-year study at Memorial Hospital. *Cancer*. 1967;20:1841–1850.
3. O'Connell JX, Renard LG, Liebsch NJ, Efird JT, Munzenrider JE, Rosenberg AE. Base of skull chordoma. A correlative study of histologic and clinical features of 62 cases. *Cancer*. 1994;74:2261–2267.
4. Stippler M, Gardner PA, Snyderman CH, Carrau RL, Prevedello DM, Kassam AB. Endoscopic endonasal approach for clival chordomas. *Neurosurgery*. 2009;64:268–277; discussion 277–278.
5. Walcott BP, Nahed BV, Mohyeldin A, Coumans JV, Kahle KT, Ferreira MJ. Chordoma: current concepts, management, and future directions. *Lancet Oncol*. 2012;13:e69–e76.
6. Zhang Q, Kong F, Yan B, Ni Z, Liu H. Endoscopic endonasal surgery for clival chordoma and chondrosarcoma. *ORL J Otorhinolaryngol Relat Spec*. 2008;70:124–129.
7. Funaki T, Matsushima T, Peris-Celda M, Valentine RJ, Joo W, Jr Rhoton AL. Focal transnasal approach to the upper, middle, and lower clivus. *Neurosurgery*. 2013;73:ons 155–190; discussion ons190–191.
8. Kawashima M, Tanriover N, Rhoton Jr AL. Ulm AJ, Matsushima T. Comparison of the far lateral and extreme lateral variants of the atlanto-occipital transarticular approach to anterior extradural lesions of the craniovertebral junction. *Neurosurgery*. 2003;53:662–674; discussion 674–675.
9. Wen HT, Rhoton Jr AL. Katsuta T, de Oliveira E. Microsurgical anatomy of the transcondylar, supracondylar, and paracondylar extensions of the far-lateral approach. *J Neurosurg*. 1997;87:555–585.
10. Di Maio S, Temkin N, Ramanathan D, Sekhar LN. Current comprehensive management of cranial base chordomas: 10-year meta-analysis of observational studies. *J Neurosurg*. 2011;115:1094–1105.
11. Park HH, Lee KS, Hong CK. Vertebral artery transposition via an extreme-lateral approach for anterior foramen magnum meningioma or craniocervical junction tumors. *World Neurosurg*. 2016;88:154–165.

67

Chondrosarcoma

Case reviewed by Peter Bullock, Franco DeMonte, Hirofumi Nakatomi, Jamie J. Van Gompel

Introduction

Skull base chondrosarcomas are rare tumors that account for 0.1% of primary intracranial neoplasms.[1] Chondrosarcomas are thought to arise from mesenchymal cells or from embryonal cartilage remnants of synchondroses, in which the majority of cranial chondrosarcomas occur at the skull base (75%) in the paraclival region, and include the petroclival, petro-occipital, spheno-occipital, and sphenopetrosal synchondroses.[1] These tumors often extend into the paranasal sinuses, middle fossa, and/or posterior fossa.[2–5] The majority of these tumors are low to intermediate grade, with slow growth and low metastatic potential, and histologically are grouped into conventional, mesenchymal, clear cell, and dedifferentiated types.[6] Primary treatment is surgical resection, in which radiation therapy, including fractionated radiation, stereotactic radiosurgery, proton beam, and heavy particle radiation, is typically used for subtotal resection and

recurrent disease.[7] In this chapter, we present a case of a patient with petroclival chondrosarcoma.

Example case

Chief complaint: right facial numbness, headaches, ataxia
History of present illness
A 72-year-old, right-handed man with a history of coronary artery disease, hypertension, and hypercholesterolemia presented with right facial numbness, headaches, and ataxia. He had a known right petroclival mass that was being followed with serial examinations. Over the past 6 months, the lesion had grown (Fig. 67.1) with increasing headaches, right facial numbness but no pain, and ataxia in which he required a walker for balance.
Medications: Aspirin, lisinopril, atorvastatin.
Allergies: No known drug allergies.

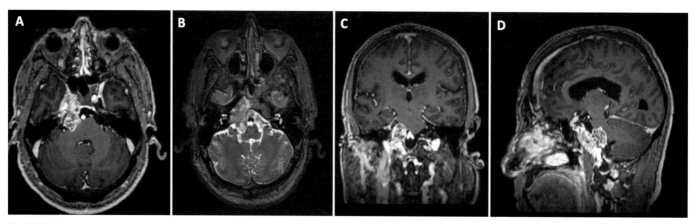

Fig. 67.1 Preoperative magnetic resonance imaging. (A) T1 axial image with gadolinium contrast; **(B)** T2 axial image; **(C)** T1 coronal image with gadolinium contrast; (D) T1 sagittal image with gadolinium contrast magnetic resonance imaging scan demonstrating a heterogeneously enhancing lesion involving the right petroclival region, with mass effect on the right cerebellopontine angle and extension into the middle fossa in Meckel cave.

Past medical and surgical history: Coronary artery disease, hypertension, hypercholesterolemia, coronary bypass, knee replacement.
Family history: No history of intracranial malignancies.
Social history: Retired military, no smoking or alcohol.

Physical examination: Awake, alert, oriented to person, place, time; Cranial nerves II to XII intact, except right V1 to V3 numbness; Moves all extremities with good strength; Cerebellar: Right to left finger-to-nose dysmetria, truncal ataxia.

	Peter Bullock, FRCS, MRCP, London Clinic, London, England	Franco DeMonte, MD, MD Anderson Cancer Center, Houston, TX, United States	Hirofumi Nakatomi, MD, PhD, University of Tokyo, Tokyo, Japan	Jamie J. Van Gompel, MD, Mayo Clinic, Rochester, MN, United States
Preoperative				
Additional tests requested	Cardiology evaluation Speech pathology with swallow evaluation Right eye tarsorrhaphy	Audiogram (BAERs) CT/CTA Speech pathology with swallow evaluation and videostroboscopy Medicine evaluation Neurology evaluation	Audiogram (PTA/SDS/BAERs) Cerebral angiogram ENT evaluation for possible biopsy, facial, and swallowing function Ophthalmology	Audiogram CTA
Surgical approach selected	Infratentorial supracerebellar	Endonasal endoscopic with right transpterygoid extension	Right suboccipital craniotomy	Right suboccipital craniotomy with endoscopic assistance and suprameatal petrosectomy
Other teams involved during surgery	None	ENT, head and neck	ENT	+/– ENT
Anatomic corridor	Infratentorial retrosigmoid anterior to and above cerebellum	Endonasal transpterygoid	Right suboccipital, paratrigeminal and lateral cerebellomedullary fissure	Right suboccipital
Goal of surgery	Maximal safe resection, brainstem decompression	Diagnosis, brainstem decompression, maximal safe resection	Stage 1–removal of CPA, Stage 2–ENT to remove parapharyngeal, Stage 3–SRS for cavernous sinus; decompress trigeminal nerve	GTR, decompress brainstem
Perioperative				
Positioning	Right lateral park bench	Supine with lateral head flexion and right rotation	Right lateral	Right lateral decubitus
Surgical equipment	Surgical navigation IOM (MEP, SSEP, BAERs, cranial nerves III–XI) Surgical microscope Ultrasonic aspirator	Surgical navigation IOM (BAERs, facial EMG) Endoscope Ultrasonic aspirator Microdebrider	Surgical navigation IOM (MEP, BAERs, facial EMG) Surgical microscope Ultrasonic aspirator Weck/AVM clips Microanastamosis set	Surgical navigation IOM (BAERs, cranial nerves V–VIII, X/XI) Surgical microscope Endoscopes with rigid arm
Medications	Steroids	None	Mannitol Steroids	Steroids
Anatomic considerations	Transverse/sigmoid sinuses, cerebellum, superior petrosal veins, cranial nerves V/VII–VIII, AICA	Sphenopalatine artery, sphenoid sinus, pituitary gland, parasellar/paraclival ICA, Eustachian tube, vidian nerve, maxillary nerve, mandibular nerve, cranial nerves VI and XII, jugular foramen	Cranial nerve V–XI and petrosal vein	ICA, cranial nerves VII–VIII
Complications feared with approach chosen	Hearing loss, facial weakness, facial numbness, corneal ulceration, facial pain, brainstem injury	Mobilizing critical neurovascular structures	Hearing decline and facial palsy	Hearing loss, facial weakness, abducens palsy, facial numbness
Intraoperative				
Anesthesia	General	General	General	General
Skin incision	Retrosigmoid lazy S	None	Retrosigmoid lazy S	Retroauricular curvilinear

(continued on next page)

	Peter Bullock, FRCS, MRCP, London Clinic, London, England	Franco DeMonte, MD, MD Anderson Cancer Center, Houston, TX, United States	Hirofumi Nakatomi, MD, PhD, University of Tokyo, Tokyo, Japan	Jamie J. Van Gompel, MD, Mayo Clinic, Rochester, MN, United States
Bone opening	Right suboccipital	+/– right middle turbinate, right anterior/posterior ethmoidectomies, right medial maxillectomy, posterior inferior turbinate, posterior septectomy, large sphenoidotomy, lateral and medial pterygoid plates, right mid and lower clivectomy, petroclival synchondrosis/petrous/clivus	Right suboccipital, foramen magnum, condylar fossa, IAC	Right suboccipital
Brain exposure	CPA	Posterior fossa dura	Cerebellum, CPA	Cerebellum, CPA
Method of resection	Tarsorrhapy prior to procedure, right suboccipital craniotomy with exposure of edge of transverse and sigmoid sinuses staying above foramen magnum, curvilinear dural opening, drain CSF from cisterna magna, identify cranial nerves IX–XI/VII–VIII/and V, work between cranial nerves, can sacrifice veins of the superior and lateral surface of the cerebellum if needed, decompress tumor, attempt to dissect from brainstem, watertight dural closure, leave remnant for proton beam radiation	Left nasoseptal flap harvest and stored in maxillary sinus, right anterior/posterior ethmoidectomies, +/– right middle turbinate removal, medial maxillectomy, removal of posterior inferior turbinate, posterior septectomy, large sphenoidotomy, exposure of right vidian canal, ligation of pharyngeal artery within palatovaginal canal, ligation of sphenopalatine artery and exposure of PPF, access the ITF through fascial incision lateral to V2 branches, detachment of the inferior head of the lateral pterygoid muscle, removal of pterygoid plates, skeletonization of V2 and V3, U-shaped mucosal incision in posterior nasopharynx and longus capitis, limited right mid and lower clivectomy, skeletonization of the paraclival and laceral ICA segments, removal of thin bony plate between ICA and superior surface of Eustachian tube, fibrocartilaginous tissue at foramen lacerum is sharply incisioned to mobilize ICA superiorly, incise lateral most Eustachian tube to expose petroclival synchondrosis/petrous apex/medial jugular foramen, removal of bone of petroclival synchondrosis/petrous bone/clivus, resection of jugular tubercle as laterally as possible, multilayer closure with nasoseptal flap	Right suboccipital craniotomy, removal of foramen magnum and condylar fossa, Y-shaped dural opening, epidural continuous suction, dissect lateral cerebellomedullary fissure to see foramen of Luschka and paratrigeminal cistern, place electrodes to monitor cranial nerves VII and VIII, devascularize tumor from petro-tentorial angle, debulk tumor, dissect from brainstem and cerebellum, open IAC and debulk tumor, reconstruct IAC	Right suboccipital craniotomy, drain cisterns, remove intracranial portion of tumor, ENT to drill suprameatal tubercle, complete bony resection with the aid of endoscopes

	Peter Bullock, FRCS, MRCP, London Clinic, London, England	Franco DeMonte, MD, MD Anderson Cancer Center, Houston, TX, United States	Hirofumi Nakatomi, MD, PhD, University of Tokyo, Tokyo, Japan	Jamie J. Van Gompel, MD, Mayo Clinic, Rochester, MN, United States
Complication avoidance	Large bony opening, decompress CSF, identify cranial nerves, work anterior to cranial nerves VII and VIII, watertight dural closure	Nasoseptal flap, exposure and mobilization of ICA by identification key landmarks (vidian nerve, V3), multilayer closure, lumbar drain if dura compromised	Large bone opening including foramen magnum and condylar fossa, cranial nerve monitoring, debulk tumor before capsular dissection	Cranial nerve monitoring, large suboccipital craniotomy, endoscopic assistance
Postoperative				
Admission	ICU	Floor	ICU	ICU
Postoperative complications feared	Swallowing dysfunction, CSF leak, facial weakness, hearing loss, facial pain, abducens weakness	Swallowing dysfunction, CSF leak, middle ear effusion, diplopia, facial weakness, hearing loss	Hearing loss, facial palsy, facial dysesthesias	Hearing loss, CSF leak, sixth nerve palsy, facial weakness, facial numbness
Follow-up testing	CT night of surgery MRI within 72 hours after surgery Speech/swallowing evaluation	MRI skull base within 24 hours after surgery Speech/swallowing evaluation Lumbar drain for 5 days if dura compromised	MRI/MRA/MRV within 72 hours after surgery	MRI 3 months after surgery
Follow-up visits	3 months after surgery	7–10 days after surgery	1 month after surgery	3 months after surgery
Adjuvant therapies recommended	Grade 1–proton beam therapy Grade 2–proton beam therapy Grade 3–proton beam therapy	Grade 1–observation Grade 2–observation if GTR, radiation for STR Grade 3–radiation +/– chemotherapy	Grade 1–observation, SRS if grows Grade 2–observation, SRS if grows Grade 3–observation, SRS if grows	Grade 1–observation if good resection Grade 2–proton beam therapy Grade 3–proton beam therapy

AICA, anterior inferior cerebellar artery; *AVM*, arteriovenous malformation; *BAERs*, brainstem auditory evoked responses; *CPA*, cerebellopontine angle; *CSF*, cerebrospinal fluid; *CT*, computed tomography; *CTA*, computed tomography angiography; *EMG*, electromyogram; *ENT*, ear, nose, and throat; *GTR*, gross total resection; *IAC*, internal auditory canal; *ICA*, internal carotid artery; *ICU*, intensive care unit; *IOM*, intraoperative monitoring; *ITF*, infratemporal fossa; *MEP*, motor evoked potential; *MRA*, magnetic resonance angiography; *MRI*, magnetic resonance imaging; *MRV*, magnetic resonance venography; *PPF*, pterygopalatine fossa; *PTA*, pure tone audiogram; *SDS*, speech discrimination scores; *SRS*, stereotactic radiosurgery; *SSEP*, somatosensory evoked potential; *STR*, subtotal resection.

Differential diagnosis and actual diagnosis

- Chondrosarcoma
- Chordoma
- Meningioma
- Skull base metastases
- Primary bone tumors

Important anatomic and preoperative considerations

For a full discussion of the cerebellopontine angle, petro-clival, and clival regions, see Chapters 51, 52, and 66, respectively. The current standard of initial treatment of skull base chondrosarcomas is surgical resection with the goal of gross total resection.[2–5] However, this may be associated with significant morbidity, in which preoperative cranial nerve deficits occur in 20% to 50% of patients, and following surgery there is an approximate 10% to 15% rate of vascular injury, 10% risk of cerebrospinal fluid leak, and 5% perioperative mortality.[2–5] In modern series, the gross total resection rate is 50% to 60%, in which the 5-year tumor recurrence and

overall survival (OS) rates are 70% to 80% and 80% to 90%, respectively, in which the rarity of this lesion has precluded definitive evidence that gross total resection as opposed to subtotal resection with radiation therapy is associated with improved recurrence-free or survival benefit.[8,9] The factors associated with worsened outcomes for patients with chondrosarcomas are tumor histology (mesenchymal and high grade) and lack of radiation therapy.[8,9]

The use of radiation therapy following surgical resection was associated with a reduction in 5-year mortality from 25% to 9%, and recurrence following surgery was decreased from 44% to 9%.[8,9] Radiation can be given by fractionated photon (55–65 Gy), particle (proton 60–79 cobalt Gy equivalents or carbon ion), or stereotactic radiosurgery, but no class 1 data exists about which modality is associated with improved outcomes.[8,9] For photon radiotherapy, the 5-year progression-free survival (PFS) and OS have been reported at 80% and 90%, respectively.[8,9] For stereotactic radiosurgery, the 5-year PFS and OS have been reported at 70% and 70%, respectively.[8,9] For proton beam therapy, the 5-year PFS and OS have been reported at 75% to 95% and 85% to 100%, respectively.[8,9] For carbon ion therapy, the 5-year PFS and OS have been reported at 89% and 98%, resepectively.[8,9] The use of chemotherapy has been ineffective for skull base chondrosarcomas, as it has with chondrosarcomas involving the axial skeleton.[8,9]

Approaches to this lesion

There are a variety of skull base and/or endoscopic approaches for petroclival chondrosarcomas, which are dictated by tumor location, patient characteristics, and/or surgeon preference.[2–5] These approaches are described in more detail in Chapter 66. For chondrosarcomas involving the petrous apex and upper third of the clivus with extension anteriorly into the Meckel cave or the cavernous sinus, the options include anterior and anterolateral cranial approaches (pterional, orbitozygomatic, middle fossa, Kawase approach, subtemporal) and anterior craniofacial approaches (endoscopic transnasal, transpterygoid, transclival, open transfacial).[2–5] For those tumors that extend posteriorly and inferiorly, approaches include retrosigmoid, extended retrosigmoid, and transpetrosal approaches.

An approach that allows concomitant posterior and middle fossa access, and is especially useful for lesions involving the cerebellopontine angle and the Meckel cave, is a retrosigmoid suprameatal approach popularized by Samii et al.[10] The advantage of this approach as opposed to transpetrosal approaches is that is minimizes surgical time and potential morbidity from hearing loss, facial weakness, and cerebrospinal fluid leaks.[10] This approach is similar to the standard retrosigmoid craniotomy but augments this approach by incorporating intradural drilling of the suprameatal area above and anterior to the internal acoustic meatus and posterior portion of the petrous apex that allows increased exposure to the Meckel cave.[10] For a description of this approach, see later text.

What was actually done

The patient was taken to surgery for a right suboccipital craniectomy with intradural suprameatal approach for a cerebellopontine angle chondrosarcoma that extends into the Meckel cave with general anesthesia, with intraoperative somatosensory evoked potentials, motor evoked potentials, and cranial nerve V, VII to VIII (with facial electromyogram), IX to XI monitoring. The patient was induced and intubated per routine. The head was fixed in pins, with two pins over left superior nuchal line and one pin over the right forehead in the midpupillary line. The patient was then placed into the right park bench position. A lazy S-incision was planned in the suboccipital region that extended above the pinna down below the lip of the foramen magnum that was about three finger breadths behind the external auditory meatus. The patient was draped in the usual standard fashion and given dexamethasone and cefazolin. The incision was made, and a myocutaneous flap was made, and the skin and muscles were retracted with a cerebellar retractor. A high-speed drill was used to thin the bone overlying the left cerebellar hemisphere and transverse and sigmoid sinuses. The bone was removed with Kerrison punches and Leksell rongeurs so that the bottom of the transverse and lateral aspect of the sigmoid sinuses were exposed. In addition, the lip of the foramen magnum was removed. The dura was opened in a cruciate fashion, with one limb being at the transverse-sigmoid junction. The cisterna magna was opened to decompress the posterior fossa. The microscope was brought in for the remainder of the

intradural portion of the case. The cerebellum was retracted medially with cottonoids and dynamic retraction. The jugular foramen cranial nerves were identified and dissected from the tumor margin. The petrosal veins were identified, coagulated, and ligated to identify the superior margin and tentorial edge. The facial nerve stimulator was used to stimulate the dorsal surface of the tumor, and the seventh and eighth nerve complex was identified on the inferior dorsal aspect of the tumor. The tumor was then debulked internally with an ultrasonic aspirator working between the lower cranial nerves and the seventh/eighth nerve complex, as well as superior to the seventh/eighth nerve complex. The tumor was fibrous as expected, and the preliminary pathology was chondrosarcoma. Alternating tumor debulking and capsular dissection was done until the trigeminal nerve was identified. Along the pontine pial boundary, the tumor appeared infiltrated, and dissection was unable to preserve this pia, and therefore this portion of the tumor was left behind. Once the cerebellopontine angle component of the tumor was removed, the tentorium with the fourth cranial nerve was identified, and the suprameatal portion of the petrous bone was drilled away over the seventh/eighth nerve complex and dorsolateral to the fifth nerve to expose the Meckel cave using a high-speed diamond drill with continuous irrigation. The tumor was followed into the Meckel cave and dissected from the trigeminal nerve. Once the tumor was removed from the Meckel cave, the dura, bone, and skin were closed in standard fashion.

The patient awoke at their neurologic baseline with symmetric facial expression and was taken to the intensive care unit for recovery. Magnetic resonance imaging was done within 48 hours after surgery and showed near total resection but with known residual along the pons (Fig. 67.2). The patient participated with physical, occupational, and speech therapy and was discharged to home on postoperative day 5 with an intact examination, except for residual right facial numbness, slight right facial weakness (House-Brackmann 2/6 with full eye closure), and slightly subjective diminished right hearing. The patient was seen at 2 weeks postoperatively with symmetric facial expression and intact hearing to finger rub. Final pathology was a chondrosarcoma. The patient was followed with serial magnetic resonance imaging at 3- to 6-month intervals, and no progression of their disease has been noted at 18 months after surgery.

Commonalities among the experts

Most of the surgeons opted for the patient to undergo vascular imaging (computed tomography angiography or cerebral angiogram) to better evaluate vascular anatomy and audiogram to establish preoperative hearing, whereas half requested formal swallow evaluation to assess for swallowing function prior to surgery. The majority of surgeons would pursue surgery through a suboccipital approach (right suboccipital in two and one supracerebellar infratentorial). Most would pursue surgery in combination with otolaryngology. Most surgeons aimed for extensive resection with decompression of the brainstem. Most surgeons were cognizant of the lower cranial nerves and petrosal vein. The most common feared complications were hearing loss and facial palsy. Surgery was generally pursued with surgical navigation, intraoperative monitoring of lower cranial nerves, surgical microscope, and ultrasonic aspirator, with

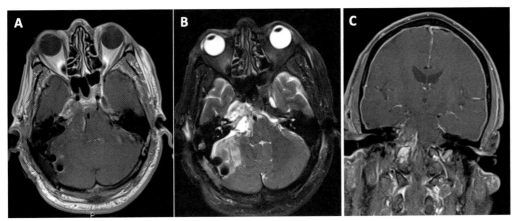

Fig. 67.2 Postoperative magnetic resonance imaging. (A) T1 axial image with gadolinium contrast; **(B)** T2 axial image; **(C)** T1 coronal image with gadolinium contrast magnetic resonance imaging scan demonstrating near total resection of the lesion, with a small rim of residual along the brainstem.

perioperative steroids. Most surgeons advocated for large boney opening, early decompression of cerebrospinal fluid, cranial nerve monitoring/identification/preservation, and decompression before capsular dissection. Following surgery, most admitted their patients to the intensive care unit and requested imaging within 72 hours to assess for extent of resection and/or evaluate for complications. Following surgery, observation versus proton beam therapy was suggested for residual grade 1 chondrosarcoma, observation versus proton beam therapy was suggested for residual grade 2 chondrosarcoma, and radiation therapy for residual grade 3 chondrosarcoma.

SUMMARY OF QUALITY OF EVIDENCE TO GUIDE SPECIFIC INTERVENTIONS FOR THIS CASE

- Retrosigmoid intradural suprameatal approach for chondrosarcomas—Class III.
- Observation of residual chondrosarcoma—Class III.

REFERENCES

1. Kitamura Y, Sasaki H, Yoshida K. Genetic aberrations and molecular biology of skull base chordoma and chondrosarcoma. *Brain Tumor Pathol.* 2017;34:78–90.
2. Gay E, Sekhar LN, Rubinstein E, et al. Chordomas and chondrosarcomas of the cranial base: results and follow-up of 60 patients. *Neurosurgery.* 1995;36:887–896; discussion 896–897.
3. Samii A, Gerganov V, Herold C, Gharabaghi A, Hayashi N, Samii M. Surgical treatment of skull base chondrosarcomas. *Neurosurg Rev.* 2009;32:67–75; discussion 75.
4. Tzortzidis F, Elahi F, Wright DC, Temkin N, Natarajan SK, Sekhar LN. Patient outcome at long-term follow-up after aggressive microsurgical resection of cranial base chondrosarcomas. *Neurosurgery.* 2006;58:1090–1098; discussion 1090–1098.
5. Zhang Q, Kong F, Yan B, Ni Z, Liu H. Endoscopic endonasal surgery for clival chordoma and chondrosarcoma. *ORL J Otorhinolaryngol Relat Spec.* 2008;70:124–129.
6. National Nosocomial Infections Surveillance System. National Nosocomial Infections Surveillance (NNIS) System Report, data summary from January 1992 through June 2004, issued October 2004. *Am J Infect Control.* 2004;32:470–485.
7. Hug EB, Loredo LN, Slater JD, et al. Proton radiation therapy for chordomas and chondrosarcomas of the skull base. *J Neurosurg.* 1999;91:432–439.
8. Bloch OG, Jian BJ, Yang I, et al. A systematic review of intracranial chondrosarcoma and survival. *J Clin Neurosci.* 2009;16:1547–1551.
9. Bloch OG, Jian BJ, Yang I, et al. Cranial chondrosarcoma and recurrence. *Skull Base.* 2010;20:149–156.
10. Samii M, Tatagiba M, Carvalho GA. Retrosigmoid intradural suprameatal approach to Meckel's cave and the middle fossa: surgical technique and outcome. *J Neurosurg.* 2000;92:235–241.

68

Vestibular schwannomas

Case reviewed by Franco DeMonte, Gerardo D. Legaspi, Robert E. Wharen, Larry B. Lundy, Gelareh Zadeh, Farshad Nassiri

Introduction

Vestibular schwannomas (VS) are also called acoustic neuromas and are benign primary intracranial tumors that form along the vestibulocochlear nerve from Schwann cells that are responsible for the myelin sheath around the nerve axons.[1] The incidence is 6 to 9 per million persons per year; however, this number is increasing as a result of widespread availability of neuroimaging.[2] Although they only account for 6% of primary intracranial tumors, they account for 85% of tumors in the cerebellopontine angle (CPA).[2] As a result of increasing diagnoses, the treatment algorithms for patients who present with VS is becoming more refined, with the goals of quality of life, facial nerve function, and hearing preservation.[3–6] These treatment options include observation, surgical resection, and/or radiation therapy.[3–6] Surgical resections vary in goal from gross total resection to planned subtotal resection, and approaches vary from retrosigmoid, middle fossa, and translabyrinthine, among others.[7–14] In this chapter, we present a case of a patient with VS.

Example case

Chief complaint: tinnitus and imbalance
History of present illness
A 53-year-old, right-handed woman with a history of diabetes, hypertension, and hypercholesterolemia presented with left-sided tinnitus and imbalance. Approximately 6 months prior, she started developing ringing in her left ear and felt as though her hearing was worse on the left side to the point in which she could not use that ear while on the telephone. In addition, she complained of progressive imbalance in which she had constant falls. Her primary care physician ordered brain imaging (Fig. 68.1).

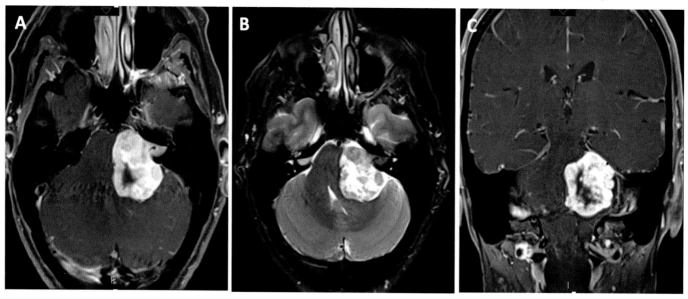

Fig. 68.1 Preoperative magnetic resonance imaging. (A) T1 axial image with gadolinium contrast; **(B)** T2 axial image; **(C)** T1 coronal image with gadolinium contrast magnetic resonance imaging scan demonstrating a heterogeneously enhancing lesion involving the left cerebellopontine angle with extension into the internal auditory canal.

Medications: Aspirin, hydrochlorothiazide, simvastatin, metformin.
Allergies: No known drug allergies.
Past medical and surgical history: Diabetes, hypertension, and hypercholesterolemia.
Family history: No history of intracranial malignancies.
Social history: Secretary, no smoking or alcohol.

Physical examination: Awake, alert, oriented to person, place, time; Cranial nerves II to XI except left V1 to V3 facial numbness, left House-Brackmann 2/6; Moves all extremities with good strength; Cerebellar: Left to right finger-to-nose dysmetria, truncal ataxia.
Audiogram: Left ear discrimination 25%, pure tone audiogram 75 dB (Gardner-Robertson class III).

	Franco DeMonte, MD, MD Anderson Cancer Center, Houston, TX, United States	Gerardo D. Legaspi, MD, Philippine General Hospital, Manila, Philippines	Robert E. Wharen, MD, Larry B. Lundy, MD, Mayo Clinic, Jacksonville, FL, United States	Gelareh Zadeh, MD, PhD, Farshad Nassiri, MD, Toronto Western Hospital, Toronto, Canada
Preoperative				
Additional tests requested	Audiogram (BAERs) Neuro-otology evaluation	None	Vestibular testing Facial EMG CT of temporal bones	CTA
Surgical approach selected	Left retrosigmoid craniotomy with opening of foramen magnum and posterior lip of IAC	Left retrosigmoid craniotomy	Left translabyrinthine with possible abdominal fat graft	Left retrosigmoid craniotomy
Other teams involved during surgery	Neuro-otologist	None	Neuro-otologist	None
Anatomic corridor	Left retrosigmoid	Left retrosigmoid	Left translabyrinthine	Left retrosigmoid
Goal of surgery	Gross total resection pending adhesion to brainstem and facial nerve	Gross total resection	Brainstem decompression, preservation of cranial nerve V and VII	Maximal safe resection with facial nerve preservation and brainstem decompression
Treatment of asymptomatic lesions surgically	Conservatively followed to assess for growth	Lesions over 2 cm adjacent to the brainstem	Lesions compressing MCP or fourth ventricle	Lesions over 3 cm and not insolated to porous
Treatment using SRS	All but largest tumors, young patients, Koos IV tumors	Patients who refuse surgery, elderly	Growth of asymptomatic lesions, tumors <2.5 cm	Lesions <3 cm that are growing on serial imaging
Perioperative				
Positioning	Left lateral, head flexed laterally to right	Left supine with right head rotation	Left supine with right head rotation	Left park bench
Surgical equipment	Surgical navigation Surgical microscope IOM (facial EMG) Nerve stimulator Ultrasonic aspirator	Lumbar drain IOM (facial nerve EMG) Surgical microscope Ultrasonic aspirator	Surgical microscope IOM (facial and trigeminal EMG) Nerve stimulator Cardiac pacer leads	Surgical microscope IOM (cranial nerve stimulator) Doppler Ultrasonic aspirator
Medications	Steroids	None	Steroids	Steroids Mannitol
Anatomic considerations	Transverse and sigmoid sinuses, petrosal vein, cranial nerves IV–XII, SCA, AICA, PICA, VA, petrous surface of cerebellum, brainstem	Cranial nerves V–XI, AICA, PICA, lateral cerebellum and pons	Cranial nerves IV–XI, posterior fossa vessels and brainstem perforators	Transverse and sigmoid sinuses, cranial nerves especially facial nerve, mastoid air cells, vertebral artery
Complications feared with approach chosen	Injury to cerebellum, facial nerve and other cranial nerve, vasculature, brainstem	Facial nerve injury	Cranial neuropathy especially facial paralysis, cerebellar and brainstem compression, CSF leak	Cranial neuropathy, venous sinus injury, brainstem injury

(continued on next page)

	Franco DeMonte, MD, MD Anderson Cancer Center, Houston, TX, United States	Gerardo D. Legaspi, MD, Philippine General Hospital, Manila, Philippines	Robert E. Wharen, MD, Larry B. Lundy, MD, Mayo Clinic, Jacksonville, FL, United States	Gelareh Zadeh, MD, PhD, Farshad Nassiri, MD, Toronto Western Hospital, Toronto, Canada
Intraoperative				
Anesthesia	General	General	General	General
Skin incision	Midline posterior cervical down to C2 and laterally to EAM above left ear	Sigmoid incision 1.5 cm lateral to mastoid extending 1 cm above transverse sinus and 5 cm below	Postauricular C-shaped incision	Sigmoid incision based on transverse-sigmoid junction
Bone opening	Occipital craniotomy exposing lower part of transverse sinus and posterior sigmoid sinus, foramen magnum	Occipital craniotomy exposing lower part of transverse sinus and posterior sigmoid sinus, IAC	Mastoidectomy and bone overlying sigmoid sinus, labyrinthectomy, removal of bone overlying middle and posterior dura	Occipital craniotomy exposing lower part of transverse sinus and posterior sigmoid sinus, foramen magnum
Brain exposure	Retrosigmoid, left cerebellar hemisphere	Retrosigmoid, left cerebellar hemisphere	Translabyrinthine, cerebellopontine angle	Retrosigmoid, left cerebellar hemisphere
Method of resection	Occipital craniotomy up to sinus margins, removal of foramen magnum and bone beneath anterior curve of sigmoid sinus, dura opened in midline over cisterna magna, CSF drained, dural incision extended to transverse-sigmoid junction, tumor exposed and queried for facial nerve with stimulator, tumor incised and centrally debulked, inferior debulking to identify flocculus/choroid plexus/lower cranial nerves, origin of facial nerve, continual debulking to identify cerebellar interface/petrosal vein/fifth nerve/upper pole of tumor, posterior IAC is drilled after cisternal portion of tumor removed, distal portion of tumor is removed to expose facial nerve in porous, removal of intermediary tumor dependent on adherence to facial nerve, watertight dural closure	Lumbar drain placement, incision carried down to periosteum, muscle flap retracted to sigmoid sinus and paramedian area, retraction held down by silk stay sutures and anchored with rubber bands, burr hole on asteroid, 3-cm keyhole craniotomy with craniotome exposing transverse and sigmoid sinuses, additional drilling down to maximize sinus exposure, air cells plugged with morselized muscle and bone wax, 5–10 cc drainage from lumbar drain, curvilinear dural opening 5 mm from edge of sigmoid sinus to transverse-sigmoid sinus, dural edge tacked up, drill 1 cm of IAC, debulk tumor if needed to visualize IAC, start IAC tumor debulking to identify location of facial nerve, arachnoid lifting before cauterization, dissect arachnoid away from tumor surface, dissect inferior pole of tumor and drain CSF as much as possible, isolate lower cranial nerves and protect with cottonoids, debulk tumor to level of IAC and test for facial nerve, superior dissection and test for facial nerve, intramural guttering in the midportion all the way to the IAC, dissect capsule from cerebellum and pons medially then laterally from the meatus, wax IAC, close in layers	Mastoidectomy with bone removal posterior to sigmoid sinus, removal of incus, amputation of malleus head, transect tensor tympani tendon, obliterate Eustachian tube with fascia and bone wax, labyrinthectomy, removal of bone overlying middle and posterior fossa dura, skeletonize IAC and identification of jugular bulb, open dura along posterior fossa and IAC, identify tumor capsule and absence of facial nerve with stimulation, protect lower cranial nerves, intratumoral debulking, identify cranial nerves VII and VIII, remove as much tumor as possible without compromising nerve function, drape bony defect with temporalis fascia, use abdominal fat to fill defect	Pericranial harvest, divide subcutaneous tissue and muscles, map transverse and sigmoid sinus based on navigation, burr hole placed inferomedial to the sinus junction, 3-cm craniotomy to level of foramen magnum and up to edge of transverse and sigmoid sinus, remove foramen magnum with rongeurs, wax mastoid air cells, Y-shaped dural opening, open cisterna magna to relax cerebellum, gentle retraction of cerebellum with telfa until superior-inferior extent of tumor identified, stimulate posterior aspect in case facial nerve present (start at 1 mA and decrease to 0.1 mA), safe entry zone identified, tumor entered, sequential debulking with internal decompression with ultrasonic aspirator and dissection of capsule from arachnoid, stimulate for facial nerve identification, remove intracanalicular portion by using diamond drill to expose dura over canal, open dura sharply, stimulate to find facial nerve, divide vestibular and cochlear nerve, roll tumor from medial to lateral and inferior to superior with direct visualization of facial nerve, reconstruct porous with fat and Tisseel, watertight dural closure with pericranium

	Franco DeMonte, MD, MD Anderson Cancer Center, Houston, TX, United States	Gerardo D. Legaspi, MD, Philippine General Hospital, Manila, Philippines	Robert E. Wharen, MD, Larry B. Lundy, MD, Mayo Clinic, Jacksonville, FL, United States	Gelareh Zadeh, MD, PhD, Farshad Nassiri, MD, Toronto Western Hospital, Toronto, Canada
Complication avoidance	Large bony opening, early drainage of CSF, identify inferior pole of tumor and lower cranial nerves, proximal and distal facial nerve identification, removal of tumor along facial nerve depends on adherence and monitoring feedback	Lumbar drain placement and drainage, avoidance of retractors, early identification of facial nerve at IAC, inferior to superior dissection	Large bone removal for exposure, stimulate to confirm absence of facial nerve, intratumoral debulking, leaving remnant on facial nerve to minimize injury	Large bone removal for exposure, drain CSF, stimulate for facial nerve, keep arachnoid plane to protect cranial nerves
Postoperative				
Admission	ICU	Floor	ICU or intermediate care	ICU
Postoperative complications feared	CSF leak, facial paralysis especially with corneal anesthesia, swallowing difficulties	Facial weakness, CSF leak	Facial nerve palsy, cranial nerves V/IX/X/XI neuropathy, brainstem stroke, CSF leak	Cranial nerve palsies namely facial, venous sinus injury, CSF leak, hydrocephalus, brainstem injury
Follow-up testing	MRI within 24 hours after surgery Ophthalmology consult if any facial weakness	MRI 6 months after surgery	CT within 48 hours after surgery Swallowing evaluation MRI 3 months after surgery	CT within 12 hours after surgery MRI within 48 hours after surgery Audiogram 12 weeks after surgery
Follow-up visits	10–14 days after surgery	1 week after surgery	2 weeks after surgery	4–6 weeks after surgery 6 months after surgery
Adjuvant therapies recommended	SRS only for clear evidence of growth	SRS only for clear evidence of growth	SRS only for clear evidence of growth	SRS or repeat resection for clear evidence of growth

AICA, anterior inferior cerebellar artery; BAERs, brainstem auditory evoked response; CSF, cerebrospinal fluid; CT, computed tomography; CTA, computed tomography angiography; EAM, external auditory meatus; EMG, electromyogram; IAC, internal auditory canal; ICU, intensive care unit; IOM, intraoperative monitoring; MCP, middle cerebellar peduncle; MRI, magnetic resonance imaging; PICA, posterior inferior cerebellar artery; SCA, superior cerebellar artery; SRS, stereotactic radiosurgery; VA, vertebral artery.

Differential diagnosis and actual diagnosis

- VS
- Meningioma

Important anatomic and preoperative considerations

For a full discussion of the CPA, petroclival, and clival regions, see Chapters 51, 52, and 66, respectively. The treatment paradigm for VS is controversial and includes observation, surgical resection, and/or radiation therapy (Fig. 68.2).[3–6] The observation option, also called the "wait and scan" approach, has been gaining more momentum, especially for smaller lesions (<1.5 cm; Koos grade I; Table 68.1) that are asymptomatic, as it is associated with avoidance of treatment-related complications (immediate hearing loss, facial nerve dysfunction, cerebrospinal fluid [CSF] leak, headaches, imbalance), identifies the subset of patients who have tumors that are growing, avoids unnecessary treatments, and sustains quality of life, including return to work and continued social well-being; however, its disadvantages include delaying necessary treatments, and is associated with increased surgical risk with increasing tumor size.[15] Some studies have reported that approximately 40% to 50% of patients who present incidentally with good hearing go on to not need surgery, in which 4% to 6% actually experience tumor shrinkage with surveillance.[15] In most "wait and scan" studies, significant growth rate was defined as an increase in the extrameatal diameter by more than 3 mm, in which VS growth rate ranges from 0.4 to 2.9 mm per year.[15] Complicating this issue is that some tumors may grow and then stop.[15] An arbitrary cutoff of 1.5 cm

Table 68.1 **Koos grading system for vestibular schwannoma location**	
Koos Grading System	
I	Intracanalicular
II	Minimal extension into CPA and not reaching brainstem
III	Reaches brainstem surface
IV	Deforming brainstem and fourth ventricular shift

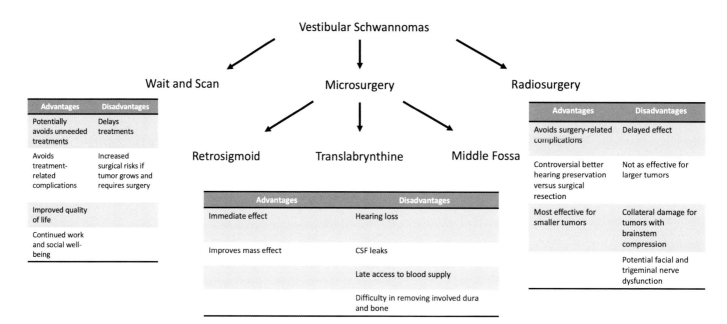

Fig. 68.2 Approaches to vestibular schwannomas. *CSF*, cerebrospinal fluid.

in diameter has been suggested by many because further growth is associated with increased intraoperative complications, namely facial paralysis and hearing loss.[15,16] Tinnitus has been suggested as a factor associated with increased risk of tumor growth.[15,16]

For those pursuing treatment, the options are stereotactic radiosurgery versus microsurgery.[6,17] The selection of which modality is dependent on several variables, including patient demographics, tumor characteristics, and institutional and surgeon preference.[6,17] Different forms of stereotactic radiosurgery exist, which include the Leksell Gamma Knife, Cyberknife, and True Beam that is typically applied to Koos grade I and II tumors because of lack of proximity to the brainstem, delayed radiation response, and concern for treatment-related toxicities with large target volumes (Table 68.1).[6,17] The typical dose is 12 to 14 Gy in a single fraction, but can be given in multiple fractions.[6,17] The 5-year tumor control rates range from 90% to 99%; hearing preservation rates range from 41% to 70% at 5 years, in which early radiation within the first 2 years of diagnosis, smaller tumor size, and pure-tone average differences <10 dB between the ears are associated with preserved hearing; facial nerve perseveration rates of 95% to 100%, and trigeminal preservations rates of 79% to 99%.[6,17] Control rates were better for radiosurgery when the tumor was small (<15 cc) and with no fourth ventricular deviation.[6,17] For tumors that were subtotally resected, tumors did not grow or regressed in 68.5% of tumors without any radiation therapy.[6,17]

Approaches to this lesion

Surgery is typically indicated for tumors that are large with significant mass effect, Koos grade III to IV.[7–14] The typical approaches for VS can be divided into retrosigmoid, middle fossa, and translabyrinthine approaches.[7–14] The retrosigmoid approach involves removing the bone inferior to the transverse sinus and medial to the sigmoid sinus, in which an extended retrosigmoid approach can extend

past these sinuses to facilitate a few more millimeters of dural opening and increased exposure.[18] The advantages of the retrosigmoid approach are that it is the conventional approach for most neurosurgeons, allows wide access and visualization of the trigeminal nerve/lower cranial nerves/posterior fossa vessels, can be used for a variety of tumor sizes, and potentially improved hearing preservation among surgical techniques for smaller tumors, but its drawbacks include decreased visualization of the internal auditory canal (IAC), cerebellar manipulation, and potentially increased risk of CSF leaks and headaches.[18–20] In a meta-analysis, the retrosigmoid approach was associated with gross total resection in 94%, good facial nerve outcomes (House-Brackmann I or II; Table 68.2) in 93% with <1.5-cm tumor, 94% in 1.5- to 3.0-cm tumors, and 70% in >3.0-cm tumors; and serviceable hearing preservation in 46% of <1.5-cm tumors, and 28% in 1.5- to 3.0-cm tumors.[21,22] The middle fossa approach involves a temporal craniotomy and approaching the seventh to eighth nerve complex from the superior surface of the temporal bone by exposing the cisternal, intracanalicular,

Table 68.2 House-Brackmann grading system for facial nerve function		
House-Brackmann Grading System		
I	Normal	Normal facial function in all areas
II	Mild dysfunction	Slight weakness on close inspection
III	Moderate dysfunction	Obvious but not disfiguring, complete eye closure with effort
IV	Moderate-severe dysfunction	Disfiguring, symmetric at rest, incomplete eye closure
V	Severe dysfunction	Asymmetric at rest, barely noticeable movement
VI	Total paralysis	No movement

labyrinthine, and proximal tympanic segment of the facial nerve.[18–20] This approach is generally most useful for small VS (<2.0 cm), primarily intracanalicular, with minimal extension into the posterior fossa.[18–20] The advantages of this approach are that it has higher rates of hearing preservation and provides good decompression of the facial nerve, but its drawbacks are that it requires temporal lobe retraction and poor posterior fossa exposure.[18–20] In a meta-analysis, the middle fossa approach was associated with gross total resection in 97%; good facial outcomes in 97% of patients with tumors <1.5 cm and 83% in patients with >1.5-cm tumors; and serviceable hearing preservation in 56%.[21,22] The translabyrinthine approach involves performing a mastoidectomy with skeletonization of the tegmen, sigmoid sinus, and posterior border of the external auditory canal, entry into the mastoid antrum and identifying the incus and lateral semicircular canal, opening the middle fossa dura in the presigmoid region with usual transection of the endolymphatic sac, identification of the vertical segment of the facial nerve, labyrinthectomy, and opening the dura over the IAC.[18] The advantages of the translabyrinthine approach is direct exposure of the facial nerve and avoiding the need for brain retraction, but its drawbacks include sacrificing of hearing and risk of CSF leak.[18–20] In a meta-analysis, the translabyrinthine approach was associated with gross total resection in 94%; good facial outcomes in 88% of patients with tumors <1.5 cm, 84% in 1.5- to 3.0-cm tumors, and 57% in patients with >3.0-cm tumors; and serviceable hearing preservation in none.[21,22]

In these meta-analyses, for hearing preservation, the middle cranial fossa approach was superior to the retrosigmoid approach for tumors <1.5 cm but not for larger tumors.[21,22] In regard to facial nerve function, the retrosigmoid approach was associated with better outcomes than the middle cranial fossa approach for intracanalicular tumors, middle cranial fossa approach was better than the translabyrinthine approach for tumors <1.5 cm, the retrosigmoid approach was better than the middle cranial fossa and translabyrinthine approaches for tumors 1.5 to 3.0 cm, and the retrosigmoid approach was superior than the translabyrinthine approach for tumors >3.0 cm.[21,22] Postoperative headaches were more significant in the retrosigmoid than translabyrinthine approach, and the incidence of CSF leak was greater in the retrosigmoid than either the middle cranial fossa or translabyrinthine approaches.[21,22] There were no differences in extent of resection, mortality, other cranial nerve dysfunctions, and tumor recurrence among the approaches.[21,22]

What was actually done

The patient was taken to surgery for a left extended retrosigmoid craniectomy with opening of the IAC for a CPA VS with general anesthesia with intraoperative somatosensory evoked potentials, motor evoked potentials, and cranial nerve V, VII to VIII (with facial electromyogram), IX to XI monitoring with neurosurgery and otolaryngology. The patient was induced and intubated per routine. The head was fixed in pins, with two pins over right superior nuchal line and one pin over the left forehead in the midpupillary line. The patient was then placed into the left park bench position. A lazy S incision was planned in the suboccipital region that extended above the pinna down below the lip of the foramen magnum that was about three finger breadths behind the external auditory meatus. The patient was draped in the usual standard fashion and given dexamethasone and cefazolin. The incision was made, a myocutaneous flap was raised, and the skin and muscles were retracted with a cerebellar retractor. A high-speed drill was used to thin the bone overlying the left cerebellar hemisphere and transverse and sigmoid sinuses. The bone was removed with Kerrison punches and Leksell rongeurs so that the entire transverse sigmoid sinuses were exposed. In addition, the lip of the foramen magnum was removed. The dura was opened in a cruciate fashion, with one limb being at the transverse-sigmoid junction. The cisterna magna was opened to decompress the posterior fossa. The microscope was brought in for the remainder of the intradural portion of the case. The cerebellum was retracted medially with cottonoids and dynamic retraction. The jugular foramen cranial nerves were identified and dissected from the tumor margin. The petrosal veins were identified, coagulated, and ligated to identify the superior margin and tentorial edge. The facial nerve stimulator was used to stimulate the dorsal surface of the tumor and confirm the facial nerve was not present. The tumor was debulked internally with an ultrasonic aspirator alternating with capsular dissection from the brainstem until the facial nerve was identified with a facial nerve stimulator from its exit from the brainstem. Preliminary pathology was consistent with a VS. At this point, otolaryngology drilled the IAC until the distal end of the tumor was reached. Dissection of the tumor continued medial to lateral and lateral to medial after identification of the facial nerve in the IAC. The facial nerve was on the anterior side of the tumor. The tumor continued to be debulked until a thin layer was present on the facial nerve, in which it took a right-angle bend to enter the IAC. The facial nerve stimulated at 0.2 mA. This thin layer of tumor was left behind, as it did not dissect easily from the facial nerve. The porous was reconstructed with bone cement. The dura was closed in standard fashion, and cement was used to fill the mastoid air cells. A cranioplasty mesh was used, and the muscle and skin were closed in standard fashion.

The patient awoke at their neurologic baseline with near symmetric facial expression and was taken to the intensive care unit for recovery. Magnetic resonance imaging was done within 48 hours after surgery and showed gross total resection even though there was known residual along the facial nerve (Fig. 68.3). The patient was tapered off dexamethasone over a 10-day period. The patient participated with physical, occupational, and speech therapy and was discharged to home on postoperative day 5 with an intact examination, except for residual left facial numbness, slight left facial weakness (House-Brackmann 2/6 with full eye closure), and absent right hearing. The patient was seen at 2 weeks postoperatively with symmetric facial expression and nearly intact facial sensation but absent hearing, as expected. Final pathology was a VS. The patient was followed with serial magnetic resonance imaging at 3- to 6-month intervals, and no progression of their disease had been noted at 36 months after surgery.

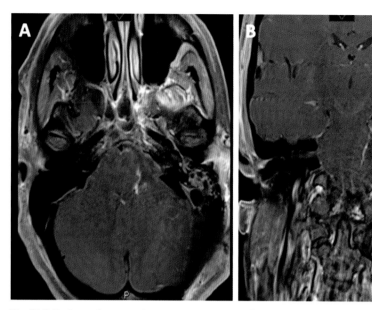

Fig. 68.3 Postoperative magnetic resonance imaging. (A) T1 axial image with gadolinium contrast; **(B)** T1 coronal image with gadolinium contrast magnetic resonance imaging scan demonstrating gross total resection of the lesion.

Commonalities among the experts

The surgeons' preoperative requests varied from audiogram to vestibular testing to computed tomography imaging for boney anatomy prior to surgery. The majority of surgeons would pursue surgery through a left retrosigmoid suboccipital approach. Half of the surgeons would pursue surgery in combination with otolaryngology. Most surgeons aimed for gross total and/or maximal safe resection with decompression of the brainstem with preservation of the facial nerve. Most surgeons were cognizant of the transverse and sigmoid sinuses, cranial nerves IV to XI, and vertebral artery. Surgery was generally pursued with a surgical microscope, intraoperative monitoring of cranial nerves, nerve stimulator, and ultrasonic aspirator, with perioperative steroids. Most surgeons advocated for large boney opening, early decompression of cerebrospinal fluid, early identification of the facial nerves, and internal debulking of tumor. Following surgery, most surgeons admitted their patients to the intensive care unit, and half requested imaging within 48 hours and the other half requested imaging several months after surgery to assess for extent of resection and/or evaluate for complications. Following surgery, all surgeons requested stereotactic radiosurgery only with definitive evidence of tumor growth.

SUMMARY OF QUALITY OF EVIDENCE TO GUIDE SPECIFIC INTERVENTIONS FOR THIS CASE

- Retrosigmoid approach for >3.0-cm VS—Class IIC.
- Near total resection and observation of residual VS—Class III.

REFERENCES

1. Chen H, Xue L, Wang H, Wang Z, Wu H. Differential NF2 gene status in sporadic vestibular schwannomas and its prognostic impact on tumour growth patterns. *Sci Rep.* 2017;7:5470.
2. Acoustic neuroma. *NIH Consens Statement Online.* 1991;9:1–24.
3. Chiluwal AK, Rothman A, Svrakic M, Dehdashti AR. Surgical outcome in smaller symptomatic vestibular schwannomas. Is there a role for surgery. *Acta Neurochir (Wien).* 2018;160: 2263–2275.
4. Daniel RT, Tuleasca C, Rocca A, et al. The changing paradigm for the surgical treatment of large vestibular schwannomas. *J Neurol Surg B Skull Base.* 2018;79:S362–S370.
5. Kaul V, Cosetti MK. Management of vestibular schwannoma (including NF2): facial nerve considerations. *Otolaryngol Clin North Am.* 2018;51:1193–1212.
6. Graham ME, Westerberg BD, Lea J, et al. Shared decision making and decisional conflict in the management of vestibular schwannoma: a prospective cohort study. *J Otolaryngol Head Neck Surg.* 2018;47:52.
7. Matthies C, Samii M. Management of 1000 vestibular schwannomas (acoustic neuromas): clinical presentation. *Neurosurgery.* 1997;40:1–9; discussion 9–10.
8. Matthies C, Samii M. Management of vestibular schwannomas (acoustic neuromas): the value of neurophysiology for evaluation and prediction of auditory function in 420 cases. *Neurosurgery.* 1997;40:919–929; discussion 929–930.
9. Matthies C, Samii M. Management of vestibular schwannomas (acoustic neuromas): the value of neurophysiology for intraoperative monitoring of auditory function in 200 cases. *Neurosurgery.* 1997;40:459–466; discussion 466–468.
10. Samii M, Gerganov VM, Samii A. Functional outcome after complete surgical removal of giant vestibular schwannomas. *J Neurosurg.* 2010;112:860–867.
11. Samii M, Matthies C. Management of 1000 vestibular schwannomas (acoustic neuromas): the facial nerve–preservation and restitution of function. *Neurosurgery.* 1997;40:684–694; discussion 694–695.
12. Samii M, Matthies C. Management of 1000 vestibular schwannomas (acoustic neuromas): surgical management and results with an emphasis on complications and how to avoid them. *Neurosurgery.* 1997;40:11–21; discussion 21–23.
13. Samii M, Metwali H, Samii A, Gerganov V. Retrosigmoid intradural inframeatal approach: indications and technique. *Neurosurgery.* 2013;73:ons53–59; discussion ons60.
14. Samii M, Tatagiba M, Carvalho GA Retrosigmoid intradural suprameatal approach to Meckel's cave and the middle fossa: surgical technique and outcome. *J Neurosurg.* 2000;92:235–241.
15. Zou J, Hirvonen T. "Wait and scan" management of patients with vestibular schwannoma and the relevance of non-contrast MRI in the follow-up. *J Otol.* 2017;12:174–184.

16. Tos M, Charabi S, Thomsen J. Clinical experience with vestibular schwannomas: epidemiology, symptomatology, diagnosis, and surgical results. *Eur Arch Otorhinolaryngol*. 1998;255:1–6.

17. Myrseth E, Moller P, Pedersen PII, Lund-Johansen M. Vestibular schwannoma: surgery or gamma knife radiosurgery? A prospective, nonrandomized study. *Neurosurgery*. 2009;64:654–661; discussion 661–663.

18. Abboud T, Regelsberger J, Matschke J, Jowett N, Westphal M, Dalchow C. Long-term vestibulocochlear functional outcome following retro-sigmoid approach to resection of vestibular schwannoma. *Eur Arch Otorhinolaryngol*. 2016;273:719–725.

19. Yates PD, Jackler RK, Satar B, Pitts LH, Oghalai JS. Is it worthwhile to attempt hearing preservation in larger acoustic neuromas. *Otol Neurotol*. 2003;24:460–464.

20. Brackmann DE, Owens RM, Friedman RA, et al. Prognostic factors for hearing preservation in vestibular schwannoma surgery. *Am J Otol*. 2000;21:417–424.

21. Ansari SF, Terry C, Cohen-Gadol AA. Surgery for vestibular schwannomas: a systematic review of complications by approach. *Neurosurg Focus*. 2012;33:E14.

22. Gurgel RK, Dogru S, Amdur RL, Monfared A. Facial nerve outcomes after surgery for large vestibular schwannomas: do surgical approach and extent of resection matter? *Neurosurg Focus*. 2012;33:E16.

69

Trigeminal schwannomas

Case reviewed by Michael R. Chicoine, William T. Couldwell, Eslam Mohsen Mahmoud Hussein, Graeme F. Woodworth

Introduction

Trigeminal schwannomas are rare benign primary intracranial tumors that arise from Schwann cells that are responsible for the myelin sheath around the nerve axons.[1] They make up 0.1% to 0.4% of all intracranial tumors and 1% to 8% of intracranial schwannomas.[1] These tumors can develop anywhere along the trigeminal nerve from the brainstem origin or the cisternal location to the peripheral divisions of the ophthalmic, maxillary, and mandibular divisions.[2–5] Depending on their origin, these tumors can be intradural, extradural, intracranial, or extracranial.[2–5] As a result, there are a variety of surgical approaches that have been developed for these tumors depending on tumor location, patient characteristics, and surgeon preference.[2–5] In this chapter, we present a case of a patient with a trigeminal schwannoma.

Example case

Chief complaint: headaches and left facial numbness
History of present illness
A 65-year-old, right-handed man with a history of hypertension, hypercholesterolemia, and depression presented with headaches and left facial numbness. For the past 3 to 6 months, he had complained of worsening headaches and numbness in the upper and lower jaw on the left side. He had undergone prior imaging, and there was notable interval growth of a left-sided brain lesion (Fig. 69.1).
Medications: Aspirin, lisinopril, atorvastatin, sertraline.
Allergies: No known drug allergies.
Past medical and surgical history: Hypertension, hypercholesterolemia, depression, appendectomy, right carpal tunnel, left meniscus.
Family history: No history of intracranial malignancies.
Social history: Nurse, no smoking or alcohol.
Physical examination: Awake, alert, oriented to person, place, time; Cranial nerves II to XI, except left V2 to V3 facial numbness; Moves all extremities with good strength.

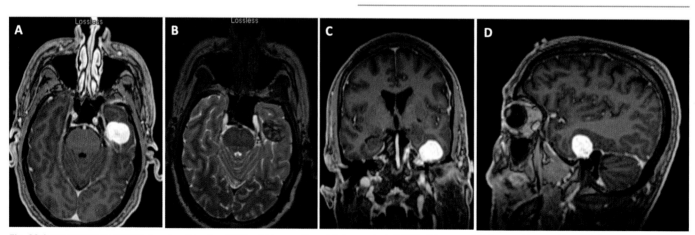

Fig. 69.1 Preoperative magnetic resonance imaging. (A) T1 axial image with gadolinium contrast; **(B)** T2 axial image; **(C)** T1 coronal image with gadolinium contrast; **(D)** T1 sagittal with gadolinium contrast magnetic resonance imaging scan demonstrating an enhancing lesion involving the left middle cranial fossa in close proximity to the Meckel cave.

	Michael R. Chicoine, MD, Washington University, St. Louis, MO, United States	William T. Couldwell, MD, PhD, University of Utah, Salt Lake City, UT, United States	Eslam Mohsen Mahmoud Hussein, MBBS, MSc, Ain Shams University, Cairo, Egypt	Graeme F. Woodworth, MD, University of Maryland, Baltimore, MD, United States
Preoperative				
Additional tests requested	CT and CTA Audiogram	CT	CT EEG Audiogram	CT
Surgical approach selected	Left middle fossa craniotomy with lumbar drain +/– abdominal fat graft	Left middle fossa craniotomy	Left temporal craniotomy with posterior petrosectomy	Left temporal and subtemporal craniotomy
Other teams involved during surgery	ENT	None	ENT	None
Anatomic corridor	Left middle fossa	Left middle fossa, extra- and intradural	Left subtemporal with posterior petrosal	Left subtemporal
Goal of surgery	Maximal resection with preservation of neurologic function, diagnosis	Gross total resection	Radical resection	Gross total resection, diagnosis, nerve preservation
Perioperative				
Positioning	Left supine with right rotation	Left lateral	Left supine with 70-degree right rotation	Left supine with lateral head position
Surgical equipment	Lumbar drain Surgical navigation IOM (SSEP, MEP, EMG of cranial nerves VII–VIII) Surgical microscope Microdoppler	Surgical navigation IOM (SSEP, MEP) Surgical microscope Ultrasonic aspirator	Surgical navigation IOM (SSEP, MEP, EMG of cranial nerves VII-VIII) Surgical microscope Ultrasonic aspirator	Surgical navigation Surgical microscope IOM (SSEP) Ultrasonic aspirator
Medications	Steroids Mannitol Antiepileptics	Steroids Mannitol	Antiepileptics Steroids	Steroids Mannitol Antiepileptics
Anatomic considerations	Superficial temporal artery, temporal bone, floor of middle fossa (arcuate eminence, GSPN, ICA, MMA, cranial nerves V/VII/VIII), vein of Labbe, left temporal lobe	Meckel cave, greater superficial petrosal nerve	Vein of Labbe, greater superficial petrosal nerve, Meckel cave	Temporal lobe, vein of Labbe, optic nerve, trochlear nerve, trigeminal nerve, PCOM
Complications feared with approach chosen	Injury to temporal lobe, vein of Labbe, petrous ICA, cranial nerves V/VII/VIII, CSF leak	Subtotal resection	Temporal lobe venous infarct	Temporal lobe injury, venous infarct
Intraoperative				
Anesthesia	General	General	General	General
Skin incision	Curvilinear preauricular	Linear	Linear	Inverted U over EAM
Bone opening	Left frontotemporal	Left temporal	Left temporal and posterior petrous	Left temporal, subtemporal
Brain exposure	Left temporal lobe	Left temporal lobe	Left temporal	Left temporal lobe

(continued on next page)

	Michael R. Chicoine, MD, Washington University, St. Louis, MO, United States	William T. Couldwell, MD, PhD, University of Utah, Salt Lake City, UT, United States	Eslam Mohsen Mahmoud Hussein, MBBS, MSc, Ain Shams University, Cairo, Egypt	Graeme F. Woodworth, MD, University of Maryland, Baltimore, MD, United States
Method of resection	Placement of lumbar drain, neck and abdomen prepped, myocutaneous flap, frontotemporal craniotomy down to zygoma, extradural dissection of middle fossa, coagulation of MMA and sectioning, identify V3 at foramen rotundum/arcuate eminence/GSPN, petrous ICA, Meckel cave, direction stimulation of GSPN, base of the tumor dissected from cranial nerve V with sharp dissection, additional drilling of petrous bone if needed, dura opened on temporal floor to separate tumor from inferior temporal lobe, tumor debulked, dural closure with dural substitute, obliterate mastoid air cells with fat if needed	Craniotomy centered over root of zygoma, bone wax to tegmen tympani, subtemporal extradural dissection identifying GSPN, enter into Meckel cave, debulk tumor, open temporal dura and debulk more tumor	Left temporal craniotomy, exposure of the Trautman triangle, opening of dura across middle cranial fossa to protect vein of Labbe, division of superior petrosal sinus, resection with tentorium cerebelli, exposure of lateral brainstem, debulking of tumor	Possible lumbar drain, inverted U-shaped incision based on EAM, temporal craniotomy based on navigation that is low to the skull base, cruciate dural opening, relax brain with CSF diversion and gentle brain retraction under microscopic visualization, biopsy and internal debulking of tumor, if frozen reveals radiosensitive tumor then less aggressive approach
Complication avoidance	Lumbar drain, identify skull base anatomy, extradural dissection, sharp dissection from nerves, leave tumor if cannot be separated from nerve, obliterate air cells with fat	Identification of GSPN, bone wax to skull base, intra- and extradural tumor removal	Protect vein of Labbe, expose middle and posterior cranial fossa	Possible lumbar drain, relax brain with CSF drainage early, care taken to avoid venous injury, goal of resection depending on frozen pathology
Postoperative				
Admission	ICU	ICU	ICU	ICU
Postoperative complications feared	Temporal lobe swelling, CSF leak, facial numbness or pain, diplopia, facial weakness, hearing loss, dry eye	CSF leak	Temporal lobe infarction, seizures	Temporal lobe edema, venous infarction, seizures
Follow-up testing	MRI 3–6 months after surgery Audiogram	MRI within 24 hours after surgery	CT immediately after surgery MRI 2 months after surgery	CT immediately after surgery MRI within 24 hours after surgery, 4–6 weeks after surgery
Follow-up visits	2–3 weeks after surgery	1 month after surgery	2 months after surgery	2 weeks, 4–6 weeks after surgery
Adjuvant therapies recommended	Observation vs. SRS	Observation, radiation if regrows	SRS	Observation for small residual, SRS for large residual

CSF, cerebrospinal fluid; CT, computed tomography; CTA, computed tomography angiography; EAM, external auditory meatus; EMG, electromyography; EEG, electroencephalogram; ENT, ear, nose, and throat; GSPN, greater superficial petrosal nerve; ICA, internal carotid artery; ICU, intensive care unit; IOM, intraoperative monitoring; MEP, motor evoked potential; MMA, middle meningeal artery; MRI, magnetic resonance imaging; SRS, stereotactic radiosurgery; SSEP, somatosensory evoked potential.

Differential diagnosis and actual diagnosis

- Trigeminal schwannoma
- Meningioma

Important anatomic and preoperative considerations

The trigeminal nerve is formed by the ophthalmic (V1), maxillary (V2), and mandibular (V3) divisions, in which V1 and V2 are purely sensory and V3 has both sensory and motor components.[6] V1 is formed by the merger of the frontal, lacrimal, nasociliary, tentorial, and dural branches that coalesce posterior to the orbital apex before entering the cavernous sinus.[6] V2 is formed by the merger of the infraorbital, zygomatic, greater and lesser palatine, posterior superior alveolar, and meningeal branches that coalesce in the infraorbital canal and pterygopalatine fossa before entering the foramen rotundum to enter the cavernous sinus.[6] The V1 and V2 divisions travel within the lateral wall of the cavernous sinus and enter the posterior aspect of the Meckel cave.[6] The sensory branches of V3 (lingual, auriculotemporal, inferior alveolar, buccal, and meningeal) merge together in the parapharyngeal space to form the V3 trunk that enters the Meckel cave through foramen ovale.[6] Within the Meckel cave, the merger of three trigeminal divisions form the trigeminal ganglion that divides into multiple individual rootlets to course through the prepontine cistern posteriorly to reach the brainstem.[6] Within the brainstem, the fibers spread out to reach the principal sensory nucleus in the pontine tegmentum for pressure and light touch sensation, the mesencephalic nucleus at the midbrain-pontine junction for proprioception, and the spinal trigeminal nucleus that extends from the pontomedullary junction to the upper cervical spine for pain and temperature sensation.[6] The motor component of the trigeminal nerve arises from the motor nucleus located in the floor of the fourth ventricle, exits the brainstem medial to the sensory components in the prepontine cistern, and enters the Meckel cave where it bypasses the trigeminal ganglion and joins the sensory component of V3 at the skull base to form the mandibular nerve.[6] The motor branch divides into masseteric, deep temporal, medial and lateral pterygoid, mylohyoid branches to innervate masticator muscles, tensor tympani, and tensor veli palatini.[6]

There have been numerous classification schemes to describe the topography of these trigeminal tumors, as they can span several different compartments, including the posterior fossa, middle fossa, and extracranial components (Table 69.1).[2–5,7] Samii et al.[5] described a four-tier system, in which type A tumors are predominantly in the middle fossa, type B in the posterior fossa, type C involves both the middle and posterior fossae, and type D the extracranial space. Yoshida and Kawase[7] had a similar topographic scheme, in which type M involves only the middle fossa, type P only the posterior fossa, type E only the extracranial space, type MP the middle and posterior fossae, type ME the middle fossa and extracranial space, and type MPE in the middle fossa, posterior fossa, and extracranial space.

Table 69.1 Common trigeminal schwannoma tumor location classification schemes

Trigeminal Schwannoma Classification System		
Samii et al.[5]	Yoshida and Kawase[7]	Tumor location
Type A	M	Predominantly middle fossa
Type B	P	Predominantly posterior fossa (CPA)
Type C	MP	Middle and posterior fossae
	E	Extracranial space
	ME	Middle and extracranial fossae
Type D	MPE	Extracranial tumor with intracranial extensions

CPA, Cerebellopontine angle.

Approaches to this lesion

There are a variety of approaches for trigeminal schwannomas because they span several different cranial compartments, and the choice of surgical approach is dependent on tumor location, patient characteristics, surgeon preference, and institutional paradigms.[2–5] Samii et al.[5] used the intradural trans-Sylvian approach for predominantly middle fossa tumors, retrosigmoid suboccipital craniotomy for posterior fossa or cerebellopontine angle tumors, combined temporal craniotomy and presigmoid approach for tumors involving both the middle and posterior fossae, and infratemporal extradural approach for tumors involving the extracranial space. Yoshida and Kawase[7] used the frontotemporal-epidural-interdural approach for isolated middle fossa, lateral suboccipital or anterior transpetrosal for isolated posterior fossa, zygomatic infratemporal for extracranial, anterior transpetrosal for middle and posterior fossae, zygomatic infratemporal or orbitozygomatic infratemporal for middle fossa and extracranial space, and zygomatic transpetrosal for multiple compartment tumors.

What was actually done

The patient was taken to surgery for a left temporal transzygomatic craniotomy for extradural approach to the Meckel cave for resection of the trigeminal schwannoma under general anesthesia, with intraoperative somatosensory evoked potentials, motor evoked potentials, and cranial nerves V, VII (with facial electromyography), and VIII monitoring. The patient was induced and intubated per routine. The head was fixed in pins, with two pins over the inion and one pin over the right forehead in the midpupillary line. The patient was then placed into the left lateral position with the right side down and with the head titled downward. A linear incision was planned from the inferior aspect of the zygoma to above the superior temporal line with the aid of surgical navigation. The patient was draped in the usual standard fashion and given dexamethasone and cefazolin. The incision was made, and an interfascial dissection was done to expose the zygoma. An ultrasonic bone-cutting device was

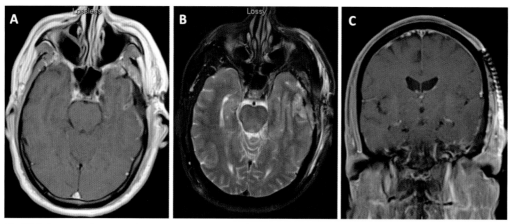

Fig. 69.2 Postoperative magnetic resonance imaging. (A) T1 axial image with gadolinium contrast; **(B)** T2 axial image; **(C)** T1 coronal image with gadolinium contrast magnetic resonance imaging scan demonstrating gross total resection of the lesion.

used to make linear cuts in the zygoma and was left attached to the temporalis muscle on the underside. The temporalis muscle was then deflected inferiorly after forming a myofascial cuff at the superior temporal line. The temporal craniotomy was made, making sure to stay near the temporal floor. The overlying bone was drilled flush with the floor. The microscope was brought in for the remainder of the case. The dura was dissected from the temporal floor, making sure to identify the greater superficial petrosal nerve and dissecting from posterior to anterior. The foramen spinosum was identified along with the middle meningeal artery that was coagulated and cut. The capsule of the tumor was identified and opened. The temporal lobe was retracted with a Greenberg retractor. The tumor was debulked with ultrasonic aspiration between the nerve fibers and removed until no tumor was visible. The temporal bone and zygoma, as well as the muscle and skin, were closed in standard fashion.

The patient awoke at their neurologic baseline with baseline left V2 to V3 numbness and was taken to the intensive care unit for recovery. Magnetic resonance imaging was done within 48 hours after surgery and showed gross total resection (Fig. 69.2). The patient was tapered off of dexamethasone over a 7-day period. The patient participated with physical and occupational therapy and was discharged to home on postoperative day 3 with an intact examination, except for residual left facial numbness. The patient was seen at 2 weeks postoperatively with nearly intact facial sensation. Final pathology was a schwannoma. The patient was followed with serial magnetic resonance imaging at 3- to 6-month intervals, and no progression of their disease had been noted at 36 months after surgery.

Commonalities among the experts

Most of the surgeons requested that the patient undergo head computed tomography to assess boney anatomy, and audiogram to assess baseline hearing prior to surgery. All surgeons would pursue surgery through a left temporal or middle fossa craniotomy with primarily an extradural approach in combination with otolaryngology. Most surgeons aimed for gross total resection. Most surgeons were

cognizant of the greater superficial petrosal nerve and vein of Labbe. Surgery was generally pursued with a surgical navigation, surgical microscope, intraoperative monitoring of cranial nerves, nerve stimulator, and ultrasonic aspirator, with perioperative steroids, mannitol, and antiepileptics. Most surgeons advocated for identification of the greater superficial petrosal nerve, preservation of the vein of Labbe, and extradural dissection. Following surgery, all surgeons admitted their patients to the intensive care unit, and most surgeons requested imaging months after surgery to assess for extent of resection and/or evaluate for complications. Following surgery, most surgeons requested observation versus stereotactic radiosurgery for residual tumor.

SUMMARY OF QUALITY OF EVIDENCE TO GUIDE SPECIFIC INTERVENTIONS FOR THIS CASE

- Middle fossa extradural approach for middle fossa trigeminal schwannoma—Class III.

REFERENCES

1. Chen H, Xue L, Wang H, Wang Z, Wu H. Differential NF2 gene status in sporadic vestibular schwannomas and its prognostic impact on tumour growth patterns. *Sci Rep.* 2017;7:5470.
2. Agarwal A. Intracranial trigeminal schwannoma. *Neuroradiol J.* 2015;28:36–41.
3. Fukaya R, Yoshida K, Ohira T, Kawase T. Trigeminal schwannomas: experience with 57 cases and a review of the literature. *Neurosurg Rev.* 2010;34:159–171.
4. Jefferson G. The trigeminal neurinomas with some remarks on malignant invasion of the gasserian ganglion. *Clin Neurosurg.* 1953;1:11–54.
5. Samii M, Migliori MM, Tatagiba M, Babu R. Surgical treatment of trigeminal schwannomas. *J Neurosurg.* 1995;82:711–718.
6. Joo W, Yoshioka F, Funaki T, Mizokami K, Rhoton Jr AL. Microsurgical anatomy of the trigeminal nerve. *Clin Anat.* 2014;27:61–88.
7. Yoshida K, Kawase T. Trigeminal neurinomas extending into multiple fossae: surgical methods and review of the literature. *J Neurosurg.* 1999;91:202–211.

70

Colloid cyst

Case reviewed by George I. Jallo, Basant K. Misra, Alessandro Olivi, Giuseppe Maria Della Pepa, Gabriel Zada

Introduction

Colloid cysts are rare intracranial tumors that are thought to be derived from an endodermal origin and represent 0.3% to 2% of all brain tumors.[1] They account for 0.5% to 2% of all intracranial tumors, typically diagnosed between the fourth and fifth decade of life, and almost always occur in the third ventricle in close proximity to the foramen of Monro, typically at the anterior roof of the third ventricle.[1-3] These lesions can present with headaches, nausea, vomiting, and some instances of sudden death from obstructive hydrocephalus, whereas a significant percentage present incidentally.[1-3] The traditional treatment of these lesions has included transcallosal or transcortical craniotomy and resection, but other options include endoscopic resection and tubular retractors with either microscopic or exoscopic visualization.[2-8] In this chapter, we present a case of a patient with a colloid cyst.

Example case

Chief complaint: headaches and vision changes
History of present illness
A 22-year-old, right-handed woman with a history of attention deficit disorder presented with headaches and vision changes. She was diagnosed with a colloid cyst 4 years prior during a workup for headaches. However, over the past 3 months, her headaches had worsened with complaints of blurry vision. Repeat imaging showed growth of the lesion from 3 to 7 mm (Fig. 70.1).
Medications: Methylphenidate.
Allergies: No known drug allergies.
Past medical and surgical history: Attention deficit disorder.
Family history: No history of intracranial malignancies.
Social history: College student, no smoking, occasional alcohol.
Physical examination: Awake, alert, oriented to person, place, time; Cranial nerves II to XII; No drift, moves all extremities with good strength.
Ophthalmology: Papilledema bilaterally.

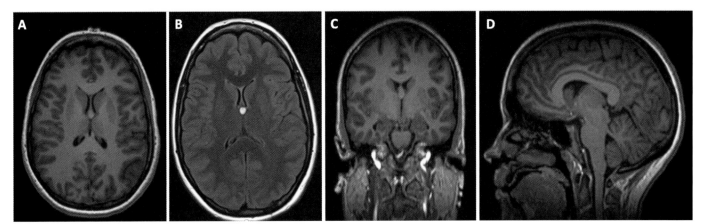

Fig. 70.1 Preoperative magnetic resonance imaging. (A) T1 axial image; **(B)** T2 axial fluid attenuation inversion recovery image; **(C)** T1 coronal image; **(D)** T1 sagittal magnetic resonance imaging scan demonstrating a hyperintense lesion involving the third ventricle near the right foramen of Monro without hydrocephalus.

	George I. Jallo, MD, Johns Hopkins All Children's Hospital, St. Petersburg, FL, United States	Basant K. Misra, MBBS, MS, Hinduja National Hospital, V. S. Marg, Mahim, Mumbai, India	Alessandro Olivi, MD, Giuseppe Maria Della Pepa, MD, Fondazione Policlinco Universitario A. Gemelli IRCSS, Catholic University of Rome, Rome, Italy	Gabriel Zada, MD, University of Southern California, Los Angeles, CA, United States
Preoperative				
Additional tests requested	Neuroophthalmology evaluation	MRV Neuropsychological assessment	Neuroophthalmology evaluation Neuropsychological assessment	DTI Neuropsychological assessment
Surgical approach selected	Right frontal endoscopic resection	Right pericoronal craniotomy and interhemispheric approach with endoscopic assistance	Right frontal endoscopic resection	Right frontal tubular retractor
Anatomic corridor	Right frontal	Right frontal interhemispheric, transcallosal, transforaminal, transchoroidal	Right frontal	Right frontal
Goal of surgery	Extensive resection, opening of foramen of Monro	Complete removal of cyst	Removal of cyst	Complete cyst removal and opening of foramen of Monro
Perioperative				
Positioning	Supine neutral	Supine neutral with 30-degree neck flexion	Supine neutral	Supine neutral
Surgical equipment	Surgical navigation Peel-away catheter Ventricular working-channel endoscope Tissue-biting device	Surgical microscope Endoscope	Ventricular endoscope	Surgical navigation Exoscope Exoscope retractor arm Tubular retractor EVD
Medications	Steroids Antiepileptics	None	Steroids	Steroids Antiepileptics
Anatomic considerations	Fornix, internal cerebral veins, thalamus, thalamostriate veins	Sagittal sinus and draining veins, pericallosal and callosomarginal arteries, corpus callosum, fornix, thalamostriate and septal veins, choroid plexus	Fornix, choroid plexus, septum pellucidum, thalamostriate veins	Fornix, internal cerebral veins, thalamus, thalamostriate veins
Complications feared with approach chosen	Short-term memory deficit, hemorrhage	Seizures, short-term memory deficit, thalamic infarct, pneumoventricle	Short-term memory deficit	Intraventricular hemorrhage
Intraoperative				
Anesthesia	General	General	General	General
Skin incision	Linear	Bicoronal curvilinear	Linear	Linear
Bone opening	Right frontal burr hole	Right fronto-parietal parasagittal $2/3$ in front of coronal suture	Right frontal burr hole	Right frontal
Brain exposure	Right frontal (MFG)	Right frontal	Right frontal (MFG)	Right frontal (MFG)

	George I. Jallo, MD, Johns Hopkins All Children's Hospital, St. Petersburg, FL, United States	Basant K. Misra, MBBS, MS, Hinduja National Hospital, V. S. Marg, Mahim, Mumbai, India	Alessandro Olivi, MD, Giuseppe Maria Della Pepa, MD, Fondazione Policlinco Universitario A. Gemelli IRCSS, Catholic University of Rome, Rome, Italy	Gabriel Zada, MD, University of Southern California, Los Angeles, CA, United States
Method of resection	Burr hole, small corticectomy, introduction of peel-away catheter into lateral ventricle under navigation, introduction of working-channel endoscope, confirm ventricular location, coagulate choroid plexus adjacent to and overlying cyst with monopolar cautery, use side-cutting tissue device to alternate between suction and biting to remove cyst with minimal spillage of cyst contents, attempt gross total resection without damaging fornix, leave EVD	Right pericoronal parasagittal frontoparietal craniotomy $2/3$ anterior to coronal suture, right dural opening based on sagittal sinus with care to preserve all cortical veins, interhemispheric dissection, identify corpus callosum based on white appearance, 1-cm incision in the corpus callosum either in-between or on the side of both pericallosal arteries, enter ventricle, identify ventricular side based on course of choroid plexus, transforaminal access of cyst, decompress cyst with needle, incise cyst wall, complete cyst decompression with avoiding spillage of contents, develop transchoroidal corridor, complete excision of cyst wall from choroid plexus, endoscope to evaluate for completeness of resection and hemorrhage, copious irrigation, watertight dural closure, subgaleal drain	Burr hole, corticectomy, insertion ventricular endoscope, intraventricular orientation and identification of landmarks, piecemeal excision	Frontal craniotomy, dural opening, confirmation of target, sulcal opening, placement of tubular retractor into ventricle, identification of foramen of Monro and colloid cyst, cauterization of choroid plexus, cyst drainage, dissection from internal cerebral veins, cyst removal, +/− EVD, port withdrawal
Complication avoidance	Endoscope, coagulate choroid plexus, EVD	No sacrifice of cortical veins, transcortical approach if interhemispheric is too narrow, interhemispheric approach, endoscope for inspection making sure complete resection and no intraventricular hemorrhage	Endoscope, piecemeal excision	Tubular retractor, cauterization of choroid plexus, dissection of internal cerebral veins
Postoperative				
Admission	ICU	ICU	ICU	ICU
Postoperative complications feared	Short-term memory deficit, hemorrhage	CSF leak, venous infarct, subdural hygroma, hydrocephalus, memory impairment, seizures	Short-term memory deficit, acute hydrocephalus	Hydrocephalus, memory loss, hemiparesis
Follow-up testing	CT immediately after surgery ICP monitoring for 24 hours MRI within 48 hours after surgery	CT within 24 hours after surgery	CT immediately after surgery	MRI within 24 hours after surgery Neuropsychological assessment if needed
Follow-up visits	14 days after surgery, MRI 3 months after surgery	10 days after surgery, MRI 3 months after surgery	10 days after surgery, CT 1 month after surgery, MRI 3 months after surgery	10 days after surgery MRI 3 months after surgery

CSF, cerebrospinal fluid; *CT*, computed tomography; *DTI*, diffusion tensor imaging; *EVD*, external ventricular drain; *ICP*, intracranial pressure; *ICU*, intensive care unit; *MFG*, middle frontal gyrus; *MRI*, magnetic resonance imaging; *MRV*, magnetic resonance venography; *SFG*, superior frontal gyrus.

Differential diagnosis and actual diagnosis

- Colloid cyst
- Central neurocytoma
- Choroid plexus papilloma
- Ependymal cyst
- Subependymal giant cell astrocytoma
- Pilocytic astrocytoma

Important anatomic and preoperative considerations

For a full discussion of the lateral and third ventricles and their approaches, see Chapters 37 and 63, respectively. In brief, the third ventricle communicates with the lateral ventricles through the foramen of Monro.[9] From superior to inferior, the roof of the third ventricle consists of the fornices and hippocampal commissure, superior membrane of the tela choroidea, internal cerebral veins and branches of the medial posterior choroidal arteries within the velum interpositum, and the inferior membrane of the tela choroidea.[9] The superior membrane of the tela choroidea extends laterally to the choroid plexus on the lateral ventricles, and the inferior membrane attaches to the lateral side of the thalamus via the stria medullaris thalami, and is where the choroid plexus along the roof of the third ventricle is attached.[9] Colloid cysts are often attached to the inferior layer of the tela choroidea, and are typically at the anterior edge in close juxtaposition to the foramen of Monro, but can also occur in the middle to posterior region of the third ventricle.[8]

Approaches to this lesion

The most common approaches for colloid cysts are microscopic and endoscopic, with hybrid approaches being more commonly used.[2–8] In the microscopic approaches, the lateral ventricle is accessed through interhemispheric transcallosal or transcortical approaches.[10] The advantages of interhemispheric transcallosal approach are that it avoids cortical injury and potentially seizures and is not dependent on ventricular size, whereas its disadvantages are potential injury to draining veins and potential morbidity from callosal injury.[10] The advantages of the transcortical approach are that it avoids need for microdissection and minimizes risk of cortical venous injury, whereas its disadvantages include dependence on large ventricles and potentially increased risk of seizures from cortical injury.[10] Once the lateral ventricle is identified and the side confirmed, surgery can take place through the foramen of Monro, or the opening can be expanded by opening the choroidal fissure.[10] The choroidal fissure is typically opened on the forniceal side of the fissure, thereby avoiding the veins of the thalamic side and proceeding medially between the internal cerebral veins.[10] In the endoscopic approach, the lateral ventricle is typically entered through a transcortical approach, and surgery takes place through the foramen of Monro.[2,3,6,7] This approach is generally limited to larger ventricles, and more recently techniques to open the choroidal fissure have

expanded the use for middle and posterior third ventricle lesions.[7,8] In comparison studies, they have found that endoscopic approaches were associated with shorter operating room times, shorter hospital stays, and less medical complications than open microscopic approaches in one study,[6] whereas less need for shunting and infections in another study.[2] More recently, a hybrid approach using tubular retractors for resection, which allow bimanual techniques and relatively minimally invasive access, have been described for colloid cysts.[4,5] Similar to endoscopic approaches, this approach is primarily transcortical and requires larger ventricles.[4,5]

What was actually done

The patient was taken to surgery for a right frontal endoscopic-guided resection of the third ventricular colloid cyst with general anesthesia without intraoperative monitoring. The patient was induced and intubated per routine. The head was fixed in neutral position, with two pins centered over the left external auditory meatus and one pin over the right external auditory meatus. The patient's head was flexed and kept neutral. A linear incision was planned in the sagittal plane over the right frontal region over the Kocher point with the use of surgical navigation. The patient was draped in the usual standard fashion and given dexamethasone, levetiracetam, and cefazolin. The incision was made, and the skin was retracted with a Weitlaner retractor. A burr hole was made over the right frontal lobe in the midpupillary line. The dura was opened in a cruciate fashion and cauterized with bipolar cautery. The cortex was cauterized with bipolar cautery, and a small corticectomy was made. A 12F peel-away catheter was placed under navigation guidance into the superficial aspect of the frontal horn of the lateral ventricle. The working channel endoscope was placed into the peel-away catheter with continuous irrigation. The right lateral ventricle was confirmed by identifying the location of the choroid plexus, septal vein, and thalamostriate vein. The colloid cyst was visualized within the foramen of Monro. The choroid plexus was cauterized over the colloid cyst with monopolar cautery. The lesion was identified and was coagulated and removed with a suction/cutting device (Myriad, NICO Corporation, Indianapolis, IN) by first debulking the center of the tumor, and then manipulating the capsule until it was removed. A septum pellucidotomy was done, and the contralateral foramen of Monro was visualized, and no residual colloid cyst was seen. The third ventricle was inspected, and no residual tumor was seen. An external ventricular drain (EVD) was passed into the third ventricle under endoscopic visualization. A burr hole cover was placed with a hole for the EVD, and the galea and skin were closed in standard fashion.

The patient awoke at their neurologic baseline and was taken to the intensive care unit for recovery. Magnetic resonance imaging was done within 48 hours after surgery and showed gross total resection (Fig. 70.2). The EVD was placed for 24 hours at a level of 10 mm Hg, clamped for 24 hours, and then removed. The patient participated with physical and occupational therapy. The

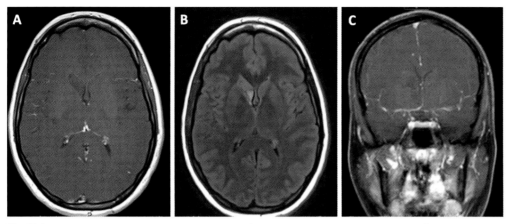

Fig. 70.2 Postoperative magnetic resonance imaging. (A) T1 axial image with gadolinium contrast; **(B)** T2 axial fluid attenuation inversion recovery image; **(C)** T1 coronal image with gadolinium contrast magnetic resonance imaging scan demonstrating gross total resection of the lesion with some edema in the right head of the caudate.

patient was discharged to home on postoperative day 4. The patient was prescribed dexamethasone that was tapered off over 5 days. The patient was seen at 2 weeks postoperatively for suture removal and remained neurologically stable with improved headaches. Pathology was a colloid cyst. The lesion was observed with serial magnetic resonance imaging examinations at 3- to 6-month intervals, and no recurrence was noted at 48 months. The patient's papilledema resolved at 3 months following surgery.

Commonalities among the experts

Most of the surgeons requested that the patient undergo a neuropsychiatry evaluation to assess baseline cognitive function, and ophthalmology evaluation to assess preoperative vision status prior to surgery. All surgeons would pursue surgery, in which the majority would choose a transcortical route through the frontal lobe (two endoscopic, one exoscopic). Most surgeons aimed for gross total removal, with removal of the obstruction of the foramen of Monro. Most surgeons were cognizant of the fornices, thalamostriate, and internal cerebral veins. The most shared feared complication was short-term memory loss and intraventricular hemorrhage. Surgery was generally pursued with a surgical navigation by half and ventricular endoscope, with perioperative steroids and antiepileptics. Most surgeons advocated for use of an endoscope to minimize brain trauma. Half of the surgeons would have left an EVD. Following surgery, all surgeons admitted their patients to the intensive care unit, and most surgeons requested imaging within 48 hours to assess for extent of resection and/or potential complications.

SUMMARY OF QUALITY OF EVIDENCE TO GUIDE SPECIFIC INTERVENTIONS FOR THIS CASE

- Endoscopic resection of colloid cysts—Class II-2.

REFERENCES

1. Beaumont TL, Limbrick Jr., DD. Rich KM, Wippold FJ 2nd, Dacey RG Jr. Natural history of colloid cysts of the third ventricle. *J Neurosurg.* 2016;125:1420–1430.
2. Horn EM, Feiz-Erfan I, Bristol RE, et al. Treatment options for third ventricular colloid cysts: comparison of open microsurgical versus endoscopic resection. *Neurosurgery.* 2008;62:1076–1083.
3. Margetis K, Christos PJ, Souweidane M. Endoscopic resection of incidental colloid cysts. *J Neurosurg.* 2014;120:1259–1267.
4. Eichberg DG, Buttrick SS, Sharaf JM, et al. Use of tubular retractor for resection of colloid cysts: single surgeon experience and review of the literature. *Oper Neurosurg (Hagerstown).* 2019;16:571–579.
5. Eliyas JK, Glynn R, Kulwin CG, et al. Minimally invasive transsulcal resection of intraventricular and periventricular lesions through a tubular retractor system: multicentric experience and results. *World Neurosurg.* 2016;90:556–564.
6. Grondin RT, Hader W, MacRae ME, Hamilton MG. Endoscopic versus microsurgical resection of third ventricle colloid cysts. *Can J Neurol Sci.* 2007;34:197–207.
7. Haider G, Laghari AA, Shamim MS. Choosing between endoscopic or microscopic removal of third ventricle colloid cysts. *J Pak Med Assoc.* 2017;67:1458–1459.
8. Iacoangeli M, di Somma LG, Di Rienzo A, Alvaro L, Nasi D, Scerrati M. Combined endoscopic transforaminal-transchoroidal approach for the treatment of third ventricle colloid cysts. *J Neurosurg.* 2014;120:1471–1476.
9. Rhoton Jr AL. The lateral and third ventricles. *Neurosurgery.* 2002;51:S207–S271.
10. Bozkurt B, Yagmurlu K, Belykh E, et al. Quantitative anatomic analysis of the transcallosal-transchoroidal approach and the transcallosal-subchoroidal approach to the floor of the third ventricle: an anatomic study. *World Neurosurg.* 2018;118:219–229.

71

Cavernoma

Case reviewed by Evandro de Oliveira, Joao Paulo Almeida, Mateus Reghin Neto, Nasser M. F. El-Ghandour, Michael T. Lawton, Isaac Yang

Introduction

Cavernous malformations, also known as cavernomas and cavernous angiomas, account for approximately 5% to 15% of all central nervous system vascular abnormalities.[1] They have an incidence that ranges from 0.2 to 0.6 per 100,000 persons per year, with an annual hemorrhage rate that ranges from 0.5% to 11% per patient-year, but they most often present with seizures (50%) as opposed to acute hemorrhage (25%).[1] They are most common among Hispanic Americans, and most are supratentorial but 10% to 25% occur in the posterior fossa.[1] Most advocate for surgical treatment after one hemorrhage for those lesions that are accessible, whereas inaccessible lesions often must have a few symptomatic hemorrhages before treatment is pursued because of the morbidity associated with treatment.[1] In this chapter, we present a case of a patient with a cavernous malformation involving the right middle cerebellar peduncle (MCP).

Example case

Chief complaint: headaches, nausea, vomiting

History of present illness

A 49-year-old, right-handed woman with a history of hypertension presented with recurrent episodes of headaches, nausea, and vomiting. Over the past 6 months, she had recurrent episodes of severe headaches, nausea, and vomiting. After the first episode, she underwent imaging and was diagnosed with a hemorrhagic right MCP cavernoma. She then had a second episode 3 months later and was diagnosed with a rebleed (Fig. 71.1).

Medications: Lisinopril.

Allergies: No known drug allergies.

Past medical and surgical history: Hypertension, hysterectomy.

Family history: No history of intracranial malignancies.

Social history: Store owner, no smoking, occasional alcohol.

Physical examination: Awake, alert, oriented to person, place, time; Cranial nerves II to XII, except slight right facial droop; No drift, moves all extremities with good strength; Right greater than left finger-to-nose dysmetria.

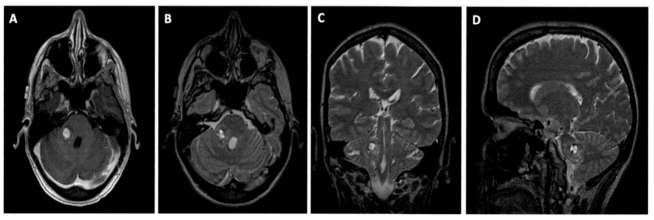

Fig. 71.1 Preoperative magnetic resonance imaging. (A) T1 axial image with gadolinium contrast; **(B)** T2 axial image; **(C)** T2 coronal image; **(D)** T2 sagittal magnetic resonance imaging scan demonstrating a heterogenous lesion within the right middle cerebellar peduncle.

	Evandro de Oliveira, MD, PhD, Joao Paulo Almeida, MD, Mateus Reghin Neto, MD, Institute of Neurological Sciences, São Paulo, SP, Brazil	Nasser M. F. El-Ghandour, MD, Cairo University, Cairo, Egypt	Michael T. Lawton, MD, Barrow Neurological Institute, Phoenix, AZ, United States	Isaac Yang, MD, University of California at Los Angeles, Los Angeles, CA, United States
Preoperative				
Additional tests requested	Transesophageal echocardiogram Anesthesia evaluation	CTA DTI CISS MRI	DTI	Cerebral angiogram MRI with gradient echo Audiogram/VEMP
Surgical approach selected	Midline suboccipital craniotomy	Right retrosigmoid craniotomy	Right retrosigmoid craniotomy for trans-MCP vs. telovelar	Right retrosigmoid craniotomy
Anatomic corridor	Right telovelar	Lateral trans-MCP	Trans-MCP vs. telovelar	Lateral trans-MCP
Goal of surgery	Gross total resection, preservation of neurologic tissue	Gross total resection, prevent future bleeding, diagnosis	Gross total resection	Minimize risk of future bleeding
Perioperative				
Positioning	Semi-sitting	Right park bench	Right lateral	Right supine
Surgical equipment	Surgical table to semi-sitting position Precordial Doppler IOM (BAERs, EMG cranial nerves) Surgical navigation Surgical microscope Brain retractors Nerve stimulator	Surgical navigation Surgical microscope IOM (BAERs, EMG cranial nerves) Nerve stimulator	Surgical navigation Surgical microscope IOM (BAERs, EMG cranial nerves) Nerve stimulator	Surgical navigation Surgical microscope IOM (MEP/SSEP/BAERs/facial EMG) Nerve stimulator
Medications	Steroids	Steroids	Steroids	Steroids
Anatomic considerations	Squamous part of occipital bone, foramen magnum, posterior arch of C1, transverse and sigmoid sinuses, cerebellum, tonsil, biventral lobule, PICA and branches, floor of fourth ventricle, lateral recess, MCP, cranial nerves VII and VIII	Cranial nerves IV–XI, AICA, SCA, vein of superior cerebellopontine fissure	Cranial nerves V–VIII	Cranial nerves VII–VIII, AICA
Complications feared with approach chosen	Injury to pyramidal tract, lateral/medial lemniscus, cranial nerves V/VII/VIII, vascular injury to PICA/AICA/branches, hydrocephalus	Cranial neuropathy, brainstem, or cerebellar injury	Cranial neuropathy, motor deficit	Facial weakness, hearing loss
Intraoperative				
Anesthesia	General	General	General	General
Skin incision	Midline suboccipital from 2 cm above inion to C4	Linear from tip of mastoid to above line connecting zygoma	Linear	Curvilinear C
Bone opening	Bilateral suboccipital including foramen magnum, posterior arch of C1	Right suboccipital	Right suboccipital	Right suboccipital
Brain exposure	Bilateral cerebellar hemispheres/tonsils	Right lateral cerebellar, CPA	Right lateral cerebellar, CPA	Right lateral cerebellar, CPA

(continued on next page)

	Evandro de Oliveira, MD, PhD, Joao Paulo Almeida, MD, Mateus Reghin Neto, MD, Institute of Neurological Sciences, São Paulo, SP, Brazil	Nasser M. F. El-Ghandour, MD, Cairo University, Cairo, Egypt	Michael T. Lawton, MD, Barrow Neurological Institute, Phoenix, AZ, United States	Isaac Yang, MD, University of California at Los Angeles, Los Angeles, CA, United States
Method of resection	Semi-sitting position with precordial Doppler, midline incision, expose fascia, create Y-shaped muscle cuff based at superior nuchal line, midline incision through avascular plane, muscle retraction, suboccipital craniotomy including posterior lip of foramen magnum and C1 lamina, Y-shaped dural opening and retraction with sutures, drain CSF from cisterna magna, dissect tonsils, identify PICA and cerebellomedullary fissure, right tonsil peduncle identified and resected, open tela choroidea and inferior medullary velum to expose ventricular floor, partial resection of biventral lobule to expose lateral recess, incise MCP at superior and lateral portion of lateral recess above seventh/eighth nerve nuclei with stimulating, carful dissection of cavernoma with minimal mobilization of parenchyma and coagulation, spare DVA	Exposure of digastric groove/posterior mastoid/asterion; craniectomy up to transverse and sigmoid sinuses; curvilinear dural opening; arachnoid open for CSF relaxation; identification of cranial nerves starting with XI, then IX and X, and then VII and VIII, followed by V and then IV; exposure of lateral MCP surface, identify and open superior limb of cerebellopontine fissure with vein preservation, identify bulge on MCP and enter sharply, remove lesion with preservation of DVA, watertight dural closure	Right suboccipital craniotomy, exposure of CPA, dissection into CPA, identification of lateral MCP, corticectomy and resection if tracks are medial on DTI, telovelar if tracks are lateral to lesion.	Burr hole over asterion, craniotomy down to mastoid, drill some of mastoid, identify transverse and sigmoid sinus, open dura toward sigmoid sinus, release CSF from cisterna magna, identify cranial nerves VII–VIII and AICA, use surgical navigation and make corticectomy lateral to seventh/eighth nerve complex and AICA and remove lesion
Complication avoidance	Semi-sitting position, protect PICA, resect tonsil and biventral lobule to increase exposure, nerve stimulation to identify corridor, minimize parenchyma manipulation and bipolar cautery	DTI, sharp dissection, identification of anatomic landmarks	DTI, approach dictated by location of tracks	Identify cranial nerves VII and VIII and AICA, corticectomy lateral and away from complex
Postoperative				
Admission	ICU	ICU	ICU	ICU
Postoperative complications feared	Cranial nerves V/VII/VIII deficit, motor/sensory deficit, CSF leak, hydrocephalus	Cranial neuropathies, CSF leak, hydrocephalus	Facial nerve dysfunction, motor deficit	Hearing loss, facial weakness, cerebellar dysfunction
Follow-up testing	MRI within 24 hours after surgery	MRI within 24 hours after surgery	MRI within 24 hours after surgery	MRI within 48 hours after surgery Audiogram 12 weeks after surgery
Follow-up visits	15 days after surgery 6 months after surgery	14 days after surgery 6 weeks after surgery	14 days after surgery 6 weeks after surgery	4–6 weeks after surgery

AICA, anterior inferior cerebellar artery; *BAERs*, brainstem auditory evoked responses; *CISS*, constructive interference in steady state; *CPA*, cerebellopontine angle; *CSF*, cerebrospinal fluid; *CTA*, computed tomography angiography; *DTI*, diffusion tensor imaging; *DVA*, developmental venous anomaly; *EMG*, electromyogram; *ICU*, intensive care unit; *IOM*, intraoperative monitoring; *MCP*, middle cerebellar peduncle; *MEP*, motor evoked potential; *MRI*, magnetic resonance imaging; *PICA*, posterior inferior cerebellar artery; *SCA*, superior cerebellar artery; *SSEP*, somatosensory evoked potential; *VEMP*, vestibular evoked myogenic potential.

Differential diagnosis and actual diagnosis

- Cavernous malformation
- Arteriovenous malformation
- Metastatic brain tumor
- Hemangioblastoma

Important anatomic and preoperative considerations

The management of cavernous malformations is controversial.[2] Symptomatic intracranial hemorrhage (ICH) is the primary concern for these lesions, and is often why many pursue treatment.[2] The recent guidelines state surgery is indicated when there is a symptomatic ICH with acute or subacute onset of symptoms accompanied by radiologic, pathological, surgical, or cerebrospinal fluid evidence of hemorrhage.[2] The 5-year ICH risk is 15.8%, in which the annual hemorrhage risk decreases over time.[2] The risk of a first-time hemorrhage for incidentally discovered lesions is 0.08% per patient-year.[2] Initial presentation with hemorrhage and brainstem location are associated with increased risk of further hemorrhages.[2] In general, the guidelines are conservative management of incidentally discovered cavernous malformations, especially those in eloquent, deep-seated areas; early surgical resection for lesions causing seizures; surgery for symptomatic lesions in accessible locations, surgical resection for deep lesions if symptomatic or after prior hemorrhage; and surgery for brainstem lesions after single disabling bleed.[2] Radiosurgery can be considered for those with symptomatic hemorrhages in eloquent areas in which there is an unacceptably high surgical risk.[2] For those considering surgery, the balance of surgical morbidity and mortality must be weighed against the anticipated survival time for living with a cavernous malformation.[2]

The MCP, also called brachium pontis, are paired structures that connect the cerebellum to the pons, in which fibers originate from the contralateral pontine nucleus, travel through the MCP to the cerebellar hemisphere, and consists of superior, inferior, and deep fasciculi.[3] The MCP conveys impulses from the cerebral cortex to the cerebellum through the corticopontocerebellar tract.[3] Symptoms of MCP injury can include vertigo, vomiting, facial palsy, ataxia, nystagmus, dysphagia, dysarthria, deafness, motor weakness, trigeminal sensory loss, pain, and temperature loss, and even locked-in syndrome.[3] The superior fasciculus is the most superficial of the fasciculi, originates from the upper transverse pontine fibers, and travel posterolaterally to the lobules on the inferior surface of the cerebellar hemisphere.[3] The inferior fasciculus originates from the inferior transverse pontine fibers, passes below the superior fasciculi, and travels posterolaterally to the folia in close proximity to the vermis.[3] The deep fasciculus originates from the deep transverse pontine fibers and travels posterolaterally to the upper anterior cerebellar folia.[3] The superior cerebellar peduncle, also called brachium conjunctivum, is involved in vestibular sensation and proprioception involving the thalamocortical pathways, and consists of paired structures that connect the cerebellum to the midbrain, and the inferior cerebellar peduncles are involved with integrating proprioceptive sensory input and postural maintenance that connects the cerebellum with medulla and spinal cord.[3]

Approaches to this lesion

The approaches to the MCP are varied and include a medial, direct posterior, and lateral approach.[4–8] The medial approach is to enter the fourth ventricle via a midline suboccipital approach with opening the tela choroidea and inferior medullary velum unilaterally or bilaterally to expose the fourth ventricle (see Chapter 13 and 31).[4–8] The pons is localized to identify the MCP, and MCP is opened at its medial aspect.[4] The lateral route involves a retrosigmoid craniotomy, dissection into the cerebellopontine angle, identification of the petrosal fissure, and entry into the MCP through the lateral transpeduncular zone.[4–8] The direct posterior approach involves going through the cerebellar hemisphere to the posterior aspect of the MCP.[4–8] Each approach is dictated by the epicenter of the tumor, in which a more medial lesion in the MCP would be best served by a medial approach as compared with a lateral-based tumor, which would be better served by a lateral approach.[4–8]

What was actually done

The patient was taken to surgery for a right suboccipital transcerebellar approach for the right MCP cavernous malformation with tubular retractor and exoscopic visualization under general anesthesia, with intraoperative monitoring of somatosensory evoked potentials, motor evoked potentials, and cranial nerves V to XII. The patient was induced and intubated per routine. The head was fixed in neutral position, with two pins centered over the left external auditory meatus and one pin over the right external auditory meatus. The patient was placed prone onto chest rolls, with the head flexed and kept in the neutral position. A right paramedian incision was then planned based on surgical navigation. The patient was draped in the usual standard fashion and given dexamethasone and cefazolin. The incision was made, and the skin and muscles were retracted with a Weitlaner retractor. A burr hole was made over the right suboccipital region and expanded to a keyhole with a high-speed drill. The dura was opened in a cruciate fashion and tacked up with sutures. The exoscope was brought in for magnified visualization. A corticectomy was made parallel to the cerebellar folia. Under the navigation and ultrasound guidance, a 65-mm tubular retractor was placed to the superficial aspect of the tumor. At intermittent depths, trajectory was confirmed with an ultrasound. The lesion was identified and removed en bloc. Hemostasis was obtained, and the retractor was withdrawn. Ultrasound was used to confirm gross total resection and no postoperative hematoma. The dura, bone, and skin were closed in standard fashion, in which the bone opening was covered with a large burr hole cover.

The patient awoke at their neurologic baseline and was taken to the intensive care unit for recovery. Magnetic resonance imaging was done within 48 hours after surgery and showed gross total resection (Fig. 71.2). The patient participated with physical and occupational therapy. The patient was discharged to home on postoperative day 3, and was prescribed dexamethasone that was tapered off over 5 days. The patient was seen at 2 weeks postoperatively for suture removal and remained neurologically intact. Pathology was a cavernous malformation. The lesion was observed

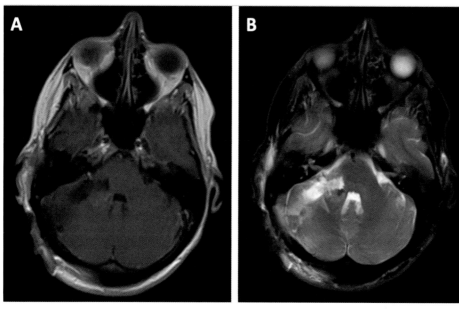

Fig. 71.2 **Postoperative magnetic resonance imaging. (A)** T1 axial image with gadolinium contrast; **(B)** T2 axial magnetic resonance imaging scan demonstrating gross total resection of the lesion.

with serial magnetic resonance imaging examinations at 3- to 6-month intervals, and no recurrence was noted at 48 months.

Commonalities among the experts

Half of the surgeons requested the patient to undergo diffusion tensor imaging to assess for location of white matter tracts prior to surgery. All surgeons would pursue surgery, in which the majority would choose a right retrosigmoid suboccipital craniotomy. Half of the surgeons would pursue surgery through a lateral MCP approach. All surgeons aimed to prevent further rebleeding, and half aimed for gross total resection. Most surgeons were cognizant of cranial nerves V to VIII and cerebellomedullary fissure. The most common shared feared complications were cranial neuropathies and motor deficits. Surgery was generally pursued with a surgical navigation, intraoperative monitoring of the cranial nerves, nerve stimulator, and surgical microscope, with perioperative steroids. Most surgeons advocated for use of diffusion tensor imaging and nerve stimulator to identify a corridor to enter the MCP. Following surgery, all surgeons admitted their patients to the intensive care unit, and all surgeons requested imaging within 48 hours to assess for extent of resection and/or potential complications.

SUMMARY OF QUALITY OF EVIDENCE TO GUIDE SPECIFIC INTERVENTIONS FOR THIS CASE

- Resection of eloquent cavernous malformations after repeated bleeds—Class III.
- Use of tubular retractors for deep-seated lesion—Class III.

REFERENCES

1. Goldstein HE, Solomon RA. Epidemiology of cavernous malformations. *Handb Clin Neurol*. 2017;143:241–247.
2. Akers A, Al-Shahi Salman R, A Awad I, et al. Synopsis of guidelines for the clinical management of cerebral cavernous malformations: consensus recommendations based on systematic literature review by the Angioma Alliance Scientific Advisory Board Clinical Experts Panel. *Neurosurgery*. 2017;80:665–680.
3. Matsushima K, Yagmurlu K, Kohno M, Jr Rhoton AL. Anatomy and approaches along the cerebellar-brainstem fissures. *J Neurosurg*. 2016;124:248–263.
4. Majchrzak H, Tymowski M, Majchrzak K, Stepien T. Surgical approaches to pathological lesions of the middle cerebellar peduncle and the lateral part of the pons: clinical observation. *Neurol Neurochir Pol*. 2007;41:436–444.
5. Abou-Al-Shaar H, Alzhrani G, Gozal YM, Couldwell WT. Retrosigmoid approach for resection of cerebellar peduncle cavernoma. *J Neurol Surg B Skull Base*. 2018;79:S420–S421.
6. Deshmukh VR, Rangel-Castilla L, Spetzler RF. Lateral inferior cerebellar peduncle approach to dorsolateral medullary cavernous malformation. *J Neurosurg*. 2014;121:723–729.
7. Russin J, Fusco DJ, Spetzler RF. Left retrosigmoid craniotomy for cavernous malformation of the middle cerebellar peduncle. *Neurosurg Focus*. 2014;36:1.
8. Wang CC, Liu A, Zhang JT, Sun B, Zhao YL. Surgical management of brain-stem cavernous malformations: report of 137 cases. *Surg Neurol*. 2003;59:444–454; discussion 454.

72

Hemangioblastoma

Case reviewed by Michael R. Chicoine, Evandro de Oliveira, Joao Paulo Almeida, Michael T. Lawton, Gerardo D. Legaspi

Introduction

Hemangioblastomas account for approximately 1.5% to 2.5% of all central nervous system tumors, and 7% to 8% of all posterior fossa tumors, but are the most common primary tumor of the cerebellar hemisphere.[1,2] The majority of posterior fossa hemangioblastomas involve the cerebellar hemispheres (70%), but other locations include the brainstem (24%), cerebellopontine angle (2%), fourth ventricle (2%), and craniocervical junction (2%).[1,2] Single tumors may appear sporadically, whereas patients with multiple tumors typically have von Hippel-Lindau disease.[1,2] Patients can present with symptoms of elevated intracranial pressure, including headaches, nausea, and vomiting, as well as cerebellar symptoms.[1,2] Surgical resection is the standard of care, but surgery can be associated with significant morbidity, including cranial nerve deficits, postoperative hemorrhage, hydrocephalus, pseudomeningocele, meningitis, and

pneumonia, among others.[1,2] In this chapter, we present a case of a patient with a right cerebellar hemisphere hemangioblastoma.

Example case

Chief complaint: headaches, nausea, vomiting
History of present illness
A 24-year-old, right-handed, female graduate student with no significant past medical history presented with headaches, nausea, and vomiting. She was in the laboratory when she developed acute onset of headaches with nausea and vomiting. She denied any loss of consciousness. She saw her primary care physician who ordered brain imaging that revealed a brain lesion (Fig. 72.1). She was started on dexamethasone.
Medications: Dexamethasone, pantoprazole.
Allergies: No known drug allergies.

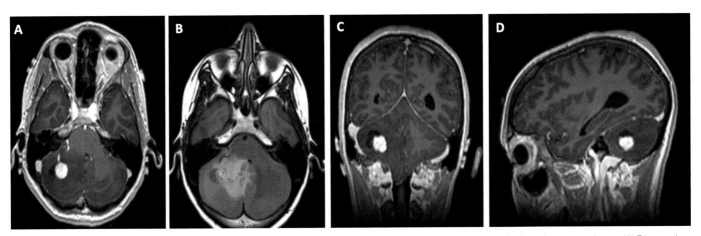

Fig. 72.1 **Preoperative magnetic resonance imaging. (A)** T1 axial image with gadolinium contrast; **(B)** T2 axial fluid attenuation inversion recovery image; **(C)** T1 coronal image with gadolinium contrast; (D) T1 sagittal image with gadolinium contrast magnetic resonance imaging scan demonstrating a homogenously enhancing lesion with perilesional cyst in the right cerebellar hemisphere.

Past medical and surgical history: None.
Family history: No history of intracranial malignancies.
Social history: PhD student, no smoking, no alcohol.
Physical examination: Awake, alert, oriented to person, place, time; Cranial nerves II to XII intact; No drift, moves all

extremities with good strength; Right greater than left finger-to-nose dysmetria.
Imaging: Retinal examination, abdominal ultrasound, and spine imaging negative for lesions.

	Michael R. Chicoine, MD, Washington University, St. Louis, MO, United States	Evandro de Oliveira, MD, PhD, Joao Paulo Almeida, MD, Institute of Neurological Sciences, São Paulo, SP, Brazil	Michael T. Lawton, MD, Barrow Neurological Institute, Phoenix, AZ, United States	Gerardo D. Legaspi, MD, Philippine General Hospital, Manila, Philippines
Preoperative				
Additional tests requested	Urine and serum metanephrines	Transesophageal echocardiogram Anesthesia evaluation	Cerebral angiogram VHL workup	None
Surgical approach selected	Right suboccipital craniotomy	Right suboccipital craniotomy	Preoperative embolization, right suboccipital craniotomy	Right suboccipital craniotomy
Anatomic corridor	Right transcerebellar	Right transcerebellar	Right transcerebellar	Right transcerebellar
Goal of surgery	Gross total resection, diagnosis	Gross total resection, preservation of neurovascular structures	Gross total resection	Gross total resection
Perioperative				
Positioning	Prone with slight left rotation	Semisitting	Right lateral	Right supine with left head rotation
Surgical equipment	Surgical navigation Ultrasound Surgical microscope Aneurysm clips	Semisitting equipment Precordial Doppler IOM (SSEP, MEP) Surgical navigation Ultrasound Surgical microscope Brain retractors	Surgical navigation Surgical microscope with ICG	Lumbar drain Surgical navigation Surgical microscope
Medications	Steroids	Steroids	Steroids	None
Anatomic considerations	Transverse and sigmoid sinuses, cerebellum brainstem, fourth ventricle, CPA	Occipital bone, foramen magnum, transverse and sigmoid sinuses, cerebellum, dentate nucleus, AICA/PICA branches	Sigmoid sinus	Dentate nucleus
Complications feared with approach chosen	Cerebral edema, hydrocephalus, brainstem, or cranial nerve injury	Injury to dentate nucleus, vascular injury to PICA or AICA and branches, hydrocephalus	Neurologic deficit	Cerebellar injury
Intraoperative				
Anesthesia	General	General	General	General
Skin incision	Linear paramedian from transverse sinus to foramen magnum	Hockey stick incision from inion to C2 with lateral extension over superior nuchal line down to mastoid tip	Linear paramedian	Linear retromastoid (~6 cm)

	Michael R. Chicoine, MD, Washington University, St. Louis, MO, United States	Evandro de Oliveira, MD, PhD, Joao Paulo Almeida, MD, Institute of Neurological Sciences, São Paulo, SP, Brazil	Michael T. Lawton, MD, Barrow Neurological Institute, Phoenix, AZ, United States	Gerardo D. Legaspi, MD, Philippine General Hospital, Manila, Philippines
Bone opening	Right retrosigmoid suboccipital	Right lateral suboccipital	Right retrosigmoid suboccipital	Right retrosigmoid suboccipital
Brain exposure	Right cerebellar hemisphere	Right cerebellar hemisphere	Right cerebellar hemisphere	Right cerebellar hemisphere
Method of resection	Right retrosigmoid craniotomy, utilize shortest trajectory to lesion, open dura, circumferential dissection around lesion with coagulation and sectioning of arterial feeders, vascular clips on larger arterial feeders, removal of lesion en bloc	Expose superficial fascia, form muscle cuff, work through avascular plane in the midline, retract muscles, right lateral suboccipital craniotomy with exposure of inferior border of transverse sinus and medial border of sigmoid sinus, inverted C-shaped dural opening near transverse and sigmoid sinus, ultrasound and navigation for localization, corticectomy, dissect tumor from surrounding parenchyma without violating tumor capsule and preserving developmental venous anomaly, watertight closure with muscle interposed	Right retrosigmoid craniotomy, transcerebellar dissection, removal of lesion with attempted en bloc	Lumbar drain placement, localize tumor with surgical navigation, linear retromastoid incision, burr hole and craniotomy, localize lesion with surgical navigation and ICG, radial dural incision, cerebellotomy based on navigation, gross total resection, closure in layers
Complication avoidance	Shortest trajectory, en bloc resection, vascular clips for larger arterial feeders	Semisitting position, ultrasound, and navigation to pinpoint location, avoid violating capsule, preserve developmental venous anomaly	Preoperative embolization, en bloc resection, ICG	ICG and navigation to pinpoint location
Postoperative				
Admission	ICU	ICU	ICU	Floor
Postoperative complications feared	Cerebellar edema, hydrocephalus, brainstem, or cranial nerve injury	Hydrocephalus, cerebellar stroke, CSF leak	Posterior fossa syndrome	Cerebellar edema
Follow-up testing	MRI 3 months after surgery	MRI within 24 hours after surgery Consider genetics referral for VHL	MRI within 24 hours after surgery	None
Follow-up visits	3–4 weeks after surgery	15 days after surgery 6 months after surgery	14 days after surgery 6 weeks after surgery	1 week after surgery

AICA, anterior inferior cerebellar artery; *CPA*, cerebellopontine angle; *CSF*, cerebrospinal fluid; *ICG*, indocyanine green; *ICU*, intensive care unit; *IOM*, intraoperative monitoring; *MEP*, motor evoked potential; *PICA*, posterior inferior cerebellar artery; *SSEP*, somatosensory evoked potentials; *VHL*, von Hippel-Lindau.

Differential diagnosis and actual diagnosis

- Hemangioblastoma
- Arteriovenous malformation
- Cavernous malformation
- Metastatic brain tumor

Important anatomic and preoperative considerations

For a full discussion of cerebellar anatomy, see Chapter 40.

Approaches to this lesion

In a patient with hemangioblastoma, the presence or absence of von Hippel-Lindau disease should be confirmed.[3] This can be done with molecular testing that is nearly 100% accurate.[3] For patients who have positive molecular testing, it is important to identify whether or not they have retinal angiomas, renal cell carcinoma, and/or pheochromocytomas, which can result in severe disability or death.[3] Screening for retinal angiomas involve annual dilated fundoscopic examinations, complete blood counts to evaluate for polycythemia vera, measurement of urinary catecholamine metabolites to detect pheochromocytomas, urinalysis for hematuria, urine cytology for renal cell cancer, and abdominal ultrasounds to evaluate the kidneys, adrenal glands, and pancreas.[3] Suspicious findings should prompt more sensitive imaging, including computed tomography and magnetic resonance imaging (MRI).

The treatment of hemangioblastomas are varied and can include some combination of embolization, surgery, and/or radiation therapy.[1,2,4–6] Angiography can help delineate vascular supply, and in some instances embolization can be done to reduce the vascularity of these lesions.[7] Various options for embolization include Onyx (ethylene-vinyl alcohol copolymer), polyvinyl alcohol, and microspheres, among others.[7] Embolization can minimize vascular feeders to decrease intraoperative blood loss and facilitate surgical resection.[7] The goal of these materials is to penetrate the smaller feeding vessels to reduce inflow to the hypervascular tumor bed.[7] Onyx, also called N-butyl cyanoacrylate, is a liquid embolic agent that polymerizes rapidly when it contacts the blood, and thereby can penetrate small vessels, but is sometimes cost prohibitive.[7] Microspheres aim to penetrate feeding arteries and occlude them before reaching the tumor bed.[7] Complications of embolization include tumoral hemorrhage, malignant edema, and unintended strokes.[7] Stereotactic radiosurgery has also been a recent option for patients with cerebellar hemangioblastomas, especially for those who are poor surgical candidates or high surgical risks.[5,6] Sayer et al.[5] treated 26 hemangioblastomas (17 cerebellar), in which 4 (15%) showed no change in volume, 14 (54%) decreased, and 8 (31%) increased, in which mean duration of tumor control was 51.9 months, and the median progression-free survival was 48.4 months. Complications in these series included hemorrhage, hydrocephalus, and tumor progression.[5] Cervio et al.[4] reported on the

outcomes of 30 patients with cerebellar hemangioblastomas (86% were sporadic cases), in which angiograms were performed in 13% and preoperative embolization in 10%. Gross total resection occurred in 93%; the 7% with subtotal resection had the resection stopped because of intraoperative bleeding, and complications included cerebrospinal fluid leak, pulmonary embolism, meningitis, urinary tract infection, and cerebellar symptoms.[4]

What was actually done

The patient was taken to surgery for a right suboccipital transcerebellar approach for resection of the hemangioblastoma, with tubular retractor and exoscopic visualization under general anesthesia without intraoperative monitoring. The patient was induced and intubated per routine. The head was fixed in neutral position, with two pins centered over the left external auditory meatus and one pin over the right external auditory meatus. The patient was placed prone onto chest rolls, with the head flexed and kept in the neutral position. A right paramedian incision was then planned based on surgical navigation. The patient was draped in the usual standard fashion and given dexamethasone and cefazolin. The incision was made, and the skin and muscles were retracted with a Weitlaner retractor. A burr hole was made over the right suboccipital region and expanded to a keyhole with a high-speed drill. The dura was opened in a cruciate fashion and tacked up with sutures. The exoscope was brought in for magnified visualization. A corticectomy was made parallel to the cerebellar folia. Under the navigation and ultrasound guidance, a 50-mm tubular retractor was placed to the superficial aspect of the tumor. The lesion was identified, coagulated from the surrounding white matter, and removed en bloc. Hemostasis was obtained, and the retractor was withdrawn. Ultrasound was used to confirm gross total resection and no postoperative hematoma. The dura, bone, and skin were closed in standard fashion, in which the bone opening was covered with a large burr hole cover.

The patient awoke at their neurologic baseline and was taken to the intensive care unit for recovery. MRI was done within 48 hours after surgery and showed gross total resection (Fig. 72.2). The patient participated with physical and occupational therapy. The patient was discharged to home on postoperative day 3, and was prescribed dexamethasone that was tapered off over 5 days. The patient was seen at 2 weeks postoperatively for suture removal and remained neurologically intact. Pathology was a hemangioblastoma. The lesion was observed with serial MRI examinations at 3- to 6-month intervals, and no recurrence was noted at 48 months.

Commonalities among the experts

Half of the surgeons requested that the patient undergo workup for von Hippel-Lindau syndrome. All surgeons would pursue surgery, and all would pursue surgery through a right retrosigmoid suboccipital craniotomy, and one would

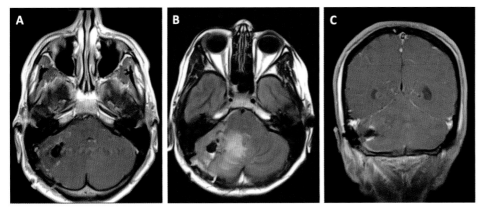

Fig. 72.2 Postoperative magnetic resonance imaging. (A) T1 axial image with gadolinium contrast; **(B)** T2 axial fluid attenuation inversion recovery image; **(C)** T1 coronal image with gadolinium contrast magnetic resonance imaging scan demonstrating gross total resection of the lesion.

pursue preoperative embolization. All surgeons aimed for gross total resection. Most surgeons were cognizant of the transverse and/or sigmoid sinuses. The most common shared feared complications were hydrocephalus and/or cerebellar injury. Surgery was generally pursued with a surgical navigation and surgical microscope with indocyanine green, as well as perioperative steroids. Most surgeons advocated for en bloc resection and indocyanine green. Following surgery, all surgeons admitted their patients to the intensive care unit, and half of the surgeons requested imaging within 24 hours to assess for extent of resection and/or potential complications.

SUMMARY OF QUALITY OF EVIDENCE TO GUIDE SPECIFIC INTERVENTIONS FOR THIS CASE

- Surgical resection of cerebellar hemangioblastomas—Class III.
- Resection of hemangioblastomas through tubular retractors—Class III.

REFERENCES

1. Slater A, Moore NR, Huson SM. The natural history of cerebellar hemangioblastomas in von Hippel-Lindau disease. *AJNR Am J Neuroradiol*. 2003;24:1570–1574.
2. Kuharic M, Jankovic D, Splavski B, Boop FA, Arnautovic KI. Hemangioblastomas of the posterior cranial fossa in adults: demographics, clinical, morphologic, pathologic, surgical features, and outcomes. A systematic review. *World Neurosurg*. 2018;110: e1049–e1062.
3. Feletti A, Anglani M, Scarpa B, et al. Von Hippel-Lindau disease: an evaluation of natural history and functional disability. *Neuro Oncol*. 2016;18:1011–1020.
4. Cervio A, Villalonga JF, Mormandi R, Alcorta SC, Sevlever G, Salvat J. Surgical treatment of cerebellar hemangioblastomas. *Surg Neurol Int*. 2017;8:163.
5. Sayer FT, Nguyen J, Starke RM, Yen CP, Sheehan JP. Gamma knife radiosurgery for intracranial hemangioblastomas—outcome at 3 years. *World Neurosurg*. 2011;75:99–105; discussion 105–108.
6. Silva D, Grabowski MM, Juthani R, et al. Gamma Knife radiosurgery for intracranial hemangioblastoma. *J Clin Neurosci*. 2016;31:147–151.
7. Akinduro OO, Mbabuike N, ReFaey K, et al. Microsphere embolization of hypervascular posterior fossa tumors. *World Neurosurg*. 2018;109:182–187.

73

Brain abscess

Case reviewed by Arturo Ayala-Arcipreste, Bernard R. Bendok, Devi Prasad Patra, Reid C. Thompson, Claudio Gustavo Yampolsky

Introduction

Cerebral abscesses are a suppurative process within the brain parenchyma owing to inflammation and infection.[1–4] The most common locations are the frontal, temporal, parietal, cerebellar, and occipital lobes, which receive the majority of cerebral blood supply.[1–4] The major predisposing factors are an associated contiguous infection in 40% to 50% (otitis media in young children and older adults, paranasal sinusitis in older children and young adults), trauma or iatrogenic in 10%, hematogenous spread in 25%, and cryptogenic in 15%.[1–4] The microbial etiology is dependent on the site of primary infection, in which the most commonly isolated are anaerobes, streptococci, Enterobacteriaceae, and *Staphylococcus aureus*, in which 30% to 60% are polymicrobial.[1–4] Successful treatment of cerebral abscess is dependent on early identification, drainage, and specific antibiotic therapy.[1–4] In this chapter,

we present a case of a patient with a deep-seated, basal ganglia cerebral abscess.

Example case

Chief complaint: headaches and left-sided weakness
History of present illness
A 33-year-old, right-handed woman with no significant past medical history presented with progressive headaches and left-sided weakness. Over the past couple of days, she noted increasing headaches with left arm and leg weakness. She complained of fevers and chills for several days prior. She was seen in the emergency room where imaging revealed a brain lesion (Fig. 73.1).
Medications: None.
Allergies: No known drug allergies.
Past medical and surgical history: None.
Family history: No history of intracranial malignancies.
Social history: Homemaker with two kids, no alcohol, no smoking, no illicit drug use.

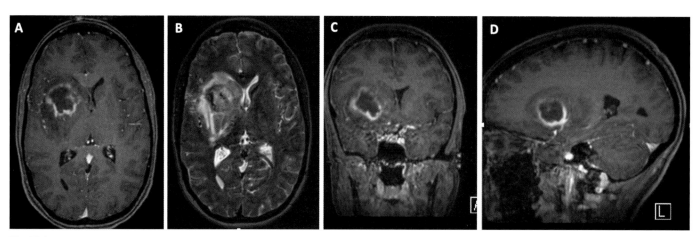

Fig. 73.1 Preoperative magnetic resonance imaging. (A) T1 axial image with gadolinium contrast; **(B)** T2 axial image; **(C)** T1 coronal image with gadolinium contrast; **(D)** T1 sagittal image with gadolinium contrast magnetic resonance imaging scan demonstrating a heterogeneously enhancing lesion within the right basal ganglia.

Physical examination: Awake, alert, oriented to person, place, time; Cranial nerves II to XII intact; Left drift, moves all extremities with good strength, except left upper and lower extremities 4/5.

Imaging: Chest/abdomen/pelvis computed tomography negative for primary lesion.

Labs: Elevated white blood cells (13K), erythrocyte sedimentation rate, C-reactive protein; Blood, urine cultures pending.

	Arturo Ayala-Arcipreste, MD, Hospital Juarez de Mexico, Mexico City, Mexico	Bernard R. Bendok, MD, Devi Prasad Patra, MD, Mayo Clinic, Phoenix, AZ, United States	Reid C. Thompson, MD, Vanderbilt University, Nashville, TN, United States	Claudio Gustavo Yampolsky, MD, Hospital Italiano de Buenos Aires, Buenos Aires, Argentina
Preoperative				
Additional tests requested	MRS DTI CSF analysis HIV serology Neuropsychological assessment	MRS fMRI DTI/DWI	Cardiac echo Panorex x-rays	MRS fMRI DTI Neurooncology evaluation Radiation oncology evaluation
Surgical approach selected	Right frontal stereotactic frame-based needle biopsy and aspiration	Right frontotemporal awake craniotomy with motor cortical and subcortical mapping	Right frontotemporal craniotomy	Right awake frontotemporal craniotomy
Anatomic corridor	Frontal transcortical	Trans-Sylvian, frontal operculum	Trans-Sylvian, transinsular	Trans-Sylvian, trans-opercular
Goal of surgery	Aspiration of purulent material and size reduction	Maximal safe resection, decompression of the lesion	Establish diagnosis, remove enhancing portion, preserve neurologic function especially CST	Maximal safe resection without affecting function
Perioperative				
Positioning	Right supine	Right supine with left head rotation	Right supine left rotation	Right supine left rotation
Surgical equipment	Surgical navigation IOM (SSEP/MEP)	Surgical navigation IOM Surgical microscope	Surgical navigation Surgical microscope Ultrasound	Surgical navigation IOM Monopolar and bipolar brain stimulator Surgical microscope Ultrasonic aspirator
Medications	Steroids Antiepileptics	Steroids Mannitol, hypertonic saline Antiepileptics	Steroids Mannitol Antiepileptics	Steroids Antiepileptics
Anatomic considerations	Frontal lobe, basal ganglia, frontal cortical veins, right lateral ventricle	Sylvian fissure vessels, M2–M3 branches, motor cortex, internal capsule	MCA branches, internal capsule, caudate	MCA M2 branches, internal capsule
Complications feared with approach chosen	Motor deficit, hemorrhage, cerebral edema	Motor deficit, MCA injury	Sylvian vascular injury, motor deficit	Motor deficits
Intraoperative				
Anesthesia	General	General	General	Awake
Skin incision	Right linear	Right pterional	Right pterional	Right pterional
Bone opening	Right frontal	Right frontotemporal	Right frontotemporal	Right frontotemporal
Brain exposure	Right frontal	Right frontotemporal	Right frontotemporal	Right frontotemporal

(continued on next page)

	Arturo Ayala-Arcipreste, MD, Hospital Juarez de Mexico, Mexico City, Mexico	Bernard R. Bendok, MD, Devi Prasad Patra, MD, Mayo Clinic, Phoenix, AZ, United States	Reid C. Thompson, MD, Vanderbilt University, Nashville, TN, United States	Claudio Gustavo Yampolsky, MD, Hospital Italiano de Buenos Aires, Buenos Aires, Argentina
Method of resection	Application of stereotactic headframe with ring parallel to skull base, acquire head CT images, check fiducials, enter coordinates into computer to get coordiantes for frame, attach frame, mark entry point, vertical incision, burr hole with high speed drill, expand burr hole, open dura, visualize cortical surface, avoid vessels, cauterize pia with bipolar, insert needle through burr hole, aspirate abscess with syringe, needle is inserted to different depths until no more purulence is aspirated, needle withdrawn	Myocutaneous flap, right pterional craniotomy with keyhole burr hole, C-shaped dural opening based on sphenoid wing, wide opening of Sylvian fissure anteriorly and posteriorly with care of MCA lenticulostriate perforators with microscopic visualization, motor mapping of frontal and temporal opercula, identify sulcus with negative mapping closest to the lesion in frontal operculum, transsulcal dissection to identify lesion capsule, decompress lesion and biopsy capsule, dissect capsule from surrounding white matter with mapping in deeper location if biopsy negative for malignancy, capsule may be adherent to MCA branches inferomedially, leave layer of capsule along Sylvian fissure if adherent, dura closure with pericranium if needed	Right pterional craniotomy (~5 cm) centered on Sylvian fissure, cruciate dural opening, Sylvian fissure split under microscopic visualization, enter mass directly, if approach unfavorable then through frontal operculum, enter mass and send specimen on nonnecrotic tissue, remove enhancing components along edges if obvious tumor, debulk until normal white matter seen but do not chase deep portions, remove organized wall only if separates easily if abscess, ultrasound and navigation to guide completeness	Scalp block, patient remains awake, right frontotemporal craniotomy, dural opening, cortical mapping for language/motor/cognitive, frontal opercular corticectomy based on negative mapping sites, expose insular cortex, identify M2 perforators and lenticulostriate arteries, resect insular portions of tumor, subcortical mapping to identify CST within internal capsule
Complication avoidance	Stereotactic headframe placement, needle aspiration, avoid sulcal vessels	Cortical and subcortical mapping, Sylvian fissure opening, careful dissection of the capsule from MCA branches	Sylvian fissure opening, intratumoral biopsy to guide further resection, ultrasound	Awake surgery, motor/language. Executive functioning, identify M2 and lenticulostriates, transopercular approach based on negative mapping
Postoperative				
Admission	ICU	Intermediate care	ICU	ICU
Postoperative complications feared	Hemorrhage, edema, motor deficit	Cerebral edema, MCA vasospasm, motor deficit, language dysfunction, meningitis, CSF leak	Hemiplegia, seizures, MCA stroke	Motor deficit
Follow-up testing	CT within 24 hours after surgery MRI 2 weeks after surgery	MRI within 72 hours and 6 weeks after surgery Culture and sensitivity testing	MRI night of surgery	MRI within 24 hours after surgery
Follow-up visits	14 days after surgery	14 days and 6 weeks after surgery	14 days and 6 weeks after surgery	7 days after surgery

5-ALA, 5-aminolevulinic acid; CSF, cerebrospinal fluid; CST, corticospinal tract; CT, computed tomography; DTI, diffusion tensor imaging; fMRI, functional magnetic resonance imaging; ICU, intensive care unit; IOM, intraoperative monitoring; MCA, middle cerebral artery; MEP, motor evoked potential; MRI, magnetic resonance imaging; MRS, magnetic resonance spectroscopy; SSEP, somatosensory evoked potential.

Differential diagnosis and actual diagnosis

- Intracranial abscess
- Metastatic brain tumor
- High-grade glioma
- Lymphoma

Important anatomic and preoperative considerations

For a full discussion of basal ganglia anatomy, see Chapter 36.

Approaches to this lesion

The management of cerebral abscess is varied and include antibiotic therapy only, surgical drainage followed by antibiotic therapy, and surgical excision followed by antibiotic therapy.[1-4] Small abscesses (<2.5 cm) and early cerebritis may respond to antibiotic therapy alone, and patients who are poor surgical candidates may respond to antibiotic therapy, which typically consists of 6 to 8 weeks of intravenous therapy with serial imaging, followed by prolonged oral antibiotics.[1-4] The imaging features typically change after clinical improvement, in which a decrease in the size of the lesion can vary from 1 to 4 weeks, and complete resolution from 1 to 11 months.[1-4] Patients who present with encapsulated lesions, tissue necrosis, multiloculated lesions, and immunocompromised patients typically require 6 to 8 weeks of intravenous antibiotics, followed by 2 to 6 months of oral therapy[1-4] For patients who undergo drainage, this antibiotic course can be shortened to 3 to 4 weeks.[1-4] Drainage can involve needle aspiration, which is typically preferred for deep-seated lesions, or open craniotomy with excision.[3,4] The inherent risk of needle aspiration is inadequate removal, whereas that of open craniotomy is surgical risk and morbidity.[3,4]

What was actually done

The patient was taken to surgery for a right frontal craniotomy for resection of the cerebral abscess with tubular retractor and exoscopic visualization under general anesthesia, with intraoperative somatosensory evoked potentials, motor evoked potentials, and electroencephalogram monitoring. The patient was induced and intubated per routine. The head was fixed in neutral position, with two pins centered over the left external auditory meatus and one pin over the right external auditory meatus. The patient was placed supine with the head neutral and flexed. A linear incision was planned in the sagittal plane over the Kocher point with surgical navigation. The patient was draped in the usual standard fashion and given levetiracetam and dexamethasone, and cefazolin was given after cultures were taken. The incision was made, and the skin was retracted with a Weitlaner retractor. A keyhole craniotomy was made over the right frontal region. The dura was opened in a cruciate fashion and tacked up with sutures. The exoscope was brought in for magnified visualization. The sulcus was opened sharply, and under navigation and ultrasound guidance a 50-mm tubular retractor was placed to the superficial aspect of the lesion. The lesion was identified, the capsule was cauterized, and the materials were cultured and drained. The top and lateral aspects of the capsule were removed, whereas the bottom aspect of the capsule was left adherent to the basal ganglia. Hemostasis was obtained, and the retractor was withdrawn. Ultrasound was used to confirm good resection and no postoperative hematoma. The dura, bone, and skin were closed in standard fashion.

The patient awoke at their neurologic baseline with left-sided weakness and was taken to the intensive care unit for recovery. Magnetic resonance imaging was done within 48 hours after surgery and showed near total resection, with expected residual at the inferior aspect of the lesion (Fig. 73.2). Cultures were positive for streptococci and sensitive for penicillin G. The patient participated with physical and occupational therapy. The patient was discharged to home on postoperative day 3 with an intact examination and a peripherally inserted central catheter and 4 weeks of intravenous antibiotic therapy. The patient was prescribed dexamethasone that was tapered off over 5 days. The patient was seen at 2 weeks postoperatively for staple removal and was neurologically intact with improved left-sided strength. The lesion was observed with serial magnetic resonance imaging at 1 and 6 months after surgery, and there was complete resolution of the cerebral abscess.

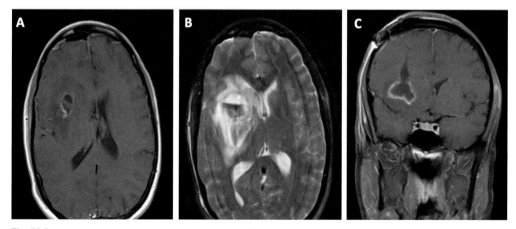

Fig. 73.2 Postoperative magnetic resonance imaging. (A) T1 axial image with gadolinium contrast; **(B)** T2 axial image; **(C)** T1 coronal image with gadolinium contrast magnetic resonance imaging scan demonstrating near total resection of the lesion with residual at the inferior aspect of the surgical cavity.

Commonalities among the experts

The majority of the surgeons requested that the patient undergo diffusion tensor imaging for evaluation of adjacent white matter tracts, and half requested magnetic resonance spectroscopy to better evaluate lesion characteristics, as well as neurooncology and radiation oncology evaluation for possible other etiologies prior to surgery. All surgeons would pursue surgery through a right frontotemporal craniotomy, the majority through a trans-Sylvian approach, and half performing awake motor and language mapping. Most surgeons aimed for maximal safe resection. Most surgeons were cognizant of the frontal and temporal opercula, Sylvian veins and middle cerebral artery vessels and perforators, and the posterior limb of the internal capsule. The most common shared feared complications were Sylvian vein and/or middle cerebral artery injury, as well as motor deficits. Surgery was generally pursued with a surgical navigation, surgical microscope, intraoperative monitoring, and ultrasonic aspirator, with perioperative steroids, antiepileptics, and mannitol. Most surgeons advocated for wide Sylvian fissure opening, monitoring of neurologic function through intraoperative monitoring or mapping, and intralesional debulking.

Following surgery, most surgeons admitted their patients to the intensive care unit, and most surgeons requested imaging within 72 hours to assess for extent of resection and/or potential complications.

SUMMARY OF QUALITY OF EVIDENCE TO GUIDE SPECIFIC INTERVENTIONS FOR THIS CASE

- Surgical resection of intracranial abscess—Class III.

REFERENCES

1. Brook I. Microbiology and treatment of brain abscess. *J Clin Neurosci.* 2017;38:8–12.
2. Calfee DP, Wispelwey B. Brain abscess. *Semin Neurol.* 2000;20: 353–360.
3. Carpenter J, Stapleton S, Holliman R. Retrospective analysis of 49 cases of brain abscess and review of the literature. *Eur J Clin Microbiol Infect Dis.* 2007;26:1–11.
4. Kao PT, Tseng HK, Liu CP, Su SC, Lee CM. Brain abscess: clinical analysis of 53 cases. *J Microbiol Immunol Infect.* 2003;36:129–136.

74

Neurocysticercosis

Case reviewed by Pablo Augusto Rubino, Román Pablo Arévalo, Javier Avendano Mendez-Padilla, Jose Hinojosa Mena-Bernal, Isaac Yang

Introduction

The primary cause of epileptic seizures in less developed countries is neurocysticercosis, which is caused when the larval stage of the pork tapeworm *Taenia solium* infects the central nervous system.[1-4] It is endemic in most of Latin America, sub-Saharan Africa, and Asia, and has become more prominent in developed countries because of migration of people from these endemic areas.[1-4] Humans typically become infected by the fecal-oral route, in which the life cycle of this tapeworm involves development of the tapeworm in the human small intestine after ingesting infected pork and eggs released in the stool, and then humans ingest stool containing the eggs of the tapeworm and the larva develops and disseminates within the human host.[1-4] The clinical presentations of patients with neurocysticercosis include seizures, headaches, and intracranial hypertension, but can occur anywhere throughout the central nervous system and lead to diverse neurologic symptoms.[1-4] The management includes surgery, drainage, and antiparasitic drugs.[1-4] In this chapter, we present a case of a patient with a fourth ventricular neurocysticercosis.

Example case

Chief complaint: headaches and vomiting
History of present illness
A 37-year-old, right-handed man with no significant past medical history presented with progressive headaches and vomiting. Over the past 3 months, he complained of progressive headaches with more frequent nausea and vomiting. He also complained of some lethargy. He went to the emergency room where imaging revealed a brain lesion (Fig. 74.1).
Medications: None.
Allergies: No known drug allergies.
Past medical and surgical history: None.
Family history: No history of intracranial malignances.
Social history: Recent immigrant from Mexico, no smoking, occasional alcohol.

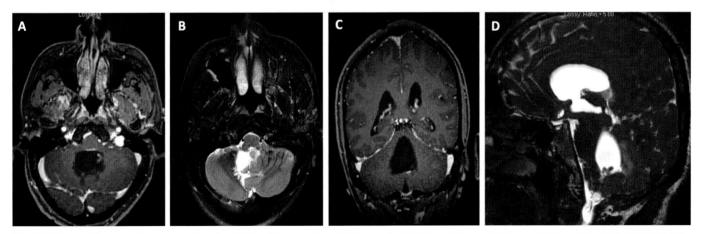

Fig. 74.1 Preoperative magnetic resonance imaging. (A) T1 axial image with gadolinium contrast; **(B)** T2 axial image; **(C)** T1 coronal image with gadolinium contrast; (D) T2 sagittal image magnetic resonance imaging scan demonstrating a lesion in the fourth ventricle with apparent scolex.

Physical examination: Awake, alert, oriented to person, place, time; Cranial nerves II to XII intact; No drift, moves all extremities with good strength; skin examination negative for lesions.

Imaging: Chest/abdomen/pelvis computed tomography negative for lesions, skeletal survey for calcified lesions.
Labs: Elevated eosinophils; blood, urine cultures pending.

	Pablo Augusto Rubino, MD, Román Pablo Arévalo, MD, Hospital El Cruce, Buenos Aires, Argentina	Javier Avendano Mendez-Padilla, MD, National Institute of Neurology and Neurosurgery, Tlalpan, Mexico	Jose Hinojosa Mena-Bernal, MD, PhD, Sant Joan de Deu, Barcelona, Spain	Isaac Yang, MD, University of California at Los Angeles, Long Angeles, CA, United States
Preoperative				
Additional tests requested	None	Western blot for neurocysticercosis PET scan MRI Spectroscopy CSF analysis	Neuroophthalmology evaluation (fundoscopy) CT head Serologic testing	CT head
Surgical approach selected	Suboccipital craniotomy	Suboccipital craniotomy and EVD placement	ETV and endoscopic intraventricular	Suboccipital craniotomy and C1 laminectomy
Anatomic corridor	Telovelar	Telovelar	Right frontal transventricular	Telovelar
Goal of surgery	En bloc removal without cyst disruption, prevent hydrocephalus	Diagnosis, relieve hydrocephalus, restore CSF flow	Removal of cyst, restoration of CSF flow	Resection of lesion, resolve hydrocephalus
Perioperative				
Positioning	Concorde	Prone	Supine neutral	Prone
Surgical equipment	IOM (SSEP, cranial nerve EMG) Surgical microscope	IOM (cranial nerve EMG) Surgical navigation Surgical microscope	Surgical navigation Endoscope with 30-degree lens	Surgical navigation Surgical microscope IOM (SSEP/EEG/MEP)
Medications	Mannitol	None	Steroids	Mannitol Steroids Antiepileptics
Anatomic considerations	Vertebral arteries, both PICA loops, floor of the fourth ventricle	Floor of the fourth ventricle, PICA	Fornix, venous system, mammillary bodies/ hypothalamus/basilar artery, mass intermedia, periaqueductal gray, mesencephalon, fourth ventricular floor and choroid plexus	Floor of fourth ventricle, facial colliculi, PICA
Complications feared with approach chosen	CSF leak	Retraction injury, cranial nerve injury from injury to floor of fourth ventricle, hydrocephalus, hematoma	Avoid posterior fossa craniotomy	Brainstem injury, PICA injury
Intraoperative				
Anesthesia	General	General	General	General
Skin incision	Midline linear	Midline linear	Linear	Midline linear
Bone opening	Midline suboccipital +/– C1 laminectomy	Midline suboccipital	Right frontal burr hole	Right frontal burr hole for EVD
Brain exposure	Cervicomedullary junction	Cervicomedullary junction, cerebellar hemispheres	Right frontal (MFG)	Cervicomedullary junction

	Pablo Augusto Rubino, MD, Román Pablo Arévalo, MD, Hospital El Cruce, Buenos Aires, Argentina	Javier Avendano Mendez-Padilla, MD, National Institute of Neurology and Neurosurgery, Tlalpan, Mexico	Jose Hinojosa Mena-Bernal, MD, PhD, Sant Joan de Deu, Barcelona, Spain	Isaac Yang, MD, University of California at Los Angeles, Long Angeles, CA, United States
Method of resection	Expose squamous part of occipital bones/posterior foramen magnum/posterior arch of C1, exposure of whole craniovertebral junction, medial suboccipital craniotomy +/– C1 laminectomy, Y-shaped dural opening, opening of inferior cerebellar cistern, telovelar opening with splitting of cerebellar amygdala, entry into fourth ventricle, handle cyst with care to not disrupt capsule, continuous irrigation, watertight dural closure	Midline opening, burr holes below transverse sinus bilaterally, craniotomy down to foramen magnum, Y-shaped dural opening, identify tonsils and cerebellomedullary fissure, open tela choroidea and inferior medullary velum, blunt dissection to dissect walls of cyst with continuous irrigation, remove en bloc, watertight dural closure	Entry of endoscope into right lateral ventricle, access to third ventricle and ETV, turn endoscope around to visualize posterior third and aqueduct, navigate to fourth ventricle, grab wall of cyst with endoscopic forceps, careful circular movements with mild retraction, and remove in single piece at same time as endoscope without working channel, visualize cavity, no EVD unless necessary. If cyst adherent, stop procedure and perform midline suboccipital craniotomy telovelar approach	EVD before surgery in supine, prone position for surgery, Y-shaped fascial opening, T-shaped muscle opening, periosteal dissection, C1 laminectomy, suboccipital craniotomy, release CSF from EVD, Y-shaped dural opening, elevate tonsils, telovelar approach, resect tumor, identify patency of aqueduct, watertight dural closure
Complication avoidance	Telovelar opening, continuous irrigation with cyst manipulation, avoid entering cyst, watertight closure	Telovelar opening, continuous irrigation with cyst manipulation, avoid entering cyst, watertight closure	ETV for hydrocephalus, gentle traction on cyst, EVD if surgical issues, stop procedure if cyst adherent	EVD before surgery, release CSF from EVD prior to dural opening, telovelar opening, evaluate patency of ventricular system
Postoperative				
Admission	ICU	ICU	ICU	ICU
Postoperative complications feared	CSF leak	Injury to fourth ventricular floor, CSF leak, arterial injury	Memory loss, injury to fourth ventricular floor	Brainstem injury, PICA injury
Follow-up testing	CT immediately after surgery	MRI within 72 hours after surgery CSF analysis	MRI 1 month after surgery Infectious disease evaluation pending excision results of cyst	CT immediately after surgery MRI within 48 hours after surgery
Follow-up visits	14 days after surgery	14 days and 1 month after surgery	7 days after surgery	3–4 weeks after surgery

CSF, cerebrospinal fluid; *CT*, computed tomography; *EEG*, electroencephalogram; *EMG*, electromyogram; *ETV*, endoscopic third ventriculostomy; *EVD*, external ventricular drain; *ICU*, intensive care unit; *IOM*, intraoperative monitoring; *MEP*, motor evoked potential; *MFG*, middle frontal gyrus; *MRI*, magnetic resonance imaging; *PICA*, posterior inferior cerebellar artery; *SSEP*, somatosensory evoked potential.

Differential diagnosis and actual diagnosis

- Neurocysticercosis
- Arachnoid cyst
- Brain abscess
- Metastatic brain tumors

Important anatomic and preoperative considerations

For a full discussion of fourth ventricular anatomy, see Chapter 13.

Approaches to this lesion

The approaches to fourth ventricular lesions are summarized in Chapter 31, and can be divided into intra- and extraaxial approaches.[5,6] The primary intraaxial approach is a transvermian approach through the vermis.[6] This approach is typically limited to the bottom half of the vermis, as an upper vermian approach is associated with a high risk of cerebellar mutism.[6] The advantages of this approach are that it minimizes potential injury to the posterior inferior cerebellar artery (PICA) vessels and allows upper and fourth ventricular access, but this approach is associated with potential cerebellar mutism and prolonged truncal ataxia.[6] As opposed to an intraaxial approach, an extraaxial approach involves unilateral or bilateral telovelar approaches through a midline suboccipital craniotomy.[5] In this approach, the cerebellar tonsils are retracted laterally, and the tela choroidea and inferior medullary velum are opened.[5] The tela choroidea forms the caudal part of the lower half of the roof of the fourth ventricle, and the inferior medullary velum is a thin sheet of tissue formed by the ependyma and the pia of the tela choroidea, and stretches from the middle cerebellar peduncle to the inferior cerebellar peduncle.[5] The advantages of this approach are that it avoids parenchymal injury and minimizes risk of cerebellar mutism, but it exposes the PICA vessels to potential injury and can have limited visualization of the fourth ventricle.[5]

What was actually done

The patient was taken to surgery for a midline suboccipital craniotomy and C1 laminectomy with bilateral telovelar approach for en bloc resection of fourth ventricular lesion, with general anesthesia and intraoperative monitoring of somatosensory evoked potentials, electroencephalography, and cranial nerves VII, VIII, and XII monitoring. The patient was induced and intubated per routine. The head was fixed in neutral position, with two pins centered over the left external auditory meatus and one pin over the right external auditory meatus. The patient was then placed prone onto chest rolls with the neck flexed and reduced. A midline incision was planned that spanned from just above the inion to the C2 spinous process. The patient was draped in the usual standard fashion and given dexamethasone and cefazolin. A midline incision was made, and dissection took place in the avascular plane between the suboccipital muscles. The skin and muscles were retracted with a cerebellar retractor, and the C1 spinous process and occipital bone with foramen magnum were identified. A suboccipital craniotomy was made below the transverse sinus and incorporated the foramen magnum, and a C1 laminectomy was completed. The dura was opened in a Y-shaped fashion, and the surgical microscope was brought in for the remainder of the case. The arachnoid between the tonsils and the cerebellar hemispheres were opened with sharp dissection, making sure to identify and protect the bilateral PICAs. The tonsils

were then retracted laterally with dynamic retraction without fixed retractors to expose the tela choroidea and inferior medullary velum on the right side followed by the left side. The cyst was encountered, and cottonoids were used to surround the area to minimize spillage of cyst contents. The cyst was dissected from the anterior wall and removed en bloc. The dura, bone, and skin were closed in standard fashion.

The patient awoke at their neurologic baseline with an intact neurologic examination and was taken to the intensive care unit for recovery. Magnetic resonance imaging was done within 48 hours after surgery and showed gross total resection of the lesion (Fig. 74.2). The patient participated with physical and occupational therapy and was discharged to home on postoperative day 2 with an intact neurologic examination. The patient was prescribed dexamethasone that was tapered to off over 10 days after surgery. Infectious disease referral stated no antiparasitic medications because lesion was removed completely and en bloc. The patient was seen at 2 weeks postoperatively for suture removal and remained neurologically intact. Pathology was neurocysticercosis. The patient was seen 3 months later, and imaging revealed no residual lesion.

Commonalities among the experts

Half of the surgeons requested that the patient undergo computed tomography to evaluate for lesion characteristics, namely calcifications, prior to surgery. Most surgeons would pursue surgery through a suboccipital craniotomy and telovelar approach for the lesion. Most surgeons aimed for complete resection of the cyst and restoration of cerebrospinal fluid flow/hydrocephalus. Most surgeons were cognizant of the floor of the fourth ventricle and PICA. The most common shared feared complications were brainstem injuries. Surgery was generally pursued with a surgical navigation and surgical microscope, with perioperative steroids and mannitol. Most surgeons advocated for telovelar opening, avoiding breach of the cyst, and continuous irrigation. Following surgery, all surgeons admitted their patients to the intensive care unit, and most surgeons requested imaging within 72 hours to assess for extent of resection and/or potential complications.

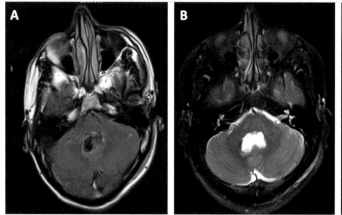
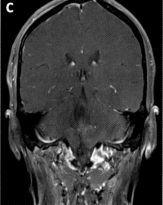

Fig. 74.2 Postoperative magnetic resonance imaging. (A) T1 axial image with gadolinium contrast; **(B)** T2 axial image; **(C)** T1 coronal image with gadolinium contrast magnetic resonance imaging scan demonstrating gross total resection of the fourth ventricular lesion.

SUMMARY OF QUALITY OF EVIDENCE TO GUIDE SPECIFIC INTERVENTIONS FOR THIS CASE

- Surgical resection of neurocysticercosis—Class III.
- Withholding of antiparasitic medications after en bloc resection and no other signs of disease—Class III.

REFERENCES

1. Coyle CM. Neurocysticerosis: an individualized approach. *Infect Dis Clin North Am.* 2019;33:153–168.
2. Del Brutto OH, Garcia HH. Neurocysticercosis. *Handb Clin Neurol.* 2013;114:313–325.
3. Garcia HH, Del Brutto OH. Cysticercosis Working Group in Peru. Antiparasitic treatment of neurocysticercosis—the effect of cyst destruction in seizure evolution. *Epilepsy Behav.* 2017;76:158–162.
4. Garcia HH, Gonzalez AE, Evans CA, Gilman RH. Cysticercosis Working Group in Peru. Taenia solium cysticercosis. *Lancet.* 2003;362:547–556.
5. Tomasello F, Conti A, Cardali S, La Torre D, Angileri FF. Telovelar approach to fourth ventricle tumors: highlights and limitations. *World Neurosurg.* 2015;83:1141–1147.
6. Deshmukh VR, Figueiredo EG, Deshmukh P, Crawford NR, Preul MC, Spetzler RF. Quantification and comparison of telovelar and transvermian approaches to the fourth ventricle. *Neurosurgery.* 2006;58:ONS-202–206; ONS-discussion ONS-206–207.

75

Epidermoid

Case reviewed by Bernard R. Bendok, Devi Prasad Patra, Michael T. Lawton, Reid C. Thompson, Gelareh Zadeh, Farshad Nassiri

Introduction

Epidermoid tumors are also called pearly tumors and cholesteatomas, and are benign tumors that account for approximately 0.1% of all intracranial tumors.[1,2] They typically arise from displaced dorsal ectodermal cell rests during neural tube closure between the third and fifth weeks of embryogenesis.[1,2] These lesions grow by accumulation of keratin and cholesterol from breakdown or desquamation of epithelial cells and tend to grow along the cisternal spaces.[1,2] This growth allows them to reach large sizes before they exert clinically significant mass effect, and typically present with cranial nerve symptoms.[1-5] The goal of surgical treatment is complete resection with preservation of neurologic function, but truly complete resection is challenging, as these lesions are typically adherent to cranial nerves, reach large sizes, and reside in difficult to visualize cisternal spaces.[1-5] The

most common locations are the cerebellopontine angle (CPA) and parasellar locations, in which approximately 40% occur in the CPA.[1,2] In this chapter, we present a case of a patient with a CPA epidermoid.

Example case

Chief complaint: headaches, nausea, imbalance
History of present illness
A 30-year-old, right-handed woman with no significant past medical history presented with progressive headaches, nausea, and imbalance. Over the past 3 months, she complained of progressive headaches with more frequent nausea without vomiting. In addition, she felt as though her coordination was off in which she felt like she was swaying (Fig. 75.1).
Medications: None.
Allergies: No known drug allergies.
Past medical and surgical history: None.

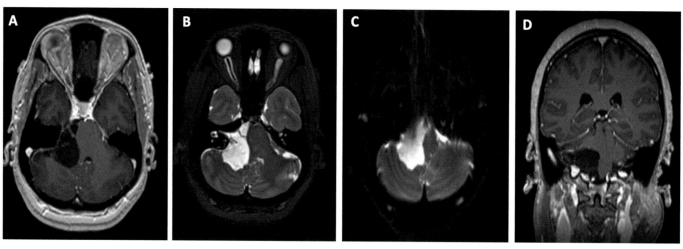

Fig. 75.1 Preoperative magnetic resonance imaging. (A) T1 axial image with gadolinium contrast; **(B)** T2 axial image; **(C)** axial diffusion-weighted image; **(D)** T1 coronal image with gadolinium contrast magnetic resonance imaging scan demonstrating a right cerebellopontine angle nonenhancing lesion that is diffusion bright consistent with an epidermoid.

Family history: No history of intracranial malignancies.
Social history: Restaurant worker, no smoking, occasional alcohol.

Physical examination: Awake, alert, oriented to person, place, time; Cranial nerves II to XII intact; No drift, moves all extremities with good strength; Right greater than left finger-to-nose-dysmetria.

	Bernard R. Bendok, MD, Devi Prasad Patra, MD, Mayo Clinic, Phoenix, AZ, United States	Michael T. Lawton, MD, Barrow Neurological Institute, Phoenix, AZ, United States	Reid C. Thompson, MD, Vanderbilt University, Nashville, TN, United States	Gelareh Zadeh, MD, PhD, Farshad Nassiri, MD, Toronto Western Hospital, Toronto, Canada
Preoperative				
Additional tests requested	Audiogram ENT evaluation Swallow and vocal cord evaluation Anesthesia evaluation	High-resolution MRI	Audiogram Neuro-otology evaluation	Audiogram Neuroophthalmology evaluation CTA/CTV
Surgical approach selected	Right far lateral retrosigmoid craniotomy	Stage 1–Right retrosigmoid craniotomy Stage 2–right pterional craniotomy	Right retrosigmoid craniotomy	Right retrosigmoid craniotomy
Anatomic corridor	Right far lateral retrosigmoid	Right retrosigmoid and right trans-Sylvian	Right retrosigmoid, CPA	Right retrosigmoid, CPA
Goal of surgery	Complete resection with preservation of cranial nerve function	Gross total resection	Maximal resection with preservation of cranial nerve function	Maximal safe resection, decompression of brainstem and neural structures, preservation of lower cranial nerves
Perioperative				
Positioning	Right lateral park bench	Stage 1–Right lateral Stage 2–Right supine	Right park bench	Right park bench
Surgical equipment	Surgical navigation IOM (EMG for facial and lower nerves, BAERs) Surgical microscope Ultrasonic aspirator Doppler	Surgical navigation IOM (EMG for cranial nerves) Surgical microscope	Surgical microscope IOM (cranial nerve VII EMG, BAERs)	Surgical navigation Surgical microscope IOM Doppler
Medications	Steroids Mannitol, hypertonic saline	Steroids	Steroids Mannitol	Steroids Mannitol
Anatomic considerations	Cranial nerves III–XII, PICA, AICA, SCA, PCA, basilar, vertebral, brainstem	Cranial nerves	Cranial nerves arterial branches off of basilar, brainstem, cerebellum	Transverse-sigmoid sinuses, cranial nerves III–XII, mastoid air cells, vertebral artery/AICA/SCA
Complications feared with approach chosen	Hearing loss, facial weakness, lower cranial nerve dysfunction, vasospasm, chemical meningitis, vascular injury to PICA/AICA/veterbral, venous sinus injury, brainstem injury, cerebellar swelling	Cranial neuropathy	Hearing loss, lack of visualization	Cranial nerve injury, venous sinus injury
Intraoperative				
Anesthesia	General	General	General	General
Skin incision	Hockey stick from 1 cm behind mastoid centered at asterion extending to above inion and then below to C2 spinous process	Stage 1–linear Stage 2–pterional	Sigmoid	Sigmoid
Bone opening	Retrosigmoid, suboccipital, right medial one-third occipital condyle, medial posterior arch of C1	Stage 1–retrosigmoid Stage 2–frontotemporal	Retrosigmoid, suboccipital	Retrosigmoid, suboccipital with foramen magnum +/– C1 lamina
Brain exposure	CPA and right cerebellum	Stage 1–CPA and right cerebellum Stage 2–frontotemporal	CPA and right cerebellum	CPA and right cerebellum

(continued on next page)

	Bernard R. Bendok, MD, Devi Prasad Patra, MD, Mayo Clinic, Phoenix, AZ, United States	Michael T. Lawton, MD, Barrow Neurological Institute, Phoenix, AZ, United States	Reid C. Thompson, MD, Vanderbilt University, Nashville, TN, United States	Gelareh Zadeh, MD, PhD, Farshad Nassiri, MD, Toronto Western Hospital, Toronto, Canada
Method of resection	Hockey stick incision, form skin flaps along paraspinal and nuchal muscles, suboccpital bone exposed inferiorly to foramen magnum laterally up to transverse/ sigmoid junction and digastric groove as well as posterior arch of C1 and C2, burr hole made medial and inferior to the asterion with navigation confirmation, second burr hole lateral to midline, craniotomy made after separating dura, bone drilled to expose edges of transverse and sigmoid sinus, coagulate mastoid emissary vein, removal of suboccipital bone and foramen magnum and posterior arch of C1 approximately 1.5 cm from midline, T-shaped dural opening based on transverse-sigmoid sinus, CSF drainage from cisterns and reverse Trendelenburg positioning, separate arachnoid layer over epidermoid with microscopic visualization starting in middle and proceeding superiorly and inferiorly, identify and separate cranial nerves VII/VIII and AICA, separate lower cranial nerves/PICA/vertebral artery from tumor, separate trigeminal nerve and SCA, as well as cranial nerve VI more medially and cranial nerve IV along tentorium, fine dissection from the brainstem with preservation of perforators and veins, careful inspection of cisterns with mirrors and endoscopes, possible intraoperative MRI or CT, primary dural closure with pericranium and fat if necessary	Stage 1–right retrosigmoid craniotomy up to sinuses, dural opening, relaxation of CSF, dissection in CPA, identify cranial nerves IX–XII/VII–VIII/V, work between nerves with resection up to tentorium Stage 2–reposition, right pterional craniotomy, open dura, trans-Sylvian opening, debulk tumor until no residual	Subperiosteal exposure to foramen magnum including transverse-sigmoid junction, suboccipital craniotomy approximately 4 cm, wax mastoid air cells, open dura, enter cisterna magna and relax CSF, minimize retraction on cerebellum but can place fixed brain retractors if necessary, remove epidermoid piecemeal under microscopic visualization, have neuro-otology on standby for tumor in IAC, early identification of cranial nerves VII and VIII, gentle microdissection away from lower cranial nerves, debulk tumor enough to see vasculature including basilar perforators, deliver rostral component if comes easily with awareness of PCA, decompress cranial nerve 5, remove tumor that delivers easily, leave small sheets of tumor along critical neurovasculature structures if difficult to dissect, dural closure with dural substitute	Subcutaneous tissue and muscles divided to expose posterior fossa to level of C2 lamina, harvest pericranial graft for closure, map transverse-sigmoid sinus with navigation, burr hole placed inferomedial to transverse-sigmoid junction and 3-cm craniotomy to level of foramen magnum and exposure of edges of transverse and sigmoid sinuses, removal of foramen magnum +/– C1 laminectomy, wax mastoid air cells, bring microscope in, Y-shaped dural opening, open cisterna magna and drain CSF, no need for retraction of cerebellum, stimulate for facial nerve starting at 1.0 mA and decreasing to 0.1 mA when closer to facial nerve, Doppler to find vertebral artery at craniocervical junction, identify safe entry zone, tumor removal with sequential intracapsular debulking and internal decompression with ultrasonic aspirator and sharp dissection of capsule from arachnoid, frequent stimulation to monitor cranial nerves, leave capsule if adherent to arachnoid, keep arachnoid plane intact, identify interface of tumor and brainstem with care to protect brainstem venous drainage system, removal of IAC component with drilling bone over canal with diamond drill, follow tumor into middle fossa based on path of tumor, identify fourth nerve near incisura, repair IAC with Tisseel, watertight dural closure with pericranium
Complication avoidance	Large bony opening, meticulous dissection of capsule from the neurovascular structures, leave portion of capsule if adherent to neurovascular structures, minimize manipulation of vessels to avoid spasm, inspection with mirrors and endoscopes, intraoperative imaging, use of fat to augment dural closure	Two-stage approach, large bony opening, identification of cranial nerves	Large bony opening, debulk tumor to find critical neurovasculature structures, remove tumor that delivers itself	Large bony opening, frequent stimulation to monitor cranial nerves, leave adherent capsule behind, keep arachnoid plane intact, follow tumor into middle fossa

	Bernard R. Bendok, MD, Devi Prasad Patra, MD, Mayo Clinic, Phoenix, AZ, United States	Michael T. Lawton, MD, Barrow Neurological Institute, Phoenix, AZ, United States	Reid C. Thompson, MD, Vanderbilt University, Nashville, TN, United States	Gelareh Zadeh, MD, PhD, Farshad Nassiri, MD, Toronto Western Hospital, Toronto, Canada
Postoperative				
Admission	Intermediate unit	ICU	ICU	ICU
Postoperative complications feared	Cranial neuropathy, vasospasm, chemical meningitis, hydrocephalus, CSF leak, brainstem injury, significant residual lesion	Cranial neuropathy, meningitis	Cranial neuropathy (facial weakness, hearing loss, dysphagia), CSF leak, chemical meningitis, delayed hydrocephalus	Cranial neuropathies (facial, lower cranial nerves), venous sinus injury, CSF leak, hydrocephalus, injury to brainstem
Follow-up testing	MRI with DWI within 72 hours, 6 months, 1 year after surgery	MRI within 24 hours after surgery	MRI with DWI night of surgery	MRI with DWI within 48 hours after surgery Audiogram 12 weeks after surgery
Follow-up visits	14 days after surgery 6 weeks, 6 months, 1 year after surgery	14 days after surgery 6 weeks after surgery	14 days after surgery 6 weeks after surgery	4–6 weeks after surgery 6 months after surgery

AICA, anterior inferior cerebellar artery; *BAERs*, brainstem auditory evoked responses; *CPA*, cerebellopontine angle; *CSF*, cerebrospinal fluid; *CT*, computed tomography; *CTA*, computed tomography angiogram; *CTV*, computed tomography venogram; *DWI*, diffusion-weighted imaging; *EMG*, electromyography; *ENT*, ear, nose, and throat; *IAC*, internal auditory canal; *ICU*, intensive care unit; *IOM*, intraoperative monitoring; *MRI*, magnetic resonance imaging; *PCA*, posterior cerebral artery; *PICA*, posterior inferior cerebellar artery; *SCA*, superior cerebellar artery.

Differential diagnosis and actual diagnosis

- Epidermoid
- Meningioma
- Schwannoma
- Arachnoid cyst

Important anatomic and preoperative considerations

For a full discussion of the CPA, see Chapter 51.

Approaches to this lesion

As with the anatomic discussion of the CPA in Chapter 51, the most common approaches to the CPA are also described in detail in the same chapter. The most common approaches to the CPA are rectosigmoid, subtemporal, and transtemporal approches.[6–9] The choice of approach to the CPA depends on several features, including lesion characteristics (size, location, extension into surrounding structures), patient characteristics (age, functional status), goals of surgery (biopsy, debulking, gross total resection), and surgeon preference.[6–9] A retrosigmoid approach involves removing the occipital bone below the transverse sinus and medial to the sigmoid sinus, and the approach is lateral to the cerebellum.[10] The advantages of the retrosigmoid approach are its versatility for the posterior fossa, wide exposure of the CPA, and ease of cerebrospinal fluid decompression, whereas its primary disadvantage include difficult to access supratentorial tumor components.[10] The subtemporal approach involves approaching the lesion from a supratentorial corridor with opening the tentorium to access the infratentorial space.[11] The advantage of the subtemporal approach is access to the supra- and infratentorial space concomitantly, whereas the disadvantages include potential injury to the temporal lobe and vein of Labbe, trochlear nerve injury, and difficulty with accessing areas below the line of the interpeduncular fossa.[11] The transtemporal approach involves performing retromastoid and temporal craniotomies, followed by removing the petrous and tympanic bone to expose the intratemporal parts of the facial nerve, petrous internal carotid artery, sigmoid sinus, and jugular bulb.[12] The advantages of this approach are that it minimizes temporal lobe retraction and provides early identification of the facial nerve, whereas its disadvantages include high risk of cerebrospinal fluid leak and loss of hearing.[12]

What was actually done

The patient was taken to surgery for a right suboccipital retromastoid craniectomy for resection of the CPA epidermoid with endoscope assistance under general anesthesia, with intraoperative somatosensory evoked potentials, motor evoked potentials, and cranial nerve V, VII, VIII, IX to XI monitoring. The goal was gross total resection unless adherence to cranial nerves prevented extensive resection. The patient was induced and intubated per routine. The head was fixed in neutral position, with two pins centered over the right external auditory meatus and one pin over the left external auditory meatus. The patient was then placed into the right park bench position. A lazy S-incision was planned in the suboccipital region that extended just above the transverse sinus to just below the foramen magnum. The patient was draped in the usual standard fashion and given dexamethasone and cefazolin. The incision was made, and a myocutaneous flap was made, and the skin and muscles were retracted with a cerebellar retractor. A right suboccipital craniotomy was done by placing a burr hole just medial and inferior to the transverse-sigmoid junction and performing a craniotomy that stayed medial to the sigmoid sinus and inferior to the transverse sinus. Additional bone was removed to expose the bone until the medial aspect of the sigmoid sinus and

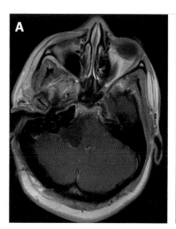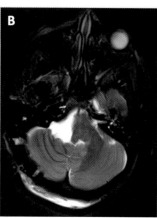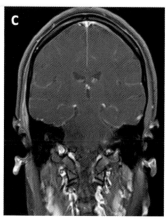

Fig. 75.2 Postoperative magnetic resonance imaging. **(A)** T1 axial image with gadolinium contrast; **(B)** T2 axial image; (C) T1 coronal image with gadolinium contrast magnetic resonance imaging scan demonstrating gross total resection of the cerebellopontine angle lesion.

inferior to the transverse sinus were exposed with a high-speed drill, and the lip of the foramen magnum was left intact. The dura was opened in a cruciate fashion, with one limb being at the transverse-sigmoid junction. The cisterna magna was opened to decompress the posterior fossa. The microscope was brought in for the remainder of the intradural portion of the case. The cerebellum was retracted medially with cottonoids and dynamic retraction. The jugular foramen cranial nerves were identified and dissected from the tumor margin. The petrosal veins were identified, coagulated, and ligated to identify the superior margin and tentorial edge. The facial nerve stimulator was used to stimulate the dorsal surface of the tumor. The tumor was then debulked internally with primarily suction, followed by capsular dissection by working above the trigeminal nerves, in between the trigeminal and facial/vestibulocochlear nerves, and between the seventh/eighth and jugular foramen nerves until no lesion was identified. Angled mirrors and endoscopes were used to confirm gross total resection. Preliminary pathology was epidermoid. The facial nerve was stimulated at 0.1 mA at the end of the case. The dura, bone, and skin were closed in standard fashion.

The patient awoke at their neurologic baseline with an intact examination with intact facial expression and preserved hearing and was taken to the intensive care unit for recovery. Magnetic resonance imaging was done within 48 hours after surgery and showed gross total resection (Fig. 75.2). The patient participated with physical and occupational therapy and was discharged to home on postoperative day 3 with an intact neurologic examination. The patient was prescribed dexamethasone that was tapered to off over 14 days after surgery. The patient was seen at 2 weeks postoperatively for suture removal and remained neurologically intact. Pathology was epidermoid. The patient was observed with serial magnetic resonance imaging examinations at 3 months, followed by 6-month intervals, and has been without tumor recurrence for 36 months.

Commonalities among the experts

Most of the surgeons requested that the patient undergo an audiogram for baseline hearing evaluation, and half requested otolaryngology evaluation for assistance prior to surgery.

Most surgeons would pursue surgery through a right retrosigmoid suboccipital craniotomy for access to the CPA for the lesion. Half of the surgeons aimed for complete resection of the lesion, whereas the other half aimed for maximal safe resection. Most surgeons were cognizant of the lower cranial nerves, posterior inferior cerebellar artery, and anterior inferior cerebellar artery. The most common shared feared complication was cranial neuropathy. Surgery was generally pursued with a surgical navigation, surgical microscope, intraoperative monitoring of the cranial nerves, and Doppler, with perioperative steroids and mannitol. Most surgeons advocated for large boney opening, internal debulking, and frequent nerve stimulation to identify cranial nerves. Following surgery, all surgeons admitted their patients to the intensive care unit, and all surgeons requested imaging within 72 hours to assess for extent of resection and/or potential complications.

SUMMARY OF QUALITY OF EVIDENCE TO GUIDE SPECIFIC INTERVENTIONS FOR THIS CASE

- Surgical resection of epidermoids—Class III.
- Use of endoscope assistance during CPA resection—Class III.

REFERENCES

1. Chowdhury FH, Haque MR, Sarker MH. Intracranial epidermoid tumor; microneurosurgical management: an experience of 23 cases. *Asian J Neurosurg.* 2013;8:21–28.
2. Kobata H, Kondo A, Iwasaki K. Cerebellopontine angle epidermoids presenting with cranial nerve hyperactive dysfunction: pathogenesis and long-term surgical results in 30 patients. *Neurosurgery.* 2002;50:276–285; discussion 285–286.
3. Kalani MYS, Couldwell WT. Retrosigmoid craniotomy for resection of an epidermoid cyst of the posterior fossa. *J Neurol Surg B Skull Base.* 2018;79:S411–S412.
4. Kunigelis K, Yang A, Youssef AS. Endoscopic assisted retrosigmoid approach for cerebellopontine angle epidermoid tumor. *J Neurol Surg B Skull Base.* 2018;79:S413–S414.
5. Vaz-Guimaraes F, Gardner PA, Fernandez-Miranda JC. Endoscope-assisted retrosigmoid approach for cerebellopontine angle epidermoid tumor. *J Neurol Surg B Skull Base.* 2018;79:S409–S410.

6. He X, Liu W, Wang Y, Zhang J, Liang B, Huang JH. Surgical management and outcome experience of 53 cerebellopontine angle meningiomas. *Cureus.* 2017;9:e1538.

7. Matthies C, Carvalho G, Tatagiba M, Lima M, Samii M. Meningiomas of the cerebellopontine angle. *Acta Neurochir Suppl.* 1996;65:86–91.

8. Roberti F, Sekhar LN, Kalavakonda C, Wright DC. Posterior fossa meningiomas: surgical experience in 161 cases. *Surg Neurol.* 2001;56:8–20; discussion 20–21.

9. Sekhar LN, Jannetta PJ. Cerebellopontine angle meningiomas. Microsurgical excision and follow-up results. *J Neurosurg.* 1984;60:500–505.

10. Liebelt BD, Huang M, Britz GW. A comparison of cerebellar retraction pressures in posterior fossa surgery: extended retrosigmoid versus traditional retrosigmoid approach. *World Neurosurg.* 2018;113:e88–e92.

11. Choque-Velasquez J, Hernesniemi J. One burr-hole craniotomy: subtemporal approach in helsinki neurosurgery. *Surg Neurol Int.* 2018;9:164.

12. Sekhar LN, Estonillo R. Transtemporal approach to the skull base: an anatomical study. *Neurosurgery.* 1986;19:799–808.

76

Choroid plexus papilloma

Case reviewed by Lucas Alverne Freitas de Albuquerque, Franco DeMonte, Vicent Quilis-Quesada, Isaac Yang

Introduction

Choroid plexus papillomas (CPPs) are rare tumors that account for less than 1% of intracranial neoplasms, but account for up to 20% of the tumors in the first year of life.[1-3] Most of these tumors arise within the ventricles, with the lateral ventricles being the most common; however, these tumors can also involve the extraventricular space.[1-3] The typical approach for these lesions is complete resection, and in some instances chemotherapy and radiation therapy.[1-3] In a single institutional experience, the 5-year local control was 84%, distal brain control was 92%, and overall survival was 97%, in which gross total resection was associated with improved local control but not overall survival.[3] Even after subtotal resection, only 50% of patients had recurrence requiring additional therapy.[3] Although these tumors are associated with favorable outcomes following complete resection, they tend to recur both locally and distally with disseminated disease along the neuraxis.[1-3] In this chapter, we present a case of a patient with a recurrent left cervicomedullary CPP.

Example case

Chief complaint: headaches, nausea, vomiting
History of present illness
A 36-year-old, right-handed woman with multiple CPPs status post temporal intraventicular gross total resection 4 years prior, and fourth ventricular subtotal resection 2 years prior, with concern of recurrence. All the prior surgeries were done at an outside hospital, and 2 years prior she underwent subtotal resection of the fourth ventricular lesion followed by radiation therapy. On serial imaging, this lesion has increased in size with increasing hydrocephalus and headaches, nausea, and vomiting, as well as imbalance (Fig. 76.1).
Medications: None.
Allergies: No known drug allergies.

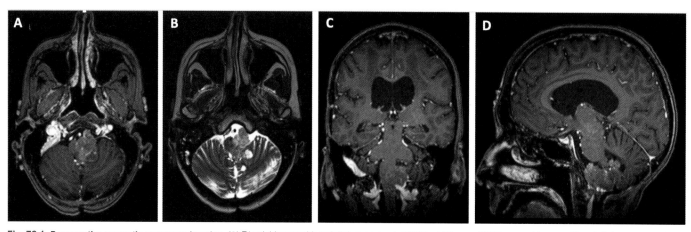

Fig. 76.1 Preoperative magnetic resonance imaging. (A) T1 axial image with gadolinium contrast; **(B)** T2 axial image; **(C)** T1 coronal image with gadolinium contrast; **(D)** T1 sagittal image with gadolinium contrast magnetic resonance imaging scan demonstrating a left cervicomedullary heterogeneously enhancing lesion that extends into the fourth ventricle and ventral aspect of the medulla.

Past medical and surgical history: Temporal horn CPP resection 4 years prior, fourth ventricular CPP 2 years prior with postoperative radiation therapy.
Family history: No history of intracranial malignancies.
Social history: Teacher, no smoking, no alcohol.

Physical examination: Awake, alert, oriented to person, place, time; Cranial nerves II to XII intact, except left House-Brackmann 2/6; No drift, moves all extremities with good strength; Left greater than right finger-to-nose dysmetria.
Spinal imaging: No evidence of drop metastases.

	Lucas Alverne Freitas de Albuquerque, MD, Hospital Geral de Fortaleza, Ceara, Brazil	Franco DeMonte, MD, MD Anderson Cancer Center, Houston, TX, United States	Vicent Quilis-Quesada, MD, PhD, University of Valencia, Valencia, Spain	Isaac Yang, MD, University of California at Los Angeles, Long Angeles, CA, United States
Preoperative				
Additional tests requested	Cerebral angiogram Audiogram Anesthesiology evaluation Ophthalmology evaluation Genetic evaluation	Spine MRI Neurooncology evaluation Radiation oncology evaluation CSF analysis Speech pathology for swallowing function	CT angiography Spinal MRI	Cerebral angiogram CT head MRI with CISS protocol
Surgical approach selected	Left extreme lateral craniotomy	Right frontal ventriculoperitoneal shunt	Left far lateral craniotomy	Left far lateral craniotomy
Anatomic corridor	Left extreme lateral	Right frontal transcortical	Left far lateral	Left far lateral
Goal of surgery	Maximal safe resection	Relief of hydrocephalus	GTR	Debulking of tumor, relief of hydrocephalus
Perioperative				
Positioning	Park bench	Right supine	Semisitting	Left lateral
Surgical equipment	IOM (SSEP, MEP, cranial nerves VII–XII EMG) Doppler Surgical microscope Ultrasonic aspirator	Shunt system with programmable valve and possible intrathecal chemotherapy	IOM (SSEP, MEP, cranial nerves EMG VII–XII) Surgical microscope Ultrasonic aspirator Echocardiogram	IOM (SSEP, BAERs, cranial nerve EMG V/VII–VIII/XI–XII) Surgical navigation
Medications	Steroids Hypertonic saline	None	Steroids	Steroids Mannitol Antiepileptics
Anatomic considerations	Vertebral artery, lower cranial nerves	Kocher point	Vertebral/basilar artery and branches, lower cranial nerves, brainstem	Left vertebral, PICA, AICA, basilar artery
Complications feared with approach chosen	Injury to lower cranial nerves, vascular injury, hemiparesis	Shunt malposition or malfunction	Vascular and cranial nerve injuries	Posterior circulation vessel injury
Intraoperative				
Anesthesia	General	General	General	General
Skin incision	Left hockey stick	Right frontal curvilinear	Fishhook shape from 5 cm below mastoid tip to superior nuchal line and 5 cm below EOP	Left hockey stick from midline C2 to inion to mastoid
Bone opening	Left suboccipital with foramen magnum, C1 hemilaminectomy, occipital condyle	Right frontal burr hole	Left suboccipital with foramen magnum, C1 hemilaminectomy, occipital condylectomy	Left suboccipital with foramen magnum, C1 hemilaminectomy, 1/3 left occipital condyle
Brain exposure	Left lateral cerebellar surface	Right frontal	Left cerebellopontine angle	Left cerebellopontine angle

(continued on next page)

	Lucas Alverne Freitas de Albuquerque, MD, Hospital Geral de Fortaleza, Ceara, Brazil	Franco DeMonte, MD, MD Anderson Cancer Center, Houston, TX, United States	Vicent Quilis-Quesada, MD, PhD, University of Valencia, Valencia, Spain	Isaac Yang, MD, University of California at Los Angeles, Long Angeles, CA, United States
Method of resection	Park bench position, convert midline linear incision into left hockey stick, muscle layers above suboccipital triangle retracted as a single flap, leave myofascial pad attached to the superior nuchal line, expose suboccipital triangle and identify vertebral artery and C1 root, lateral suboccipital craniotomy, left C1 hemilaminectomy, extradural transcondylar resection to expose anterior craniocervical junction, resection 2/3 to 1/2 of occipital condyle, dural opening, identify cranial nerves, vascular inspection with Doppler, resection tumor, watertight dural closure, subcutaneous drain	Right frontal burr hole, tunneling of catheter in subcutaneous space, insertion into frontal horn of lateral ventricle, placement of distal catheter into peritoneum	Dissection of suboccipital triangle with vertebral artery exposure, left suboccipital craniotomy from midline to sigmoid sinus, opening of foramen magnum with C1 hemilaminectomy, dural opening following sigmoid sinus, cisterna magna opening and release of CSF, posterior fossa relaxation, exposure of tumor and dissection of lower cranial nerves/vertebral artery/PICA, total resection of cisternal part of tumor prior to fourth ventricle	EVD before surgery, position in left lateral, C1 laminectomy, suboccipital craniotomy, drill 1/3 of left occipital condyle, open dura toward left, debulk tumor and decompress brainstem and fourth ventricle, watertight dural closure
Complication avoidance	Extreme lateral transcondylar approach, resect less than 1/2 of occipital condyle	Avoiding surgery for disseminated disease	IOM, dissection of suboccipital triangle for identification of vertebral artery, cisterna magna opening, dissection of critical neurovascular structures from tumor	EVD prior to surgery, IOM, far lateral craniotomy, debulk tumor
Postoperative				
Admission	ICU	Floor	ICU	ICU
Postoperative complications feared	Dysphagia, facial paresis, vascular injury, CSF leak, hydrocephalus	Shunt malfunction or malposition, infection	Vascular and cranial nerve injury	Posterior circulation injury, inadequate decompression of brainstem, hydrocephalus
Follow-up testing	MRI within 48 hours after surgery Speech therapy	CT and shunt survey after surgery	MRI within 48 hours after surgery	MRI within 48 hours after surgery
Follow-up visits	14 days, 1 and 3 months after surgery	7–10 days after surgery	4–6 weeks after surgery	3–4 weeks after surgery
Adjuvant therapies recommended	STR–radiosurgery GTR–observation	Chemotherapy +/− reirradiation	STR–+/− radiation GTR–observation	STR–fractionated radiotherapy GTR–observation

AICA, anterior inferior cerebellar artery; *BAERs*, brainstem auditory evoked responses; *CISS*, constructive interference in steady state; *CSF*, cerebrospinal fluid; *CT*, computed tomography; *EMG*, electromyogram; *EOP*, external occipital protuberance; *EVD*, external ventricular drain; *GTR*, gross total resection; *ICU*, intensive care unit; *IOM*, intraoperative monitoring; *MEP*, motor evoked potential; *MRI*, magnetic resonance imaging; *PICA*, posterior inferior cerebellar artery; *SSEP*, somatosensory evoked potential; *STR*, subtotal resection.

Differential diagnosis and actual diagnosis

- CPP
- Ependymoma
- Metastatic brain tumor

Important anatomic and preoperative considerations

For a full discussion of the cervicomedullary anatomy, see Chapter 54.

Approaches to this lesion

As discussed in Chapter 54, the approaches to foramen magnum lesions can be categorized into posterior, posterolateral, anterolateral, and anterior approaches.[4–7] The posterior approach is a midline suboccipital craniotomy with or without cervical laminectomies, in which this approach is familiar to most surgeons, minimizes pain by dissecting in the avascular plane, and is minimally destabilizing, whereas its disadvantages are limited access to the lateral and ventral aspects of the cervicomedullary junction, potential need for cervicomedullary manipulation, and potential difficulty in identifying the vertebral artery, especially where it enters the dura at the V2/V3 junction.[4] The posterolateral approach is the far lateral transcondylar approach, in which this approach provides more posterolateral access to the cervicomedullary junction with bone removal to minimize cervicomedullary manipulation, and identifies the V2/V3 segment of the vertebral artery early for vascular control, but can be associated with potential vertebral artery injury, spinal instability, and cervical pain from muscular dissection.[8] The anterolateral approach is an extreme lateral transcondylar approach, in which this approach provides good lateral and anterolateral visualization of the cervicomedullary junction and minimizes the need for retraction and manipulation, but can be an unfamiliar approach, with potential vertebral artery injury, especially with transposition, and spinal instability.[9,10] The anterior approach is the transoral-transclival approach, in which this approach obviates the need for brain retraction and keeps critical neural and vascular structures laterally and posteriorly, but is associated with increased risk of wound dehiscence, cerebrospinal fluid leak, unfamiliarity, and small working corridors.[10]

What was actually done

Spinal magnetic resonance imaging (MRI) was done and showed no drop lesions. The patient was taken to surgery for midline suboccipital craniotomy with left far lateral transcondylar extension for resection of the cervicomedullary recurrent CPP, with general anesthesia and intraoperative motor evoked potentials, somatosensory evoked potentials, and cranial nerve VII to XII monitoring. The patient was induced and intubated per routine. The head was fixed with two pins over the left external auditory meatus and one pin over the right external auditory meatus. The patient was then placed into the prone position on chest rolls. The prior midline linear incision was identified and extended from the inion down to the C2 spinous process. The patient was draped in the usual standard fashion and given dexamethasone and cefazolin. The incision was made, and the suboccipital muscles were dissected in the avascular plane. The skin and muscles were retracted with a cerebellar retractor. A high-speed drill was used to extend the prior suboccipital defect to include the foramen magnum and a C1 laminectomy. A left far lateral transcondylar extension was done by identifying the vertebral artery at the sulcus arteriosus with Doppler ultrasound and drilling the occipital condyle until the bone was removed lateral to the lateral margin of the dura at the cervicomedullary junction. The dura was opened in the midline and angled to the left at the superior and inferior aspects of the opening to allow the dura to retract to the left. The microscope was brought in for the remainder of the intradural portion of the case. The nerve stimulator was used to identify cranial nerve XI, which was dorsal to the lesion. The dentate ligament and dorsal C1 nerve roots were identified and sectioned to allow access to the tumor. The tumor was debulked internally with an ultrasonic aspirator, followed by capsular dissection. Preliminary pathology was CPP. Alternating tumor debulking and capsular dissection was done until the tumor was removed. There was a portion of the tumor adherent to the pial medullary surface and was cauterized and left in place. The dura, bone, and skin were closed in standard fashion.

The patient awoke with an intact neurologic examination and was taken to the intensive care unit for recovery. An MRI was done within 48 hours after surgery and showed subtotal resection of the tumor, with known residual adherent to the medulla (Fig. 76.2). The patient participated

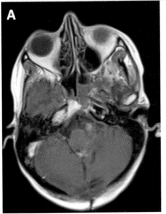 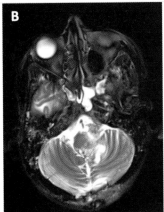 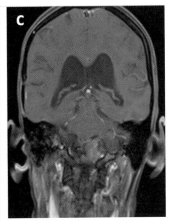

Fig. 76.2 Postoperative magnetic resonance imaging. **(A)** T1 axial image with gadolinium contrast; **(B)** T2 axial image; **(C)** T1 coronal image with gadolinium contrast magnetic resonance imaging scan demonstrating subtotal total resection of the cervicomedullary lesion with residual along the ventral aspect of the medulla.

with physical, occupational, and speech therapy and was discharged to home on postoperative day 5 with an intact neurologic examination. The patient was prescribed dexamethasone that was tapered to off over 10 days after surgery. The patient was seen at 2 weeks postoperatively for suture removal and remained neurologically intact. Pathology was an atypical CPP (World Health Organization grade II). The patient underwent postoperative radiation therapy of the residual lesion at 4 weeks after surgery. The patient was observed with serial MRI examinations at 3 months, followed by 6-month intervals, and has been without tumor recurrence for 36 months.

Commonalities among the experts

Most of the surgeons requested that the patient undergo vascular imaging to better characterize vascular supply and vascularity of the lesion, and half requested spinal MRI to evaluate for drop lesion prior to surgery. Most surgeons would pursue surgery through a left far lateral transcondylar approach. Most surgeons aimed for maximal safe resection and relief of hydrocephalus. Most surgeons were cognizant of the lower cranial nerves, as well as the vertebral and basilar arteries. The most common shared feared complications were lower cranial neuropathy and vascular injury. Surgery was generally pursued with a surgical microscope, intraoperative monitoring of the cranial nerves, and ultrasonic aspirator, with perioperative steroids and diuretics. Most surgeons advocated for large boney opening with far lateral transcondylar approach and internal debulking. Following surgery, most surgeons admitted their patients to the intensive care unit, and most surgeons requested imaging within 48 hours to assess for extent of resection and/or potential complications.

SUMMARY OF QUALITY OF EVIDENCE TO GUIDE SPECIFIC INTERVENTIONS FOR THIS CASE

- Surgical resection of recurrent CPP—Class III.
- Radiation for residual atypical CPP—Class III.

REFERENCES

1. Bettegowda C, Adogwa O, Mehta V, et al. Treatment of choroid plexus tumors: a 20-year single institutional experience. *J Neurosurg Pediatr.* 2012;10:398–405.
2. Cannon DM, Mohindra P, Gondi V, Kruser TJ, Kozak KR. Choroid plexus tumor epidemiology and outcomes: implications for surgical and radiotherapeutic management. *J Neurooncol.* 2015;121:151–157.
3. Krishnan S, Brown PD, Scheithauer BW, Ebersold MJ, Hammack JE, Buckner JC. Choroid plexus papillomas: a single institutional experience. *J Neurooncol.* 2004;68:49–55.
4. Bernard F, Lemee JM, Delion M, Fournier HD. Lower third clivus and foramen magnum intradural tumor removal: the plea for a simple posterolateral approach. *Neurochirurgie.* 2016;62:86–93.
5. Bruneau M, George B. Foramen magnum meningiomas: detailed surgical approaches and technical aspects at Lariboisiere Hospital and review of the literature. *Neurosurg Rev.* 2008;31:19–32; discussion 32–33.
6. Leon-Ariza DS, Campero A, Romero Chaparro RJ, Prada DG, Vargas Grau G, Rhoton Jr AL. Key aspects in foramen magnum meningiomas: from old neuroanatomical conceptions to current far lateral neurosurgical intervention. *World Neurosurg.* 2017;106:477–483.
7. Flores BC, Boudreaux BP, Klinger DR, Mickey BE, Barnett SL. The far-lateral approach for foramen magnum meningiomas. *Neurosurg Focus.* 2013;35:E12.
8. Pai SB, Raghuram G, Keshav GC, Rodrigues E. Far-lateral transcondylar approach to anterior foramen magnum lesions: our experience. *Asian J Neurosurg.* 2018;13:651–655.
9. Liu JK. Extreme lateral transcondylar approach for resection of ventrally based meningioma of the craniovertebral junction and upper cervical spine. *Neurosurg Focus.* 2012;33:1.
10. Sen CN, Sekhar LN. An extreme lateral approach to intradural lesions of the cervical spine and foramen magnum. *Neurosurgery.* 1990;27:197–204.

77

Ependymoma

Case reviewed by William T. Couldwell, Evandro de Oliveira, Joao Paulo Almeida, James Rutka, Reid C. Thompson

Introduction

Ependymomas are relatively rare intracranial tumors that account for 1% to 5% of central nervous system tumors and arise from ependymal lining of the ventricular system or spinal canal.[1-4] They account for 5% of central nervous system tumors in children and adolescents, but only 1.9% in adults.[1-4] The overall 10-year survival rate for all patients with ependymomas is 79.2%; however, these tumors can occur anywhere along the neuroaxis, and therefore prognosis is different for different locations.[1-4] Among ependymomas, a relatively common location is within the fourth ventricle, in which increasing extent of resection is associated with better overall and progression-free survival.[5,6] However, surgical morbidity remains relatively high and ranges from 10% to 30% in several series, in which the most significant morbidity is owing to injury of cranial nerve nuclei along the fourth ventricular floor.[5,6] In this chapter, we present a case of a patient with a fourth ventricular ependymoma.

Example case

Chief complaint: headaches, nausea, vomiting

History of present illness

A 38-year-old, right-handed woman with a history of asthma presented with headaches, nausea, and vomiting. Over the past 2 to 3 days, she complained of increasing bifrontal headaches that were recently accompanied by nausea and vomiting. She was seen by her primary care physician in which imaging revealed a brain lesion (Fig. 77.1).

Medications: Albuterol inhaler.

Allergies: No known drug allergies.

Past medical and surgical history: Asthma.

Family history: No history of intracranial malignancies.

Social history: Engineer, no smoking, no alcohol.

Physical examination: Awake, alert, oriented to person, place, time; Cranial nerves II to XII intact; No drift, moves all extremities with good strength; No finger-to-nose dysmetria.

Spinal imaging: No evidence of drop metastases.

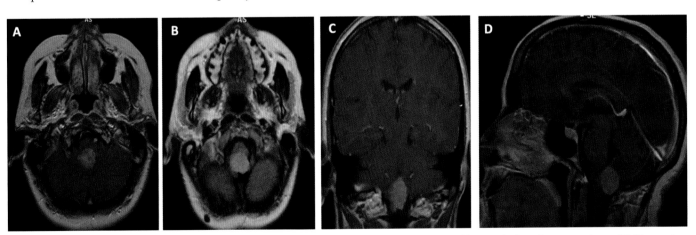

Fig. 77.1 Preoperative magnetic resonance imaging. (A) T1 axial image with gadolinium contrast; **(B)** T2 axial fluid attenuation inversion recovery image; **(C)** T1 coronal image with gadolinium contrast; **(D)** T1 sagittal image with gadolinium contrast magnetic resonance imaging scan demonstrating a fourth ventricular enhancing lesion.

	William T. Couldwell, MD, PhD, University of Utah, Salt Lake City, UT, United States	Evandro de Oliveira, MD, PhD, Joao Paulo Almeida, MD, Institute of Neurological Sciences, São Paulo, SP, Brazil	James Rutka, MD, PhD, University of Toronto Sick Kids, Toronto, Canada	Reid C. Thompson, MD, Vanderbilt University, Nashville, TN, United States
Preoperative				
Additional tests requested	Swallowing evaluation	Transesophageal echocardiogram Anesthesia evaluation	Neuroophthalmology evaluation Neuropsychological assessment Complete MRI brain and spine	Swallow evaluation
Surgical approach selected	Midline suboccipital craniotomy	Midline suboccipital craniotomy, C1 laminectomy	Midline suboccipital craniotomy	Midline suboccipital craniotomy, C1 laminectomy
Anatomic corridor	Telovelar	Telovelar	Telovelar	Telovelar
Goal of surgery	GTR	GTR, preservation of neurovascular structures	GTR	GTR, preservation of neurologic function
Perioperative				
Positioning	Prone	Semisitting	Prone	Prone
Surgical equipment	Surgical navigation IOM (SSEP, MEP low cranial nerve EMG) Ultrasonic aspirator	Semisitting equipment Surgical navigation Precordial Doppler IOM (SSEP/MEP, EMG of cranial nerves V–XII) Brain retractors	Surgical microscope IOM Ultrasonic aspirator Brain stimulator	Surgical microscope Weck vascular clips
Medications	Steroids Mannitol	Steroids	None	Steroids Mannitol
Anatomic considerations	Brainstem, PICA	Occipital bone and foramen magnum, posterior arch of C1, cerebellar hemisphere, tonsils, cerebellomedullary fissure, inferior medullary velum, tela choroidea, PICA, floor of fourth ventricle, upper spinal cord	Obex, floor of fourth ventricle, brainstem (medulla)	Medulla, lower cranial nerves, obex, PICA
Complications feared with approach chosen	Brainstem injury	Cerebellar/brainstem injury, floor of fourth ventricle damage, PICA stroke	Brainstem injury, cranial nerve injury (IX–XII), cerebellar injury	Brainstem injury, swallowing dysfunction, CSF leak, hydrocephalus
Intraoperative				
Anesthesia	General	General	General	General
Skin incision	Linear	Linear from 2 cm above inion to C4	Linear	Linear from inion to C3
Bone opening	Midline suboccipital	Midline suboccipital and C1 laminectomy	Midline suboccipital +/– C1 laminectomy	Midline suboccipital and C1 laminectomy
Brain exposure	Cerebellar hemispheres, cervicomedullary junction	Cerebellar hemispheres, cervicomedullary junction	Cerebellar hemispheres, cervicomedullary junction	Cerebellar hemispheres, cervicomedullary junction

	William T. Couldwell, MD, PhD, University of Utah, Salt Lake City, UT, United States	Evandro de Oliveira, MD, PhD, Joao Paulo Almeida, MD, Institute of Neurological Sciences, São Paulo, SP, Brazil	James Rutka, MD, PhD, University of Toronto Sick Kids, Toronto, Canada	Reid C. Thompson, MD, Vanderbilt University, Nashville, TN, United States
Method of resection	3 x 3 cm lower suboccipital craniotomy with foramen magnum, Y-shaped dural opening, drain CSF from cisterna magna, open tela choroidea at cerebellomedullary fissure, identify tumor and PICA, dissect tumor from roof of ventricle and PICA branches, avoid damage to brainstem floor, watertight dural closure with Alloderm	Semisitting position with precordial Doppler, expose fascia, Y-shaped muscle cuff above superior nuchal line, midline incision through avascular plane, muscle retraction, suboccipital craniotomy with removing lip of foramen magnum and C1 lamina, Y-shaped dural opening, drain CSF from cisterna magna, open tela choroidea at cerebellomedullary fissure, identify tumor and PICA, dissect tumor from roof of ventricle and PICA branches, attempted en bloc resection with preservation of ventricular floor, watertight dural closure with interposed muscle	Midline scalp incision from inion to C2, craniotomy of occipital bone +/− C1 laminectomy, Y-shaped dural opening, identify tumor below tonsils, dissect around tumor laterally, debulk with ultrasonic aspirator, identify floor of fourth ventricle and leave tumor if transgresses floor, remove tumor up to aqueduct, dural closure with graft, supplement with Tisseel	Midline incision, subperiosteal exposure of posterior fossa to foramen magnum and C1 lamina, keep musculature on C2 intact, posterior fossa craniotomy with inclusion of foramen magnum, drill laterally to widen exposure, palpate for vertebral arteries along C1 and laminectomy medially, Y-shaped dural opening to C1 with Weck vascular clips if circular venous sinus encountered, establish planes between tumor and brainstem with microscopic visualization, devascularize tumor capsule and internally debulk, mobilize tumor from cerebellar tonsils with protection of PICA, determine feasibility of removal if component stuck to brainstem, watertight dural closure with dural substitute
Complication avoidance	Dissect tumor from roof, preserve floor of fourth ventricle	Semisitting position, dissect tumor from roof, protect floor of fourth ventricle	Identify floor of fourth ventricle, do not transgress floor, dissect around lateral edges	Identify floor of fourth ventricle, intraoperative decision to remove completely based on adherence to the brainstem and plane of separation
Postoperative				
Admission	ICU	ICU	ICU	ICU, keep intubated over night
Postoperative complications feared	Brainstem injury, swallowing dysfunction	Hydrocephalus, injury to floor of fourth ventricle (lower cranial nerve deficits, motor/sensory deficits, decreased consciousness)	CSF leak, hydrocephalus, brainstem injury, cranial nerve nuclei injury	Brainstem injury, swallowing dysfunction, CSF leak, hydrocephalus
Follow-up testing	MRI within 24 hours after surgery	MRI within 24 hours after surgery	MRI within 24 hours after surgery	MRI night of surgery Complete spine MRI Swallowing evaluation 1 day after surgery
Follow-up visits	1 month after surgery	15 days after surgery 6 months after surgery	4–6 weeks after surgery	14 days after surgery 6 weeks after surgery
Adjuvant therapies recommended	GTR–radiation STR–radiation	GTR–observation STR–reoperation, radiation if repeat surgery does not achieve GTR Grade III–radiation	GTR–observation vs. focal radiation therapy STR–possible repeat surgery if possible or radiation therapy	GTR–radiation therapy STR–possible repeat surgery if possible or radiation therapy

CSF, cerebrospinal fluid; EMG, electromyography; GTR, gross total resection; ICU, intensive care unit; IOM, intraoperative monitoring; MEP, motor evoked potentials; MRI, magnetic resonance imaging; PICA, posterior inferior cerebellar artery; SSEP, somatosensory evoked potentials; STR, subtotal resection.

Differential diagnosis and actual diagnosis

- Ependymoma
- Choroid plexus papilloma
- Meningioma
- Metastatic brain tumor

Important anatomic and preoperative considerations

For a full discussion of the fourth ventricular anatomy, see Chapters 13 and 31. The fourth ventricle consists of a roof, floor, and two lateral walls.[7] The superior portion of the roof is formed by the superior medullary velum that connects the bilateral superior cerebellar peduncles, whereas the inferior portion is formed by the inferior medullary velum that comes from the cerebellum itself.[7] The inferior portion of the roof has three recesses consisting of the center foramen Magendie and the lateral foramina of Luschka, and has a posterior prominence referred to as the fastigium where the fastigial nucleus lies immediately superior to the roof of the fourth ventricle.[7] The floor is also known as the rhomboid fossa, in which it is demarcated by several prominent sulci.[7] The median sulcus extends the length of the floor from the aqueduct to the central canal and divides the floor into halves, in which each half is further divided by a parallel sulcus called the sulcus limitans that bifurcates into the superior fovea rostrally and the inferior fovea caudally.[7] Sensory neurons reside medial to the sulcus limitans, whereas motor neurons reside lateral.[7] The pons is anterior to the middle and superior portion of the ventricular floor, and is where the facial colliculus can be identified looping around the abducens nucleus within the inferior pontine region.[7] The medulla is anterior to the inferior portion of the floor, and is where the hypoglossal nucleus bulges into the floor to create the hypoglossal trigone located superiorly to the inferior fovea within the median eminence, and the dorsal nucleus of vagus that also bulges into the floor to create the vagal trigone that is inferior to the inferior fovea.[7] The medullary stria also can be seen in the floor of the fourth ventricle at the medullary level, where they emerge from the median sulcus and run transversely to become part of the inferior cerebellar peduncle.[7] The inferior cerebellar peduncles form that lateral walls of the fourth ventricle.[7]

Approaches to this lesion

The approaches to the fourth ventricle are summarized in Chapter 31. These approaches can be divided into intra- and extra axial approaches.[8] The primary intraaxial approach is a transvermian approach through the inferior vermis, in which an upper vermian approach is associated with a high risk of cerebellar mutism.[8] The primary extraaxial approach is unilateral or bilateral telovelar approaches through a midline suboccipital craniotomy.[8] The advantages of the transvermian approach are that it minimizes potential injury to the posterior inferior cerebellar artery (PICA) vessels and allows upper and fourth ventricular access, but can be associated with cerebellar

mutism and prolonged truncal ataxia.[8] The advantages of the telovelar approach are that it avoids parenchymal injury and minimizes risk of cerebellar mutism, but it exposes the PICA vessels to potential injury, and can have limited visualization of the entire fourth ventricle without retraction.[8]

What was actually done

The patient was taken to surgery for a midline suboccipital craniotomy for bilateral telovelar approach for resection of the fourth ventricular tumor with general anesthesia. The goal was complete resection. The patient was induced and intubated per routine. Intraoperative monitoring was used to monitor somatosensory evoked potentials, as well as cranial nerves V, VII, IX, X, XI, and XII. The head was fixed in neutral position, with two pins centered over the left external auditory meatus and one pin over the right external auditory meatus. The patient was then placed prone onto chest rolls with the neck flexed and reduced. A midline incision was planned that spanned from just above the inion to the C2 spinous process. In addition, a Frazier burr hole site was planned in case it was needed for an external ventricular drain. The patient was draped in the usual standard fashion and given dexamethasone and cefazolin. A midline incision was made, and dissection took place in the avascular plane between the suboccipital muscles. The skin and muscles were retracted with a cerebellar retractor, and the C1 spinous process and occipital bone with foramen magnum were identified. A suboccipital craniotomy was made below the transverse sinus with incorporation of the foramen magnum. In addition, a C1 laminectomy was done to facilitate dural opening and closure. The dura was then opened in a Y-shape that extended down the midline to C1 and tacked up to the surrounding muscles. The microscope was brought in, and the arachnoid between the tonsils and the cerebellar hemispheres were opened with sharp dissection, making sure to identify and protect the bilateral PICAs. The cerebellar tonsils were retracted laterally with dynamic retraction without fixed retractors to expose and open the tela choroidea and inferior medullary velum bilaterally. The spinal canal was protected with cottonoids to minimize potential tumor seeding. The tumor was debulked until the ventricular walls were seen on all edges. A small attachment to the floor of the fourth ventricle was identified and sharply removed after brainstem mapping to confirm no facial nerve involvement. No residual tumor was seen. A synthetic dural graft was used for watertight dural closure, and the bone and skin were closed in standard fashion.

The patient awoke at their neurologic baseline with intact speech, full strength bilaterally, and intact cranial nerves, and was taken to the intensive care unit for recovery. Magnetic resonance imaging was done within 48 hours after surgery and showed gross total resection (Fig. 77.2). The patient participated with physical and occupational therapy and was discharged to home on postoperative day 3 with an intact neurologic examination. The patient was prescribed dexamethasone that was tapered to off over 7 days after surgery. The patient was seen at 2 weeks postoperatively for suture removal and remained neurologically intact. Pathology

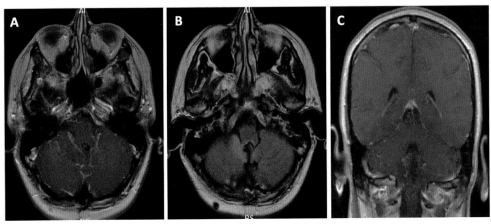

Fig. 77.2 Postoperative magnetic resonance imaging. (A) T1 axial image with gadolinium contrast; **(B)** T2 axial fluid attenuation inversion recovery image; **(C)** T1 coronal image with gadolinium contrast magnetic resonance imaging scan demonstrating gross total resection of the fourth ventricular lesion.

was a World Health Organization grade II ependymoma. Radiation was deferred because of the gross total resection. The lesion was observed with serial magnetic resonance imaging examinations at 3 months including spinal imaging, followed by 6-month intervals, and has been without recurrence for 24 months.

Commonalities among the experts

Half of the surgeons requested that the patient undergo swallowing evaluation to assess baseline function prior to surgery. All surgeons would pursue surgery through a midline suboccipital craniotomy and telovelar approach, and half would supplement with C1 laminectomy. All surgeons aimed for gross total resection. Most were the floor of the fourth ventricle and PICA. The most common shared feared complications were cranial neuropathy and brainstem injury. Surgery was generally pursued with a surgical microscope, intraoperative monitoring of the cranial nerves, and ultrasonic aspirator, with perioperative steroids and mannitol. Most surgeons advocated for identification of the floor of the fourth ventricle and to avoid transgressing the floor. Following surgery, all surgeons admitted their patients to the intensive care unit, and all surgeons requested imaging within 48 hours to assess for extent of resection and/or potential complications. For gross total resection, most surgeons would observe the lesion. For subtotal resection, most surgeons advocated for repeat surgery and/or radiation therapy.

SUMMARY OF QUALITY OF EVIDENCE TO GUIDE SPECIFIC INTERVENTIONS FOR THIS CASE

- Surgical resection of fourth ventricular ependymoma—Class II-2.
- Deferral of radiation for gross total resection of intraventricular ependymoma—Class III.

REFERENCES

1. Gerstner ER, Pajtler KW. Ependymoma. *Semin Neurol.* 2018;38:104–111.
2. Hubner JM, Kool M, Pfister SM, Pajtler KW. Epidemiology, molecular classification and WHO grading of ependymoma. *J Neurosurg Sci.* 2018;62:46–50.
3. Pajtler KW, Mack SC, Ramaswamy V, et al. The current consensus on the clinical management of intracranial ependymoma and its distinct molecular variants. *Acta Neuropathol.* 2017;133:5–12.
4. Wu J, Armstrong TS, Gilbert MR. Biology and management of ependymomas. *Neuro Oncol.* 2016;18:902–913.
5. Healey EA, Barnes PD, Kupsky WJ, et al. The prognostic significance of postoperative residual tumor in ependymoma. *Neurosurgery.* 1991;28:666–671; discussion 671–672.
6. Lyons MK, Kelly PJ. Posterior fossa ependymomas: report of 30 cases and review of the literature. *Neurosurgery.* 1991;28:659–664; discussion 664–665.
7. Ribas EC, Yagmurlu K, de Oliveira E, Ribas GC, Rhoton A Jr. Microsurgical anatomy of the central core of the brain. *J Neurosurg.* 2018;129:752–769.
8. Tomasello F, Conti A, Cardali S, La Torre D, Angileri FF. Telovelar approach to fourth ventricle tumors: highlights and limitations. *World Neurosurg.* 2015;83:1141–1147.

Index

Page numbers followed by a *b* indicate boxes; those followed by an *f* indicate figures; those followed by a *t* indicate tables.